D1712252

G. W. KORTING and R. DENK

Differential Diagnosis in Dermatology

Differential Diagnosis in Dermatology

with 786 illustrations, 720 in color

by

G. W. KORTING

Professor and Director of Dermatology,
University Hospital, Mainz

R. DENK

Chief Physician in Dermatology,
University Hospital, Mainz

Translated and Adapted by

HELEN O. CURTH, M. D.

Special Lecturer in Dermatology,
College of Physicians and Surgeons, Columbia University

WILLIAM CURTH, M. D.

Assistant Clinical Professor of Dermatology (retired),
New York Medical College

W. B. SAUNDERS COMPANY · Philadelphia · London · Toronto · 1976

W. B. Saunders Company : West Washington Square
Philadelphia, PA 19105

12 Dyott Street
London, WC1A 1DB

833 Oxford Street
Toronto, Ontario M8Z 5T9, Canada

Authorized English Edition. All rights reserved.

Original German Edition : Dermatologische Differentialdiagnose
© 1974 by F. K. Schattauer Verlag, Stuttgart

English Edition published 1976 by W. B. Saunders Company,
Philadelphia, London, Toronto

Differential Diagnosis in Dermatology   ISBN 0–7216–5488–6

Preface

Diagnosis as well as its counterpart, differential diagnosis, belongs to the great medical tradition. Differential diagnosis is of prime importance because a wrong diagnosis based on faulty judgment of phenomenologic criteria indicates an error in the differential diagnosis. In addition, it happens, especially in dermatology, that the same signs can have many etiologic bases. Concerning differential diagnosis: WICHMANN (1740–1802), to whom we owe our knowledge of infantile eczema and pemphigus, has written: "This great and difficult art, which is a part of nosology, involves careful comparison, examination, and differentiation of individual diseases that resemble each other, searching especially for signs that separate one from the other. This is diagnosis." The need for differential diagnosis in dermatology is answered in the literature by only a few attempts, such as those of W. SCHOLTZ (S. Hirzel, Leipzig, 1930) or FITZPATRICK and WALKER (1962, Year Book Medical Publishers), besides certain paragraphs in various textbooks. The reader, however, should not expect too much from the following treatise. The task, and I refer you to volumes of our former and present textbooks, can be only a partial attempt, especially if the compilation is aimed at practical use. For this reason the material has been organized, not according to a nosologic system, but by cutaneous manifestations or important dermatologic symptoms such as pruritus or sweating. According to this plan of dermatologic differential diagnosis no detailed clinical description of each disease has been given, but, assuming some knowledge of the reader of its manifestations, differential diagnostic points will be discussed. In some disorders, as for example in chapters dealing with eczema and tumors, topographically oriented listings could not be avoided. In addition, the reader will find a basic compendium of ophthalmological findings. It is the relatively frequent, not the rare, dermatoses that will be fully discussed.

The photography was, as always, in the hands of the photographer of the Hospital, Mr. Faber, whose excellent technique is well known. Several illustrations were given to us by the following colleagues, whom we want to thank again: Dr. CARRIE, Dortmund (Figs. 627 and 711); Prof. Dr. DENDEN, Göttingen (Figs. 636 and 637 [Klin. Monatsbl. Augenheilk. 156:49, Enke, Stuttgart, 1970]), Prof. Dr. FISCHER, Mainz (Fig. 734); Prof. Dr. JÄGER, Heidelberg (Fig. 219); Prof. Dr. KÖTTGEN, Mainz (Fig. 334); Prof. Dr. MISGELD, Berlin (Figs. 170c, 446, 743, 744, and 780); Prof. Dr. NASEMANN, Frankfurt (Figs. 475 and 476); Prof. Dr. NÖDL, Homburg/Saar (Figs. 179a, 444, 445, and 536); Prof. Dr. NOVER, Mainz (Fig. 531); Prof. Dr. PARTSCH, Homburg/Saar (Fig. 365); Prof. Dr. REICH, Münster (Fig. 53); Prof. Dr. STAHL, Heidelberg (Fig. 77); Prof. Dr. STÜTTGEN, Berlin (Fig. 206a); Prof. Dr. WOLF, Freiburg (Fig. 76, [Humangenetik 2:165, Springer; Berlin, Heidelberg, New York, 1966]). The histologic slides for Figs. 69a and b, and 562 were kindly put at our disposal by Prof. Dr. POPP, Porto Alegre, Brazil. We have to thank Mrs. Ass and Prof. Dr. R. GEBHARDT for the compilation of the references. The typing of the manuscript was done by the indefatigable Mrs. G. MORITZ and Mrs. R. RÖHRIG. The Schattauer Publishing House, especially Prof. Dr. P. MATIS and Director Ph. REEG, have shown their generosity again, making the present excellent technical appearance of the book possible.

Mainz, March, 1974

G. W. KORTING and R. DENK

Translators' Foreword

Translating from one language into another requires a thorough knowledge of both languages. It is a challenging task, but the adaptation of a medical text from one language to another makes additional special demands.

Not all aspects of the practice of dermatology in Germany and America are similar. Footnotes have been added when, in the opinion of the translators, these differences are significant enough to warrant them. For example, poison ivy dermatitis, which is a great hazard for American lovers of the outdoors, is virtually unheard of in Germany. On the other hand, the nettle producing immediate wheals is unknown in the United States. Similarly, procedures for diagnosing certain dermatoses may vary in the two countries. Incisional biopsies of melanomas, not recommended in Germany, are considered justified in the United States if an excisional biopsy would be mutilating.

The authors' experience sometimes runs counter to that of the translators: for example, the hypothesis that circumscribed senile hyperplasia of the sebaceous glands occurs in people with seborrhea and rhinophyma.

To facilitate use of the book in this edition we have translated into English many of the Latin phrases so common in the European literature. For certain German drugs not available in this country, American drugs with similar actions were substituted.

We hope we have met the formidable challenge that translation of the book presented, and that it will prove to be as useful to the English-speaking physician as it has been to its audience in its original German edition.

WILLIAM and HELEN O. CURTH

New York, July, 1975

Contents

1. Fever

Changes in body temperature are of interest to the dermatologist since the blood supply as well as transpiration through the skin is affected.

Among the first thermometric medical experiments was the measurement of his urethra by HUNTER (1728–1793), who is known to us by his self-infliction of a syphilitic primary lesion. Other venereologists, such as BOORHAVE, also studied the effect of fever in this early period. Systematic measurements of body temperature in German hospitals, however, began with TRAUBE, WUNDERLICH, and LIEBERMEISTER, but most of all with the dermatologist BAERENSPRUNG (1822–1864).

A. Disorders with Insufficient Sweat Delivery

Disturbed regulation of the temperature may result from exogenous, physical, and chemical causes as well as from personal vegetative-endocrine conditions.[6] Hyperpyrexia from faulty or absent thermoregulation owing to diminished or absent sensible perspiration has been noted in the following dermatoses.

1. Anhidrotic ectodermal dysplasia (anhidrosis hypotrichotica). This disorder is known by the triad: hypohidrosis or anhidrosis, hypotrichosis, and oligodentia. Other nonessential signs are frontal bossing, small projecting ears, and malformations of the mammary glands, as well as follicular changes of keratinization, primarily of the cheeks and temporal areas. Sometimes there are various disturbances in the growth of nails.

The diminished anatomic substrate of sweat glands causes the appearance of etiologically unclear fevers after physical effort, sometimes in infancy but also in later life. Insensible perspiration of these patients, however, is undisturbed.

2. Angiokeratoma corporis diffusum (Fabry's disease). This lipid storage disease is based on a deficiency of the enzyme ceramide-trihexosidase, which leads to thesaurismosis of ceramide-trihexoside and ceramide-dihexoside, primarily in the autonomic nervous system in smooth and cardiac muscle. Cutaneous manifestations are represented by blackish or dark bluish papules, which are rarely keratotic and measure a few millimeters in diameter. They favor the lower abdomen and the buttocks. Of diagnostic importance is the involvement of the umbilical fossa. The first manifestations usually occur around the age of puberty. Heterozygous carriers of Fabry's disease (women), who do not always show any cutaneous lesions, can be recognized by split-lamp examination, which discloses yellow-brown corneal lines (cornea verticillata). Furthermore, these patients often show hyperhidrosis, which rapidly changes into hypo- or anhidrosis. This is accompanied by bouts of fever, which usually provoke crises of joint pains. The elevations in temperature can be explained by severely delayed or diminished delivery of sweat secretion, but as a rule, lipoid sediments are not observed histologically in the sweat duct apparatus. The cause of this disturbance of the sweat gland secretion seems to originate in innervation which has been altered by the lipoid sediment. Parenthetically, one can also elicit the pain in the extremities caused by higher temperatures by immersion of the extremities in warm (38° C) or cold (below 22° C) water.[1, 2, 4]

3. Incontinentia pigmenti (Franceschetti-Jadassohn type). This second form of incontinentia pigmenti affects children of both sexes, who develop reticular pigmentation without preceding inflammatory signs. A characteristic manifestation that should be mentioned here is the diminution or even lack of sweat glands. This leads to an inability to perspire and, if the outer temperature increases or if the patient is subjected to physical strain, to an immediate increase in body temperature.

(1) BISCHOFF, A., U. FIERZ, F. REGLI und J. ULRICH: Peripher-neurologische Störungen bei der Fabryschen Krankheit (Angiokeratoma corporis diffusum universale). Klin. Wschr. *46:* 666–671 (1968).

(2) DENDEN, A.: Über die diagnostische Bedeutung der Cornea verticillata für die Erkennung des Morbus Fabry-Anderson. Klin. Mbl. Augenheilk. *156:* 49–62 (1970).

(3) FRANCESCHETTI, A., et W. JADASSOHN: À propos de l'« incontinentia pigmenti »; délimitation de deux syndromes différents figurant sous le même terme. Dermatologica (Basel) *108:* 1–28 (1954).

(4) KORTING, G. W., und R. DENK: Über die klinischen Unterschiede zwischen Fabry-Krankheit und M. Osler. Med. Welt *17:* (N. F.): 851–855 (1966).

(5) PERABO, F., J. A. VELASCO und A. PRADER: Ektodermale Dysplasie vom anhidrotischen Typus; 5 neue Beobachtungen. Helv. paediat. Acta *11:* 604–639 (1956).

(6) VOIT, K., und W. TILLING: Zur Pathogenese fieberhafter Zustände. Med. Klin. *57:* 1511–1514 (1962).

B. Erythemas

1. Among the prodromas as a whole, fever as well as mild sore throat or headache plays a relatively minor role in **pityriasis rosea.** The patient is hardly aware of a possible rise in temperature but may feel somewhat chilly. After the rash has erupted, the body temperature subsides.[2]

2. In **erythema scarlatiniforme desquamativum recidivans** preeruptive fever varies from case to case. High temperatures and chills, however, rarely occur. Occasionally, cutaneous manifestations with no fever have been observed.[7]

3. In **erythema annulare rheumaticum** the febrile course is caused by the basic rheumatic-cardiac disease.

4. In **pityriasis rubra pilaris** preeruptive bouts of fever may precede the cutaneous manifestations even in recurrences and may occasionally persist temporarily in the presence of the exanthem.[4]

5. Erythema multiforme. This disease has many causes, and its chief manifestations are round spots, which, because of varying concentric-zonal exudations, soon assume a peculiar iris form. A favorite site is the extensor surface of the upper extremities. Prodromal or initial subfebrile temperatures have been noted. There are, however, deviations in both directions: erythema multiforme may occur with no increase in temperature, but some variants, especially the Stevens-Johnson syndrome in children, are almost always accompanied by a very high fever. In this latter febrile mucocutaneous syndrome the high temperatures may last several days or up to three weeks. A possible viral etiology is indicated by occasionally occurring fever curves with two peaks (dromedary curves).[8]

6. Erythema nodosum affects the lower extremities especially, in the form of either highly painful, superficial, and plaquelike nodules or more nodose and deeper infiltrations. Like erythema multiforme, erythema nodosum can be explained as a reaction to many possible causes. According to the particular cause, muscular and articular pain as well as a febrile course may be part of the clinical picture. When the onset is acute, these symptoms and signs are accompanied by headache, chilliness, and fatigue. If the nodose erythemas have been present for some time, fewer constitutional signs and, therefore, no fever, are present.

Erythema nodosum is a frequent sign of *rheumatic fever*, which it is important to recognize early. In infants fever and cardiac involvement are predominant; in schoolchildren, adolescents, and adults, however, polyarthralgias prevail. Laboratory tests show high ESR values and a rise in the antistreptolysin titer. Often distinct anemia and hyposideremia exist.

If the acute onset of erythema nodosum is accompanied by a fever of up to 40° C, *Löfgren's syndrome* must be considered. This syndrome, which shows enlargement of both sides of the hilar lymph nodes, is often observed in individuals 20 to 40 years old as the initial manifestation of sarcoidosis. Some erythema nodosum statistics show that up to 70 per cent of cases were secondary to sarcoidosis (Boeck's disease).[1, 6, 10]

7. Periodic fever with skin lesions. Subsepsis allergica and acute febrile neutrophilic dermatosis (Sweet's syndrome). This periodic fever occurring at irregular intervals leaves no particular impairment of the patient even if it lasts for years. Different forms (arthralgic, abdominal, cardiovascular) of periodic fever are known. The exanthematic variety shows skin lesions of urticarial or multiform-erythematous character. Usually, the skin lesions are restricted to "fixed" predilection sites and develop only episodically, although they increase during a bout of fever. Arthralgia is almost always present. An elevated ESR and a shift to the left are other common changes. On

rare occasions the latex and antiglobulin consumption tests become positive. Blood cultures always remain negative. The therapeutic effect of corticosteroids and the ineffectiveness of antibiotics are characteristic. This disorder has been rarely observed in adults, but occurs in children in the form of subsepsis allergica.

Febrile neutrophilic dermatosis is an acute and almost always febrile disorder. The skin shows asymmetric nodular or plaquelike, often tender, infiltrations on the face, neck, hands, arms, and legs. The mucous membranes are always unaffected, and there is no involvement of the regional lymph nodes. Neutrophilic leukocytosis of up to about 25,000 cells is found in the blood and, histologically, polymorphic cellular infiltrations without essential vascular changes predominate. Other characteristics are the exclusive involvement of females, the lack of a scarring facility of the skin lesions, and a readiness to respond to corticosteroid therapy. In the differential diagnosis, chronic lupus erythematosus, erythema elevatum diutinum, and erythema nodosum must be considered. The skin lesions of lupus erythematosus differ mostly by their firmly attached follicular hyperkeratoses and the fact that they heal with scars. Fever and leukocytosis do not accompany the skin changes of lupus erythematosus. In systemic lupus erythematosus the presence of antinuclear factors should be proved. Further differences are apparent in the histological picture. Characteristic of Sweet's syndrome but not of erythema elevatum diutinum are: an acute onset with fever, asymmetric skin lesions, accompanying leukocytosis, and an elevated ESR. In addition, the single lesions of erythema elevatum diutinum do not show the same intensive red color as those of Sweet's syndrome; they tend to be located near joints and on the distal parts of the extremities.

Histologically, in erythema elevatum diutinum, vasculitis and a hyaline degeneration with subsequent fibrosis of the connective tissue are very important. If the cutaneous changes in Sweet's syndrome occur on the extremities exclusively, clinical differentiation from erythema nodosum can become difficult. Evidence of panniculitis, however, is a point in favor of erythema nodosum.[3, 4, 9, 11]

(1) BEHREND, H., T. BEHREND und M. WILCKENS: Zur Differentialdiagnose des Erythema nodosum. Z. Rheumaforsch. *26:* 65–73 (1967).

(2) BJÖRNBERG, A., and L. HELLGREN: Pityriasis rosea, a statistical, clinical and laboratory investigation of 826 patients and matched health controls. Acta derm.-venereol. (Stockh.) *42*, Suppl. 50 (1962).

(3) CROW, K. D., F. KERDEL-VEGAS and A. ROOK: Acute febrile neutrophilic dermatosis, Sweet's syndrome. Dermatologica (Basel) *139:* 123–134 (1969).

(4) GAY PRIETO, J.: Beziehungen zwischen Psoriasis und Pityriasis rubra pilaris. Act. dermo-sifiliogr. (Madr.) *26:* 345–352 (1934), ref. Zbl. Haut- u. Geschl.-Kr. *49:* 141 (1935).

(5) GOLDMAN, G. C., and S. L. MOSCHELLA: Acute febrile neutrophilic dermatosis (Sweet's syndrome). Arch. Derm. (Chic.) *103:* 654–660 (1971).

(6) ROTNES, P. L.: Untersuchungen über Erythema nodosum im Erwachsenenalter. Acta derm.-venereol. (Stockh.) *17*, Suppl. 3 (1936).

(7) RIEGEL, K., und G. W. KORTING: Zur Kenntnis viscerocutaner Wechselwirkungen mit hoher Bluteosinophilie unter dem Bilde des Löfflerschen Lungeninfiltrates und des Erythema scarlatiniforme desquamativum recidivans. Arch. klin. exp. Derm. *205:* 235–244 (1957).

(8) STRÖM, J.: Febrile mucocutaneous syndromes (ectodermosis erosiva pluriorificalis, Steven-Johnson's syndrome etc.) in adenovirus infections. Acta derm.-venereol. (Stockh.) *47:* 281–286 (1967).

(9) SWEET, R. D.: An acute febrile neutrophilic dermatosis. Brit. J. Derm. *76:* 349–356 (1964).

(10) WEBER, S., und W. SIEGENTHALER: Das Löfgren-Syndrom (akuter Morbus Boeck). Dtsch. med. Wschr. *92:* 1356–1357 (1967).

(11) WISSLER, H.: Subsepsis allergica. Ergebn. inn. Med. Kinderheilk. N. F. *23:* 202–220 (1965).

C. Erythematosquamous Dermatoses and Eczemas

1. Psoriasis non vulgaris. In its vulgar manifestation this erythematosquamous skin disease most probably represents an irregularly dominant hereditary disorder with a threshold effect. This is illustrated by the obvious dependence of manifestations upon changes in the internal as well as in the external conditions of the patient. In contrast to psoriasis vulgaris, which is consistently without fever, psoriasis non vulgaris in its ectodermal *(erythrodermic)*, mesenchymal *(arthropathic)*, and exudative *(pustular)* forms, representing maximal variants, is often accompanied by fever.

In particular, *generalized pustular psoriasis*, i. e., psoriasis of von Zumbusch's type (Fig. 1), differs from benign psoriasis with pustules by its extent and its grave and prolonged clinical picture. It is characterized by high temperatures. The high fever usually starts shortly before the onset of an eruption of pustules and for some time shows a periodic rhythm of remittent temperatures (Fig. 2). As a rule, no bacterial or other "infectious" causes can be found for the "psoriasis fever." The contents of the pustules are initially always sterile until germs from the outside settle in the lesions secondarily. If the intensity of the disease increases, the fever-free intervals become shorter and the fever phases longer, so that when confluent areas of pustules are present, high fever is finally present continuously.

In the course of morphologic regression, which corresponds step by step to the regression of the fever, exfoliating and (rarely) epidermolytic manifestations may occur. It has, however, been noted that the final restitutio ad integrum leads from a full expression of signs to normal skin conditions via the usual picture of psoriasis vulgaris. The palmoplantar form (Barber type) of pustular psoriasis usually has no accompanying fever. *Psoriasis arthropathica*, however, tends to show elevations of temperature in about 30 per cent of patients, mostly at the time of acute polyarticular progression. In such cases temperatures may reach 39° C.[1, 4, 9]

2. Reiter's disease (urethro-oculosynovial syndrome). This disorder, starting almost always with a monarthritis, is characterized by the triad of abacterial urethritis, conjunctivitis, and arthritis. In about 30 per cent of cases the characteristic skin changes – the so-called blenorrhagic keratoses – develop, as well as pustular, exudative-psoriasiform lesions. Balanitis circinata parakeratotica may also be present. A light and oligosymptomatic course usually involves no elevation of temperature; in severe cases and in those with acute onsets as well as in those with

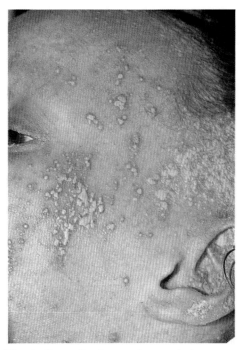

Fig. 1. Generalized pustular psoriasis.

polyarthritic manifestations, however, sepsislike intermittent temperatures up to 40° C occur. At the same time, a high ESR of up to 100 mm. in the first hour as well as

Fig. 2. "Periodical" fever in generalized pustular psoriasis.

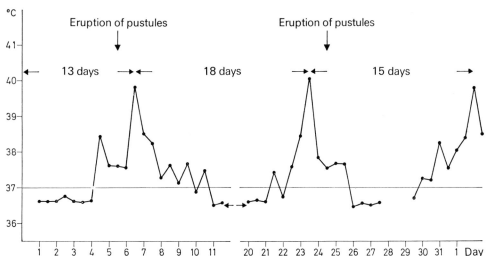

pronounced leukocytosis with an "inflammatory" shift to the left[3, 6, 8] are
observed.

3. Atopic erythroderma. In the course of
this maximal variant of endogenous eczema
of the infant, periods of fever may appear,
especially when secondary infections caused
by general failure of resistance set in.
Other forms of erythroderma in childhood
do not show the severe itching, generalized
lymph node enlargement, and marked
eosinophilia of atopic erythroderma (see
Chapter 22, B2).

The so-called *acute death from eczema* as a
consequence of tightly applied dressings
with salves or of severe resorption of toxin
and caused in most cases by interstitial
myocarditis is characterized before death
by steep and steady hyperpyrexias.[2, 5, 7]

(1) BAKER, H., and T. J. RYAN: Generalized
    pustular psoriasis. Brit. J. Derm. *80:*
    771–793 (1968).
(2) BERNHEIM-KARRER, I.: Ekzemtod und
    Myokarditis. Z. Kinderheilk. *35:* 120–126
    (1923).
(3) CSONKA, G.: Reiter's syndrome. Ergebn.
    inn. Med. Kinderheilk. N. F. *23:* 125–189
    (1965).
(4) FEHR, K.: Die Psoriasis-Arthritis. Docu-
    menta Geigy, Folia rheumatologica, H. *15*
    (1967).
(5) GARSCHE, R.: Der plötzliche Tod im
    Kindesalter. Ergebn. inn. Med. Kinder-
    heilk. N. F. *1:* 139–175 (1949).
(6) HAUSER, W.: Zur Diagnostik der Reiter-
    schen Krankheit. Med. Welt *15* (N.F.):
    2404–2409 (1964).
(7) HILL, L. W.: Nomenclature, classifica-
    tion, and pathogenesis of "eczema" in
    infancy. Arch. Derm. Syph. (Chic.) *66:*
    212–222 (1952).
(8) SCHUERMANN, H., und W. HAUSER:
    Reitersche Krankheit. Med. Klin. *44:*
    1269–1274 (1949).
(9) SCHUPPENER, H. J.: Ausdrucksformen
    pustulöser Psoriasis. Derm. Wschr. *138:*
    841–854 (1958).

D. Thesaurismoses

1. Uric arthritis. In gout the onset of a
severe attack can begin with chills, acute
fever, and, above all, profuse sweat secretion. Another sign of the inflammatory
process is a distinct leukocytosis. This may
often be important in the differential
diagnosis from acute arthralgic lupus
erythematosus, which, however, would
be accompanied by leukopenia.

2. In **interstitial calcinosis** some attacks
may lead to more or less distinct elevations
of temperature, among other constitutional
signs.

3. Scleredema adultorum. At the present
time this disorder is considered to be a
mucopolysaccharide thesaurismosis and
not a connective tissue disease. Its course is
without fever, but its classic manifestations are initiated by prodromal diseases
accompanied by fever.

4. Angiokeratoma corporis diffusum. See
Chapter 1, A 2.

E. Virus Infections of the Skin

1. Herpes simplex virus. The formerly
frequently used term *febris herpetica*
(herpetic fever) proves that a herpes
simplex virus infection with its manifold
manifestations may under certain conditions be accompanied by fever. This is of
short duration, lasting as a rule only one
day, and is accompanied by unexpected
chills. Occasionally, however, normal temperatures are not reached until the third
day. With the onset of fever herpetic
blisters develop around the mouth and
nose or on the oral mucous membrane. In
exceptional cases, however, all skin manifestations are lacking and the correct
diagnosis can be made only serologically.

The prognosis of such herpetic fever, which affects mostly 20- to 30-year-old persons, is favorable, but occasionally complications such as headaches, vertigo, tinnitus of the ears, fleeting meningism, proteinuria, or splenomegaly accompany the disease.

If, however, these CNS complications gain the upper hand, *herpetic meningo-encephalitis* must be considered. This grave disease, if not fatal, can be ascertained by isolation of the virus from blood and cerebrospinal fluid and a fall in the antibody titer. The classic picture of the primary infection of the herpes simplex virus, *herpetic gingivostomatitis*, begins rapidly with high fever, among other constitutional signs. Formerly, this disease was almost exclusively seen in infants; in the past few years, however, it has been observed more often in adolescents. The diagnosis can be made from the clinical picture if the numerous but seldom regularly grouped, aphthous lesions, which begin simultaneously and are located in the anterior oral cavity and on the gingiva, are present, as well as tender regional lymphadenopathy, fetor ex ore, and salivation. Deeper or larger aphthous ulcerations, which are characteristic of the usually singular habitual aphthae, are not found in this disorder.

Eczema herpeticum is present if the herpes simplex virus spreads rapidly over wide areas. This occurs almost exclusively in the region of a manifest endogenous eczema (infantile eczema or neurodermatitis disseminata). The blisters are smaller than those of *eczema vaccinatum* and are unilocular. The incubation period of eczema herpeticum, which occurs in children in 75 per cent of cases, is significantly shorter than that of eczema vaccinatum — only two to five days. It is lethal in 10 per cent of adults and 20 per cent of infants. In eczema herpeticum the fever is extremely high from the beginning and remains so continuously for seven to ten days. It disappears rather dramatically, not gradu-ally. It should be noted further that each new eruption of lesions is accompanied by elevation of temperature.[1, 3]

2. Herpes zoster (shingles). Herpes zoster, caused by the varicella zoster virus located in a spinal ganglion, is today considered a secondary infection projected to a certain dermatome in partially immune persons. The development of the segmentary groups of blisters on a light reddish, not rarely edematous base occurs with or without constitutional prodromas. Distinct elevations of temperature are usually not seen, although initially higher, preeruptive peaks of fever do not rule out an early diagnosis. Such a preeruptive fever tends to disappear again after one to two days. In the later course pronounced attacks of fever occur only with obviously considerable secondary infection.

3. Variola virus. Regular cyclic *smallpox* appear after an incubation period of 8 to 14 days, which in the case of varioloid is shortened to 8 days. The beginning is peracute owing to the generalization of the causative organism, with sharply mounting fever and simultaneously severe general manifestations following an uncharacteristic preliminary exanthem. Three to four days later the organotropic virus has become fixed, this stage being accompanied by abatement of the fever and subsequent development of the real smallpox exanthem. This becomes vesicular on the sixth day, pustular on the eighth day, and dries up on the eleventh to twelfth day. The development of the exanthem is characterized by a new elevation of temperature in the form of a septic suppurative fever. If the disease is not severe, the fever ends as early as the fourteenth to the sixteenth day. The severe forms show toxic signs at the suppurative stage and loss of consciousness, so that the patient dies from general exhaustion without regression of the high body temperature.

Eczema vaccinatum develops if the smallpox virus becomes generalized in a patient with endogenous eczema following vaccination against smallpox or after contamination from a smallpox infection from a neighboring source. The mortality rate from *eczema vaccinatum* may reach 30 per cent. In contrast to *generalized vaccinia*, the primary virus inoculation and its spread are completely exogenous. The appearance of the pustules within the eczematous areas and later also on unaffected skin is accompanied by temperatures of up to 41° C. As in variola vera the fever, which is constantly high for 7 to 12 days, gradually abates.

4. Varicella (chicken pox). In this highly contagious, typical children's disease, small red spots, which change into small papules and soon afterward into thin-walled blisters, appear with moderate general manifestations 7 to 12 days after infection. Because of repeated bouts of the disease, many lesions in different stages of development are present next to each other, forming the well-known "map of stars."

Before the typical varicella exanthem appears, uncharacteristic moderate fever, which may rise higher in association with new crops, is evident. More vigorous feverish attacks usually occur only in adults, in whom the rash is usually more severe and sometimes similar to varioloid.

5. Hand-foot-mouth exanthem. This epidemic virus disease (Coxsackie virus A 5, 10, and 16) shows vesicular-pustular eruptions on the hands and feet as well as aphthous lesions in the oral cavity. The usual general signs (headaches, diarrhea, and so on) may be accompanied by bouts of moderate fever. On the other hand, a completely feverless course is possible.

6. Acrodermatitis papulosa eruptiva infantilis (Gianotti-Crosti syndrome) appears as a lichenoid-papular rash in children and

adolescents. The lymph nodes close to the eruption are regularly affected; hepatopathia as well as lymphomonocytosis in the hemogram is constantly encountered, with occasionally mildly elevated temperatures.

(1) NASEMANN, TH.: Die Infektion durch das Herpes simplex-Virus. Fischer, Jena 1965.
(2) TAPPEINER, J., und K. WOLFF: Zoster. Fischer, Jena 1968.
(3) WEISSE, K.: Die Herpes simplex-Virus-Infektionen. Ergebn. inn. Med. Kinderheilk. N. F. *14:* 390–481 (1960).

F. Acute Bacterial Infectious Diseases of the Skin

1. Erysipelas. Erysipelas, especially in its first attack, is initially accompanied by high fever and other constitutional signs such as chills, headaches, and nausea. Fever usually precedes the development of the characteristic flamelike, sharply circumscribed, and later less sharp and confluent erythema. Without modern therapy the remittent fever may persist for a few days with peaks in the evening until the skin manifestations have regressed. A characteristic type of fever, however, is not present. Relapses, which occur a few days after the end of the first attack, are likewise accompanied by fever. Recurrences after a longer interval, however, especially those of recurrent forms of the disease, tend to have mitigated temperatures or even an afebrile course.

2. Erysipeloid. Erysipeloid, together with erysipelas and erythema migrans, belongs to the group of migrating erythemas. When the causative organism *(Erysipelothrix insidiosa)* enters through the skin, the disease may appear with general manifestations and elevated temperatures of up to about 38.5° C. Most of the erysipeloids, however, are mild and harmless, and are accompanied by only slight fever.

3. The primary lesion of **anthrax** is a sharply limited, edematous infiltration, which soon changes into a pustule and forms a coal-black eschar (Fig. 3). Occasionally, the edema of anthrax appears about two to three days after infection, already accompanied by generalized septic signs. Fever is irregular and remains unspecific. Especially at onset, temperatures can reach 39° C and above. There are no infallible rules about the fever in cases of anthrax; completely feverless courses are possible and, on the other hand, cases with mild findings may be accompanied by high fever.

(1) CALLOMON, FR. T.: Das Erysipeloid. In: Hdb. Haut- u. Geschlkrh. Hrsg. J. JADAS-SOHN. Erg.-Werk IV/1A, S. 239–261. Springer, Berlin, Heidelberg, New York 1965.
(2) DELBANCO, E., und F. CALLOMON: Erysipel. In: Hdb. Haut- u. Geschlkrh. Hrsg. J. JADASSOHN. Bd. IX/1, S. 1–92. Springer, Berlin 1929.

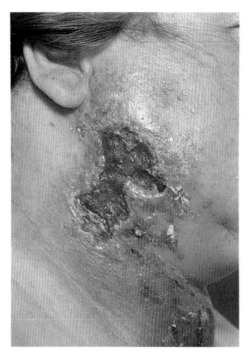

Fig. 3. Anthrax.

G. Chronic Bacterial Infectious Diseases and Mycoses of the Skin

1. Leprosy. The main types of leprosy are, first, highly infectious, malignant *lepromatous leprosy*, and second, benign *tuberculoid leprosy*, formerly called the maculoanesthetic form. Remittent or intermittent elevations of temperature with many other general signs accompany lepromatous leprosy initially. The subsequent course shows that the development of skin manifestations is always initiated by recurrent peaks of fever, especially in the evening. Therefore, a rise in temperature in chronic leprosy signifies the outbreak of new eruptions lasting over many years. In the major type of

tuberculoid leprosy (neural leprosy) there are always also initial general signs, among them rising temperatures.

Another type of fever in leprosy accompanies the *lepra reaction*. This is most probably an allergic phenomenon showing lepromatous exacerbation. The manifestations consist mainly of specific erythema nodosum or multiple necrotizing erythemas. This serious condition is associated with headaches, fatigue, and chills and high fever that are remittent in the morning. After about 9 to 12 days the fever suddenly abates completely. There are, however, lepra reactions lasting for months with only moderate elevations of temperature.[2]

2. Sarcoidosis. The *Löfgren syndrome* has been mentioned earlier in the section on erythema nodosum (see Chapter 1, B6). Another dermatologically important manifestation is the *Heerfordt syndrome*, which is characterized by subfebrile temperatures for a relatively long period of time. The main signs are nodular iritis and a characteristic, hard enlargement of the parotid and lacrimal glands, and, occasionally, the other salivary glands also.[1, 3]

3. Mycoses. Fever in dermatomycoses is almost entirely limited to systemic mycoses, although these do not invariably have a febrile course. In particular, the bronchopulmonary forms of septic *Candida mycosis* will show elevated temperatures. Pulmonary *cryptococcosis* and South American blastomycosis, however, are accompanied by subfebrile temperatures. In *sporotrichosis* any fever which may be present remains fairly steady and is pronounced only at the beginning of the generalization of the fungus into the body organs. The flu-like beginning of *coccidioidomycosis* is accompanied by moderate temperatures. In extensive involvement, however, chills and more pronounced hyperpyrexia are common.

(1) SCADDING, J. G.: Sarcoidosis. Erye & Spottiswoode, London 1967.
(2) SCHALLER, K. F.: Krankheiten durch Mykobakterien: »Lepra«. In: Infektionskrankheiten. Hrsg. O. GSELL u. W. MOHR. Bd. II/2, S. 887–932. Springer, Berlin, Heidelberg, New York 1968.
(3) WEBER, G.: Zur Teilsymptomatologie der Boeckschen Sarkoidose: das Heerfordtsche Syndrom. Derm. Wschr. *144:* 925–933 (1961).

H. Venereal Diseases

1. Owing to modern epidemiologic conditions and the range of therapeutic possibilities available for the treatment of the venereal infectious diseases, one need not expect fever even in the eruptive secondary stage of **syphilis.** Perhaps the explanation for the often noted evening elevations of temperature of syphilitics in the secondary stage during wars in this century, which the authors have also observed, is that poor nutrition, overexertion, and unaccustomed exposure to strong sun are responsible. After the war we rarely saw remittent fever at the time of the early tertiary stage eruption, or in cases with pronounced pustular eruptions, and only occasionally in congenital syphilis. Recurrent roseola associated with recent generalized lymph node swellings and bouts of fever is very rare, but may lead to diagnostic errors.

A different situation is found, however, with the *Jarisch-Herxheimer reaction.* In this suddenly beginning, rapid, and therapeutic destruction of many spirochetes, fever is one of the cardinal signs. It starts a few hours after the beginning of the treatment (Fig. 4). In the salvarsan era this reaction was mainly limited to the beginning of treatment of the florid secondary period. Today the Jarisch-Herxheimer reaction can occasionally be observed even in the primary (seropositive) stage of syphilis if the patient has been treated with strongly treponemicidal penicillin. Even if prophylactic cortisone is given, all signs cannot always be prevented.[5]

2. The septic complications of **gonorrhea** (epididymitis, prostatitis, arthritis, and endocarditis), formerly often dramatic and occasionally associated with continuous fever for several weeks, are extremely rare today. The diagnosis of gonorrheal sepsis must be ascertained by a positive blood culture inoculated during a bout of fever.[1, 2]

3. On the other hand, **lymphogranuloma inguinale** is more frequently associated with fever as a sign of generalized involvement even if other complications are lacking. Fever lasts generally only a few days after the development of the buboes and falls again when they have softened

Fig. 4. Herxheimer (Jarisch-Herxheimer and Krause) reaction in seropositive primary syphilis. Peak of fever after the first penicillin injection in spite of simultaneous intravenous cortisone.

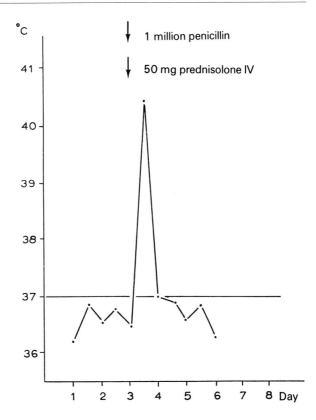

(Fig. 5). Infrequently, we observe protracted intermittent fever curves, occasionally even without accompanying signs of the skin or joints. In such cases lymphogranulomatosis may be considered. In the late stages of the disorder subfebrile temperatures exist; more pronounced fever in these phases, however, is limited to secondary infections or id-reactions.[3, 4]

(1) BURCKHARDT, W.: Die Klinik der Gonorrhoe des Mannes. In: Hdb. Haut- u. Geschlkrh. Hrsg. J. JADASSOHN. Erg.-Werk VI/1, S. 103–122. Springer, Berlin, Göttingen, Heidelberg 1964.

(2) DAVIS, J. S.: Diagnosis and treatment of gonorrheal septicemia and gonorrheal endocarditis. Arch. intern. Med. *66:* 418–440 (1940).

(3) HELLERSTRÖM, S.: A contribution to the knowledge of lymphogranuloma inguinale. Stockholm 1929.

(4) HENSCHLER-GREIFELT, A., und H. SCHUERMANN: Klinik des Lympho-
granuloma inguinale. In: Hdb. Haut- u. Geschlkrh. Hrsg. J. JADASSOHN. Erg.-Werk VI/1, S. 545–619. Springer, Berlin, Göttingen, Heidelberg 1964.

(5) LÖHE, H.: Wesen und Verlauf der Frühsyphilis im einzelnen. In: Die Haut- u. Geschlkrh. Hrsg. L. ARZT u. K. ZIELER. Bd. IV, S. 165–260. Urban & Schwarzenberg, Berlin, Wien 1934.

I. Groups of Collagenoses or Diffuse Connective Tissue Diseases

For practical nosologic reasons we shall deal mainly with systemic lupus erythematosus, dermatomyositis, and progressive scleroderma in this group of diseases.

1. Clinically, patients with **systemic lupus erythematosus** present with poor general condition, polyserositis and, above

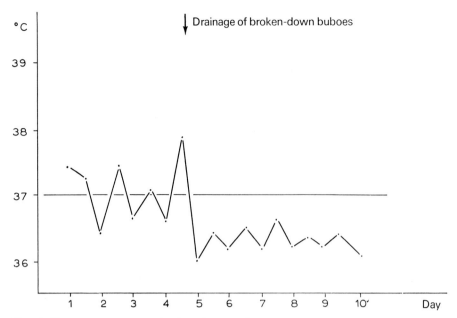

Fig. 5. Temperature curve in lymphogranuloma inguinale: disappearance of fever after drainage of buboes.

all, elevation of temperature. In about 85 per cent of cases specific cutaneous lesions are recognizable. In association with few characteristic signs in the joints, transient subfebrile elevations of temperature may sometimes occur. On the other hand, in a generally stormy course or during an acute exacerbation, high remittent or intermittent peaks of fever are encountered. In any case, fever associated with a poor general condition is one of the most frequent (about 90 per cent) initial signs of the disorder. Intercurrent paroxysms of fever suggest a secondary infection or a hyperergic therapeutic side effect (drug fever) with high temperatures.[2, 4]

2. The diagnosis of **dermatomyositis** is based on the findings from an electromyogram and skin-muscle biopsy as well as on the determination of creatinuria and the serum enzymes (GOT, GPT, aldolase, CPK, and myokinase). The diagnosis is greatly aided if the well-known cutaneous

changes, such as the strange wine-red to violet coloring of the face and upper trunk, follicular papular lesions of the neck, and hardening of the cuticle are present. In a distinctly acute onset of the disease flabby weakness of the muscles and elevation of temperature, which may even be of a septic character, prevail. However, in clinically doubtful cases general experience would indicate that paroxysmal steep febrile episodes are attributable to systemic lupus erythematosus rather than to dermatomyositis.[3]

3. Fever in **progressive scleroderma** is also, according to our own observations, extremely rare. It is "theoretically" possible that in later stages subfebrile temperatures occur owing to atrophy of the sweat glands.

4. In the course of **polychondritis chronica atrophicans** ("relapsing polychondritis") elevations of temperature also occur.

These may be caused by the basic disorder itself and are, therefore, associated with the simultaneously occurring inflammatory changes in the nasal and otic cartilage, trachea, and joints. The rapid regression of such an episode of inflammation in response to symptomatic glucocorticosteroid therapy is typical. On the other hand, the rises in temperature may be caused by intercurrent bronchopneumonia subsequent to involvement of the smaller bronchi and in such cases they respond better to treatment with antibiotics. In addition to the inflammatory changes of the cartilage just mentioned, ocular involvement occurs in about 50 per cent of cases (conjunctivitis, iritis, and scleritis) as well as disorders of the inner ear (25 per cent of cases) with hearing difficulties, vertigo, and others. Damage to the myocardium and multiple recurrent superficial thrombophlebitides are rarer. Among the laboratory findings, excessively elevated ESR values and a distinct leukocytosis are noteworthy. The antistreptolysin titer and the rheumatic factors are not increased.

(1) NITZSCHNER, H., O. PETTER und K. SCHLENTHER: Polychondritis recidivans et atrophicans. Derm. Mschr. *156:* 789–797 (1970).

(2) SCHÖLMERICH, P., und H. DEICHER: Der Lupus erythematodes visceralis. In: Klinik der Gegenwart, Hdb. prakt. Med. Hrsg. R. COBET, K. GUTZEIT u. H. E. BOCK. Bd. VI, S.639–684. Urban & Schwarzenberg, München, Berlin 1963.

(3) SCHUERMANN, H.: Dermatomyositis. Ergebn. inn. Med. Kinderheilk. N. F. *10:* 427–480 (1958).

(4) SIEGENTHALER, W., und R. HEGGLIN: Der viscerale Lupus erythematosus (Kaposi-Libman-Sacks-Syndrom). Ergebn. inn. Med. Kinderheilk. N. F. *7:* 373–428 (1956).

(5) THURSTON, M. C. S., and A. C. CURTIS: Relapsing polychondritis; report of a patient with "beefy" red ears and severe polyarthritis. Arch. Derm. (Chic.) *93:* 664–669 (1966).

K. Vascular Diseases of the Skin

The group of angiitides, which probably have a hyperergic etiology and are characterized by a tendency to multiple-discontinuous spreading, include several special forms, i. e., hypersensitivity angiitis, giant cell angiitis, giant cell granulomatous angiitis (Wegener-type), and many others.

1. In **panarteritis nodosa** of the classic type, the skin is affected in 15 to 60 per cent of cases. Even more often, in about 75 per cent of cases, the disease starts with insidious elevations of temperature. Definite septic temperatures with chills or continuous fever as in typhoid are encountered less often. Only exceptionally is a completely afebrile course observed.[6, 10]

2. Giant cell arteritis favors the temporal **(temporal arteritis)** and ophthalmic arteries. Patients complain of severe unilateral headaches and sudden deterioration of vision. Among the general complaints are fatigue and inability to work, and subfebrile temperatures, which in view of the signs and symptoms are not especially conspicuous. The other leukocytoclastic vasculitides, mainly the so-called *arteriolitis "allergica" cutis,* usually develop entirely without fever.[4, 8]

3. In rare instances **pityriasis lichenoides et varioliformis acuta,** which is today considered one of the arteriolitides, can have an acute and ulceronecrotic onset. It then would be accompanied by fever, which persists for some time.[2, 3]

4. The classic eruptions of **Schönlein's purpura** are associated with mild elevations of temperature only in cases with abdominal involvement. Fever, together with painful joint swellings (Fig. 6), occurs mostly in children as a premonitory sign in the first days of illness.

5. In **Wegener's granulomatosis,** however, fever occurs in about 10 per cent of

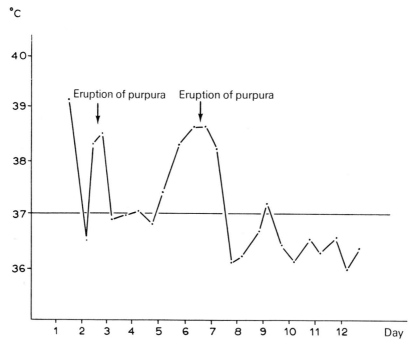

Fig. 6. Schönlein-Henoch purpura with peaks of fever during single eruptions of exanthems.

cases, mainly in the initial phase of the disease, when the nasal sinuses or the middle ear have a serous-purulent discharge. In the generalized and terminal stages subfebrile fever or bouts of fever are observed. Transitory or persistent, mainly purpura-like or papulonecrotic lesions are the typical cutaneous manifestations of this disease.[5]

In *lethal midline granuloma* (granuloma gangraenescens), which is closely related to Wegener's granulomatosis, bouts of irregularly high fever occur in the stage of overt manifestations after an unspecific prodromal stage, which is marked by inflammatory changes in nose and sinuses and watery-purulent coryza. The fever curve is either high and continuous or shows septic peaks. In spite of this the patients remain* in a relatively good general state. For details of the clinical picture see p. 524.[1]

_____

* Temporarily. (Tr.)

6. In **thrombo- and varicophlebitis** the body temperature is normal or only slightly elevated in spite of severe, local, and painful inflammation. If considerable elevation of temperature should occur in thrombophlebitis, and especially, if it is associated with chills, this would be indicative of a septic course. Previously, an increase in the pulse frequency with the same (subfebrile) temperature (Mahler's sign) was regarded as a sign of deeply located *phlebothrombosis*.

7. **Phlebitis migrans** (saltans) points in some cases to analogous correlations in the arterial vessels or alarming situations such as pancreatitis or pancreatic carcinoma. The body temperature may stay constantly within normal limits but with a new attack it may rise for a short time.

8. In **phlegmasia caerulea dolens,** which is considered a fulminant massive thrombosis of veins of the smallest to the widest caliber, elevations of temperature occur in the later stages as an expression of resorption fever. Based on the impressive clinical picture one can adopt a diagnostic rule: The local skin temperature overlying a thrombosed vein or in phlebothrombosis is elevated, whereas in the dramatically sudden onset of phlegmasia caerulea dolens it is definitely lowered.[11]

9. The so-called **thrombotic thrombocytopenic purpura** (in which, in combination with hemolytic anemia, thrombocytic thromboses of the small arteries lead to cerebral, cardial, renal, or gastrointestinal signs) shows, in contrast to Werlhof's disease, petechial and partly necrotizing purpuric skin manifestations. Also important are subungual hemorrhages on fingers and toes with accompanying trophic disturbances. One of the clinical signs of this disorder, which may be influenced by the ovaries or may represent mostly postinfectious manifestations or those of a drug allergy, is a sudden elevation of fever. This is an important differential diagnostic sign in regard to leukocytoclastic-hemorrhagic microbids (Schönlein's purpura). Histologically, one should examine the perilymphonodular skin areas especially, not only for characteristic occlusion of vessels (mentioned before) but also for aneurysmatic formations at the sites of transition of arterioles to capillaries. It may seem strange that the involved vessels are not accompanied by inflammatory reactions in the neighboring area.[7, 9]

(1) ALTENBURGER, K., und K. PFEIFFER: Beitrag zum Krankheitsbild Granuloma gangraenescens. Med. Klin. 57: 1940–1946 (1962).
(2) BURKE, D. P., R. M. ADAMS and F. D. ARUNDELL: Febrile ulceronecrotic Mucha Habermann's disease. Arch. Derm. (Chic.) 100: 200–206 (1969).
(3) DEGOS, R., B. DUPERRAT et F. DANIEL: Le parapsoriasis ulcéro-nécrotique hyperthermique. Ann. Derm. Syph. (Paris) 93: 481–496 (1966).
(4) EULEFELD, F.: Zur Pathogenese der Hortonschen Riesenzellarteriitis. Dtsch. med. Wschr. 90: 255–258 (1965).
(5) KESSELRING, F., und H. U. ZOLLINGER: Die Wegenersche Granulomatose. Ergebn. inn. Med. Kinderheilk. N. F. 16: 41–78 (1961).
(6) KORTING, G. W.: Über cutane Periarteriitis nodosa unter besonderer Berücksichtigung begleitender Leberstörungen und der sogenannten Thrombophlebitis migrans. Arch. Derm. Syph. (Berl.) 199: 332–349 (1955).
(7) KREY, W.-D., und F. LEYH: Beitrag zur Klinik und Pathogenese der thrombotischen thrombopenischen Purpura (Moschcowitz). Med. Welt (N. F.) 18: 2355–2360 (1967).
(8) LÜBBERS, P.: Larvierte Arteriitis temporalis. Dtsch. med. Wschr. 90: 2246–2251 (1965).
(9) MOSCHCOWITZ, E.: An acute febrile pleiochromic anemia with hyaline thrombosis of the terminal arterioles and capillaries. Arch. intern. Med. 36: 89–93 (1925).
(10) PORTWICH, F.: Periarteriitis nodosa. Ergebn. inn. Med. Kinderheilk. N. F. 12: 428–485 (1959).
(11) RAU, H.: Die Phlegmasia coerulea dolens. Münch. med. Wschr. 108: 2012–2016 (1966).

L. Urticaria and Toxic-Allergic Exanthems

1. In "ordinary" **urticaria**, which has a definitely polyetiologic background, fever is usually not among the typical accompanying signs. It is, in any case, observed as often as is a decrease in basophils in the blood or the occurrence of gastrointestinal disturbances. The typical skin lesions may be associated with normal or even shortened ESR values as well as with medium-high to high ESR values.

If urticaria is associated with an elevated ESR, high fever is occasionally noted. Food and drug allergies (drug fever) are primarily suspected as the cause of such a febrile urticarial eruption. Such suspicion is supported if the questionable drug eruption is associated with other signs of shock such as eosinophilia, cytopenia, hemolysis, or arthralgias and if the temperature falls immediately after discontinuance of the drug. The example of penicillin urticaria, however, which in most cases appears as the "exanthem of the ninth day" demonstrates that such febrile drug allergies can persist irregularly and intermittently for weeks.

2. Toxic epidermal necrolysis (Lyell's disease) (see also Chapter 22, B3 and Chapter 25, A8) is the life-threatening maximal variant of a bullous-epidermolytic exanthem. In infants and children it is probably of staphylogenous origin; in adults, however, it represents an allergic drug reaction. Temperatures in such widespread epidermolyses occur as a premonitory sign and are characterized by steep and high elevations (Fig. 7) in all cases at the onset. If no special complications in inner organs are present, the rise in temperature subsides to subfebrile values on the sixth to the eight day, if the patient survives. Renewed attacks of fever are caused preponderantly by secondary

infections (such as those from widespread burns) and require immediate special antibiotics. A course of the disease without fever is exceptional.[1, 4]

(1) KORTING, G. W., und H. HOLZMANN: Universelle Epidermolysis acuta toxica. Arch. klin. exp. Derm. *210:* 1–13 (1960).
(2) LYELL, A.: A review of toxic epidermal necrolysis in Britain. Brit. J. Derm. *79:* 662–671 (1967).
(3) MISGELD, V., U.-M. GROSS, J. KRATZER und K.-D. ROSENSTIEL: Zum Lyell-Syndrom (Toxic Epidermal Necrolysis). Med. Klin. *68:* 398–404 (1973).
(4) PETTER, O., und E. SÜSS: Die pemphigoide Allergodermie unter dem Bild der toxic epidermal necrolysis (Morbus Lyell). Dtsch. Gesundh.-Wes. *23:* 2318–2322 (1968).

M. Reticulogranulomatoses and Reticuloses

1. In **malignant lymphogranulomatosis cutis** (Paltauf-Sternberg disease and Hodgkin's disease) loss of weight, itching, enlarged lymph nodes, and eosinophilia of

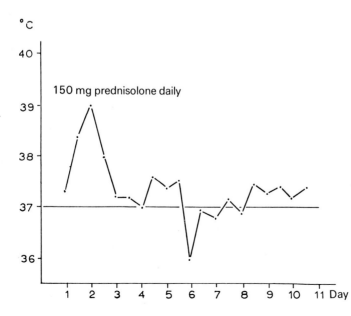

Fig. 7. Initial peak of fever in toxic acute epidermolysis.

the blood as well as high, continuous, or undulating elevations of temperature ("chronic relapsing fever") constitute the main signs (Fig. 8). In the middle stages of lymphogranulomatosis, however, the rise in temperature is often interrupted by fever-free phases, although toward the end the fever can remain continuous. The explanation for the character of the attacks of fever in lymphogranulomatosis must take into account the flooding of malignant, reticular, and cellular elements into the blood stream. In any case, long-lasting fever is as characteristic of the disease as itching.[3, 5]

2. In contrast, neither pruritus nor fever are regularly present in **mycosis fungoides,** the sister disease. Even the eruptive phases of the tumors are unaccompanied by fever. Only if fungoid granulomas change into pyodermas, or if extensive ulcerative areas develop, are septic temperatures encountered. If present, they are often accompanied by uncontrollable gastrointestinal signs and bronchopulmonary infiltrations.

3. **Reticuloses** in the narrow sense of the word consist of irreversible autonomous proliferations of the reticuloendothelial system. They sometimes simulate leukemias. In the chronic types, even with the development of preponderantly multicentric granulations which tend to form neoplasias in certain systems, elevated temperatures as a rule are lacking. However, in the previously mentioned reticulogranulomatosis cutis, especially shortly before death, high peaks of fever are observed. In the course of acute and subacute reticuloses, distinct attacks of fever that sometimes seem almost septic develop without any intercurrent secondary infections or therapeutic reactions that could be held responsible. If during this period of fever, which may be undulating, pronounced liver, spleen, or lymph node swellings develop, the picture may for a while simulate that of malignant lymphogranulomatosis.[2, 6]

4. Similar conditions prevail in the lipoid storage reticuloses such as **Letterer-Siwe disease** and **Hand-Schüller-Christian**

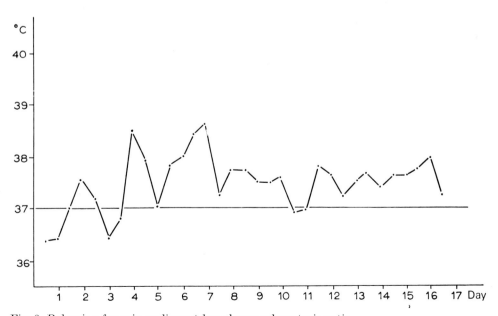

Fig. 8. Relapsing fever in malignant lymphogranulomatosis cutis.

lipoid granulomatosis. Here also there are only occasional hikes in temperature, which in exceptional cases may reach 39° C, or there may be undulating fever, if attacks of eruptions closely follow each other.

5. In **mast cell reticulosis** but apparently not in urticaria pigmentosa, high fever, sometimes initiated by chills and lasting up to 30 minutes with continous hyperemia, has been observed following dissemination of mast cells. This is in contrast to the flushes that occur with the carcinoids. In this condition only very short attacks of hyperemia are observed in the beginning, which, however, later tend to initiate a persistent pellagroid.[1]

6. **Multiple reticulohistiocytoma** ("lipoid dermatoarthritis") is only rarely accompanied by severe or recurrent bouts of fever.[4]

(1) BRINKMANN, E.: Mastzellenreticulose (Gewebsbasophilom) mit histaminbedingtem Flush und Übergang in Gewebsbasophilen-Leukämie. Schweiz. med. Wschr. *89:* 1046–1048 (1959).

(2) GERTLER, W.: Nosologie und Klinik der kutanen Retikulosen. Derm. Mschr. *155:* 621–638 (1969).

(3) HOERNI, B., J. CHAUVERGNE et M. PARSI: La fièvre de la maladie de Hodgkin. Presse méd. *78:* 1317–1319 (1970).

(4) HOLUBAR, K., und K. MACH: Histocytosis giganto-cellularis. Hautarzt *17:* 440–445 (1966).

(5) KNOTH, W., P. BREITWIESER und D. KLEINHANS: Zur Kenntnis unspezifischer Begleitdermatosen bei Lymphogranulomatose. Med. Welt. (N. F.) *19:* 170–177 (1968).

(6) MUSGER, A.: Hautretikulosen. Med. Klin. *62:* 1157–1160 (1967).

N. Panniculitis

1. Only nodular nonsuppurative **panniculitis** (Weber-Christian disease) among the various types of panniculitis is characterized by fever. The recurrent attacks of fever are usually associated with the development of nodes, which are typically painful when pressed but usually do not break down. They are located in the subcutaneous fat tissue. With single peaks of up to 39° C, periods of fever can recur for weeks and months. For further details see Chapter 22, A.[1]

(1) BAUMANN, R.: Die Panniculitisformen unter besonderer Berücksichtigung der Spontanpanniculitis Rothmann-Makai. Ärztl. Wschr. *8:* 609–613 (1953).

O. Diseases of the Sebaceous Glands

1. In patients with long-lasting and pronounced acne vulgaris or **acne conglobata,** papulopustular infiltrations can change into torpid ulcerations accompanied by sudden high fever. The cutaneous infiltrates, which are covered by a thin bluishred epidermis, discharge a gelatin-like material before they burst open. Fever and joint pains are present, simulating a septic picture. Antibiotics do not influence the course of the disease. Doses of corticosteroids, however, quickly improve the general condition. If topical treatment is added, the ulcerations heal rapidly. The etiology and pathogenesis of this disorder are still not clear.[1, 2]

(1) KELLY, A. P., and R. E. BURNS: Acute febrile ulcerative conglobate acne with polyarthralgia. Arch. Derm. (Chic.) *104:* 182–187 (1971).

(2) WINDOM, R. E., J. P. SANFORD and M. ZIFF: Acne conglobata and arthritis. Arthr. and Rheum. *4:* 632–635 (1961).

We have learned that no dermatosis can be recognized by "fever" or a special course of fever as is possible by observing Wunderlich's curve in typhus fever, continuous fever in abdominal typhoid, or a Pel-Ebstein curve in malignant lymphogranulomatosis of the skin (Hodgkin's disease). We know, however, that "ill-defined," elevated temperatures may occur in anhidrosis hypotrichotica, whereas pustular psoriasis is characterized by usually pronounced hyperpyrexia. Generally speaking, subfebrile temperatures or predominantly nightly elevations of temperature point to an infection secondary to the cutaneous changes or to a related complication in the inner organs. The occurrence of fever before death in rapidly progressive dermatoses of semimalignant character ("specific" erythrodermias or terminal mycosis fungoides) has the same significance. Finally, elevations of temperature belong to the many manifestations of primary infectious or "allergicly" conditioned skin reactions, as in the "toxic-allergic" exanthems, penicillin urticaria, Lyell's syndrome (in cases of "drug fever"), or infectious-hyperergic mechanisms such as the Jarisch-Herxheimer reaction.

2. Pruritus

The sensation of itching similar to that of tickling is usually considered a subthreshold pain perception, and because its definition has varied historically, it cannot be precisely defined. Therefore, "pruritus" cannot be objectively described except by occasional concomitant symptoms or signs such as shivering, goose pimples (cutis anserina), or the secondary results of scratching. They are caused by mechanical defense reactions against the "categorical imperative" of itching. Generally speaking, factors favoring the development of pruritus are changes of the circulatory volume such as dilatation of blood vessels, the liberation of proteases and occasionally also of biogenic amines, or changes of the potassium calcium quotient. Besides such peripheral or local factors a center located in the thalamus or hypothalamus has been postulated.

The subthreshold pain perceptions of itching or tickling are absent in skin without epidermis; the threshold of pruritus is elevated in analgesic areas which occur in, for instance, leprosy or syringomyelia. Vegetative nerve fibers may take part in the process of itching, but the existence of specific vegetative nerve elements causing pruritus is improbable. Nevertheless, pruritus and pain can occur synchronously or they can be perceived separately, as proved by the wheal caused by morphine injection. This results in a diminution of pain but an increase in the sensation of itching. It is possible to produce pain but not itching in mucous membranes adjacent to the skin. However, individuals with congenital analgesia do not experience itching.

As mentioned before, so-called natural pruritogenic substances exist, such as proteases and biogenic amines; in addition, there are chemicals that cause a precursory pain perception (for instance, some inorganic and organic acids, a 10 per cent sodium chloride solution, or methylbromide). For a long time clinicians felt that bile acids were responsible for the itching in obstructive jaundice; however, intravenous injection of bile acids does not provoke itching or, if it is already present, its exacerbation. From a psychic point of view the cause of itching may be attributed to aggressive tendencies, excessive clean-liness, or eroticism.

Dermatologists emphasize the role of special local tissue changes resulting in lichenification as a prerequisite to favoring, triggering, or maintaining itching. Lichenification is the result of a defense mechanism against pruritus that requires a great deal of effort. The change of originally normal skin into the coarseness of lichenified skin is brought about by about 100,000 scratches. Different kinds of scratching – i. e., rubbing, pressing, squeezing, or kneading – are used to stop itching or tickling. Not infrequently, stubborn pruritus leads to the removal or actual digging out of small pieces of skin ("prurits biopsiants" of the French); this happens especially in patients with chronic papular urticaria or prurigo simplex. In contrast, the patient with urticaria is content with rubbing or brushing the lesions; only exceptionally will he lacerate urticarial wheals.

Intensification of itching during the night or in hot surroundings occurs not only in scabies patients, but in any patient with a diminished threshold of itching. Beyond this, there are differences in the intensity of itching and hyperpathic or hypopathic responses to itching from patient to patient even with the same underlying disease or the same dermatosis. Dry air indoors during the winter months plus frequent bathing, especially in patients with an ichthyosiform skin condition, favors the development of itching (pruritus hiemalis).* Another factor for the (obese) person predisposed to itching is the removal of pressure on the skin upon undressing at night, especially the removal of constricting corsets, girdles, brassieres, and so on. Finally, a vicious circle of itching

_____
* Pruritus hiemalis even without an ich-thyosiform disposition is common in the United States owing to prolonged hot baths and overheated apartments or offices. (Tr.)

and scratching can turn into a fixation lasting for some time even after the pruritogenic agent has been removed. In addition, the presence of dead **Acarus scabiei** organisms, even after successful scabies treatment, results in a slowly decreasing antigen activity. The well-known sign of a shiny, highly polished nail of the patient suffering from itching (Fig. 9) is observed only after the scratching has gone on for some time. When this sign is present, statements of the patient about the degree of his subjective sensation of itching are superflous. (As von Hebra said, "Only those will scratch thoroughly who really suffer from itching.")[1, 2]

(1) BRACK, W.: Über die Entstehung des Juckens. Hautarzt *13:* 541–543 (1962).
(2) HENSEL, H.: Allgemeine Sinnesphysiologie, Hautsinne, Geschmack, Geruch. Springer, Berlin, Heidelberg, New York 1966.

A. Pruritus Without Obvious Cause or Essential Pruritus

Pruritus without an obvious cause or esential pruritus serves as a working diagnosis until a final elucidation has been made of a dermatosis, so far invisible, as for instance lichen planus before it has become manifest. Pruritus without visible skin changes, if one disregards endocrine causes (hypo- or hyperthyroidism), pregnancy, or menopause, is primarily due to liver disease.

1. Hepatic pruritus occurs in patients suffering from liver disease with or without jaundice as the result of cholestasis, and occasionally also as a cholestatic side effect of some medications (methyltestosterone, chloroquine, phenothiazine, and similar substances). Therefore, pruritus is absent in anhepatic hemolytic jaundice.

Fig. 9. Shiny nails in chronic pruritus; at right for comparison a normal fingernail.

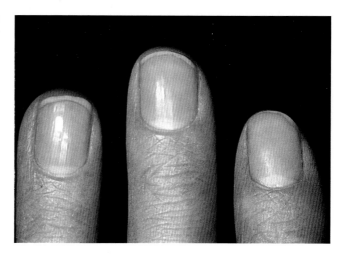

About one-fifth of patients with cirrhosis of the liver develop either generalized or localized pruritic crises unless they suffer from hepatic prurigo. In about 10 to 40 per cent of cases of acute hepatitis, and more frequently in adults than in children, pruritus will occur, not infrequently even before the appearance of jaundice, and nearly synchronously with the elevation of biliary acids in the blood serum. Almost always after some time has elapsed, hepatic pruritus becomes manifest through excoriations, pyodermas, and eczematization. A common finding is pruritus in xanthomatous biliary cirrhosis.

2. The statistics of the frequency of essential pruritus in diabetics, called **pruritus diabeticorum,** range widely from 2 to 40 per cent. Younger diabetic patients seem to suffer less from itching than older ones; this points to unspecific factors (age, dry skin, hypertension, mycotic or bacterial infections). Pruritus may persist even after control of the diabetes. Hypoglycemic shock is only very infrequently accompanied by itching. Usually, pruritus of the diabetic patient is generalized; more rarely, it may be localized in the genitoanal region.[1]

3. Pruritus and the erythemas are leading symptoms and signs of **renal dysfunction:** uremic conditions do not cause dermatoses. Such renal pruritus may have several causes, as shown during the last few years by patients undergoing dialysis. Itching is definitely caused by the retention of substances ordinarily excreted with the urine; it quickly stops once dialysis has been started. If patients continue to itch after dialysis treatment one must look for secondary hyperparathyroidism. Elimination of parathyroid glandular dysfunction often results in quick disappearance of itching. A third group of patients with kidney disease have increased itching only while undergoing dialysis; therefore, while uremia cannot be the cause of their itching, other, so far unknown, factors must be held responsible. An increase of uremic substances in the skin or an elevated calcium level in the serum does not necessarily result in pruritus. Uremic prurigo belongs to a type of prurigo which is extremely rare.[2, 3, 5]

4. According to the experience of the last few years, **hyperuricemia** has to be considered more frequently as a cause of pruritus. If a normally nonpruritic dermatosis is accompanied by itching (for instance, psoriasis vulgaris), an elevated serum uric acid level must be considered. Occasionally, pruritus can precede an attack of gouty arthritis.

5. Older patients with **arteriosclerotic hypertension** have an increased tendency toward itching. An apoplectic attack may be preceded by premonitory attacks of pruritus. Patients with polycythemia suffer from primarily nocturnal itching caused by warmth.

6. Furthermore, visceral **neoplasias** (such as bronchial cancers) show pruritus universally in the beginning; however, localized pruritus of the vulva and perianal region are much more frequently seen in cases of genital or rectal cancers. Chronic *leukemia* often shows very troublesome and therapy-resistant itching as a striking initial sign; very often such blood dyscrasias are accompanied by uncharacteristic cutaneous lesions caused by itching. Leukemic *pruritus*, one of the chronic leukemias, is usually considered to have a "central" origin; chronic myeloses commonly present itching with a concomitant hyperuricemia. Typically, acute, subacute, or chronic reticuloses are not accompanied by itching, but the plasmocytomas may occasionally present crises of itching.

7. Pruritus is the inevitable accompaniment of the two reticulogranulomatoses, **malignant lymphogranulomatosis** and mycosis fungoides. Pruritus lymphogranulomatosis is an almost invariable, continuous, or paroxysmal prodromal sign. Its intensity runs synchronously with the progression of the disease. In the beginning the pruritus of lymphogranulomatosis is localized primarily on the extremities; later it has a more or less diffuse involvement, sometimes for one to two years before the development of skin lesions. The itching of patients suffering from lymphogranulomatosis is a partial expression of their vegetative impairment (excessive hunger, disturbance of sleep, fever, and so on), and leads to persistent reactions to scratching, such as typical melanodermic ichthyosiform changes resembling vagabond skin; subsequent to this condition the typical eruption of itching, *prurigo lymphogranulomatosa*, will result.

8. In contrast to lymphogranulomatosis, pruritus of the closely allied **mycosis fungoides** is an optional sign; in some cases, however, it can be extremely recalcitrant. On the one hand, itching may be completely absent during the entire course of the disease, or it may be only a part of a many-faceted oversensitivity of the skin (such as burning), similar to that observed in dermatitis herpetiformis.

9. The so-called **senile pruritus,** which is the most frequent kind of generalized itching, is explained by the venous stasis that is observed in advanced age, increasing cardiac decompensation, senile lack of digestive acids and enzymes, and the general decrease of function of internal organs. Other factors that should be considered are urinary retention due to prostatic hypertrophy and the high rate of malignancies, even if the dryness of the skin so common to the older age group is disregarded. In addition, one has to think of undiagnosed tabes in older patients suffering from localized itching, especially in segmentary distribution (lumbosacral, periocular, perianal, for instance).

10. The **generalized anhidrosis** usually associated with this disease, not just dry skin, may account for pruritus. Clinical observations show pruritus in congenital ectodermal defects, in anhidrosis due to atabrine, and in Sjögren's syndrome, among others.[4]

(1) BREHM, G., und M. SANEI: Dermatologische Erkrankungen bei Diabetes mellitus. Med. Klin. *63:* 201–208 (1968).
(2) GROSSHANS, E., J. MALEVILLE und H. JAHN: Histopathologie und Pathogenese der Kalkablagerungen in der Haut bei Haemodialysis. Z. Haut- u. Geschl.-Kr. *47:* 467–473 (1972).
(3) HAMPERS, C. L., A. I. KATZ, R. E. WILSON and J. P. MERRILL: Disappearance of "uremic" itching after subtotal parathyroidectomy. New Engl. J. Med. *279:* 695–697 (1968).
(4) KAY, D. M., and H. I. MAIBACH: Pruritus and acquired anhidrosis. Arch. Derm. (Chic.) *100:* 291–293 (1969).
(5) MASSRY, S. G., M. M. POPOVTZER, J. W. COBURN, D. L. MAKOFF, M. H. MAXWELL and C. R. KLEEMAN: Intractable pruritus as a manifestation of secondary hyperparathyroidism in uremia. New Engl. J. Med. *279:* 697–700 (1968).

B. Pruritus of the Anogenital Region

The prototype of localized pruritus is the variety seen in the genital, anal, and perianal regions. It may present either as dermatitis, eczema, or typical lichenification.

1. The patient with **pruritus ani** should be examined for hemorrhoids, anal fissures, and the presence of intestinal parasites (especially pinworms). Diseases of the rectal area such as prostatitis, adenomas, cancers, constipation, or dyspeptic stools should also be considered. Rarely will pruritus ani be an early sign of diabetes mellitus or leukemia.

2. Formerly, **genital pruritus** was frequently caused not only by local dermatoses (eczema, kraurosis vulvae, for example), but also by many extracutaneous diseases such as diabetes, kidney and liver disease, or as a warning sign of cancer of the uterus; today, monilia infections of the vagina occupy first place in the etiology of genital pruritus.

The main symptom of *colpitis* or *vulvitis candidamycetica* is mild continuous itching and at times a burning pain in the lower vagina. Vaginal discharge is always present but the intertriginous, scaly, monilial dermatitis with satellite spreading is not. Small erosions with almost velvety granules also suggest moniliasis. Usually or for a long time, the small labia form a barrier to vaginal monilial infection. An inguinal intertriginous monilial mycosis, which also affects the vulva, may be a partial manifestation of a thrush infection of other sites of the skin.

Smear preparations showing dermatophytes of mucous membranes suffice for the diagnosis of a yeast infection since the mucosa is not invaded by trichophytons. To establish a diagnosis of candida mycosis of the skin, however, it is necessary to perform culture studies. *Trichomonal vaginitis* is characterized by the absence of the yellowish-white, spilled milk-like spongelets of thrush. The vaginal discharge of trichomonas is foamy, the vaginal mucosa is highly red and eroded, and the peri-urethral region shows dusky-red inflammation.

3. The diagnosis of "essential" pruritus vulvae, with the exception of that caused by urinary infections, has been difficult to narrow down by the ambiguity of so-called **kraurosis.** Today, kraurosis vulvae (or kraurosis of the glans penis) is recognized as a most characteristic end-stage of shrinkage, with stenosis of the meatus and flattening of the genital profile. Various basic conditions can cause this, particularly lichen sclerosus et atrophicus, less often lichen planus, morphea guttata, or senile atrophy. Therefore, if evidence of "primary" dermatoses at the periphery of other body areas is not forthcoming, kraurosis vulvae, together with "essential" pruritus of the vulva, remains unexplained, at least for the time being.

(1) KORTING, G. W.: Über einige »anonyme« Krankheitszustände der Haut. Münch. med. Wschr. *108:* 973–978 (1966).

C. Urticaria and Prurigo

Not only laymen consider itching a concomitant or predominant symptom of many skin diseases. This symptom is especially prevalent in the nosologically related *urticaria-strophulus – prurigo* group.

1. Urticaria itches not only before it becomes visible but also when it presents evanescent, reddish, or porcelain-white patches, and later annular or gyrate welts, depending on the degree of filtration pressure. The patient may become conscious (in a "mnemodermic" way) some time afterwards of circumscribed pruritus involving different cutaneous areas, corresponding to former urticarial wheals. Characteristic of urticaria is the fact that the lesions hardly ever show scratch effects because the patient may rub or press but not scratch.

The *angioneurotic edema* of *Quincke* (or *Milton*), which should be diagnosed only when it has a somewhat symmetric distribution, shows large swellings involving the deep cutaneous or subcutaneous layers, especially of the face, and presents tightly distended tissue which is less pruritic than markedly painful.

Itching in combination with other anaphylactoid fragments of shock (fever, for example), characterizes either *cold urticaria*, which is restricted to the area of cold exposure, or cold reflex urticaria, which shows wheals distant from the site of the cryogenic action. The numerous types of urticaria do not differ with regard to the qualities of itching.

Following a bath in cold water, especially in the open air, after a free interval of about fifteen hours a widespread outbreak of wheals appears accompanied by unusually severe itching and sometimes mild general symptoms such as headache and fever. Such an attack of urticarial wheals is restricted to those parts of the skin which were in contact with water. The cause is the penetration of the skin by the *cercariae of schistosomes.* The individual wheals persist for about three to four days, and after changing into hard infiltrated papules, they heal during the following weeks. The blood smear shows eosinophilia during the first phases of the disease. The trigger for this hypersensitive reaction to avian schistosome-dermatitis is repeated contact with the cercariae. The wheals are not a direct reaction to the penetration of the cercariae but are the result of sensitization. Careful histologic examination of an excised wheal shows cercaria in the epidermis.[2, 12]

Urticaria after streaking or other local triggering mechanisms is called *urticaria factitia* or red dermographism which can be provoked mainly on the upper half of the body, whereas the lower half shows white dermographism; both types are accompanied by little itching. Such dermographism is frequently observed as a somatic stigma in vagotonic individuals; generally speaking, this occurs with a diminution of the threshold of itching or in a minimal diffuse pruritus. Urticaria, therefore, is the response of the patient to itching.

2. In this connection mention should be made of **erythropoietic protoporphyria,** which gives rise to burning pruritus within a few minutes after solar exposure. It is followed by erythema, urticarial wheals, or vesicles. Of diagnostic importance is the finding of fluorescent erythrocytes* in a fresh smear with the aid of the fluorescent microscope (lamp: HBO 22; interference filter: BG 2 mm; barrier filter: 500 mm).[8, 10]

---

* Fluorocytes. (Tr.)

3. Strophulus is a descriptive term for a cutaneous disease; it is synonymous with lichen urticatus, papular urticaria, or acute prurigo simplex; the primary lesion is defined as an acute, small, nodular, papulovesicular, urticarial papule (histologically, a "serous papule"), characterized by compulsive, special itching. The result is persistent, intense pruritus with exoriation of the center of numerous papules scattered indiscriminately over the entire body. The almost unavoidable result is the development of impetigolike secondary infections. In young people suffering from strophulus, violent itching occurs particularly on palms and soles; these areas are rubbed so intensively that pyodermic infections result, leading to the picture of typical bullous staphylodermic "impetigo." However, the appearance of itching lesions on the midface, axillae, or genito-anal area contraindicates a diagnosis of strophulus, which however, may show in the teething child a few more nodules cn the face than centrally vesicular single lesions. Attacks of strophulus with eosinophilia and vesicles with central hemorrhagic points suggest insect bites ("piqûre").* Intestinal parasites are another factor in strophulus, but food allergies play only a minor role. Typical of strophulus are nocturnal attacks of itching and improvement with a change of environment ("sanatio spontanea nosocomialis" **). In contrast to strophulus, varicella (chickenpox) seldom shows pronounced itching. After an evanescent preexanthem, clear vesicles that later become turbid appear and new crops erupt, resulting in a polymorphic picture (resembling a navigational "chart of stars"). Although chickenpox favors the trunk, it also frequently involves the face, head, and, especially, the oral mucosa, with lentil-sized, erythema-tous lesions having central vesiculation. More difficult is the differential diagnosis against scabies, because the saclike burrows (which affect adults as well as children) are located on palms and soles as well as on anterior axillary folds, nipples, glans penis, and scrotum. Early scratching soon transforms these lesions into vesicular or papulovesicular lesions, with a resulting resemblance to strophulus lesions with palmoplantar location.[13]

4. The **prurigo papule** is characterized as a "réaction cutanée," which means a certain specific type of reaction of the skin of some individuals toward various etiologic factors. The average primary lesion may reach lentil-size and is a more or less skin colored, brownish-red, deep-lying nodule which is better felt than seen. The nodule causes severe itching, and for this reason is frequently excoriated; following such a scratch effect pruritus disappears

Fig. 10. Excoriated papules of prurigo.

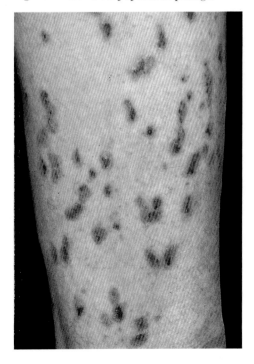

---

* Ninety per cent of which is caused by bedbugs. (Tr.)

** Healing upon hospitalization. (Tr.)

(Fig. 10). Later, deep-lying linear scratch marks appear as characteristic typical accessory lesions; these have unavoidable secondary infections which cause swelling of the regional lymph nodes. When such adenitis is marked it is called the bubo of prurigo. Histologically, such buboes present only the unspecific picture of dermatopathic lymphadenitis. The prurigo papule heals as it atrophies. Frequently, a patient with prurigo shows dry skin and an increase of the action of the arrectores of the hair, which gives the appearance of gooseflesh; in cases of endogenous eczemas especially, the prurigo stage usually constitutes the last cutaneous reaction, the final stage. There is no special pattern of distribution of the prurigo nodules, except the preponderance of those on the extensor aspects of the extremities, regardless of whether the disease is "prurigo Hebra" or prurigo vulgaris (or symptomatic prurigo). In cases of the now rather rare prurigo ferox Hebra, and especially the large nodular type of prurigo, dense dissemination of numerous lesions is seen on the extensors of the extremities, prurigo ferox favoring the inner aspects of the upper thighs.

Prurigo nodularis presents as semispherical or oval nodes of up to 1.0 cm in diameter, with superficially loosened horny layers. It is always accompanied by intense pruritus. Histologically, in the older type of prurigo nodularis, papillomatosis and irregular, almost pseudoepitheliomatous hyperplasia of the epidermis occur, as well as an abundance of nerve elements in the cutis within the area of infiltration; these findings are different from those of the other types of prurigo. There is hardly any other itching dermatosis which shows such an increase of nerve elements and the presence of schwannoma-like corpuscles. However, such nerve elements cannot be found in every case of typical prurigo nodularis. In my opinion *keratosis verrucosa* should not be identified with prurigo nodularis. Ordinarily, keratosis verrucosa is characterized by the close aggregation of large horny or obtuse lichen simplex papules. The differential diagnosis must consider the more pruritic multiple eruptive keratoacanthomas, which resemble keratosis verrucosa in their appearance. However, in contrast to prurigo nodularis these acanthomas are almost always limited to light exposed regions; they show the Koebner phenomenon and are frequently seen in the presence of an underlying malignant disease.[1, 11]

The diagnosis of *multiform chronic prurigo* is made when eczematization or lichenification caused by pruritus develops into typical prurigo papules, unless family or personal history put such lesions into the group of endogenous eczemas. Flexural eczema is an integral part of such a dermatosis, whereas the patient with prurigo shows a softness and pliability of the skin on the elbows and knees; even "palpation in a dark room" of such skin would lead to a diagnosis of prurigo.

Prurigo characterized by premenstrual exacerbation may be caused by hypersensitivity to an increase in the serum level of progesterone.[4, 5] Likewise, *chronic papular urticaria* is observed more often at menopause than at menarche.

Summer prurigo is a solar dermatosis presenting transitory polymorphic lesions with urticarial or vesicular components. *Prurigo gestationis* seems to be a form of the prurigo type of herpes gestationis rather than of dermatitis herpetiformis in pregnancy. *Melanotic prurigo*, which occurs mainly in women, shows atypical prurigo papules with widespread melanotic hyperpigmentations that vary in their duration and itch uniformly. Within the prurigo group leukodermas have been observed, not only in melanotic prurigo but also in *leukodystrophic* diathetic prurigo.[9] In any case, the diagnosis of prurigo in the adult must lead to a search for a number of possible causes, such as intestinal parasites, anacidity of the stomach, metabolic disturbances, liver diseases, and sometimes leukemias or systemic reticulo-granulomatoses. It cannot be stated whether prurigo, especially symptomatic prurigo vulgaris, will begin as pruritus followed later by the development of typical prurigo papules, or whether, in reverse, the existence of prurigo papules will stimulate pruritic crises. Frequently, the typical prurigo papule will give rise to a tormenting stinging itch, causing the patient not only to excoriate the center of the lesion but to remove the entire papule with his fingernail. The absence of the Koebner phenomenon in the patient with prurigo argues against precursory or preeruptive pruritus and more in favor of the primacy of the prurigo papule in the causation of the pruritus.[3, 6, 7, 13, 14]

(1) COWAN, M. A.: Neurohistological changes in prurigo nodularis. Arch. Derm. (Chic.) 89: 754–758 (1964).

(2) DÖNGES, J.: Hautreaktionen bei Schistosomeninvasion. Dtsch. med. Wschr. 89: 1512–1516 (1964).

(3) GREITHER, A.: On the different forms of prurigo, pruritus-prurigo. Current Problems in Dermatology 3: 1–30 (1970).

(4) HOISCHEN, W., und G. K. STEIGLEDER: Überempfindlichkeit gegen Progesteron bei Prurigo mit prämenstrueller Exazerbation. Dtsch. med. Wschr. 91: 398–399 (1966).

(5) JONES, W. N., and V. H. GORDON: Auto-immune progesterone eczema. Arch. Derm. (Chic.) 99: 57–59 (1969).

(6) KOGOJ, F.: Die morphologischen Aspekte der Prurigo. Z. Haut- u. Geschl.-Kr. 31: 37–49 (1961).

(7) LENNERT, K.: Lymphknoten. In: Hdb. der spez. pathol. Anatomie u. Histologie. Hrsg. E. UEHLINGER. Bd. I/3 A, S. 392–402. Springer, Berlin, Göttingen, Heidelberg 1961.

(8) LYNCH, P. J., and L. J. MIEDLER: Erythropoietic protoporphyria. Report of a family and a clinical review. Arch. Derm. (Chic.) 92: 351–356 (1965).

(9) PIERINI, L. E., and J. M. BORDA: Prurigo melanotica. Hautarzt 11: 104–107 (1960).

(10) SUURMOND, D., J. VAN STEVENINCK and L. N. WENT: Some clinical and fundamental aspects of erythropoietic protoporphyria. Brit. J. Derm. 82: 323–328 (1970).

(11) THIES, W.: Neurohistologische Studie zur Differentialdiagnose der Prurigo nodularis Hyde und anderer Formen umschriebener Lichenifikation. Arch. klin. exp. Derm. 201: 539–555 (1955).

(12) VOGEL, H.: Hautveränderungen durch Cercaria ocellata. Derm. Wschr. 90: 577–581 (1930).

(13) WINKLER, M.: Prurigo, Strophulus, Pruritus, In: Hdb. Haut- u. Geschl.-Krh. Hrsg. J. JADASSOHN. VI/1, S. 301–370. Springer, Berlin 1927.

(14) ZAUN, H., und D. ATHANASSIADIS: Prurigo simplex subacuta. Eine charakteristische Hautreaktion bei Störungen anderer Organe. Fortschr. Med. 87: 1017–1023 (1969).

D. Groups of Eczemas

The eczemas, which can easily be subdivided into common, seborrheic, and endogenous eczemas, are excellent representatives of dermatoses associated with itching.

1. Common eczema is a response to external conditions, whereas seborrheic and endogenous eczemas are based on constitutional factors and affect different age groups. Dermatitis or contact dermatitis (dermatitis venenata) represents a cutaneous reaction, which with regard to time and place is distinctly dependent on a noxious agent. For the most part, it has a monotonous erythematous appearance, whereas common eczema is characterized by ever changing lesions. Papular vesicular lesions characterize an intermediate stage. Common eczema may, therefore, represent a nodular dermatosis.

2. Patients with **dermatitis** complain in general of stinging, burning, or sore sensations, limited by the extension of the eruption. In contrast, common eczema apparently depends on the acuity of the eruption and is characterized by intense itching. At the papulovesicular stage, the characteristic intermediate lesions of common eczema convey a rather tense sensation, which at the stage of chronic morphologic eczematization – i. e., with distinct lichenification and a squamous component – reverts again to intense itching. The patients are forced to scratch and excoriate, which leads to harmful effects and the intensification of the eczematous process.

3. The patient with **endogenous eczema** experiences a characteristic change of reaction sites and reaction modes. At the stage of torpid chronic lichenification of flexures and wrists especially, or when disseminated, common, eczematous lichen simplex-like reactions occur, the patient is tormented and persecuted by violent itching.

4. The same can be said about **lichen simplex chronicus** (also called neurodermatitis circumscripta), which is related to endogenous eczema but should be separated from it. The long oval lesions of lichen simplex chronicus are almost always accompanied by stubborn pruritus. They can be recognized by a characteristic division into three zones: (1) a round, level, pinhead-sized (rarely slightly larger), obtuse papule, (2) a centrally flat, primary, lichenified zone, and (3) toward the periphery, a dirty brown pigmented edge.

5. Lichen amyloidosus is also accompanied by violent itching. Most often affected are the legs or the extensor surfaces of the forearms, usually symmetrically. A differential diagnosis from lichen simplex chronicus may be difficult. However, the latter's characteristic three-zone structure is missing, and the papule of lichen amyloidosus has a definite brownish-red hue. The decisive factor, however, is the optic polarization evidence of pericollagenous amyloid in the lesion itself.[1, 2]

Lichen planus, which tends to become verrucous, especially on the legs, must also be excluded. In general, the diagnosis of lichen planus is confirmed by the presence of oral or genital mucous membrane lesions or the visualization of Wickham's striae within a flat polygonal papule. If this is not possible, the histologic examination will help. It would show a widening of the granular layer, hyperkeratosis, and a bandlike infiltrate of lymphocytes bordering on the epidermis. Parakeratotic features are always lacking to some extent, and if at the same time regular uniform acanthosis and spongiosis with a loose, chronically inflamed infiltrate exist, the diagnosis indicates lichen simplex chronicus.

6. Seborrheic eczema hardly ever itches, except in intertriginous areas combined with a relatively more pronounced, acute, common eczematization ("acutely eczematized seborrheic eczema"), or if there is a tendency toward an acute eruptive dissemination, or if pronounced thick dry scales form on the scalp. Of the two maximal variants of seborrheic eczema, *erythrodermia desquamativa*, occurring in childhood, apparently does not itch. The so-called *seborrheic erythrodermia of the aged*, however, greatly torments the cachectic patient, who will almost always soon develop generalized dermopathic lymphadenitis.

7. Fox-Fordyce disease is, more than any other dermatosis, characterized by vehement, almost tormenting, itching. Because of its clinical lichenoid aspect, it is considered by some dermatologists to be

Fig. 11. Fox-Fordyce dis-
ease; pronounced desquamation with lumen of an apocrine sweat gland. HE stain,
400×.

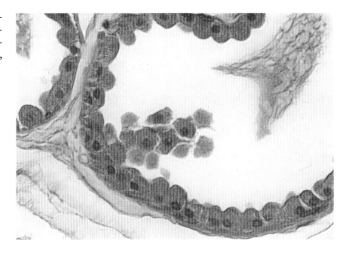

identical with lichen simplex chronicus, although the location of the grouped nodules in the axillas and around the nipples, the umbilical region, and the genital and perianal regions justifies a certain special classification of this disorder. The individual pinhead-sized, lichen simplex-like, flat but semispherically protuberant nodules, which simulate papules of prurigo, develop mostly in connection with an exceptionally severe attack of itching. In contrast to lichen simplex, however, Fox-Fordyce disease lacks the central confluence and flat extensions of lichenification. Also different from classic prurigo is the continuous itching which persists even after excoriation of the single lesions and in spite of no eruption of nodules. The symptom of localized pruritus is, therefore, in Fox-Fordyce disease much more pronounced and significant than in prurigo vulgaris. Other peculiarities of the itching in this disease, which is distinctly dependent on female hormones, are the tendency toward premenstrual exacerbation and its association with paroxysmal hyperhidrosis, i. e., localized attacks of sweating, in the areas in which Fox-Fordyce disease is located. Today one can hardly consider the disorder a syndrome limited to apocrine

sweat retention (Fig. 11) because the characteristic histologic changes are neither uniform nor unequivocal from case to case.[1, 2]

(1) BROWNSTEIN, M. H., and E. B. HELWIG: The cutaneous amyloidoses; I. Localized forms. Arch. Derm. (Chic.) *102:* 8–19 (1970).

(2) SCHNEIDER, W., und H. P. MISSMAHL: Lichen amyloidosus als Beispiel der perikollagenen, primären, hautbeschränkten und vorwiegend umschriebenen Amyloidose. Arch. klin. exp. Derm. *224:* 235–247 (1966).

E. Papular Dermatoses

1. In **lichen planus,** another lichenoid dermatosis, pruritus may again precede the development of polygonal primary lesions on the flexor aspect of the wrists, forearms, and legs ("prurit lichénien sans éruption cutanée" or "invisible dermatosis"). Pruritus may, however, also be felt only in the neighborhood of the lichen planus eruption, or may, as already described in the section on urticaria, persist after the regression of the papular lesions. In any case, there are types with severe, mostly paroxysmal, itching, as well as others in which the patients have only insignificant itching or no itching at all. There are still other patients with the disease in whom pruritus, which is undoubtedly the most characteristic symptom of the disorder, is subject to great variations. Mild itching almost always occurs in genital locations, whereas it is completely lacking in the oral mucosa. Involvement here occurs before or together with that on the rest of the body but is often discovered only by chance.

Patients with lichen planus of the oral mucosa have a rather strange burning sensation, the same sensation that patients with acute lichen planus feel on the skin of the entire body in the early stages before the outbreak of a massive eruption. Patients suffering from *lichen ruber pemphigoides* who have a denuded oral mucosa complain of pain when they eat or drink highly seasoned food.

The extent and severity of the itching in a patient with lichen planus can always be recognized by observing the presence of scratch effects and streaks of lesions in the scratch effects adjacent to the eruption; these scratch effects are apparently due to an isomorphic response.

This Koebner's phenomenon is characteristic of lichen planus, but can also be observed in eruptive psoriasis vulgaris, certain eczemas that spread hematogenously, juvenile or plane warts, lichen sclerosus et atrophicus, and also in rare cases of multiple-eruptive keratoacanthomas.

2. Pityriasis rubra pilaris, which some dermatologists incorrectly identify with lichen ruber acuminatus, is characterized by closely agminated and acuminated papules which are confined to the hair follicles, especially on the fingers and the shaft of the penis. Initial complaints are vague, but sometimes mild burning and moderate itching occur. The itching almost never reaches the extent of that of lichen planus. *Lichen nitidus*, likewise, is not an itching dermatosis. Some dermatologists identify it with lichen planus; it presents, however, no Wickham's striae, no Koebner's phenomenon, and, in contrast to lichen planus, no morphologic changes of the papule.

F. Acanthosis Nigricans Group

Pruritus may serve as a crude differentiation between benign and malignant acanthosis nigricans, since it has been more frequently observed and is more intense in malignant acanthosis nigricans[1] than in other types.

(1) FLADUNG, G., und H.-J. HEITE: Häufigkeitsanalytische Untersuchungen zur Frage der symptomatologischen Abgrenzung verschiedener Formen der Acanthosis nigricans. Arch. klin. exp. Derm. *205:* 282–311 (1957).

G. Zoonoses

1. Pruritus is a leading symptom in all animal parasitoses. It behaves, however, differently in each dermatozoonosis. Even in **scabies,** itching varies from case to case and does not occur in proportion to the extent of the existing rash. This is proved by the strongly parakeratotic but also markedly anesthetic crusted or *Norwegian scabies* (Fig. 12), since the mites which create the parakeratotic shell of crusts are not prevented from doing so by the patients, who are run-down and less sensitive to itching. Apparently, scabies causes greater itching in the beginning than after the patients have become accustomed to it. In contrast to other epizoonoses, the patient with scabies is plagued by itching, especially at the site of the invading mite. This results in excessive excoriation at the site of the burrows and in marked pyoderma. The patient with scabies suffers from nightly increases of itching as in every other pruritus. In scabies, however, this seems to result from the nightly increased activity of the parasites and not only from the warmth of the bed. I learned this by questioning men working by day in a hot place. We observed in a film, however, that the scabies mite becomes conspicuously more active in the heat given by the light cone of the klieg light. The diagnosis of scabies is based in part on the manifestations just mentioned, but primarily on the presence of burrows and the finding of the mite (Fig. 13) in the interdigital folds of the fingers, the wrists, and the axillary folds (Fig. 14), or on the shaft of the penis (Fig. 15).[1, 3, 4]

2. In **pediculosis corporis,** in contrast to scabies, the sensation of itching is not fixed to the site of the invading body louse (Fig. 16) or to developing erythematous hives or nodular reactions. Patients soon become indifferent to the itching caused by the lice. Pruritus is, however, present within the whole infested area. Therefore, characteristic long excoriation marks caused by nails are present over the entire integument; these together with the pigmentations and depigmentations that occur create the so-called *vagabond's* skin (Fig. 17). In contrast, a massive infestation

of head lice *(pediculosis capitis)* is often tolerated for a long time on the neck and scalp without any response. People of low intelligence may note an agreeable soft sense of warmth and hardly notice any itching. Similar observations are made by patients with pediculosis pubis (crab lice, Fig. 18). Itching, if present, is so mild that the after effects of scratching, eczematization, or pyoderma are usually lacking, even if distinct maculae caeruleae (Fig. 19) are already present.

The bite of the *bedbug* usually produces violently itching wheals (Fig. 20), which may be transformed like the wheal of Culicinae *(mosquitoes,* Fig. 21) into a nodule even after a long time. Such a nodule of urticaria from bedbug bites can cause itching when touched. On the other hand, prolonged contact with bedbugs produces an increasing acclimatization to bites with a corresponding decrease in the sequence of reactions. In general, hives from bedbugs are usually located on skin not covered by nightwear. The distribution of bedbug wheals resembling footprints is also characteristic (Fig. 20).

3. Itching from **flea bites** (pulicosis) is, like that of lice bites, not confined to the site of the bite. The sensation from a flea bite has been occasionally described as a painfully radiating "light" or "biting." Not only does the degree of involvement from flea bites vary from individual to individual according to disposition, but the mode of reaction also differs greatly (gigantic urticaria, purpura pulicosa).

4. One should think of **trombiculiasis** (chigger bite, "harvest bug," "août̂at") if severe itching with lesions like those of "chronic papular urticaria" (and, to a lesser extent, of strophulus) occur, depending on the season (July to September), climatic conditions (warm and dry weather), and occupation of the patient (harvest workers, workers in forests, or

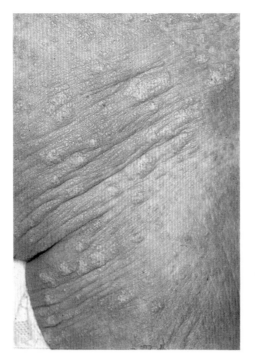

Fig. 12. Norwegian scabies.

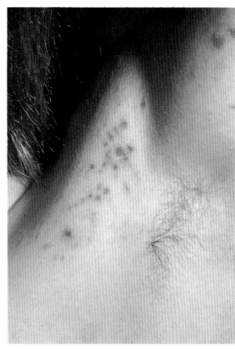

Fig. 14. A favorite localization of scabies in the anterior axillary fold.

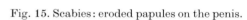

Fig. 15. Scabies: eroded papules on the penis.

Fig. 13. *Sarcoptes scabiei*.

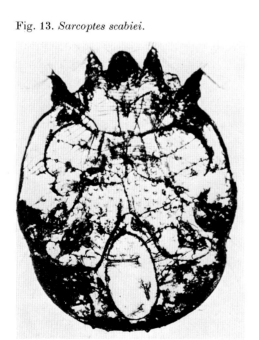

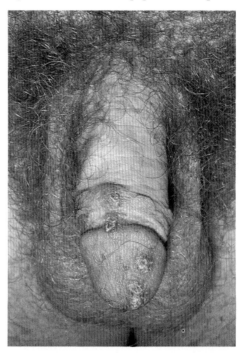

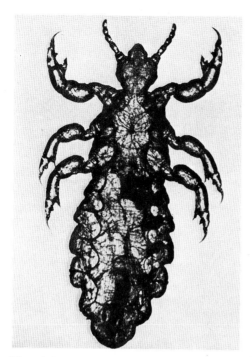

Fig. 16 *Pediculus vestimentorum*.

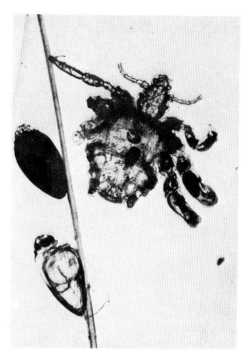

Fig. 18. *Pediculus (Phthirus) pubis* with nits.

Fig. 19. Tâches bleues (maculae caeruleae) in
pediculosis corporis.

Fig. 17. Vagabond's skin.

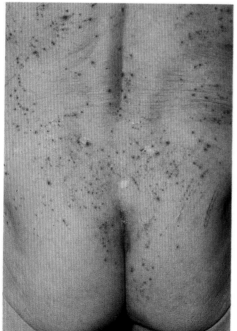

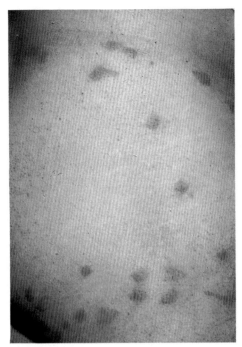 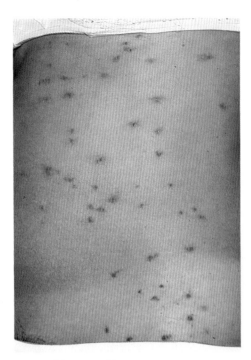

Fig. 20. Linear distribution of bites from bedbugs. They follow each other like footprints.

Fig. 21. Mosquito bites.

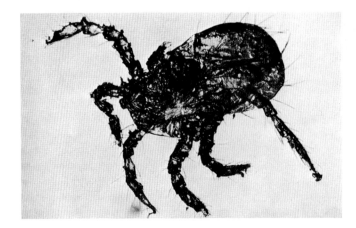

Fig. 22. *Trombicula autumnalis*.

pickers of gooseberries or currants). In Germany it is usually caused by the mite *Trombicula* (or *Leptus*) *autumnalis* (Fig. 22).* Suspicion is increased if about three to four hours after the questionable exposure pruritus, which is mild in the beginning, develops into intense itching, especially in the popliteal areas and in places with tight clothing (garters, suspenders, and brassières). After 24 to 48 hours, lentil-sized lesions, which sometimes develop into hemorrhagic or vesicular hempgrain-sized papules lasting a fortnight, can be observed, although itching may be present for only one week (Fig. 23). If the distribution on sites of contact favors trombiculiasis rather than purpura pulicosa, proof of the presence of the parasite is feasible only immediately after the development of the strophuluslike lesion. (In scabies the mite can be demonstrated at later stages.) Only rarely can a small red point be scraped with the scalpel and identified under the microscope as the larva of the mite. *Leptus autumnalis* itself remains always on the surface of the skin and soon falls off. Reexposure may cause new eruptions, but otherwise, even three to four weeks after the leptus invasion, residual pigmentations or a few deeply cutaneous nodes point to the previous infestation, as we have also often observed in scabies. In summary, in trombiculiasis the diagnosis rests not so much on the individual lesion but rather on the predilection of the location and the typical history.[2]

In **grain** or **wheat itch** caused by *Pyemotes ventricosus* of the family Tarsonemidae, proof of the presence of the parasite is almost never successful. The mite reaches the skin by contact with grain or straw. A search of the dust of the grain or straw sacks may prove successful.

* In North America it is caused by *Trombicula alfreddugèsi*. (Tr.)

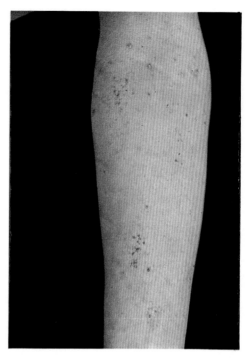

Fig. 23. Trombiculiasis.

A few hours after exposure violent pruritus and an urticarial eruption occur, which increase in the following days and are transformed into papulovesicular or purpuric lesions, gradually regressing within two weeks. In sensitive patients and those with intense infestation, general signs (fever, tachycardia, enlargement of the lymph nodes, edema, proteinuria, eosinophilia, and asthma) develop. Characteristic is the intensity of lesions at the sites of immediate contact, such as the backs of sack-carriers.

In **gamasoidosis** or bird mite "eczema," caused by *Dermanyssus avium*, nightly itching and micropapular lesions which are soon excoriated, or, less frequently, urticarial or eczematized lesions, predominate. The cutaneous changes are usually located on uncovered skin areas, in persons who handle bird cages, hen- and pigeon-houses, and thus come in contact with these blood-sucking mites. As in the previously mentioned epizoonoses, the mites usually cannot be found on the skin of the infested individuals.

Finally, **grocer's itch** should be mentioned. It also shows severely itching, micropapular or papulovesicular eruptions, which, however, may be complicated by asthma. It occurs on uncovered areas or sites of contact. If infested cheese is the cause, a tyroglyphic mite is responsible.*

---

* If the parasites are from infested fruit, such as dates and raisins, this mite is *Carpoglyphus passularum*. (Tr.)

The eruption, also called "copra itch" or "gale des épiciers," will have to be diagnosed by the history of contact with the above-named substances rather than by the morphology of the lesions.

(1) HEILESEN, B.: Studies on acarus scabiei and scabies. Acta derm.-venereol. (Stockh.) *26*, Suppl. 14 (1946).
(2) FUSS, S., und R. HANSER: Über Trombidiosis. Arch. Derm. Syph. (Berl.) *167:* 644–658 (1933).
(3) MISGELD, V.: Differentialdiagnostisches Problem: impetiginisierte ekzematisierte Skabies-Lues II-Psoriasis vulgaris. Med. Klin. *64:* 2189–2192 (1969).
(4) NÜRNBERGER, F.: Skabies. Med. Welt *19* (N. F.): 575–576 (1968).

3. Disturbances of Sweating

A. Hyperhidrosis

From a neurologic point of view one can distinguish between cortical-emotional thermoregulatory, subcortical, gustatory-bulbar, and spinal-sensory causes of sweating.

The innervation of the eccrine sweat glands runs through the sympathetic chain, although the transmission of the nervous impulse is due to cholinergic substances and can be inhibited only by atropine or allied substances. Depending upon which level of the pathway responsible for sweating is interrupted, different kinds of cessation of sweat gland secretion will result. Severance of the route proximal to the sympathetic ganglia will result in

an absence of sweating after central physiologic stimulation, while peripheral irritation will cause undiminished or excessive reactions. An interruption beyond the spinal ganglion (distal from the sympathetic chain or within the ganglion itself) will cause interruption of any response to stimuli and also to cholinergic substances. At first, the sweat glands will show reversible atrophy, but when the interruption is prolonged, irreversible atrophy will occur.

Accordingly, in several diseases a deficiency in or a dysfunction of the central or the peripheral nervous system regulation will result in a disturbance of the sweat secretion in certain areas of the skin. This is of diagnostic importance (i.e., unilateral

Fig. 24. Hyperhidrosis of the palm after contact with cold wave fluid.

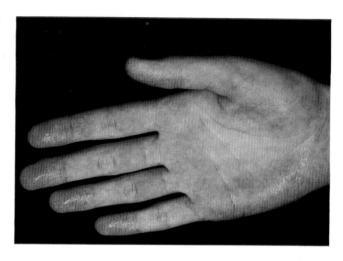

alteration of sweat gland function due to paralysis of one side of the body, such as that observed in hemiplegia, unilateral abscesses, or tumors of the hemispheres). Radiculitis of a spinal nerve may lead to segmentary disturbance of sweat secretion. Substances causing hyperhidrosis are cholinergic drugs such as pilocarpine, muscarine, cocaine, nicotine, and some poisons of snakes and fishes. Clinically important is the increased sweating which occurs after treatment with salicylic acid, penicillin, or cortisone. Palmar hyperhidrosis has been observed after repeated contact with hair-waving preparations (Fig. 24) or calcium chloride. [6]

Insensible perspiration, the insensible loss of water vapor through the skin, takes place through transepidermal diffusion without action of the sweat glands; in many dermatoses this loss of water is increased within the affected areas as compared to nonaffected skin. Corresponding to the physically passive character of insensible perspiration, such an increase will take place within skin areas which are covered with loose keratinous structures (scales) and which tend to dry out more readily, whereas cutaneous conditions involving a thickened structure of tissue

(scleroderma) will show diminution of aglandular loss of water. [3]

1. Horner's syndrome in particular shows zonal anhidrosis; **auriculotemporal** or **Frey's syndrome** presents a red area on the cheek with sweating and disturbance of the taste sensation after operative procedures on the parotid gland. There are other **taste-linked hyperhidroses** occurring in the submental region after injury to the chorda tympani and on the upper arm after sympathectomy of the cervical ganglia. [1, 2, 7, 10]

Paradoxically, sympathectomy may result in thermoregulatory hyperhidrosis; such an event requires a cautious approach to sympathectomy for the treatment of palmoplantar hyperhidrosis. [7]

2. There is a close connection between sweat gland secretion and the endocrine system; it is well known that **hyperthyroidism** presents an increase in sweating while the dry skin of **myxedema** shows diminution of perspiration. So-called **vegetative dystonia** shows irregular anhidrotic cutaneous areas with generalized pronounced hyperhidrosis. The distribution of the disturbed sweating pattern sometimes varies greatly at short intervals, but if cutaneous changes are present, the disturbance persists for a relatively long time.

3. Quantitative disturbance of sweat gland activity as a dermatosis *sui generis* is known as **idiopathic universal hyperhidrosis.** This may occur in families and may also be increased by obesity, vegetative-emotional hypersensitivity, and other factors. Symptomatic hyperhidroses are observed as an accompaniment of inner foci of infection, tuberculosis, eruptive secondary syphilis, tetanus, trichinosis, and in the form of the acid sweat of rheumatic patients and in those with gout. In addition, women in the premenstruum, during pregnancy, or around the climacterium suffer from increased universal sweating.

4. Among the most important ephidroses are **hyperhidrosis of the feet and hands** and **hyperhidrosis of the axilla,** which usually occur in combination with osmi- or bromhidrosis. Increased sweat secretion on the palms is also observed in persons who handle calcium chloride or cold wave solutions. On the feet, however, unsuitable footwear which does not absorb perspiration (such as rubber boots or stockings made from polyamide textiles) is to be blamed. Symptomatic hyperhidroses accompany **palmoplantar keratoses,** which form a nosologic entity. Even before the development of hyperkeratosis, i.e., in the preceding erythematous phase which is later evident as a red margin around the yellow-brownish keratinization, excessive hyperhidrosis limited to the involved skin plays an important role.

It is possible that the presence of increased keratoplastic amino acids in the sweat favors the formation of hyperkeratoses. In some cases of severe keratinization, however, there is an absence of hyperhidrosis, which can be explained partly by

the absorption of the sweat in the especially severe horny masses, which then appear somewhat macerated. In general, hyperhidrosis of the palmoplantar keratoses is characterized by the valerianlike smell of sweat decomposition. Striking palmoplantar hyperhidrosis occurs, however, only in the diffuse keratodermas, less regularly in the circumscribed and striated forms, and hardly at all in the forms with multiple small lesions or in the dissipated palmoplantar keratodermas. The rare poriform losses of substance on palm and sole, which are not regularly bound to the openings of the sweat glands as in *periporal keratoma,* are usually not accompanied by a distinct local increase in sweat secretion. Likewise, other palmoplantar, maculopapular manifestations with increased keratinization (such as those caused by arsenic, secondary syphilis, palmar and plantar psoriasis vulgaris, tinea hyperkeratotica, and others) hardly ever show an obvious palmoplantar increase in sweat such as that characteristic of the genetically determined, mostly diffuse, palmoplantar keratoses.

Accordingly, in other universal skin dysplasias or polydysplasias with considerable palmoplantar changes, such as *pachonychia congenita* or *dyskeratosis congenita,* obvious palmoplantar hyperhidrosis is noted.

5. Of the hereditary epidermolyses only the **recurrent bullous eruption of the feet** (Cockayne disease), a special type of epidermolysis bullosa simplex, involves noticeable hyperhidrosis of the palms and soles. [4]

6. The general significance of the findings (mostly precursory) on hyperhidrosis in early **endangiitis obliterans** in zones of disturbed blood supply is unknown. Vasomotor prodromas in the form of disturbances of the sweat secretion in progressive scleroderma are also hard to evaluate.

7. Among the hamartomas and tumors, circumscribed increases of sweat are found in the isolated and often painful **glomus tumors** or in the angiomas of Maffucci's syndrome. Here especially, attention should be paid to the unusual sweat formation on the surface of the cavernous hemangiomas (Fig. 25) because, histopathologically, they apparently resemble the sweat gland structures in hidroangioma cutis. [5, 8, 9]

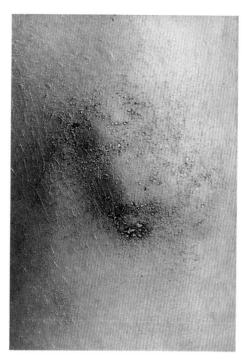

Fig. 25. Hidroangioma. Increased activity of the sweat glands is shown with starch powder.

(1) FEGELER, F.: Zur Kenntnis des auriculotemporalen Syndroms mit Bemerkungen zur nervösen Schweißversorgung des Gesichts. Hautarzt *3:* 178–180 (1952).

(2) HERXHEIMER, A.: Gustatory sweating and pilomotion. Brit. med. J. *1958/I:* 688–689.

(3) HOLZMANN, H., G. W. KORTING und CH. OEHMICHEN: Vergleichende Messungen der Feuchtigkeitsabgabe von Herdbezirk und unveränderter Haut bei verschiedenen Hautkrankheiten. Arch. klin. exp. Derm. *212:* 312–318 (1961).

(4) KORTING, G. W.: Zur Kenntnis der sog. rezidivierenden Blasen-Eruption an den Füßen bei heißem Wetter (Weber-Cockayne). Z. Haut- u. Geschl.-Kr. *17:* 36–40 (1954).

(5) KORTING, G. W., und G. BREHM: Hidroangioma cutis. Z. Haut- u. Geschl.-Kr. *38:* V – VIII (1956).

(6) SCHLIACK, H.: Zum Problem der Schweißdrüseninnervation. Nervenarzt *33:* 421–423 (1962).

(7) SHELLEY, W. B., and R. FLORENCE: Compensatory hyperhidrosis after sympathectomy. New Engl. J. Med. *263:* 1056–1058 (1960).

(8) SÖLTZ-SZÖTS, J.: Bericht über einen Fall von Schweißdrüsennaevus kombiniert mit einem Angiom. Z. Haut- u. Geschl.-Kr. *24:* 189–192 (1958).

(9) VILANOVA, X., J. PIÑOL AGUADÉ et A. CASTELLS: Hamartome angiomateux sudoripare sécrétant. Dermatologica (Basel) *127:* 9–16 (1963).

(10) YOUNG, A. G., and G. E. STEIN: A further report on the chorda tympani syndrome. Brit. med. J. *1960/I:* 620–621.

B. Anhidroses and Hypohidroses

1. Anhidroses caused anatomically. Complete anhidrosis can be expected only if the sweat glands are entirely absent. This absence is only a part of a generalized malformation of *anhidrotic ectodermal dysplasia*. It becomes evident soon after birth when attention is called to "unexplained" bouts of fever caused by disturbed heat regulation.

In *incontinentia pigmenti* (Franceschetti-Jadassohn type) hypohidrosis is also caused anatomically. It usually becomes evident as late as the second year of life, as does the anhidrosis in patients with *Fabry's disease*. Here, most probably anhidrosis develops by deposits of the disease-specific ceramide trihexoside in the nerves regulating the sweat glands. Degeneration of sweat glands occurs after the administration of atabrine and chloroquin. After doses of atabrine hypohidrosis develops with a lichenoid dermatitis. [2, 3]

2. Segmentally arranged anhidrotic areas are sometimes observed in the course of **diabetic neuropathia.** According to the extent of the skin area for which the regulation of sweat has been shut off, these patients experience disturbances of general well-being and even bouts of fever, which often remain unnoticed. This happens especially when the external temperature is high. A compensatory regulation of body temperature then causes increased hyperhidrosis in skin areas which have not been affected by anhidrosis.

3. Similar dissociated disturbances of sweat secretion will also be observed after **nerve injuries,** exclusion of the spinal ganglia, or **metastatic lesions** in the spinal marrow between T 3 and L 3. A typical disturbance of sweat secretion of the postganglionic type occurs in **Pancoast's tumors.** Anhidrosis extends ipsilaterally to the face, neck, shoulder, arm, and hand and ends below in the fourth to eight cervical dermatome. [1, 8]

4. Functionally conditioned anhidroses and hypohidroses. Primarily functional *anomalies of the distribution of sweat* which occur in dermatoses that are associated with hyperkeratosis and parakeratosis and with acanthosis are important in the differential diagnosis. These include especially *common eczema* and *psoriasis vulgaris,* which are characterized by suppression of sweat in the involved areas; this may be preceded for several days *in loco* by circumscribed hyperhidrosis. Secretion of sweat may also be stopped in *hypertrophic lichen planus* and in some *erythrodermas.*[5]

Pharmacologically, parathormone can revive the sweating which has ceased in such affected areas. This hormonal effect

can be stopped by the sedation of the brain stem.

Cessation of sweat secretion or a blocked pilocarpine effect is also present within an erythema from ultraviolet light. Sweat secretion is also nonfunctioning in an area of vitiligo but not within a nevus depigmentosus.

The profile of the type of sweating in the patient with *endogenous eczema* is characteristic: the site of visibly increased water secretion is at the same time the site of actual or potential skin manifestations. This can be proved at the stage of eczema of the flexor sites if one subjects the patient to a centrally regulated trial of sweating. Increased sweating of the flexures and on the face results, although the general sweat delivery is diminished or delayed. On the other hand, in seborrheic eczema diffusely distributed sweat is present, with a preference for the middle body line corresponding to its predilection sites. [6, 7]

A dermatosis directly connected with the function of the sweat glands is cholinergic *perspiration urticaria,* which affects small areas. It usually spares the areas of the apocrine sweat glands, which produce less acid sweat. The phenomenon of perspiration urticaria, moreover, occurs as an axon reflex or by stimulation with acetyl choline.

Symptomatic oligohidroses are sometimes observed around an *ozenanose,* in *renal hydrops, diabetes insipidus,* and massive *diarrhea.* The skin of the patient with hypothyroidism should again be mentioned. It lacks the moisture from perspiration. *Postinfectious anhidroses* are present following typhoid and typhus. *Drugs* such as thallium, lead, arsenic, or salvarsan may have the same aftereffect. Even more infrequent are oligohidroses due to hypertension, tumors of the hypothalamus, or psychic traumas. "Tropic anhidrosis" means disturbed heat regulation as in heat stroke or in connection with bouts of miliaria rubra or chloroquine medication.

(1) BECK, K.: Die Bedeutung des vegetativen Syndroms, insbesondere der Schweiß-störungen, für die Frühdiagnose der sog. Pancoasttumoren. Nervenarzt 25: 373 bis 378 (1954).

(2) BISCHOFF, A., U. FIERZ, F. REGLI und J. ULRICH: Peripher-neurologische Stö-rungen bei der Fabryschen Krankheit (Angiokeratoma corporis diffusum universale). Klin. Wschr. 46: 666–671 (1968).

(3) FRANCESCHETTI, A., et W. JADASSOHN: A propos de l' « Incontinentia pigmenti », délimitation de deux syndromes différents figurant sous le même terme. Dermatologica (Basel) 108: 1–28 (1954).

(4) GOODMAN, J. I.: Diabetic anhidrosis. Amer. J. Med. 41: 831–835 (1966).

(5) JOHNSON, C., and S. SHUSTER: Eccrine sweating in psoriasis. Brit. J. Derm. 81: 119–124 (1969).

(6) KORTING, G. W.: Zur Pathogenese des endogenen Ekzems. Thieme, Stuttgart 1954.

(7) ROVENSKÝ, J., und O. SAXL: Die Rolle der Schweiß-Sekretion beim atopischen Ekzem im Kindesalter. Dermatologica (Basel) 129: 245–256 (1964).

(8) SCHLIACK, H., und R. SCHIFFTER: Anhidrose der Fußsohle: Symptom retroperitonealer Tumorinvasion. Dtsch. med. Wschr. 96: 977–979 (1971).

4. Color and Odor of Sweat

A. Chromhidrosis

1. Chromhidrosis is caused primarily by occupational contact with substances such as copper, ferrous oxide, pyrocatechin (catechol), hexachlorcyclohexane, or by external application of Castellani's paint.

Discoloration of originally colorless sweat is known as **trichomycosis palmellina** of axillary hair (Fig. 26). Usually, patients observe staining of their underwear from colored sweat in regions with apocrine sweat glands. Such stained secretory products are lipopigments, which vary in their final color according to the amount of secreted granules of lipofuscin and the stage of oxidation.

2. Pseudochromhidrosis plantaris has been observed in young people active in sports; the horny layer of the heel region presents an aggregation of dark brown to bluish-black points. At first, a diagnosis of tattooing or satellites of a melanoma may be considered, but these grouped pigmentations associated with marked hyperkeratosis are probably deposits of blood pigments from ruptured capillaries of the papillae. Rarely, these uniform cutaneous lesions develop into hemorrhagic bullae. [1, 2, 3]

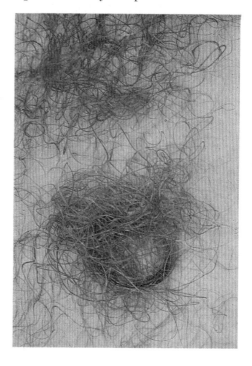

Fig. 26. Trichomycosis palmellina.

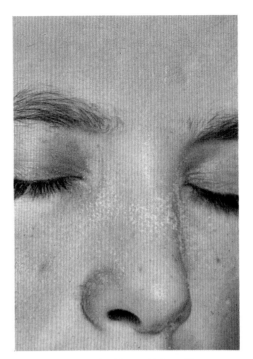

Fig. 27. Urhidrosis ("uremic frost").

(1) BAZEX, A., A. DUPRÉ et J. FERRÉRE: La pseudo-chromidrose plantaire. Ann. Derm. Syph. (Paris) *94:* 169–185 (1967).

(2) CRISSEY, J. T., and J. C. PEACHEY: Calcaneal petechiae. Arch. Derm. (Chic.) *83:* 501 (1961).

(3) DUPRÉ, A.: Une « forme majeure » de pseudo-chromhidrose plantaire, phlycténulaire et hémorragique – Association à

des troubles thrombocytaires – Essai pathogénique. Dermatologica (Basel) *140:* 178–185 (1970).

B. Bromhidrosis

Bromhidrosis or osmidrosis is rarely characteristic of a distinct disease. Body or sweat odors are present in rheumatic fever, measles, chronic pemphigus (odor of macerated skin); the mousy smell of favus and the rancid odor of some kinds of acne are other examples. Transitory special odors of sweat restricted to the time of medication can be caused by valerians, turpentine, or garlic.

C. Urhidrosis

Urhidrosis (sudor urinosus or uremic "frost") was first described in epidemic cholera; it is due to secretion and deposits of urinary substances, uric acid, and especially, sodium chloride on the skin, particularly on the tip of the nose, the forehead, and temporal areas; this phenomenon is observed in patients with prolonged terminal azotemia (Fig. 27).

5. Dermatologic Pain Sensations

In Chapter 2 the relationship between itching and pain was extensively discussed. With regard to dermatologic conditions causing pain sensations, it can be said that the objective cause of a painful sensation comes from certain noxae or injuries to the tissue. Every local "inflammation" of the skin is an example. But the intensity of the pain sensation does not always run parallel with the cause triggering it. It depends, as we all know, on the subjective sensitivity of the affected person. Mechanical, thermic, or chemical contacts triggering pain will, under certain conditions, be felt very strongly, and the victim does not become accustomed to them even if they last a long time, as experience with herpes zoster shows. The phenomenon of pain can even persist or become more intense after the apparent disappearance of its cause.

The intensity and the quality of the sensation of pain have created a special vocabulary, which characteristically describes the phenomena of pain in such terms as "stinging," "burning," "sharp," and others. A "bright" pain describes superficially located pain sensations, whereas a "dull" pain occurs mostly in deep or subcutaneous areas. It can also be said that the "bright" pain describes circumscribed sensations, whereas the "dark, dull" pain applies to more diffusely felt sensations.

Today, the presence of pain-conducting intraepithelial nerves and the existence of nerves in the epithelium of human skin have been proved by electron microscopy. Thus it is not strange that besides itching other abnormal sensations as well as anesthesias and hyperesthesias are symptoms of a multitude of dermatoses. [3, 4, 5]

A. Hypesthesias and Anesthesias

Lowered or missing pain sensations lead to unusually extensive, localized and often recurrent trauma, which results in mutilations. The dermatologist may first see the sequelae of loss of pain but must then arrive at the diagnosis of the exact primary cause.

1. Congenital total analgesia is extremely rare. It constitutes one of the possible diagnoses of absent pain sensation. The patients are indifferent to pain from the time of birth, but have no other neurologic or psychic deficits. Pathologically, there are no deviations from the normal, either in the CNS or in the peripheral nerves. [1, 2]

2. In contrast, in **congenital sensory neuropathia** myelinated nerve fibers in the sensory nerves and nerve fibers in the skin are missing (absent cholinesterase-positive nerves). Still present are "cutaneous islands" with intact pain sensation. Electrophysiologically, absence of thick sensory nerve fibers (A delta-fibers) is characteristic in this condition. [9]

3. The two disorders just mentioned are not hereditary, but familial sensory neuropathy – **familial acroosteolysis,** the Thévenard syndrome – is inherited dominantly with little penetrance and variable expressivity. The first signs of the disease are seldom observed before the second year of life. Located mainly in the lower extremities are symmetrically distributed sensory disturbances, varying in intensity, of temperature, touch, and pain. Motor and proprioceptive deficits (without ataxia) are rare, but the tendon reflexes of the legs are absent or diminished. The mutilating acroosteolyses are characteristic clinical signs. There are no sensory nerves containing myelin. In the differential diagnosis, neuropathic familial amyloidosis (Andrade type) and especially, syringomyelia must be ruled out. [6, 7, 8]

4. Ulcerations which occur symmetrically on the upper extremities and especially on the hands suggest, above all, **syringomyelia** (Fig. 28). Characteristic of this disease is a dissociated sensory disturbance, with absent or lowered pain and temperature sensations but normal sensation to touch. In the beginning there may be transitory increased pain perception. Quite often there are simultaneous motor nerve deficits, which lead to muscular atrophies with pseudosclerodermiform features. In the myelogram the spinal canal in the thorax and lumbar region is widened following disintegrating vegetations of glia. Dermatologically, hyperhidrotic or anhidrotic disturbances of sweat secretion and

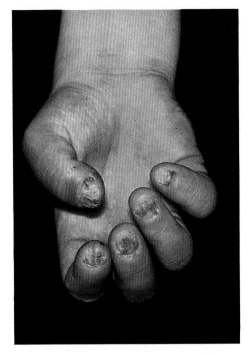

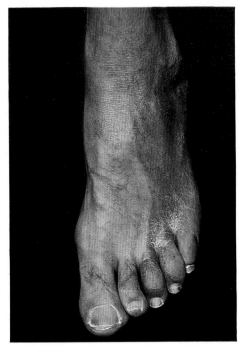

Fig. 28. Changes of the terminal phalanges of fingers in syringomyelia.

Fig. 29. Tuberculoid leprosy.

acrocyanoses or succulent edema of the dorsa of the hands occur at the beginning of the disease. Soon afterward rhagades, remnants of blisters, and especially, scars which are the sequelae of burns that the patient did not notice, occur.

Trophic nail changes and warty keratoses on the palms are also not infrequent. If in the final stage of the disorder definite mutilations develop, differential diagnosis is mandatory from leprosy, tabes dorsalis, or, especially, familial acroosteolysis, which at times simulates syringomyelia.

5. The dermatologist is familiar with sensibility disturbances, especially those of leprosy and tabes dorsalis. In **maculo-anesthetic leprosy** dissociated sensibility disturbances occur, usually manifesting themselves first in an increased sensitivity to touch. Such sensations are not all confined to the immediate vicinity of visible skin changes. The duration of the neuritic or neuralgiform disturbances varies: they may persist for days or start repeatedly anew every day. Sometimes there are lancinating pains which considerably curtail the movements of the patient. If there are changes in the nerves themselves, especially in the great auricular or the ulnar nerves in the form of characteristic nodes or thickenings like a string of pearls, classification of such hyperesthetic symptoms is easy (Figs. 29, 30, 31 and 240).

If the disorder becomes pronounced, anesthesia of circumscribed areas of skin – for instance, the distal phalanges of the fingers or the border of the ulnar bone – becomes distinct. It is, however, worth mentioning that the anesthetic skin areas do not always correspond to the anatomic distribution of nerves.

Fig. 30. Tuberculoid leprosy:
perineural sarcoidal granulomas. HE stain, 100×.

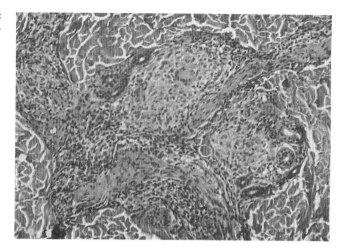

6. In **tabes dorsalis,** especially in the so-called algetic stage, i.e., before the atactic and pseudoparalytic phases, painful sensations characterized by a lightninglike beginning and lancinating, stabbing pain with a beltlike tightening predominate. The tabetic patient with gastric crises complains of a dull, internal, painful sensation of fullness. Some patients vomit incessantly. In some cases genuine gastrointestinal ulcerations are present. Finally, lancinating attacks of pain can be triggered by fever attacks. On the skin "mal perforant" and uncharacteristic pigment shiftings, suggillations, attacks of itching, and occasionally, eczematous reactions at the site of lancinating belt-pain occur. Anesthesias over the Achilles tendon or the ulnar nerve are suggestive. An objective sign which is almost pathognomonic of tabes dorsalis is the Argyll Robertson pupil phenomenon, i.e., a miotic pupil that responds to accommodation but not to light. In other late neurologic disorders an absolute fixed pupil is usually present, often associated with miosis.

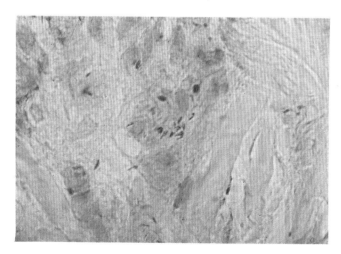

Fig. 31. Tuberculoid leprosy:
bacteria in the tissue section.
Ziehl-Neelsen stain, 1000×.

Adie's syndrome, which is a pseudo-Argyll Robertson phenomenon, is accompanied by reflectory disturbances of the extremities and must be differentiated from tabes dorsalis.

In addition to these disorders with diminished pain perception a bout of **schizophrenia** can occasionally be associated with a complete loss of reaction to painful stimuli. Furthermore, tumors of the CNS as well as **toxic** or **infectious** peripheral **neuropathies** may show circumscribed hypesthetic or anesthetic zones.

(1) BAXTER, D. W., and J. OLSZEWSKI: Congenital universal insensitivity to pain. Brain *83:* 381–393 (1960).

(2) FANCONI, G., und F. FERRAZZINI: Kongenitale Analgie (kongenitale generalisierte Schmerzindifferenz). Helv. paediat. Acta *12:* 79–115 (1957).

(3) HENSEL, H.: Allgemeine Sinnesphysiologie, Hautsinne, Geschmack, Geruch. Springer, Berlin, Heidelberg, New York 1966.

(4) HENSEL, H.: Die Spezifität der Hautsinne. Studium Generale *17:* 471–478 (1964).

(5) KANTNER, M.: Morphologische Beiträge zu den Empfindungen des Schmerzes, der Berührung, des Juckens und des Kitzels. Studium Generale *17:* 493–500 (1964).

(6) MOSCHELLA, S. L., and G. E. WIRE: Sensory radicular neuropathy of the hereditary type. Arch. Derm. (Chic.) *94:* 449–453 (1966).

(7) PARTSCH, H.: Ulceromutilierende Neuropathien der unteren Extremitäten. Zum Krankheitsbild der »Acropathie ulcéromutilante«. Hautarzt *22:* 283–289 (1971).

(8) WADULLA, H.: Familiäre neuro-vaskuläre Dystrophie. Dtsch. Z. Nervenheilk. *160:* 413–438 (1949).

(9) WINKELMANN, R. K., E. H. LAMBERT and A. B. HAYLES: Congenital absence of pain. Arch. Derm. (Chic.) *85:* 325–339 (1962).

B. Hyperesthesias

1. Herpes zoster (shingles) can be accompanied by extremely severe attacks of pain. They may suggest in the preeruptive stage, according to their localization, appendicitis, cholecystitis, and urolithiasis, among others. Intensity and duration of the pain vary from case to case, but it is safe to say that older people will experience more intense pain. In the preeruptive stage up to two weeks prior to the eruption, 10 to 20 per cent of patients experience segmentally projected neuralgias or irradiating pain. The patient with herpes zoster may have persistent pain for several months (or rarely, years) after the regression of the cutaneous lesions. This seems to happen when intense pain or persistent grouped blisters have been observed from the beginning (Fig. 32). Compared to these zosterneuralgias, hypesthesias or analgesias in affected zoster areas do not play any role. [13, 16]

2. Raynaud's syndrome involves an acral changing rhythm which is felt, preponderantly by young women, as increased sensitivity to cold or painful numbness and blanching of one or more fingers. This spasm of the blood vessels is followed by dilation before normal blood supply is restored. In a typical case the second to fourth fingers of both hands are affected, whereas the thumbs and palms almost always remain unaffected. If an attack of Raynaud's syndrome involves only one side, a special etiology such as a cervical rib or the scalenus syndrome must be considered. Occasionally, similar angiospastic attacks occur in the areas of the nose, cheeks, and tongue. Even if there are in the beginning purely functional vascular disturbances, the search for a basic systemic disorder (e. g., progressive scleroderma,

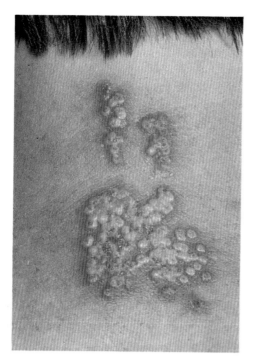

Fig. 32. Herpes zoster.

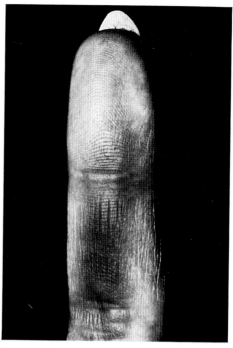

Fig. 33. Paroxysmal hematoma of a finger.

dermatomyositis, lupus erythematosus, endangiitis obliterans, periarteritis nodosa, ergotism, cold agglutinin disturbance, polycythemia, exposure to polyvinyl-chloride, and others) should not be omitted under any circumstances. The diagnosis of Raynaud's disease sui generis should be made only after several years and if the disorders mentioned above can be ruled out. [11, 15]

3. Pain beginning abruptly in one or more fingers characterizes the **paroxysmal finger hematoma.** It occurs mostly in women over 30 who feel such pain during their daily work with their hands. About 15 to 60 minutes after the onset of the stabbing pain a hematoma appears at the site of the finger joint (Fig. 33). This may lead to the full picture of a "dead finger" due to vascular compression. Apparently,

strictly localized damage to the vascular wall is responsible. [1, 10]

4. Erythromelalgia differs from the varying symptoms of pain in Raynaud's syndrome; it shows a continuous pathological dilatation of the terminal part of the blood vessels (arterioles, venules, and capillaries) accompanied by an increase in temperature within the diseased areas. Erythromelalgia is not infrequently a secondary sign of other systemic vascular or nervous disorders (for instance, endangiitis obliterans). In contradistinction to Raynaud's syndrome such attacks of pain are triggered by an increase in the temperature of the environment (such as warmth of the bed). Patients are well aware of this dependence on environmental temperature; they try to avoid the tormenting burning attacks of pain by lowering their skin temperature.

This means that differentiation between erythromelalgia and Raynaud's syndrome is not difficult because blanching is absent; furthermore, the hepatogenic painless palmar erythemas do not present any swelling. [12]

5. It is easy to differentiate vascular pain that is either caused or increased by impairment of the arterial circulation of the extremities– it is due to walking or to elevation of the lower extremities. Painful sensations due to venous impairment (varicose veins) are felt primarily while standing. Considerable pain is caused by **acute thrombophlebitis** when an area of erythema overlying an inflamed varicose vein develops. This is accompanied by an increase in the temperature of the skin. Quite frequently, a painful thickened vein can be palpated within the inflamed swollen area. It may become almost impossible to rule out erysipelas because palpation is difficult owing to edematous swelling, and there may also be an increase in the body temperature. Nocturnal paroxysms of pain in the legs are primarily symptomatic cramps caused by hypocalcemia or acute concentration of blood volume, enteric water loss due to diarrhea, or powerful saluretics.*

6. The symptom of **burning feet** is observed on soles and palms. These sensations do not correspond to the distribution of peripheral nerves and do not present a glove or stocking pattern. Such burning sensations characteristically improve in a cold environment or when the legs are hanging down, whereas "**restless legs**" ("tibial anxiety") occur in the prone position. The cause of distal burning pain may be manifold and requires the elimination of peripheral nervous disorders, posterior spinal tract disease, and spinal ganglion

---

* Diuretics causing loss of sodium and chloride ions in the urine. (Tr.)

involvement of the gelatinous substances of the spinal cord or the thalamus. The most frequent cause is a metabolic "myelosis" (vitamin B_{12} deficiency; diabetes mellitus); tumors and spinal angiomatoses, however, must not be overlooked. [3]

7. Erythema nodosum is especially painful; the diagnosis is doubtful if typical pain on pressure is absent (see Chapter I, B6, and Chapter 18, G1).

8. Circumscribed hyperesthesias of the thigh may be the result of peripheral nerve irritation. In **meralgia paresthetica,** a neuralgia located on the external aspect of the thigh and involving the region supplied by the external cutaneous femoral nerve, such painful paresthesias are aggravated by walking. Occasionally, this region may present pemphigoid, "glossy skin"-like eczematous reactions or scleroderma-like conditions by disturbances of the above-named nerve supply.[17]

9. The **ilioinguinalis syndrome** is characterized by pain caused by compression of the ilioinguinal nerve with dysesthesias of the inguinal region. The patient walks bending forward; when lying down the lower extremity is held in a position of adduction and inward rotation. There are typical pressure points along the anterior iliac superior spine. Contraction of the abdominal muscles and stretching of the lower extremity increase the pain.[14]

10. The **Melkersson-Rosenthal syndrome** is characterized by facial swelling, recurrent episodes of facial paralysis, and fissured tongue accompanied by neurovegetative signs such as premonitory unilateral retroauricular neuralgias of the neck, dysesthesias of one side of the face, tinnitus of the ears, or migrainous painful sensations felt deeply within the skull. Such "headaches" may alternate with the other typical chief manifestations of the Melkersson-Rosenthal syndrome.[9]

11. Within the facial region headaches with an extracranial vascular cause are part of the disease known as **temporal arteritis,** which affects the terminal branches of the external or internal carotid artery. Initially, severe unilateral headaches or pains of the face almost always predominate. The patients are all over 50 years old; they show edematous swelling of the temporal region accompanied by fever, an increased sedimentation rate (after one hour more than 40 mm), and leukocytosis. There is also an increase of the alpha-2 and beta globulin fractions of the serum, whereas the gammaglobulins are normal or at most slightly increased. Retention of bromsulphalein is regularly increased. The temporal arteries show nodular thickening and tenderness. Ocular symptoms are arterial occlusion causing sudden blindness or colliquative necrosis of the optic nerve near the papilla. A cutaneous sign seen occasionally is a circumscribed necrosis of the scalp.[2, 8]

12. At times, Bing's **erythroprosopalgia** may resemble temporal arteritis quite closely because it also involves paroxysms of unilateral pain of the temples and facial swelling of the same side. Accompanying these attacks are unilateral lacrimation, nasal secretion, and acute facial perspiration. The painful attacks occur quite suddenly, usually at night or when lying down, and last only a few minutes. The differential diagnosis against trigeminal neuralgia is based on the following points: trigeminal neuralgias seldom occur when lying down; they affect the entire region of the trigeminal nerve; the attack has a wavelike pattern and lasts continually as in erythroprosopalgia. The latter condition is not triggered by external stimuli, whereas these stimuli play an important role in trigeminal neuralgia. It is possible to produce a typical attack of pain in erythroprosopalgia within 30 to 50 minutes by a sublingual dose of 1 mg of nitrolingual,* provided the patient is in a free interval.

13. Pain can be used as an aid to diagnose papular or lichenoid **syphilids;** a single lesion, especially on the palms and soles, when pressed with a dull probe will elicit pain.**

14. Such focal hyperesthesia triggered by a mechanical stimulus is observed with some regularity in areas of **chronic lupus erythematosus;** touching an affected area with the edge of a tongue depressor will be felt by the patient as distinctly painful. Occasionally, such painful sensations caused by touch or pressure can be experienced even in the atrophic stage of lupus erythematosus.

15. Preeruptive local sensation are more constant and therefore more pathognomonic in **dermatitis herpetiformis.** Attacks of pruritus are not the leading subjective symptom but patients often complain of painful sensations of heat or burning.

16. Priapism or the protracted painful erection of the penis requires in every case a diagnostic evaluation of its pathogenic mechanism, which may be cerebral, spinal, or peripheral (thrombotic cavernitis). Twenty to 30 per cent of all cases of priapism are caused by leukemia, but other possible causes are poisoning with illuminating gas or lead, compressions or contusions of the spine, sickle cell anemia, mumps, tularemia, thrombosis of the pelvic veins and, last but not least, constant abuse of aphrodisiacs.

---

* The corresponding American drug is Nitro-Bid (Marion), 2.5 mg. (Tr.)

** The so-called Ollendorff probe test described by Helen Ollendorff Curth. (Tr.)

17. Severe pain can be present in general adiposity. Such **adiposis dolorosa** (Dercum's disease) predominates in women in the menopause and must be precisely differentiated from lipomatosis dolorosa (see Chapter 38, A5). Adiposis dolorosa presents diffuse increases of fatty tissue, frequently around joints, accompanied by spontaneous paroxysms of pain and intense sensitivity to pressure. Occasionally, patients complain simultaneously of arthritic pain and nose bleeds (hypertension?). General lassitude and psychic complaints occur almost regularly.[4, 5, 6]

18. Painful tumors are discussed separately in Chapter 38, A.

(1) ACHENBACH, W.: Das paroxysmale Handhämatom. Med. Welt (Stuttg.) *1958:* 2138–2140.

(2) ANDREWS, J. M.: Giant-cell ("temporal") arteritis. A disease with variable clinical manifestations. Neurology *16:* 963–971 (1966).

(3) BALZEREIT, F.: Die »brennenden Füße« – "burning feet". Dtsch. med. Wschr. *94:* 35–36 (1969).

(4) BLOMSTRAND, R., L. JUHLIN, H. NORDENSTAM, R. OHLSSON, B. WERNER and J. ENGSTRÖM: Adiposis dolorosa associated with defects of lipid metabolism. Acta derm.-venereol. (Stockh.) *51:* 243–250 (1971).

(5) DERCUM, F. X., and D. J. McCARTHY: Autopsy in a case of adiposis dolorosa. Amer. J. med. Sci. *124:* 994–1006 (1902).

(6) GÜNTHER, H.: Die Lipomatosis und ihre klinischen Formen. Arbeiten aus der Med. Klinik zu Leipzig, H. 5. Fischer, Jena 1920.

(7) HEYCK, H.: Über das Bingsche Kopfschmerzsyndrom (Erythroprosopalgie). Dtsch. med. Wschr. *87:* 1942–1947 (1962).

(8) HOIGNÉ, R., U. LATSCHA, M. MUMENTHALER, P. NIESEL und J. LAISSUE: Arteriitis temporalis oder Riesenzellarteriitis. Schweiz. med Wschr. *99:* 392–397 (1969).

(9) HORNSTEIN, O., und H. SCHUERMANN: Das sogenannte Melkersson- Rosenthal-Syndrom. Ergebn. inn. Med. Kinderheilk. N. F. *17:* 190–263 (1962).

(10) JUNG, E. G.: Das paroxysmale Fingerhämatom. Schweiz. med. Wschr. *94:* 458–460 (1964).

(11) KORTING, G. W., und H. HOLZMANN: Die Sklerodermie und ihr nahestehende Bindegewebsprobleme. S. 20. Thieme, Stuttgart 1967.

(12) KREBS, A., und H. U. ANDRES: Zum Krankheitsbild der Erythromelalgie. Schweiz. med. Wschr. *99:* 344–349 (1969).

(13) MOLIN, L.: Aspects of the natural history of herpes zoster. Acta derm.-venereol. (Stockh.) *49:* 569–583 (1969).

(14) MUMENTHALER, A., M. MUMENTHALER, G. LUCIANI und J. KRAMER: Das Ilioinguinalis-Syndrom. Dtsch. med. Wschr. *90:* 1073–1078 (1965).

(15) RATSCHOW, M.: Angiologie. Thieme, Stuttgart 1959.

(16) TAPPEINER, J., und K. WOLFF: Zoster. Fischer, Jena 1968.

(17) WAGNER, W.: Hautveränderungen bei Schädigung des Nervus cutaneus femoris lateralis. Derm. Wschr. *136:* 971–976 (1957).

6. Fetor ex ore and Halitosis

Fetor ex ore (offensive oral smell) and **halitosis** (bad odor of the breath) are caused by caries, gingivitis, dirty dental protheses, decomposing tumors of the oral cavity and its surroundings, fetid sore throats, remnants of blood, and, not infrequently, a long period without food or an acute sympatheticotonic excitement, or in other words, a state similar to that of taking belladonna preparations. In cases of halitosis one should think first of all of fetid disorders of the respiratory tract (bronchiectasis, pulmonary abscess, and pulmonary gangrene), dammed-up material in the diverticula, and decomposing neoplasms of the gastrointestinal tract. A patient does not notice his own fetor ex ore, but halitosis is disagreeable to the patient himself. Most characteristic is the fruitlike smell of acetone in diabetic coma; the urinous breath of the patient with uremia,

which results from the bacterial reduction of urea and the development of ammonia on the mucous membranes; the liverlike breath of patients with coma hepaticum; and the garliclike odors caused by arsenic, phosphorus, sodium tellurate, and recently, by the percutaneous use of DMSO (in the breath as sulfuric-smelling dimethylsulfide). Much rarer is fetor resembling bitter almonds, which occurs after the use of ether, chloroform, carbolic acid, and so on. Seldom observable except in a sanitarium is the odd, unpleasant liquorlike smell of paraldehyde. After doses of medications containing vitamin B_2, besides the changed smell of the skin a slight nutlike oral smell may be noticed.[1]

(1) DEMLING, L.: Foetor ex ore, Halitosis, belegte Zunge. Med. Klin. *59:* 1916–1918 (1964).

7. Arthropathias and Myopathias

A. Erythemas

1. Arthropathy is part of the typical general picture of polyetiologic **erythema nodosum**, regardless of the etiology of the individual case. In **Löfgren's syndrome** arthropathias are the second most frequent sign. The polyarthralgic disturbances, which favor the big joints in this syndrome, usually follow a mild course. Only if the condition is more severe do redness and swelling of the joints occur. Furthermore, Löfgren's syndrome, if part of sarcoidosis, is prognostically favorable. In the beginning, owing to accompanying fever, it may be misdiagnosed as rheumatic fever. Radiologic evidence of bilateral enlarged hilar lymph nodes permits the correct differential diagnosis.

Laboratory tests will show an increased ESR and leukocytosis corresponding to the stage of the acute inflammation. In contrast to rheumatic fever and rheumatoid arthritis, the antistreptolysin titer, the Waaler-Rose test, and the so-called rheumatoid factors are always negative. If in doubt, the outcome of the Kveim test which in Löfgren's syndrome is 85–92 per cent positive, will clinch the diagnosis.[3, 4]

2. Arthropathias are also found in **erythema multiforme**, although milder and in fewer cases than in erythema nodosum. The knee and ankle joints are primarily affected. Hydrarthrosis is usually absent and the temperature is not increased. Occasionally, the overlying muscles are also affected and this can be recognized in the laboratory by an increased activity of creatine phosphokinase.[5]

3. Behçet's syndrome. Inhabitants of the Mediterranean countries and Japan are the primary sufferers of this uveo-aphthous syndrome.* The patients suffer from chronically recurrent attacks of aphthous lesions on the mucous membranes and the skin (scrotum)** and from recurrent hypopyoniritis. Also important are nodose erythemas, ulcerated pyodermas, and phlebothromboses. Large veins, including even the vena cava, may become involved. In some cases the CNS, the gastrointestinal tract, the heart, and the blood vessels become affected. During an attack the patient may give the impression of a severely ill person because of the ocular pain, myalgias, and arthralgias of many sites. About 35 per cent of cases show involvement of the joints, which are red, inflamed, edematous, and painful to pressure. This picture may repeat itself during the protracted course of the disorder. Spontaneous regression and complete healing are the rule. The large joints, such as the knees and elbows, or those of the hands and feet are predominantly affected. Even in this form of arthritis an increased ESR, moderately increased alpha-2 and gammaglobulins are present but there is no evidence of rheumatoid factors in the serum.[1, 2]

(1) MASON, R. M., und C. G. BARNES: Behçet-Syndrom mit Arthritis. Schweiz. med. Wschr. *98:* 665–671 (1968).

---

* There are many cases of Behçet's syndrome in the United States and other parts of America. Some black people are among the victims of the disorder. (Tr.)

** Not only the scrotum but other sites on the skin of the male and female genitals and the region of the anus may show ulcerations. (Tr.)

(2) NASR, F. W.: Les manifestations articulaires de la maladie de Behçet. Rev. Rhum. *36:* 81–83 (1969).

(3) PAVELKA, K., C. FARNER, A. BÖNI und F. I. WAGENHÄUSER: Gelenksarkoidose. Z. Rheumaforsch. *28:* 340–350 (1969).

(4) ROTNES, P. L.: Untersuchungen über Erythema nodosum im Erwachsenen-Alter. Acta derm.-venereol. (Stockh.) *17* Suppl.3 (1936).

(5) WOENCKHAUS, J. W., und D. KLEMM: Muskuläre Beteiligung beim Erythema exsudativum multiforme majus (Stevens-Johnson-Syndrom). Med. Klin. *61:* 1423–1424 (1966).

B. Erythematosquamous Dermatoses

1. As early as the last century the relationship between psoriasis and arthritis had led to the recognition of **psoriasis arthropathica.** The two main signs, psoriasis and chronic deforming arthritis, each occur in the population with a frequency of 1 to 2 per cent. Among patients with psoriasis a combination with arthritis is present in 10 per cent of cases. Whereas rheumatoid arthritis occurs about three times more often in women than in men, psoriasis arthropathica does not favor one sex over the other. Therefore, psoriasis arthropathica does not represent a chance association of psoriasis vulgaris with seronegative rheumatoid arthritis. In the psoriasis-arthritis combination the cutaneous changes usually precede the arthritis by years, but arthropathy may be the first manifestation. In about half of the cases in later stages bouts of progressive manifestations occur simultaneously. The cutaneous manifestations in the arthropathic patient, furthermore, behave atypically: they favor an inverse location and have a tendency to erythrodermic spreading and pustulation. Moreover, the affected flexural or intertriginous areas of psoriasis arthropathica may show increasing resistance to therapy, even to the usual systemic drugs. Generalized pruritus is present more

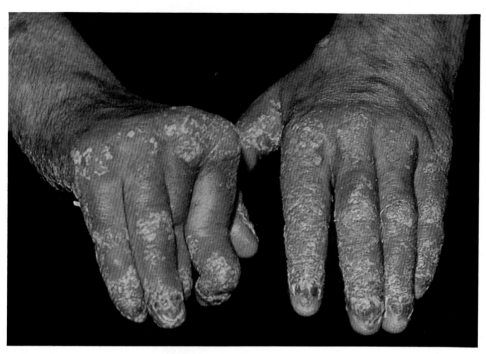

Fig. 34a

Fig. 34. Psoriatic arthropathy of the hands (a) and of the feet (b) with pronounced formation of crumbly nails.

Fig. 34b

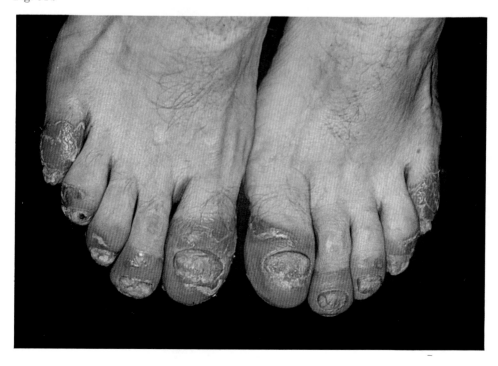

often than in psoriasis vulgaris, but this may be explained by the high content of uric acid in the serum. An association with usually severe nail disturbances occurs in about 85 per cent of cases compared to a similar association of about 15 per cent in psoriasis vulgaris. The picture is more or less that of a crumbling nail (Fig. 34 a, b).

The disease of the joints in psoriasis arthropathica begins predominantly with mono- to oligoarticular forms (60 per cent), in which the joints of the end phalanges of the fingers are affected in 6 per cent of the cases, and those of the toes in 10 per cent. The continuous involvement of a chain of phalanges or of several end phalanges is typical. The distal interphalangeal joints of hands and feet are affected most. The changes are well defined, often not very painful, and tend to become osteolytic and ankylosing. Most important, the ilio-sacral joints are affected at an early stage on one or both sides.

The differential diagnosis by x-rays between psoriasis arthropathica and rheumatoid arthritis is difficult. Fairly characteristic of psoriasis arthropathica are osteolyses and ankyloses of finger and toe joints and the wearing out of the tuberosities of the distal phalanx and periostitides, i.e., the simultaneous existence of osteodestructive and osteoproliferative processes. Characteristic roentgenologic findings of arthritis of the ileosacral joints and the cervical intervertebral joints are also part of the picture. Psoriatic spondylarthritis differs from spondylarthritis ankylopoetica* (Bechterew's disease) by its tendency to hyperuricemia, simultaneous and frequent peripheral arthritides, mild subjective difficulties, and the relatively late onset and more favorable prognosis in general.

The patient with psoriatic spondylarthritis complains of pains in the heel at an earlier date and more regularly than the patient with Bechterew's disease. One

---

* Marie-Strümpell ankylosing spondylitis. (Tr.)

should, of course, not overlook the fact that occasionally Bechterew's disease and psoriasis vulgaris may occur by chance together in the same patient. New findings point to the presence of myopathia, which can be diagnosed only by electromyography and the occasional occurrence of an unspecific myocarditis. As signs of an acute inflammation, tests will show changes in the ESR, electrophoresis, and the C-reactive protein. An increased ESR in clinical psoriasis should suggest the onset of a mesenchymal extension of the disorder. As in rheumatoid arthritis, diminishing hemoglobin and iron and an increase in copper are found in the serum. An increase of uric acid in the serum occurs only in pruritic psoriasis arthropathica. The rheumatoid factors in the serum (Waaler-Rose test, latex fixation test) are all negative in psoriasis arthropathica in contrast to rheumatoid arthritis. A similar statement can be made with regard to the determination of the so-called antinuclear factors, whereas the antistreptolysin titer is increased in about 25 per cent of the cases. Because in childhood the so-called rheumatoid factors are absent in rheumatoid arthritis, this rather important differential diagnostic possibility versus psoriasis arthropathica cannot be utilized (see Table 1).[2, 4-9, 11, 13]

2. Reiter's disease. This urethro-oculosynovial syndrome, occurring mostly in men, is characterized by arthritis in addition to the exudative-psoriasiform manifestations. This makes it mandatory to differentiate this disease from psoriasis arthropathica.

Several joints are more often affected than a single joint. Favorite locations are the joints of the knees, ankles, shoulder, and hand – i.e., the large joints. The iliosacral joints may show radiologic changes following the first attack.

Clinically, either mildly pronounced arthralgias or joint effusions are present;

Table 1. Differential Diagnosis of Psoriatic Arthropathy

Psoriasis Arthropathica	Reiter's Disease	Progressive Chronic Polyarthritis	Gonorrheic Arthritis
Sex ratio 1:1	Very rare in women	More women than men (3:1)	Sex ratio 1:1
Successive attacks, mono- or oligoarticular; asymptomatic to subacute course	Tendency to recurrences; preponderantly monoarticular; subacute to acute course	Successive attacks; as a rule polyarticular; usually lingering, subacute course	First manifestation 3 weeks after infection; preponderantly monoarticular; subacute to acute course
Asymmetric involvement of joints	Asymmetric involvement of joints	Mostly symmetric involvement of joints	Asymmetric involvement of joints
Distal finger and toe joints often distinctly affected	Distal finger and toe joints usually free	Distal finger and toe joints rarely affected	Distal finger and toe joints usually free
Ulnar deviation rare; predominantly indiscriminate deviation	Ulnar deviation absent	Early ulnar deviation	Ulnar deviation absent
Iliosacral joints almost regularly involved. Always simultaneous signs of ankylosis, sclerosis, and destruction	Iliosacral joints affected early	Iliosacral joints very rarely involved; signs of sclerosis usually absent	Iliosacral joints usually free
Rheumatoid factor almost always negative	Rheumatoid factor negative	Rheumatoid factor positive in 80% of cases	Rheumatoid factor negative
Balanitis occasionally present	Characteristic balanitis circinata hyperkeratotica	Balanitis is absent	Erosive balanitis may be present
Urethritis absent	History of unspecific urethritis preponderant	Urethritis absent	Urethritis gonorrheica
Ocular changes lacking	Recurrent conjunctivitis and iritis frequent		Conjunctivitis gonorrheica and iritis can be present
Joint punctate: rheumatoid factor negative; a few histiocytes; sterile punctate	Joint punctate: rheumatoid factor negative; histiocytes rare, polynuclear cells; virologically positive finding: Bedsonia	Joint punctate: rheumatoid factor first negative, later positive; histiocytes in changing numbers; sterile punctate	Joint punctate: polynuclear cells; bacteriologically positive evidence of gonococci

these contain either clear fluid or leukocytes. Sometimes the tendons are affected, especially as calcaneus spurs (fasciitis plantaris, tendinitis calcanea, or others). Besides the completely different signs of arthritis (different predilections of joints in the two diseases) conjunctivitis, which often occurs at the same time, and unspecific urethritis help to differentiate Reiter's disease from psoriasis arthropathica. One should not forget that the so-called Reiter triad (arthritis, conjunctivitis, and urethritis) may occur scattered over a long period of time. The manifestations of palmoplantar keratodermia with small lesions that are interrupted by pustules and parakeratotic balanitis also lead to a diagnosis of Reiter's disease.

Various tests point to an inflammation, as could be expected. The serologic rheumatoid factors are usually negative, as in psoriasis arthropathica. This is unfortunate and prevents a clear distinction between the two. In later stages, moreover, the picture also resembles Bechterew's disease (ankylosing spondylitis). [1, 3, 10, 12]

(1) CSONKA, G.: Reiter's Syndrome. Ergebn. inn. Med. Kinderheilk. N. F. *23:* 125–189 (1965).

(2) DIHLMANN, W.: Zur Differentialdiagnose der Gelenkerkrankungen bei Psoriatikern. Dtsch. med. Wschr. *96:* 557 (1971).

(3) HAUSER, W.: Zur Diagnostik der Reiterschen Krankheit. Med. Welt *15:* 2404–2409 (1964).

(4) HOLZMANN, H., G. SOLLBERG und I. ELGAMILI: Zur Kenntnis der psoriatrischen Myopathie. Arch. klin. exp. Derm. *230:* 329–335 (1967).

(5) HORNSTEIN, O.: Zur nosologischen Stellung der Psoriasis arthropathica. Arch. klin. exp. Derm. *214:* 622–651 (1962).

(6) PETRES, J., A. KLÜMPER und P. MAJERT: Zur Differentialdiagnose der psoriatischen Arthropathie auf Grund röntgenmorphologischer Befunde. Hautarzt *21:* 26–32 (1970).

(7) RECORDIER, A.-M., G. SERRATRICE, H. ROUX, R. AQUARON, D. DUBOIS-GAMBARELLI, G. DE BISSCHOP et J. BARET: Les atteintes musculaires au cours du psoriasis arthropathique. Rev. Rhum. *36:* 91–104 (1969).

(8) SCHACHERL, M., und F. SCHILLING: Röntgenbefunde an den Gliedmaßengelenken bei Polyarthritis psoriatica. Z. Rheumaforsch. *26:* 442–450 (1967).

(9) SCHATTENKIRCHNER, M.: Zur Symptomatologie der Arthritis psoriatica. Med. Klin. *65:* 1360–1363 (1970).

(10) SCHILLING, F., A. GAMP und M. SCHACHERL: Das Reiter-Syndrom und seine Beziehungen zur Spondylitis ankylopoetica. Z. Rheumaforsch. *24:* 342–353 (1965).

(11) SCHILLING, F., und M. SCHACHERL: Röntgenbefunde an der Wirbelsäule bei Polyarthritis psoriatica und Reiter-Dermatose: Spondylitis psoriatica. Z. Rheumaforsch. *26:* 450–459 (1967).

(12) SCHIRMER, A., und A. BÖNI: Kritische Stellungnahme zur Diagnostik des Reiter-Syndroms. Z. Rheumaforsch. *26:* 142–152 (1967).

(13) THEISS, B., A. BÖNI, F. WAGENHÄUSER, U. W. SCHNYDER und K. FEHR: Psoriasis-Spondylarthritis. Z. Rheumaforsch. *28:* 93–117 (1969).

C. Storage Diseases

1. In **angiokeratoma corporis diffusum** (Fabry's disease) there are occasionally painful swellings, especially of the finger, but also of the elbow, shoulder, and knee joints. Such arthropathy of the distal interphalangeal finger joints may lead to persistent diminishing mobility of the fingers. In some cases aseptic necrosis of the femoral head is noted. Of practical significance is the possibility of mistakenly diagnosing the articular signs as rheumatic fever. In patients with Fabry's disease these signs are accompanied by fever and an increased ESR. Changes in the muscular system are rarely well defined and enzymes in the serum do not have any characteristic deviations. But the electromyogram is pathologic, showing such criteria of myopathy as definite shortening of the duration of the action potential, increased polyphases, and lessening of the tension potentials of a motor unit.[3, 16]

2. In **pericollagenous amyloidosis** abnormal deposits in bones and joints also occur but usually remain undetected. Enlarged joints, sometimes caused by an effusion, are extremely rare. More frequent are deposits of paramyloid in the muscles, which cause muscular weakness or pain.[2]

3. Scleredema adultorum only rarely causes articular changes. Involvement of the muscles, however, in the form of discrete myopathias occurs more frequently.

4. In **scleromyxedema** sclerodactylia may occur, but in other forms of the **mucinoses,** including its various tumorous, nodose, or lichenoid variants, involvement of the bones and skeletal muscles does not occur. There are, however, instances of scleromyxedema in which a simultaneous myeloma causes deposits in the joints.[14]

5. In the **xanthomatoses** involvement of the supporting framework is limited to the tendons. Xanthomas of the tendons occur more often in primary hypercholesterinemia than in connection with primary hypertriglyceridemia. Articular swellings or pain are extremely rare in the xanthomatoses, and, if they occur, will probably be observed in hypercholesterinemic xanthomatosis (Fig. 35). The increased incidence of rheumatic fever in patients with primary hypercholesterinemia, however, is striking.[6, 10]

6. Alkaptonuria or endogenous ochronosis is characterized by the storage of homogentisic acid in "cartilage and bonelike structures" (Virchow). By means of

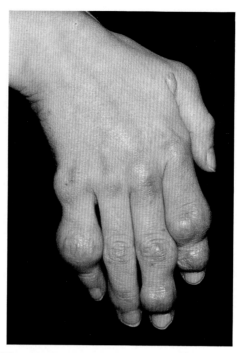

Fig. 35. Xanthomatosis of the joints.

radioscopy of the auricle alone loss of transparency of the cartilage can be proved. In these areas it is irregularly thickened and inelastic. In the x-ray picture small spots or marginal deposits of calcium are visible. As in the cartilage of the ear, polymerized homogentisic acid is stored in the cartilage of the joints and causes pronounced pain. In general, however, arthropathias caused by destruction of the cartilage (osteoarthrosis deformans alcaptonuria) occur only after years of latency. Radiologically, the most frequent changes of the intervertebral disks are thinning and calcification. Larger joints show narrowing of the articular space and floating articular bodies.[5, 9]

7. In **primary gout,** which is characterized by multiple buttercreamlike tophi of the auricles or the tips of the fingers, an acute attack of arthritis is often the first sign of the disorder (Figs. 36 and 37). Men have

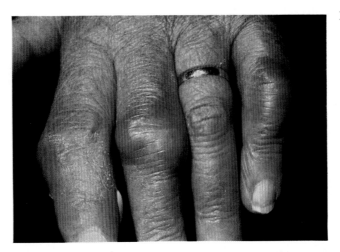

Fig. 36. Uratic arthritis.

gout about 20 times more often than women. An acute attack of gout is preceded by various auralike symptoms such as tachycardia, insomnia, and meteorism. The dreaded acute articular pain is brought about by the suddenly appearing joint effusion and the likewise acute development of periarticular edema.

Sometimes the inflammatory process also involves the lymph vessel system surrounding the joint and consequently a phlegmonous condition appears to be present. The skin covering the gouty joint is dusky red and glossy because of the tight tension (Fig. 36). An acute involvement of the bursa or tendons (tenontagra) is rare.

The favorite location of arthritis urica is the proximal joint of the big toe, but theoretically other joints may also be affected. In addition to evidence of hyperuricemia, formation of tophi, and attacks of arthritis with complete remission, decisive radiologic criteria offer help in reaching the correct diagnosis. Besides irregularly formed osteolyses (so-called punch hole defects), which may extend to the diaphysis, there are near the joints a halberd form of the head of the first metatarsal, an osteophytic thorn, and cuplike mutilations of gout.[4, 8, 11, 15]

In **secondary gout,** which is familiar to the dermatologist among other possible signs in psoriasis or mycosis fungoides, and which is known to the internist in chronic myelosis, the signs just described cannot be differentiated from those of primary gout.[7]

8. Painful and doughy-edematous swellings, especially of the joints of the hands and feet, occur in **Farber's disease.** This is a disorder in the storage of mucopolysaccharides and abnormal glycolipoids that begins in early childhood and, combined with disturbances of nutrition (vomiting and refusal to eat), leads to dystrophy. Soon hoarseness and the just mentioned articular swellings appear. The affected joints themselves are very tender to the touch and greatly limited in their mobility; they form early contractures. Afterwards, subcutaneous and submucous nodes slowly appear, in the beginning near the joints and later near pressure points of the skin. Such cutaneous granulomas do not ulcerate or break down with necroses. Enlargement of liver, spleen, and lymph nodes

Fig. 37. Great toe affected by
an acute attack of gout with
erysipelatoid redness.

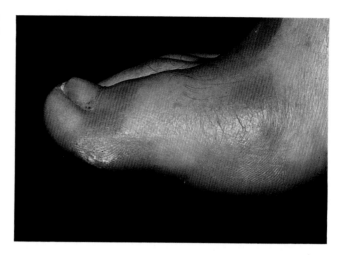

follows and, owing to chronic pulmonary
infiltrations, death ensues, apparently
from cardiorespiratory insufficiency. Neurologically important are the findings of
muscular weakness, hypotonia, and loss of
reflexes.

It is important to differentiate this form
of disease from the rest of the mucopoly-
saccharidoses. Such a diagnosis is helped
by the extremely early onset of the
disease, the involvement of the vocal
cords and joints, and the absence of
corneal opacities and changes of the
osseous structure.[1, 12, 13]

(1) BATTIN, J., C. VITAL et X. AZANZA:
    Une neuro-lipidose rare avec lésions
    nodulaires souscutanées et articulaires:
    la lipogranulomatose disséminée de
    Farber. Ann. Derm. Syph. (Paris) *97:*
    241–248 (1970).

(2) BERNHARD, G. C., and G. T. HENSLEY:
    Amyloid arthropathy. Arthritis Rheum.
    12: 444–453 (1969).

(3) DENK, R., und G. SOLLBERG: Skelet-
    muskelbefunde beim Angiokeratoma
    corporis diffusum. Hautarzt *17:* 248–252
    (1966).

(4) DIHLMANN, W., und H. J. FERNHOLZ:
    Gibt es charakteristische Röntgen-
    befunde bei Gicht? Dtsch. med. Wschr.
    94: 1909–1911 (1969).

(5) FRIDERICH, H., und W. NIKOLOWSKI:
    Endogene Ochronose. Arch. Derm.
    Syph. (Berl.) *192:* 273–289 (1951).

(6) GAÁL, A. M.: Untersuchungen über
    Cholesterinstoffwechsel bei Xantho-
    matosis essentialis. Z. klin. Med. *113:*
    349–361 (1930).

(7) GEBHARDT, R., und H. HOLZMANN:
    Sekundäre Gicht bei Hautkrankheiten.
    Arch. klin. exp. Derm. *230:* 146–152
    (1967).

(8) GOTTRON, H. A., und G. W. KORTING:
    Chronische Hautgicht. Arch. klin. exp.
    Derm. *204:* 483–499 (1957).

(9) LAGIER, R., I. BOUSSINA, W. TAILLARD,
    A. SASFAVIAN, M. CHAFIZADEH et G. H.
    FALLET: Etude anatomo-radiologique
    d'une arthropathie ochronotique du
    genou. Schweiz. med. Wschr. *101:*
    1585–1590 (1971).

(10) LORENZ, K., und K. HINKEL: Familiäre
    Hypercholesterinämie mit polyarthri-
    tischem Verlauf beim Kind. Dtsch. Ge-
    sundh.-Wes. *24:* 1471–1474 (1969).

(11) MISGELD, V.: Primäre Hautgicht. Eigene
    Beobachtung und Beitrag zur Klinik
    der Gicht. Hautarzt *19:* 299–304 (1968).

(12) MOSER, H. W., A. L. PRENSKY, H. J. WOLFE and N. P. ROSMAN: Farber's lipogranulomatosis. Report of a case and demonstration of an excess of free ceramide and ganglioside. Amer. J. Med. *47:* 869–890 (1969).

(13) RAMPINI, S., und J. CLAUSEN: Farbersche Krankheit (disseminierte Lipogranulomatose). Klinisches Bild und Zusammenfassung der chemischen Befunde. Helv. paediat. Acta *22:* 500–515 (1967).

(14) RAVAULT, P.-P., E. LEJEUNE, M. BOUVIER et J. GAUTHIER: Les manifestations articulaires paranéoplasiques. In: Les syndromes paranéoplasiques. Rapp. présent. XXXV Congr. franç. Méd., Paris 1965. S. 149–190.

(15) TALBOTT, J. H.: Die Gicht. Hippokrates, Stuttgart 1967.

(16) WISE, D., H. J. WALLACE and E. H. JELLINEK: Angiokeratoma corporis diffusum. A clinical study of eight affected families. Quart. J. Med. *31:* 177–206 (1962).

Fig. 38. Spindleform enlargement of the proximal phalanges in sarcoidosis: osteopathia cystoides multiplex.

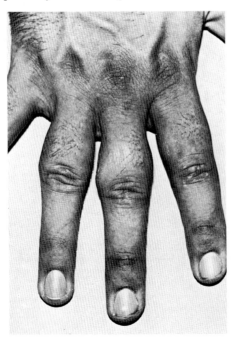

D. Acute Infectious Dermatoses

1. Occasionally, although not too rarely, **erysipeloid** involves adjacent joints with redness and swelling owing to its slowly migratory nature. Besides the usual cutaneous form of this disease there exists a predominantly articular form; it is confined to the vicinity of the port of entry of the bacillus *Erysipelothrix insidiosa*. The affected joints are extremely painful; movements may become so difficult that immobility and sometimes even deformity may result.[1]

(1) AXHAUSEN, G.: Zur Diagnostik der Fingergelenkserkrankungen. Klin. Wschr. *2:* 2197–2198 (1923).

E. Chronic Infectious Dermatoses

1. Sarcoidosis of the joints, which affects 5 to 30 per cent of all patients with sarcoid, favors the younger age group. Not infrequently, the articular location may be the first manifestation of sarcoid. Its course is variable and shows transitory arthralgias corresponding to Löfgren's syndrome (combined with erythema nodosum and fever); it may involve deforming articular changes, which clinically cannot always be differentiated from rheumatoid arthritis. The most frequent sites of disease are the joints of the ankles, elbows, knees, hands, and feet. The diagnosis can be facilitated by other manifestations of sarcoid such as those in lungs, liver, and skin. When in doubt, biopsy of a joint would show sarcoidal granulomas.

Radiographs of the hands of about 5 to 10 per cent of all sarcoid patients show cystic rarefactions, the so-called *osteitis cystoides multiplex* (Fig. 38). They are found in the bones of the phalanges, metacarpals, and carpals. However, these findings have no connection with the extent or duration of the underlying sarcoidosis; they cannot be influenced therapeutically. There is some doubt whether these osseous changes really belong to Boeck's disease because of the absence of other specific changes and because such cysts are observed with equal frequency in persons not suffering from sarcoidosis. During the course of sarcoidosis about 30 to 50 per cent of all cases will show muscular involvement. Such myopathy remains asymptomatic as a rule and will seldom progress to acute myositis or chronic myopathia. Muscular involvement takes place preponderantly during the first two years of sarcoidosis; muscle or liver biopsies will verify the diagnosis.[1-4]

2. Acrodermatitis chronica atrophicans may present inflammatory changes of articular capsules and concomitant arthritis. Later, the mobility of the affected joints will be impaired.[5]

(1) BALTZER, G., H. BEHREND, T. BEHREND und H. DOMBROWSKI: Zur Häufigkeit zystischer Knochenveränderungen (Ostitis cystoides multiplex Jüngling) bei der Sarkoidose. Dtsch. med. Wschr. *95:* 1926–1929 (1970).

(2) NICKLING, H. G.: Lymphadenopathien bei Tuberkulose und Morbus Boeck. Dtsch. med. J. *16:* 693–696 (1965).

(3) PAVELKA, K., C. FARNER, A. BÖNI und F. I. WAGENHÄUSER: Gelenksarkoidose. Z. Rheumaforsch. *28:* 340–350 (1969).

(4) RUDOLF, G.: Die Muskelsarkoidose (Morbus Boeck) in der Differentialdiagnose neuromuskulärer Erkrankungen. Dtsch. med. Wschr. *96:* 1605–1607 (1971).

(5) SCHILLING, F.: Die symptomatischen Arthritiden. Heilkunst *83:* 1–6 (1970).

F. Venereal Diseases

1. Syphilitic arthropathy is today much rarer than formerly. Its manifestations are many-faceted and it can be diagnosed only within the framework of the entire clinical picture. In the early stages of syphilis joints may be painful without special objective findings. It is well known that such arthralgias are mainly present during the night; the patient tries to get relief by walking around. As in gonorrhea the knee joint is the preferred site; there is a bland specific effusion. Elbow and hip joints may be involved also, but the migration from one joint to another observed in rheumatoid arthritis is absent. Arthropathy in the early stages of syphilis, in spite of frequent febrile episodes, differs from rheumatic polyarthritis because there is no cardiac involvement and no response to salicylates, but simultaneously specific syphilitic exanthems are present. A history of recent infection, the clinical findings, and a serological test are additional indications for the diagnosis of syphilitic arthritis. The presence of rheumatoid factors in the serum offers additional help because they are not found in luetic arthropathia. However, there is no doubt that a definite differential diagnosis between a specific syphilitic mono- or polyarthritis as opposed to rheumatoid arthritis can be more difficult.

Neurosyphilis should be called "metasyphilis" only if its immunopathological genesis is to be emphasized. Among the neurosyphilitic manifestations the **tabetic arthropathy** may become severe. Although occasionally spirochetes have been demonstrated, it is in the trophic spinal centers that degeneration causing the tabetic changes of the affected joints takes place. This can be proved by the fact that syphilitic arthropathy of the recent or tertiary period will react quickly to specific therapy while tabetic joint disease, in spite of such treatment, usually progresses. Protracted use of tabetic joints especially subject to static stress and the fact that these joints are insensitive to pain finally brings about a degenerative end-stage. In any case, in the presence of a painless chronic deforming arthropathy other cardinal signs of tabes dorsalis such as lancinating pains, pupillary and reflex abnormalities, and an ataxic gait should be looked for. Because the classical sero-diagnosis of late syphilis is negative in about 40 per cent of cases it is necessary when in doubt to perform the fluorescent treponemal antibody absorption test.

2. Even today, there is a possibility that monarthritis, especially of the knee joint, that occurs after urethritis might be **gonorrheic monarthritis.** Usually this happens around the third week after a specific urethritis; such arthritis may present either a plain effusion, or an inflammatory serofibrinous, purulent, or even phleg-monous exudate. Clinically, severe pains of the joint are predominant, as well as local signs of inflammation. In addition, gon-orrheic arthritis has a tendency to heal with bony ankylosis. Because occasionally a specific iridocyclitis may be present, it can be difficult to exclude Reiter's syn-drome. Definite proof is the finding of gonococci in the intraarticular fluid. In contrast to Reiter's syndrome there is no involvement of the ileosacral joints.[1]

(1) KEISER, H., F. L. RUBEN, E. WOLINSKY and I. KUSHER: Clinical forms of gono-coccal arthritis. New Engl. J. Med. *279:* 234–240 (1968).

G. Collagenosis Group (Generalized Connective Tissue Diseases)

1. Systemic lupus erythematosus is ac-companied by articular and periarticular involvement in up to 90 per cent of the patients. These polyarthritic, sometimes myalgic pains are felt mostly as stiffness in the morning; they present a most common clinical sign of this disease. Besides such indefinite arthralgias one also observes acute migratory polyarthritis. Later on, there may be transitions to a chronic progressive type of arthritis; however, deformities and more severe changes of the bones are absent. Such articular manifestations may be present long before the first signs of cutaneous changes appear.

Frequently, muscular changes that are refractory to salicylates and resemble dermatomyositis are superimposed on the arthritic joints. The affected groups of muscles are extremely sensitive to pressure; the swelling is more indurative than doughy. There is slightly less pain when movements are performed very carefully. Besides the painful sign of a muscular "hangover" a pronounced muscular weak-ness also exists; it can be mistaken for a sign of general infirmity and later may be confused with dermatomyositis. Such myoparesis cannot be differentiated by electromyography from the same findings obtained in typical dermatomyositis. Histo-logically, the main feature is parenchyma-tous damage to the fibers; the damage may range from myelosis of single fibers to complete destruction, the same changes seen in acute dermatomyositis. In lupus erythematosus, myopathy may either in-volute spontaneously or recur with a new bout of activity, regardless of whether it manifests itself as myalgic, myasthenic, or myoparetic. In the presence of systemic lupus erythematosus the myopathy that manifests itself as generalized muscle weakness can also be caused by prolonged therapy with chloroquine or corticosteroids.

As shown by laboratory tests, about one-fifth of patients with systemic lupus erythematosus or with rheumatoid arthritis present common serologic findings. Twenty per cent of patients with rheumatoid arthritis show positive reactions to tests for lupus erythematosus or other antinuclear factors, while about the same percentage of lupus erythematosus patients present positive rheumatoid factors.[2, 3, 8, 12]

2. Arthropathies seen with **progressive scleroderma** cannot always be differentiated with certainty from rheumatoid arthritis even in the absence of rheumatic nodules and ulnar deviations of the fingers and even if pronounced sclerodactylia is present. In addition to the polyarthritic changes of scleroderma resembling rheumatoid arthritis, cutaneous indurations simulating pseudoarthropathies may also be seen. However, sclerodermic arthropathies are not always mild arthritic types but can also be mutilating destructive conditions with a tendency to calcification of the surrounding interstitial tissue. Radiographs show an absence of cystic translucent areas and proliferative osseous changes in destructive sclerodermic arthropathies; these lesions are seen in rheumatoid arthritis. However, epiphyseal osteoporosis and osteolysis of the distal extremities are quite frequent.

As in systemic lupus erythematosus sclerodermic polyarthralgias or arthritis may not too rarely precede the cutaneous changes for some time, with the result that the differentiation against rheumatoid arthritis may become extremely difficult. As a rule, however, Raynaud's phenomena precede symmetric polyarthralgias by one or more years in progressive scleroderma. Muscular participation produces no clinical signs and can be discovered only by electromyography.

Laboratory tests show a considerable difference in the rheumatoid and antinuclear factors between progressive sclero-

derma on the one hand and rheumatoid arthritis and systemic lupus erythematosus on the other hand. Antinuclear factors are seldom found in progressive scleroderma. Our own observations of 12 patients suffering from progressive scleroderma showed rheumatoid factors in only two cases.[1, 4, 5, 9, 10]

3. Involvement of the joints in **dermatomyositis** plays a minor role as compared with that in progressive scleroderma and systemic lupus erythematosus; sometimes muscular pain is mistakenly attributed to afflictions of the joints. In any case, 10 to 20 per cent of patients with dermatomyositis present rheumatoid arthritic signs which do not favor any particular region of the joint. Paraneoplastic dermatomyositis occurring together with malignant tumors does not show any conspicuous involvement of the joints.[6, 11]

4. Sjögren's syndrome, mostly seen in women, is also called the sicca syndrome, as it shows characteristic dryness and keratosis of the mucous membranes. The cardinal clinical signs are xerostoma, swelling of the parotid gland, dry shiny tongue, rhinolaryngotracheitis sicca, vulvitis, and ichthyosiform condition of the skin with subsequent eczematization, sometimes showing pellagroid or sclerodermiform aspects. Ophthalmologically, the typical changes are filamentous keratitis, absence of tears, and conjunctivitis sicca. Additional findings can be dysproteinemia, hepatosplenomegaly, increase of lymphoid reticulum cells in the bone marrow, and also presence of antinuclear factors and the so-called rheumatoid factors.

One of the main signs of the syndrome is the articular involvement which corresponds in every respect to rheumatoid arthritis. This associated polyarthropathy has become such an essential part of the syndrome that its absence should make one reluctant to consider a diagnosis of the sicca syndrome.

Abortive symptoms of Sjögren's syndrome have been observed in the other important members of the collagenoses group, especially in progressive scleroderma.[7]

(1) BOCHU, M., et P. BUFFARD: Les manifestations ostéo-articulaires au cours de la sclérodermie. J. Radiol. Electrol. *50:* 415–418 (1969).

(2) ERBSLÖH, F., und W. D. BAEDEKER: Lupusmyopathie. Dtsch. med. Wschr. *87:* 2464–2470 (1962).

(3) KAESER, H. E., und R. KOCHER: Iatrogene Muskelsymptome und Myopathien. Ther. Umsch. *27:* 387–393 (1970).

(4) KORTING, G. W., und H. HOLZMANN: Die Sklerodermie und ihr nahestehende Bindegewebsprobleme. Thieme, Stuttgart 1967.

(5) MEYER ZUM BÜSCHENFELDE, K. H., H. TALKE und H. HOLZMANN: Zur Frage immunbiologischer Beziehungen zwischen Lupus erythematodes disseminatus und progressiver Sklerodermie. Arch. klin. exp. Derm. *228:* 396–407 (1967).

(6) PEARSON, C. M.: Rheumatic manifestations of polymyositis and dermatomyositis. Arthr. and Rheum. *2:* 127–143 (1959).

(7) SEIFERT, G., und G. GEILER: Speicheldrüsen und Rheumatismus. Dtsch. med. Wschr. *82:* 1415–1417 (1957).

(8) SIEGENTHALER, W., und R. HEGGLIN: Der viscerale Lupus erythematosus (Kaposi-Libman-Sacks-Syndrom). Ergebn. inn. Med. Kinderheilk. N. F. *7:* 373–428 (1956).

(9) SOLLBERG, G., R. DENK und H. HOLZMANN: Neurologische und elektrophysiologische Untersuchungen bei progressiver Sklerodermie und Morphea. Arch. klin. exp. Derm. *229:* 20–32 (1967).

(10) SCHACHERL, M., und H. HOLZMANN: Zur Polyarthritis bei progressiver Sklerodermie. Fortschr. Röntgenstr. *107:* 485–493 (1967).

(11) SCHUERMANN, H.: Dermatomyositis. Ergebn. inn. Med. Kinderheilk. N. F. *10:* 427–480 (1958).

(12) SCHULTEN, H., H. H. HENNEMANN und W. KUHN: Praktische Hinweise zur Diagnostik und Therapie des Lupus erythematodes visceralis. Med. Welt *13:* 993–1001 (1962).

H. Urticaria and Toxic Allergic Exanthems

1. Acute urticaria, Quincke's **angioneurotic edema,** and **serum sickness** may present in up to 20 per cent of cases either arthritis, arthralgia, or painful joints without objective findings. Occasionally, bland swelling of joints known as **intermittent hydrarthrosis** may occur repeatedly. This appears as, a rule as periodic "idiopathic" articular effusion. After a few days without any other local manifestations except impaired function and pain the fluid disappears spontaneously. The most frequent site of such transient effusions is the knee joint, but there may be involvement of one or several other joints. [1]

2. Dermatitis herpetiformis may occasionally show urticaria, either as a transient sign or as articular hydrops, an equivalent urticarial manifestation. [2]

(1) BERGER, H.: Intermittent hydrarthrosis with allergic basis. J. Amer. med. Ass. *112:* 2402–2405 (1939).

(2) ZAUN, H.: Hydrops articularis als Symptom der Dermatitis herpetiformis. Z. Haut- u. Geschl.-Kr. *43:* 797–800 (1968).

I. Reticuloses

1. Multiple reticulohistiocytoma ("lipid dermatoarthritis") is characterized by arthritis, among other manifestations. This reticulohistiocytoma is a systemic disease, presenting solitary or, more frequently, multiple cutaneous nodules of distinct histologic composition with special reticulohistiocytes. The disease takes a protracted chronic course, interrupted by systemic signs such as fever, lassitude, and loss of weight; the articular changes usually precede the appearance of the cutaneous nodules but rarely, this sequence is reversed. Initially, the clinical signs are arthropathy with swelling and painful immobilization; later mutilating arthritis and marked bony destruction follow. Less frequently there is isolated involvement of the synovia alone. The osseous changes usually occur in the distal interphalangeal joints; however, all other joints of the extremities can be symmetrically involved. The phalanges show characteristic rarefaction, with the resultant picture of a "lorgnette" or "telescopic" hand. Although the clinical appearance of the joints may resemble rheumatoid arthritis for some time, in the long run the unusually severe osteolysis surpasses that observed in typical arthritis. Another finding that helps in the differential diagnosis against rheumatoid arthritis is the absence of rheumatoid factors in the serum of such patients. There is no increase in the antiglobulin consumption test or the antistreptolysin titer. Development of multiple brownish to bluish-red nodules in the vicinity of the joints is a clue to the diagnosis of the progressive character of the joint disease; this was discussed in the chapter on juxta-articular nodes. [1-4]

(1) EHRLICH, G. E., I. YOUNG, ST. Z. NOSHENY and W. A. KATZ: Multicentric reticulohistiocytosis (lipoid dermatoarthritis). A multisystem disorder. Amer. J. Med. 52: 830–840 (1972).

(2) FANTINI, F., I. CARUSOe F. SOLAZZI: Caso di artrite mutilante da reticoloistiocitosi multicentrica (Dermatoartrite lipidea). Reumatismo 21: 381–390 (1969).

(3) HOLUBAR, K., und K. MACH: Histiocytosis giganto-cellularis. Hautarzt 17: 440–445 (1966).

(4) LYELL, A., and A. J. CARR: Lipoid dermato-arthritis (reticulohistiocytosis). Brit. J. Derm. 71: 12–21 (1959).

K. Diseases of Fat Tissue

1. Patients with **nodular nonsuppurative panniculitis** (Weber-Christian syndrome) often have recurrent attacks of fever and rheumatoid arthritis. Rarely, however, do they have articular swellings at the same time. The combination of fever attacks and articular changes first suggests rheumatic fever. Nodular panniculitis is occasionally accompanied by muscular weakness or dystrophic muscular arthropathies. Symptomatic "poststeroid panniculitis" does not differ clinically and histologically from nodular panniculitis. In *idiopathic panniculitis* of the Rothmann-Makai type, however, arthropathies are lacking.

2. In "symptomatic Pfeifer-Weber-Christian disease," **the syndrome of metastasizing exocrine pancreatic adenoma,** articular swellings are pronounced. This disorder is characterized by the triad of polyarthritis, panniculitis, and blood eosinophilia. The associated polyarthritic changes occur almost always in the joints of the lower extremities. Whereas in genuine nodular panniculitis young women are preponderantly affected, manifestations of the syndrome of metastasizing pancreatic adenoma favor men in the fourth decade of life or older. [1]

3. Arthropathies associated with **adiposis dolorosa** are discussed in Chapter 5, B 17.

(1) WUKETICH, ST., und F. PAVLIK: Syndrom des metastasierenden lipase-bildenden Pankreasadenoms. Arch. klin. exp. Derm. 216: 412–426 (1963).

L. Hemorrhagic Diatheses

1. The frequent association of **Schönlein-Henoch purpura** with articular changes explains the historic name of so-called purpura rheumatica. The coincidence of "rheumatism" in the strict sense of the word with Schönlein-Henoch purpura must be regarded, however, as a very rare event. The age distribution reaches a peak in childhood, but adults can have this disease at any age. Clinically, the disease manifests itself in cutaneous attacks which are in the beginning maculopapular, and raised, and later rather macular and intrafocally petechial. They are only rarely transformed into bullous or necrotizing lesions. Favorite locations of this leukocytoclastic-hemorrhagic microbid are the extensor surfaces of the extremities, the buttocks, and the sides of the trunk. If occasionally abdominal signs occur, they are caused by intestinal mucosal or renal bleedings (purpura abdominalis). In general, involvement of the mucosal surfaces is rare. The associated arthropathies affect the joints of the feet and knees most of all.

2. Among the hemorrhagic diatheses the greatest involvement of the joints occurs in the **hemophilias** with their readiness to respond to the slightest traumatic provocation with bleeding. These bleedings may cause extensive mucsular hematomas or massive intraarticular bleeding, which, if recurrent, may lead in the end to irreversible articular changes. Other manifestations are extraarticular, cystic osseous bulges, which are caused by subperiostal or endostal bleeding. Such pseudotumors (Fig. 39) can eventually cause rarefaction and destruction of the osseous structure. [1]

3. Among the forms of purpura accompanied by thrombocytopenia, **thrombotic thrombocytopenic purpura** shows fatigue, dizziness, headaches, and articular pain, mostly in the afebrile prodromal phase. Affirming the diagnosis are the signs of thrombocytopenic purpura with hemolytic anemia, which begin with the sudden onset of elevated temperatures. At the same time multiple organs (heart, liver, kidney, and CNS) show disturbances caused by the closure of arterioles and capillaries by fibrin and thrombocytic thrombus formations.

Fig. 39. Pseudotumor in hemophilia.

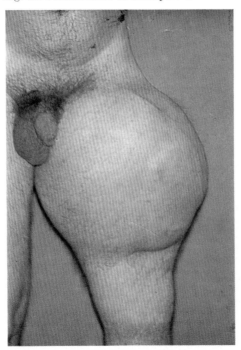

(1) FISCHER, M., P. FUCHSIG, K. LECHNER, H. W. PILGERSTORFER, M. SALZER und K. STEINBEREITHER: Erfolgreiche Operation eines Pseudotumors nach Oberschenkelfraktur bei Hämophilie B. Dtsch. med. Wschr. *94:* 2145–2148 (1969).

M. Diseases of the Connective and Supporting Tissues

1. Cutis hyperelastica (Ehlers-Danlos syndrome), if fully developed, is rare. It comprises overextensibility and abnormal vulnerability of the skin and hyperextensibility of the joints (Fig. 40). Even minor traumas cause subcutaneous hematomas or elliptically gaping wounds (Fig. 41). An additional stigma of such hypoplasia and hypotonia of the system of supporting tissue is the characteristic compressibility of the thenar and hypothenar when pressing hands. Because the joints have a propensity to become easily dislocated, effusions, sometimes hemorrhagic, develop in the joints. In many cases flat feet and kyphoscoliosis exist.

2. Among the manifestations of **idiopathic pachydermoperiostosis** (Touraine-Solente-Golé syndrome) are painless articular thickenings, clubbed fingers, nails like watch-crystals, and thickening of the skin of the hands and fingers (as well as of the feet and toes) and the scalp. In most cases the disorder begins at puberty and distinctly favors the male sex. Besides the enlargement of skin and periosteum there is also a tendency toward hyperhidrosis.

Radiologically, destructive signs of the joints in general are lacking, but the distal bones of the extremities, including the phalanges, show distinct periarticular peri-

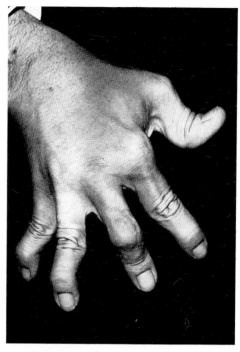

Fig. 40. Ehlers-Danlos syndrome. Bizarre hyperextensibility of joints.

ostal reactions, making the bones appear generally thickened. In contrast to acromegaly there is never evidence of a tumor of the hypophysis. [6, 8]

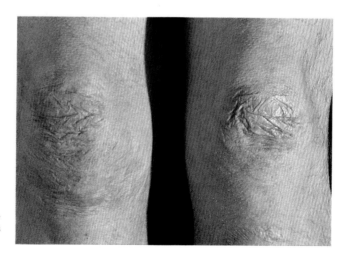

Fig. 41. Ehlers-Danlos syndrome: finely atrophic folds over molluscoid tumors.

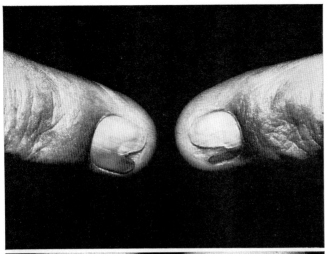

Fig. 42a

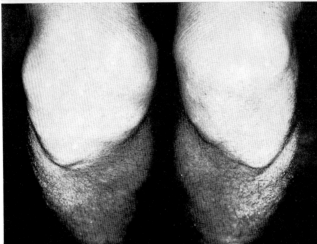

Fig. 42b

3. Associated with chronic pulmonary disease or malignant pulmonary tumors as a paraneoplastic syndrome, hypertrophic osteoarthropathy (Marie-Bamberger syndrome) represents a form of **secondary pachydermoperiostosis** and cannot be distinguished from the idiopathic form. Clinically, there is a difference inasmuch as joint involvement in hypertrophic osteoarthropathy occurs as distinctly painful polyarthritis. Also the manifestations appear in the fourth decade of life instead of at puberty. In idiopathic pachydermoperiostosis as well as in hypertrophic osteoarthropathy, typical disturbances in the calcium-phosphorus metabolism are missing. Alkaline phosphatase is also not increased. [1, 5, 7, 8]

Another special form of secondary pachydermoperiostosis is "**thyroid acropachy,**" which neither clinically nor morphologically can be distinguished from the idiopathic form. Its accompanying enlargements first begin as a rule after successful treatment of hyperthyroidism. In a large number of cases they are accompanied by exophthalmos and pretibial myxedema circumscriptum. In contrast to thyroid hyperfunction, which favors the female sex, more men than women suffer from "thyroid acropachy." The osseous changes, which are evident roentgenologically, are almost exclusively limited to the diaphyses of the metacarpal or metatarsal bones as well as the proximal phalanges of fingers and toes. Changes of the bones in joints have never been observed.

In the differential diagnosis these two just named syndromes involving enlargements must be distinguished from osteitis deformans (Paget's disease), the Camurati-Engelmann syndrome, and acromegaly. In **osteitis deformans** differentiation is possible because the age at which manifestations begin is later, rarely before the fortieth, and usually as late as the sixtieth year of life. In addition, there are typical radiologic changes of the osseous structure, with a honeycomblike, fibrous and loosened but also sclerotic and thickened cortex. Usually, alkaline phosphatase in the serum is increased. If in doubt, a biopsy of the bone can determine the diagnosis. In the Camurati-Engelmann syndrome, however, the first signs appear before puberty and are accompanied by myopathy. Among other radiologic signs, generalized symmetrical hyperostoses of the diaphyses of the long bones occur, but the epiphyses and metaphyses are spared. Characteristic cutaneous manifestations are not known. **Acromegaly** can occur at any age and is often accompanied by pachyderma. In most cases the sella turcica is widened. Often diabetes mellitus, hyperphosphatemia, and an increased growth hormone level in the serum coexist. The most important differential diagnostic criterion is the presence of an eosinophilic adenoma of the hypophysis.

4. Hereditary arthro-onychodysplasia align with pelvic horns, the **nail-patella syndrome,** shows characteristic nail changes (Fig. 42a and b) which are regularly present on the nails of the thumbs and index fingers, whereas the nails of the other fingers are rarely affected and the toenails always remain free. The disturbance of the nail is characterized by furrows and splitting of the nails, which have become loose in the nailbed, and the so-called lunulae triangulares. Occasionally, only rudimentary remnants of nails can be found. Besides the already mentioned exostosis-like pelvic horns there may be aplasia or hypoplasia of the patella, often with lateral luxation (Fig. 42b), and in the elbow joint a hypoplastic head of the radius. A number of patients have proteinuria and microhematuria as well, but a definite classification of the renal disorder has not yet been achieved. Genetically, the disease is linked with the locus of the ABO blood groups. [3, 4]

(1) Höfer, R., und E. Ogris: Akropachie – eine seltene Komplikation der Basedowschen Erkrankung. In: Wachstumshormon und Wachstumsstörungen, S. 226–232. 11. Symp. dtsch. Ges. Endokrinologie. Hrsg. E. Klein. Springer, Berlin, Heidelberg, New York 1965.
(2) Korting, G. W.: Fehlbildungen der Haut und Hautveränderungen bei Fehlbildungssyndromen. In: Hdb. Haut- u. Geschlkrh. Hrsg. J. Jadassohn. Erg.-Werk III/1. S.375–493. Springer, Berlin, Göttingen, Heidelberg
(3) Laur, S., und W. Haberlandt: Hereditäre Onycho-Osteo-Dysplasie (HOOD) in einer schwäbischen Familie. Arch. klin. exp. Derm. 240: 278–300 (1971).
(4) Lucas, G. L., and J. M. Opitz: The nail-patella-syndrome. Clinical and genetic aspects of 5 kindreds with 38 affected family members. J. Pediat. 68: 273–288 (1966).
(5) Richter, G.: Ein weiterer Fall von EMA-Syndrom (Exophthalmus-prätibiales Myxödem) – Akropachy. Dtsch. Gesundh.-Wes. 26: 250–253 (1971).
(6) Schubert, E., H. Vetter und R. Juchems: Pachydermoperiostose, Touraine-Solente-Golé-Syndrom. Münch. med. Wschr. 112: 229–235 (1970).
(7) Steiner, H., O. Dahlbäck und J. Waldenström: Ectopic growth-hormone production and osteoarthropathy in

carcinoma of the bronchus. Lancet *1968/I:* 783–785.

(8) UEHLINGER, E.: Paraneoplastische Syndrome. Almanach f. d. Ärztl. Fortb. München *1966*, S. 17–44.

N. Diseases of the Sebaceous Glands

For a discussion of polyarthralgias in **acne conglobata** see Chapter 1, Ol.

8. Nodes Near Joints

A. Juxta-Articular Nodes

1. Juxta-articular nodes were apparently first observed in tropical treponematoses **frambesia** and **pinta** and in **syphilis.** Clinically, these are formations of nodes which are located symmetrically mainly on the extensor surfaces of the elbow and knee joints. Other sites of predilection are the joints of the feet and the hips. The forehead may relatively frequently be the site of similar nodose eruptions. Other characteristics are slow development and, almost without exception, painlessness. These globular nodes may reach the size of pigeon eggs, or they may be much smaller, only rice corn to lentil-sized. Usually, several nodes are present at the same time, and solitary lesions are the exception. They have the consistency of tense, elastic, or hard swellings, and they usually represent nodes in the cutis. The overlying skin is slightly streched but shows no change in color. Usually the nodes can be easily moved in the underlying skin. Regular fixations to the periosteum or the bursa do not occur.

Histologically, juxta-articular nodes are granulomas with three zones and are, especially in the early stages of development, very cellular with lymphocytes, plasma, and epithelioid cells and, occasionally, Langhans' giant cells. There are also thickened blood vessels, which are surrounded by dense conglomerations of plasma cells. Such an outer granulomatous zone in older bones borders on the inside on a fibrous layer of a few cells. In the center, there is a fibrinized or hyaline connective tissue, which is under certain conditions

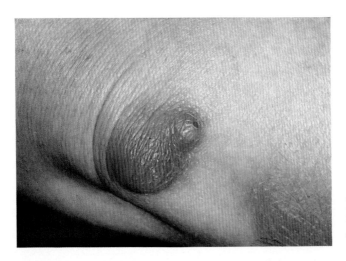

Fig. 43. Acrodermatitis chronica atrophicans: fibroid, juxta-articular nodes on the elbow and along the ulna.

Fig. 44. Heberden's nodes.

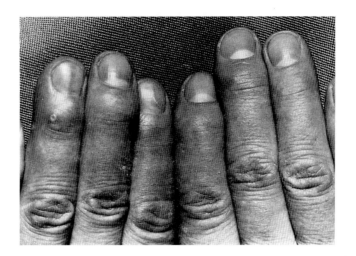

"cystically widened." Occasionally, cholesterol can be found in the cavities. Therefore, the juxta-artivular nodes lack any aspect of a rheumatoid condition.

Neither the macroscopic nor the microscopic picture offers any clues to the etiology of these nodes. This is also true with regard to the differences between juxta-articular nodes in frambesia and those in tertiary syphilis. Since even modern serologic aids for syphilis (FTA absorption test, among others) do not help, clinical criteria, especially the behavior of the skin, must be used as a basis for a diagnosis. [4, 5, 6]

2. Acrodermatitis chronica atrophicans plays an important role in the differential diagnosis. In about 20 per cent of cases juxta-articular nodes may exist simultaneously. Their relationship to acrodermatitis chronica atrophicans seems well founded since they usually occur in the same areas along the ulna and tibia (Fig. 43). Moreover, they as well as the surrounding skin are covered by atrophically changed skin. Such nodes are often replaced by a ropelike sclerotic swelling.

Histologically, acrodermatitis chronica atrophicans, fibroid nodes, and the ropelike scleroses are characterized by an area

of complete absence of elasticity. These findings are generally considered important in the differential diagnosis against circumscribed scleroderma. In addition, the juxta-articular nodes associated with acrodermatitis chronica atrophicans show a distinct acceleration of the ESR and an increase of the gammaglobulin in the serum, as well as occasionally a swelling of the regional lymph nodes. [1, 2, 3]

(1) ARNOLD, W., und F. NÜRNBERGER: Akrodermatitis chronica atrophicans mit geschlossen-strangförmiger Wulstbildung über der Ulna. Arch. klin. exp. Derm. *232:* 225–232 (1968).

(2) HAUSER, W.: Akrodermatitis chronica atrophicans. Ergebn. inn. Med. Kinderheilk. N. F. *22:* 58–89 (1965).

(3) KORTING, G. W., N. HOEDE und H. HOLZMANN: Zur Frage des Elasticaverhaltens bei einigen sklerosierenden und atrophisierenden Hautkrankheiten. Hautarzt *20:* 351–361 (1969).

(4) ROSSOW, A. W.: Zur Klinik und Diagnostik der Nodosités juxta-articulaires. Arch. Derm. Syph. (Berl.) *157:* 677–684 (1929).

(5) STERN, F.: Über juxtaartikuläre Knotenbildung bei Syphilitikern. Derm. Wschr. *90:* 677–682 (1930).

(6) WELTI, M. H.: Über Nodositas juxtaarticularis. Arch. Derm. Syph. (Berl.) *159:* 541–550 (1930).

B. Heberden's Nodes

1. Heberden's nodes, small nodes near the joints, represent a peculiar form of polyarthrosis of the hands. These nodes, located on the bases of the distal phalanges of the fingers (Fig. 44), are swellings about pea-sized which are rarely tender to the touch. The skin over the nodes is easily movable, and a deviation of the affected distal phalanges from the straight axis is present. Radiologically, the proximal ends of the distal phalanges show spur formation, and there are nodose enlargements of the distal ends of the middle phalanges, if the location of the disease is typical. Patients with idiopathic Heberden's nodes often have osteoarthroses of several joints. Localized or generalized signs of inflammation are always absent. As a matter of principle, **traumatic Heberden's nodes,** which are limited to a few fingers and occur mostly in men, should be distinguished from *idiopathic Heberden's nodes.* The latter affect women in the thirtieth to sixty-fifth year of life and are obviously transmitted by a single autosomal factor. This is inherited recessively in the female sex. [2, 3, 4]

Fig. 45. Dorsal finger cyst.

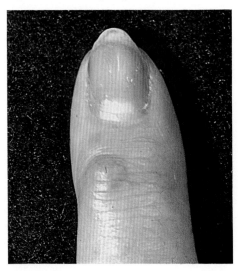

2. The occurrence of Heberden's nodes is preceded by the formation of a cyst in the para-articular tissue. This lesion is known to the dermatologist as a **synovial cyst** or so-called dorsal cyst (Fig. 45). The epidermis over these hazelnut-sized cysts is usually unchanged. Occasionally, one may be able to feel fluctuation; spontaneous perforations, however, do not occur. These peculiar cysts are predominantly located on the extensor surface of the interphalangeal, metacarpophalangeal, or metatarsophalangeal joints. Since an essential wall is absent, they are actually pseudocysts, whose jellylike contents seem to consist of hyaluronic acid. Radiologically, a bony spur formation regularly occurs below these cysts on the dorsal aspect of the fingers. [1, 3]

(1) GÖTZ, H., und R. KOCH: Zur Klinik, Pathogenese und Therapie der sogenannten »Dorsalcysten«. Hautarzt 7: 533–537 (1956).
(2) SCHILLING, F.: Die Polyarthrose. Diagnostik 4: 350–353 (1971).
(3) STECHER, R. M., und A. AUSENBACHS: Heberdensche Knoten. Die Besonderheit der Osteoarthrose der Finger. Z. Rheumaforsch. 13: 65–85 (1954).
(4) WEBER, G.: Zur Klinik der Heberdenschen Knoten. Derm. Wschr. 135: 162–165 (1957).

C. Clavi

1. Some clavi (calluses or tyloses) are located near joints. **Occupational clavi** in violinists or cellists are found on the tips of the second to fifth left fingers and are produced by the pressure of the strings. Especially well known, and likewise resulting from long-lasting mechanical maneuvers, are genuine milker's clavi (tylositas pollicis) (Fig. 46). Clinically, they represent two bilateral symmetrical lentil-sized flat clavi. They are located on the dorsum of the terminal phalanx of the thumb and develop only if the thumb is folded in

Fig. 46. Milker's clavi.

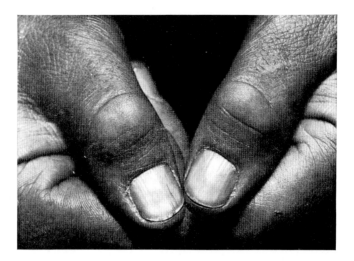

when milking so that pressure on the extensor surface of the terminal phalanx is exerted. These milker's clavi should not be confused with *milker's nodules* (para-vaccinia nodules) (Fig. 47) or *milker's granulation nodules* (caused by penetrating cow's hairs). Also, occasionally thickened

clavi *(clavi from sucking)* develop in small children on the extensor surface of the thumb's proximal joint (Fig. 48) from constant sucking of the finger.[1, 2]

2. In contrast to the regularly diffuse hyperkeratosis of such a callus, a **clavus**

Fig. 47. Milker's nodule.

Fig. 48. Clavus from sucking.

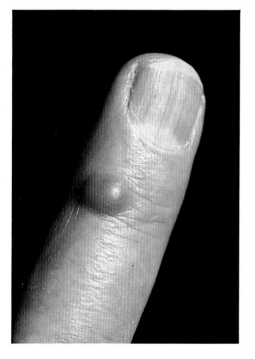

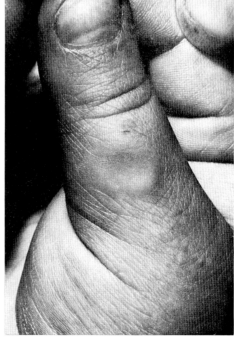

(corn) possesses a single central horny plug. This, however, is not the sole cause of the special tenderness of such a modified hyperkeratosis, since often a multiform nerve hyperplasia originates beneath a clavus. Corns develop usually over the distal heads of the metatarsal bones, toe joints, and exostoses, i. e., the sites of increased, unphysiologic pressure on the foot. In addition, in contrast to vulgar warts the surface is always smooth.

(1) HABERMANN, R.: Die in land- und forstwirtschaftlichen Betrieben vorkommenden beruflichen Hautveränderungen. In: Die Schädigung der Haut durch Beruf und gewerbliche Arbeit. Hrsg. K. ULLMANN. Bd. II. S. 447–468. Leipzig 1926.
(2) RONCHESE, F.: Knuckle pads and similar-looking disorders. Giorn. ital. Derm. *107:* 1227–1236 (1966).

D. Knuckle Pads

1. Knuckle pads represent relatively rare, sharply circumscribed, cutaneous thicken-

Fig. 49. Knuckle pads.

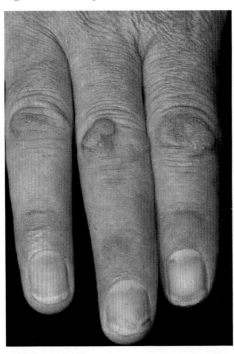

ings over the extensor surfaces of the joints of the fingers. The folds over the joints are obliterated and the joint surface is pinched or granularly rough (Fig. 49). Clinically, noticeable hyperkeratosis is absent. Knuckle pads, in contrast to Heberden's nodes, are freely movable over the joint and are not associated with arthritic changes. Moreover, these "cushions" are absent on the thumbs. The preference for the fingers of the left hand is noteworthy. It should not be overlooked that these knuckle pads, which almost without exception cause no complaints, are often associated with Dupuytren's contracture and induratio penis plastica (Peyronie's disease), or, in other words, they express a hereditary polyfibromatosis. There is a familial frequency in the occurrence of knuckle pads, but its mode of heredity has not yet been elucidated. An occasional family history shows an inter-relationship of knuckle pads, leukonychia, and deafness, indicating a dominantly inherited disorder.

Histologically, the important features are hyperkeratosis, acanthosis, or an increase of sclerosis of the cutaneous connective tissue or all of these. Occasionally dilated vessels at places associated with proliferations of the intima are conspicuous. [1, 2, 4, 5]

2. In connection with knuckle pads the term "**helodermia simplex (et anularis)**" seems superfluous, since the subsequent references hardly mention it and its application is contradictory. In 1911 Vörner described under this designation, "on the flexor side of the hands and fingers and also on the sides and the back, inconspicuous, almost regularly pitted nodules, which occur either as singular or multiple lesions." The term is mentioned only because occasionally these "helodermas" were later considered the same as the cushionlike thickenings of the distal phalanges of the fingers.[6]

Fig. 50. Erythema hyper-
keratoticum supra-articulare
dyspepticum of the fingers.

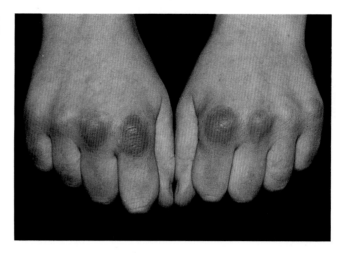

3. More attention should be paid to certain cutaneous changes near the joints in
patients with disorders of the gastrointestinal tract. **Erythema hyperkeratoticum
dyspepticum supra-articulare digitorum**
is located on the extensor surface of the
interphalangeal or the proximal phalangeal finger joints (Fig. 50). Exceptionally,
these nail-sized, pale lilac erythemas with
a more or less horny surface are situated
on the palms. In any case, within these
supra-articular keratoses the lines of the
skin of the fingers remain intact although
somewhat thickened.[3]

(1) BART, R. S., and R. E. PUMPHREY:
Knuckle pads, leukonychia and deafness.
A dominantly inherited syndrome. New
Engl. J. Med. *276:* 202–207 (1967).
(2) BURCKHARDT, W.: Die Fingerknöchel-
polster, eine häufige Hautveränderung.
Dermatologica (Basel) *88:* 192–197 (1943).
(3) CSILLAG, J.: Erythema hyperkeratoticum
dyspepticum supraarticulare digitorum.
Zbl. Haut- u. Geschl.-Kr. *60:* 476–477
(1938).
(4) GOSSRAU, G., und W. SELLE: Zur Koin-
zidenz der Induratio penis plastica, der
Dupuytrenschen Kontraktur und der
Knuckle pads. Derm. Wschr. *151:*
1039–1043 (1965).
(5) KRANTZ, W.: Über die »Fingerknöchel-
polster« (»Knuckle pads«). Derm. Wschr.
107: 945–949 (1938).
(6) VÖRNER, H.: Helodermia simplex et
anularis. Arch. Derm. Syph. (Wien,
Leipzig) *108:* 161–200 (1911).

E. Granuloma Annulare

1. The lesions of **granuloma annulare** are
nodular and arranged in grouped beadlike
rings. They may remain isolated even after
long duration. On the other hand, confluence of the lesions with formation of flat
patches is possible (Fig. 51 a), with the
result that the single pathologic lesion that
originally had a cartilagelike consistency
is no longer distinctly demarcated. A
single nodule usually is whitish-yellow,
and the surrounding skin is a pale red
color. The surface of the lesions becomes
so smooth that the cutaneous lines
disappear. Larger areas of infiltration in
time may show central regression, which
results in another kind of ring formation
(Fig. 239 b). Granuloma annulare generally
is a disease of early childhood but older
persons may well be affected. The fact that
typical granuloma annulare shows a
predilection for the extensor aspects of the
joints is of definite help in the differential
diagnosis. The first eruption in about four-
fifths of all cases is located on the joints of

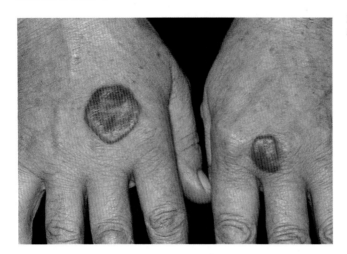

Fig. 51 a. Granuloma annulare.

fingers and hands. The joints of the feet are more often affected in children than in adults (Fig. 51 b).

Granuloma annulare generalisatum is a very rare multilocular eruption involving the entire skin. There is less tendency to

Fig. 51 b. Granuloma annulare.

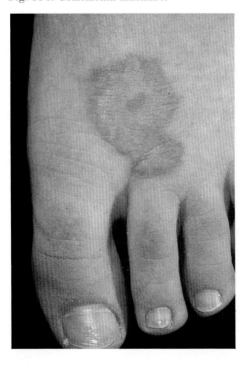

group formation of the nodules in such cases. Frequently there is a simultaneous diabetic metabolic disorder. If such disseminated annular granulomas are not ring-shaped and show central pitting, one may at first consider multiple mollusca contagiosa. A single lesion may resemble a spontaneous keloid or annular lichen planus; if the lesions are larger and form extensive patches, a differential diagnosis of necrobiosis lipoidica should be considered.

Histologically, it is necessary to separate necrobiosis lipoidica because this disease shows a very similar collagenous degeneration in the middle of the cutis. However, granuloma annulare lacks more pronounced vascular changes, accumulation of lipid material, and giant cell reaction to a foreign body. The subcutaneous nodules of acute and chronic rheumatoid arthritis as a rule show more massive degeneration of the connective tissue. The histologic decision in a single case may be difficult; this is shown by the fact that histopathologists frequently group all these periarticular nodes together as "palisading granulomas".[1, 3]

2. Erythema elevatum diutinum, which occurs mainly between the third and sixth decades of life without preference as to sex, can be grouped nosologically halfway between erythema multiforme and granuloma annulare. It also favors the extensor aspects, especially of the smaller joints of the extremities. At these locations subacute globular or polycyclic knotty infiltrates of a bluish-red hue, frequently with a central depression, develop slowly. The lesions of erythema elevatum diutinum may change their consistency, a feature absent in granuloma annulare. Some patients suffering from this nodular erythema complain about stinging pains or burning sensations. *Extracellular cholesterosis* represents a variant of erythema elevatum diutinum with secondary lipid inclusion.[2, 3, 4]

The torpid clinical appearance of erythema diutinum shows rather surprising histologic findings, with marked fibrosis permeated by chronic inflammatory cells and in the same section, highly acute polynuclear and leukocytoclastic infiltrates.

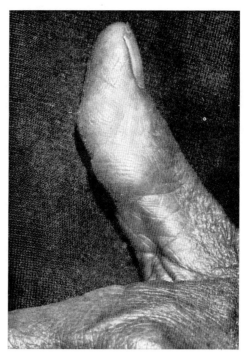

Fig. 52. Rheumatoid nodules on the ulnar side of the thumb.

(1) DICKEN, CH. H., ST. G. CARRINGTON and R. K. WINKELMANN: Generalized granuloma annulare. Arch. Derm. Syph. (Chic.) *99:* 556–563 (1969).

(2) HABER, H.: Erythema elevatum diutinum. Brit. J. Derm. *67:* 121–145 (1955).

(3) HEITE, H.-J., und H. X. SCHARWENKA: Erythema elevatum diutinum, Granuloma anulare, Necrobiosis lipoidica und Granulomatosis disciformis Gottron-Miescher. Arch. klin. exp. Derm. *208:* 260–290 (1959).

(4) HERZBERG, J. J.: Die extracelluläre Cholesterinose (Kerl-Urbach), eine Variante des Erythema elevatum diutinum. Arch. klin. exp. Derm. *205:* 477–496 (1958).

F. Rheumatic Nodules

Rheumatoid nodules, formerly known as nodose rheumatism, are formed in long drawn out and far advanced cases of polyarthritis as nongrouped hard nodes. They lie deeper than the solitary nodes of granuloma annulare and are often attached to tendons and fasciae. This means that visible rheumatoid nodules protrude only slightly above their surroundings, with the exception of especially large single nodes. Usually multiple ipsilateral cherry-stone-sized lesions develop rapidly; they become hard only through secondary calcification (Fig. 52). They can be moved only with difficulty on their base; however, the overlying skin, which does not show any color change, can easily be lifted. Sites of preference of such mostly non-tender nodes are the small joints at the extremities, the elbow joint, the galea aponeurotica of the scalp, and the spinous processes of the vertebrae. After a period ranging from a few days to months the rheumatoid nodules regress into scar tissue consisting of connective tissue. Perforation into the open occurs very rarely. It should be emphasized that in arthropathic psoriasis such extra-articular subcutaneous formation of nodules does not take place.

Histologically, rheumatoid nodules present a central zone of necrosis surrounded by an intermediate zone of histiocytes. Electron-microscopic examination, however, seems to show that histiocytes occur in a rheumatic granuloma only sporadically. The cells of the granulomatous wall of the rheumatic nodule are said to derive from the intima of blood vessels; one type of these granuloma cells originates from smooth muscle cells, the second type from proliferating endothelial cells. A third peripheral zone of such rheumatoid nodules shows a chronic inflammatory infiltrate. In critical approach to the evaluation of the fibroid damage to the tissue, one should consider that the histologic and histochemical findings depend to a large degree on the duration of this alteration. The histologic differentiation from erythema elevatum diutinum should take into account the pronounced exudative to leukocytoclastic infiltration and the simultaneous tendency to fibrosis. Granuloma annulare, however, presents necrobiosis as its main histologic feature, and necrobiosis lipoidica shows in addition marked thickening of the walls of the vessels.[1, 2, 3]

(1) GAMP, A., und A. SCHILLING: Extra-artikuläre Manifestationen der chronischen Polyarthritis am Bewegungsapparat: Sehnen-, Sehnenscheiden-, Schleimbeutelentzündung, subkutane Knoten. Z. Rheumaforsch. 25: 42–56 (1966).

(2) GIESEKING, R.: Das feinmikroskopische Bild des Rheumatismus nodosus. Beitr. path. Anat. 138: 292–320 (1969).

(3) KERL, H.: Knotige rheumatische Hautmanifestationen und ihre Differentialdiagnose. Z. Haut- u. Geschl.-Kr. 47: 193–208 (1972).

G. Reticulohistiocytomas

Multiple reticulohistiocytomas ("lipoid dermatoarthritis") occur as cutaneous nodules located typically on the distal interphalangeal joints. They are found also on the face, trunk, and arms; they vary from pinhead-to pea-size. The semi-spherical, protuberant, mostly multiple nodules have a consistency that ranges from elastic to a firmly fibrous state, and have a certain similarity to xanthomas and histiocytomas, somewhat less so to large lichen planus papules. This similarity extends also to the pruritus which is elicited by such growths. Sometimes the combination of an elevated serum cholesterol level with reticulohistiocytomas indicates a similarity to hypercholesterolemic xanthomatosis. But reticulohistiocytosis affects the joints, in contrast to the xanthomatoses, as discussed previously (Chapter 1, C5). In addition, the nodules of multiple reticulohistiocytomas are hardly tender on pressure; they are covered by atrophic skin and are relatively firmly attached to the underlying tissue.

Histologically, the multiple eruptive cutaneous nodules show an accumulation of histiocytes and giant cells with pink-staining and sometimes finely granulated cytoplasm. There are also infiltrations of round cells and an absence of a more pronounced tissue reaction against the giant cell — reticulohistiocytic infiltrate. Another characteristic is the capacity of the histiocytes to store substances supposed to represent mucoproteins with a lipoid component. Synonyms like *multicentric reticulohistiocytosis* or *histiocytosis gigantocellularis* are an attempt to describe these histologic criteria. A cellular analysis of the histiocytes of multicentric reticulohistiocytosis shows that they are capable of considerable variation, so it is understandable that the observations made thus far will have a certain divergence from case to case.[1-3]

(1) EHRLICH, G. E., I. YOUNG, S. Z. NOSHENY and W. A. KATZ: Multicentric reticulo-histiocytosis (lipoid dermatoarthritis). A multisystem disorder. Amer. J. Med. *52:* 830–840 (1972).
(2) FLAM, M., S. C. RYAN, G. L. MAH-POY, K. F. JACOBS and K. H. NELDNER: Multicentric reticulohistiocytosis. Report of a case, with atypical features and electron microscopic study of skin lesions. Amer. J. Med. *52:* 841–848 (1972).
(3) HOLUBAR, K., und K. MACH: Histiocytosis giganto-cellularis. Ein Beitrag zur Klinik und Histologie. Hautarzt *17:* 440–445 (1966).

H. Maffucci's Syndrome

Maffucci's syndrome is characterized by multiple subcutaneous cavernous hemangiomas and asymmetrical dyschondroplasia. This combination of signs does not occur in families and is seen more frequently in males.

Enchondromas resembling juxta-articular nodes occasionally develop after birth, especially on the phalanges. Noteworthy is the high frequency of malignant degeneration and also the occasional combination with vitiligo or pigmented nevi (a variant described by Kast and von Recklinghausen).

I. Interstitial Calcinosis

In **calcinosis interstitialis (Teutschländer syndrome),** nodules appear mainly in the vicinity of the joints of the extremities (Fig. 53). Other preferred locations are the buttocks and the trunk, but the face and scalp are almost always spared. The eruption of such calcified nodes may be accompanied by high temperature and general signs. The originally small, tender, hard nodules can develop into large nodes through apposition and can then perforate through the inflamed skin which has become atrophic through pressure. After the viscous and partly calcified contents have been discharged, a painful ulceration showing a tendency to poor healing will remain. In contradistinction to the other diseases of this group, internal organs remain free of calcium deposits. Abnormalities of the blood, except for occasional eosinophilia and sometimes an increased sedimentation rate, are absent; in addition, there are no changes in calcium or phosphate metabolism. In the diseased regions of the body, radiographs show characteristic, small macular, aggregated shadows without definite structure. It is generally accepted today that this is not a disorder of the calcium metabolism but involves second-

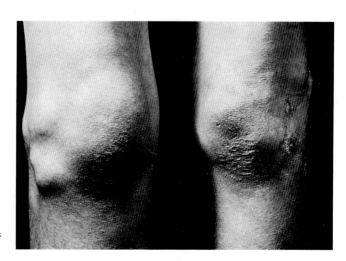

Fig. 53. Interstitial calcinosis (Teutschländer syndrome).

ary calcifications of previously damaged connective tissue. Accordingly, in some cases there may be present either a prior or simultaneous dermatomyositis, progressive scleroderma, or endangiitis obliterans. However, there is no definite relationship between these diseases and interstitial calcinosis. It should be noted that interstitial calcinosis as well as progressive scleroderma is observed preponderantly in women. In the differential diagnosis of myositis ossificans and calcinosis interstitialis, the former presents ankylosis of the joints and calcifications along the distribution of the muscles; radiographs show smooth osseous bands connected with the skeleton. Gout would show elevation of uric acid and areas of roentgenologic osseous rarefaction. Calcifications similar to those in calcinosis interstitialis can be seen as post-traumatic deposits of calcium in hematomas and scars, in lipomas, in tuberculous lymph nodes, in parasitoses (toxoplasmosis, trichinosis), at sites of injections, as postphlebitic subcutaneous calcinoses, and in hyperparathyroidism, rickets, overdosage of vitamin D, and hypercalcemic sarcoidosis.[1, 2]

(1) JESSERER, H.: Erkrankungen und Probleme aus den Grenzgebieten der Inneren Medizin. XVII. Calcinosis interstitialis (Kalkgicht). Med. Klin. 55: 2229–2234 (1960).
(2) REICH, H.: Das Teutschlaender-Syndrom. Hautarzt 14: 462–468 (1963).

K. Cutaneous Cysticercosis

In the course of **cutaneous cysticercosis** cutaneous or subcutaneous nodes located usually near joints may be observed in rare instances. Such often fluctuant nodes develop in recurring crops without marked general signs and very rarely give rise to local inflammation. The diagnosis can be established by opening the nodes and examining their contents (for the presence of cysticerci). Examination of antibodies through complement fixation tests or tests of the intracutaneous cyst are uncertain. Eosinophilia, which is present in other parasitoses, is found only rarely.[1]

(1) SCHMORANZER, H., und H. PAASCH: Kasuistischer Beitrag zur Hautzystizerkose und ihrer Differentialdiagnose. Derm. Wschr. 154: 1225–1232 (1968).

9. Deafness and Dermatoses

1. Of the group of dermatoses associated with pigment anomalies **partial albinism,** accompanied by deaf-mutism, should be mentioned first. This combination of manifestations may represent autosomal dominant (Tietz's syndrome) or x-chromosomal heredity. A special form of partial albinism occurs in the **Klein-Waardenburg syndrome,** which involves congenital deafness of the inner ear and other dysplasias of the skull. As a hereditary syndrome *total albinism* is occasionally associated with deaf-mutism. Further details on these three disorders can be found in Chapter 24, A1 and 3.[4, 15, 19, 32, 33]

Vitiligo, which is not infrequently a hereditary disease, can be accompanied by deafness if inherited recessively (see Chapter 24, A.)[19]
Congenital inner ear deafness associated with lentiginosis profusa is an essential sign of the **leopard syndrome** (see Chapter 24, E2).[5, 14]

2. Malformations of the nails or hairs can be associated with disturbances of hearing. Thus, congenital inner ear deafness can be combined with **onychodystrophies.** In these patients the nail plates either are missing or are present only in a rudimentary form. Hair anomalies, disturbances of the function of the sweat glands, and pigmentary disturbances, however, do not occur. Heredity of this condition is either autosomal dominant or recessive.[8, 10, 15]

The combination of **knuckle pads, leukonychia, and deafness** is transmitted as an autosomal dominant trait. The leukonychia applies to the entire nail plate, making the lunula no longer recognizable. Loss of hearing is caused by a combination of sensorineural and conduction deafness. In one case palmoplantar keratoses were also present.[1, 15, 29]

Pili torti associated with sensorineural deafness may occur as a hereditary and congenital syndrome.[3, 25]

The joint occurrence of deafness and malformations of the cutaneous appendages suggests that congenital deafness also occurs in **ectodermal dysplasias.** This is observed in the anhidrotic as well as in the hidrotic variants.[12, 24]

3. The association of **ichthyosis congenita** and deafness, which has been reported, may have been coincidental. There have also been reports of families with congenital deafness, ichthyosis, and **struma.** A single observation has been recorded of congenital deafness with **pigmented hyperkeratoses** of articular folds near the trunk as well as on elbows and extensor surfaces of the fingers. Such hyperkeratoses have also been observed in association with diffuse keratoses of palms and soles and **absence of hair** on the entire skin. Such disturbances of keratinization are preponderantly expressed in thornlike follicular hyperkeratoses. The relationship of these disorders to congenital ichthyosiform erythroderma has not yet been elucidated. Relatively frequent, however, are ichthyosiform dermatoses and inner ear deafness in **Refsum's syndrome** (for details see Chapter 24).[6, 11, 12, 21, 31]

4. Hereditary inner ear deafness occurs in the various **palmoplantar keratoses.** In some families there are also ainhum-like **constrictions** of fingers and toes. In families with **endogenous eczema** cases of hereditary congenital deafness have occurred, but one cannot simply conclude that a genetically determined relationship between the two disorders exists.[16, 24]

5. However, the combination of recurrent **urticaria, amyloidosis,** and progressive neurogenic deafness constitutes a definite syndrome. The diagnosis can easily be ascertained by a rectal biopsy. Occasionally, **mucopolysaccharidosis** of the Pfaundler-Hurler type shows a disturbance in the conduction of sounds.[17, 22, 30]

6. A few patients with **xeroderma pigmentosum** suffer from congenital deafness. This is not surprising since xeroderma pigmentosum is associated with a number of neurologic deficits, including disturbances of reflexes and coordination. For diagnosis of this skin condition see Chapter 24, E13).[7, 25]

7. In **Cockayne's syndrome,** a genetic familial disorder, disproportionate dwarfism, increased disposition to caries, retinitis pigmentosa, and deafness are the cardinal signs. With regard to the skin, a peculiar facies is present, comprising deep-lying eyes, dysplastic auricles, prognathism, and, above all, a hypersensitivity to light, which causes the development of blisters and bullae.

8. The classic late triad of **congenital syphilis** includes inner ear deafness as well as Hutchinson's teeth and keratitis parenchymatosa. It usually starts around the tenth year of life and begins with labyrinthine vertigo. This is followed by a progressive loss of hearing starting at the upper tonal range; it may be unilateral or bilateral. If loss of hearing occurs soon after birth, the child becomes a deaf-mute.

The slowly developing disturbances of hearing follow almost exclusively the sequence of periostitis or gummatous osteitis. Suddenly beginning loss of hearing in the course of **secondary syphilis,** however, is caused by a direct specific involvement of the CNS. This can be concluded from its good therapeutic response to penicillin.[9, 20, 27]

9. In the course of **relapsing polychondritis** inner ear deafness as well as fever occurs in a high percentage of cases (see Chapter 1, I4).[23]

10. Patients with an atypical course of **erythrokeratodermia variabilis** may also have associated deafness. In these cases there are usually other cerebral disturbances as well and, in exceptional cases, involvement of the muscles.[2, 28]

(1) BART, R. S., and R. E. PUMPHREY: Knuckle pads, leukonychia and deafness. New Engl. J. Med. *276:* 202–207 (1967).

(2) BEARE, J. M., N. C. NEVIN, P. FROGGATT, D. C. KERNOHAN and I. V. ALLEN: Atypical erythrokeratoderma with deafness, physical retardation and peripheral neuropathy. Brit. J. Derm. *87:* 308–314 (1972).

(3) BJÖRNSTAD, R.: Pili torti and sensory-neural loss of hearing. Proc. Fenno-Scand. Ass. Derm. *1965:* 3–12.

(4) CAMPBELL, B., N. R. CAMPBELL and S. SWIFT: Waardenburg's syndrome. Arch. Derm. (Chic.) *86:* 718–724 (1962).

(5) CAPUTE, A. J., D. L. RIMOIN, B. W. KONIGSMARK, N. B. ESTERLY and F. RICHARDSON: Congenital deafness and multiple lentigines. Arch. Derm. (Chic.) *100:* 207–213 (1969).

(6) DERAEMAEKER, R.: Congenital deafness and goiter. Amer. J. hum. Genet. *8:* 253–256 (1956).

(7) ELSÄSSER, G., O. FREUSBERG und F. THEML: Das Xeroderma pigmentosum und die »xerodermische Idiotie«. Arch. Derm. Syph. (Berl.) *188:* 651–655 (1950).

(8) FEINMESSER, M., and S. ZELIG: Congenital deafness associated with onychodystrophy. Arch. Otolaryng. *74:* 507–508 (1961).

(9) FIUMARA, N. J., and S. LESSELL: Manifestations of late congenital syphilis. An analysis of 27 patients. Arch. Derm. (Chic.) *102:* 78–83 (1970).

(10) GOODMAN, R. M., S. LOCKAREFF and G. GWINUP: Hereditary congenital deafness with onychodystrophy. Arch. Otolaryng. *90:* 474–477 (1969).

(11) HARDERS, H., und H. DIECKMANN: Heredopathia atactica polyneuritiformis. Klinik und Diagnostik des Refsum-Syndroms. Dtsch. med. Wschr. *89:* 248–254 (1964).

(12) HAXTHAUSEN, H.: Hyperkeratosis ichthyosiformis? Acanthosis nigricans? in a 4-year-old girl with congenital deafness. Acta derm-venereol. (Stockh.) *35:* 191–192 (1955).

(13) HELWIG-LARSEN, H. F., and K. LUDVIGSEN: Congenital familial anhidrosis and neurolabyrinthitis. Acta derm.-venereol. (Stockh.) *26:* 489–505 (1946).

(14) HORNSTEIN, O. P., und F. WEIDNER: Systematisierte Lentiginosis mit kongenitaler Taubheit und diskretem Status dysrhaphicus. Dermatologica (Basel) *143:* 79–83 (1971).

(15) KONIGSMARK, B. W.: Hereditary childhood hearing loss and integumentary system disease. J. Pediatr. *80:* 909–919 (1972).

(16) KONIGSMARK, B. W., M. B. HOLLANDER and C. I. BERLIN: Familial neural hearing loss and atopic dermatitis. J. Amer. med. Ass. *204:* 953–957 (1968).

(17) LAGRUE, G., J. P. VERNANT, J. REVUZ, R. TOURAINE et B. WEIL: Syndrome de Mückle et Wells. Cinquième observation familiale. Nouv. Presse méd. *1:* 2223–2226 (1972).

(18) LUCHSINGER, R., und E. HANHART: Über erhebliche Manifestationsschwankungen rezessiver Taubheit bei drei eineiigen Zwillingspaaren. Arch. Klaus-Stift. Vererb.-Forsch. *24:* 417–436 (1949).

(19) MARGOLIS, E.: A new hereditary syndrome – sexlinked deaf-mutism associated with total albinism. Acta genet. (Basel) *12:* 12–19 (1962).

(20) MAYER, O.: Zur Kenntnis der pathologischen Veränderungen im Gehör-
organ bei der Lues congenita tarda. Z.
Hals-, Nas- u. Ohrenheilk. *37:* 2–30
(1934).

(21) MORRIS, J., A. B. ACKERMAN and P. J.
KOBLENZER: Generalized spiny hyperkeratosis, universal alopecia, and deafness. Arch. Derm. (Chic.) *100:* 692–698
(1969).

(22) MÜCKLE, T. J., and M. WELLS: Urticaria, deafness, and amyloidosis: a new
heredo-familial syndrome. Quart. J.
J. Med. *31:* 235–248 (1962).

(23) NITZSCHNER, H., O. PETTER und K.
SCHLENTHER: Polychondritis recidivans
et atrophicans. Derm. Mschr. *156:* 789–
797 (1970).

(24) NOCKEMANN, P. F.: Erbliche Hornhautverdickung mit Schnürfurchen an Fingern und Zehen und Innenohrschwerhörigkeit. Med. Welt *1961/II:* 1894–
1900.

(25) REED, W. B., V. M. STONE, E. BODER
and L. ZIPRKOWSKI: Hereditary syndromes with auditory and dermatological manifestations. Arch. Derm. (Chic.)
95: 456–461 (1967).

(26) ROBINSON, G. C., J. R. MILLER and
J. R. BENSIMON: Familial ectodermal
dysplasia with sensori-neural deafness

and other anomalies. Pediatrics *30:*
797–802 (1962).

(27) SCHNEIDER, S., und B. BOLTE: Plötzliche Hörminderung bei Lues II. Med.
Welt *23* (N. F.): 319–321 (1972).

(28) SCHNYDER, U. W., H. WISSLER und
G. G. WENDT: Eine weitere Form von
atypischer Erythrokeratodermie mit
Schwerhörigkeit und cerebraler Schädigung. Helv. paediat. Acta *23:* 220–230
(1968).

(29) SCHWANN, J.: Keratosis palmaris et
plantaris cum surditate congenita et
leuconychia totali unguium. Dermatologica (Basel) *126:* 335–353 (1963).

(30) SMITH, E. B., T. C. HEMPELMANN, S.
MOORE and D. P. BARR: Gargoylism
(dysostosis multiplex): two adult cases
with one autopsy. Ann. int. Med. *36:*
652–667 (1952).

(31) WINTERNITZ, R.: Ichthyosis congenita.
Zbl. Haut- u. Geschl.-Kr. *26:* 345 (1928).

(32) ZIPRKOWSKI, L., and A. ADAM: Recessive total albinism and congenital deaf-
mutism. Arch. Derm. (Chic.) *89:* 151–
155 (1964).

(33) ZIPRKOWSKI, L., A. KRAKOWSKI, A.
ADAM, H. COSTEFF and J. SADE: Partial
albinism and deaf mutism. Arch. Derm.
(Chic.) *86:* 530–539 (1962).

10. Recurrent and Persistent Edemas

A. Transitory and Recurring Edemas

1. Quincke's edema is a typical example of an edema with an acute onset. It is a special form of urticaria in that it presents a widespread bilateral swelling almost completely confined to the face; it can also involve mucous membranes and the deeper parts of the soft tissue (Fig. 54). In addition to the appearance of separate

wheals, the main feature is a diffuse, often pale edema which seldom itches. The main danger of Quincke's edema is the sudden development of life-threatening edema of the glottis. Allergy to food or drugs is the chief cause, but occasionally an insect sting may be the inciting factor.

2. Hereditary angioedema represents a special form of Quincke's edema. The mode

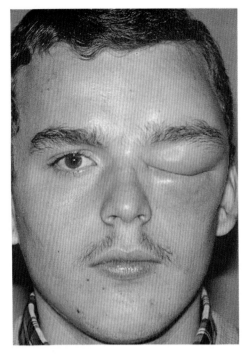

Fig. 54. Quincke's edema.

of inheritance is autosomal dominant and only heterozygotic individuals are affected; homozygosity is probably a lethal factor. Clinically, urticarial lesions are replaced by circumscribed, lightly pruritic, pale edematous areas on the extremities and face, and above all, within the larynx. Similar edemas affect the gastrointestinal tract,

causing such severe abdominal pain that failure to recognize the true character of this condition may raise the question of surgical intervention. Hereditary angioedema manifests itself first in early infancy with edema of the extremities and abdominal crises. With increasing age, edema of the face or larynx becomes more frequent. Many patients succumb to acute laryngeal edema before the age of 40. Quincke's edema has a multiplicity of different causes, but hereditary angioedema has only one well-known etiologic factor – the absence of the C_1-esterase inhibitor (an alpha 2-neuroaminoglycoprotein) normally found in everyone. It is present in an amount that is either too small or is normal but functionally inactive. The diagnosis can be established in special laboratories by finding either a diminished concentration of the C_1-inhibitor or by demonstrating its enzymatic inactivity. It is simpler to make the diagnosis by establishing a definite reduction of the C_2, C_3, and C_4 components of complement during an acute attack of edema.[3, 8, 12, 14]

3. Recurrent unilateral facial edema is part of the **Melkersson-Rosenthal syndrome.** This entity is more common in women than in men; when fully devel-

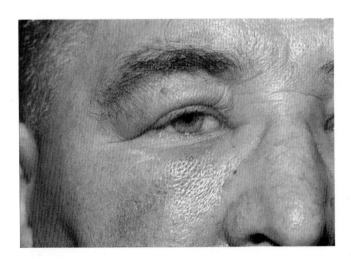

Fig. 55a. Melkersson-Rosenthal syndrome: granulomatous blepharitis.

Fig. 55 b. Melkersson-Rosenthal syndrome: recurrent
swelling of lips.

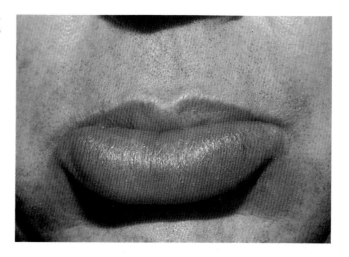

oped it presents recurring facial paresis, scrotal tongue, and cheilitis granulomatosa (Fig.55 b, c). Besides additional neurovegetative signs, involvement of the buccal mucosa (pareiitis granulomatosa) and of the palate (uranitis granulomatosa) occurs with transitory manifestations at first which later become more and more persistent. The palate presents in its final stage cobblestone-like, confluent, granulomatous, and elevated lesions. As a rare localization granulomatous swellings around the eye (blepharitis granulomatosa) have been observed (Fig.55 a). According to the stage of the disease there are histologically transudations at first, and later more cellular proliferations of either sarcoid or tuberculoid structure. The differential diagnosis must consider chronic recurrent erysipelas without fever and the previously mentioned Quincke's edema. A persistent swelling and enlargement of the lips (macrocheilia) may be caused by lymphangiomas, hemangiomas (Fig.56), and deeply situated diseases such as tuberculosis, tertiary syphilis, leprosy,

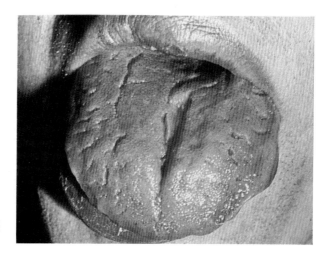

Fig. 55 c. Melkersson-Rosenthal
syndrome: fissured tongue.

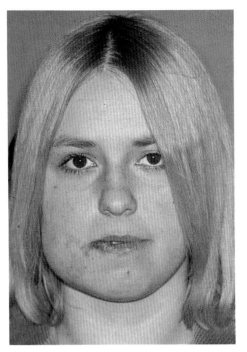

Fig. 56. Facial hemihypertrophy caused by subcutaneous hemangiomas in the area of the right cheek.

fungal granuloma, an otherwise typical sarcoidosis (Fig.57), and the different kinds of glandular cheilitis. All of these fail to show the tendency to spontaneous remission typical of the Melkersson-Rosen-

thal syndrome. Granulomatous thickenings of the buccal mucosa similar to those in pareiitis granulomatosa may be observed also in malignant acanthosis nigricans (Fig.58). The diagnosis depends in such cases on the presence of the typical cutaneous changes of acanthosis nigricans. The diagnosis of *morsicatio buccarum** (Fig.59) is made as a chance observation because the physician usually is not consulted for this condition. The buccal mucosa presents as a rule only a few elevated lesions, which run parallel to the dental line of closure. These lesions are caused by habitual sucking and chewing of these regions of the mucosa. The surface almost always shows cloudiness of the epithelium, small, partly detached pieces of mucosa, and areas of bleeding and erosions.[1, 5, 10, 11]

4. The lips of young girls may show recurrent edematous erythemas as a **premenstrual syndrome:** this has a corresponding dependence on the beginning of the menstrual period. Sometimes an abortive *herpes simplex* is also present,

---

* Caused by neurotic chewing of the buccal mucosa. (Tr.)

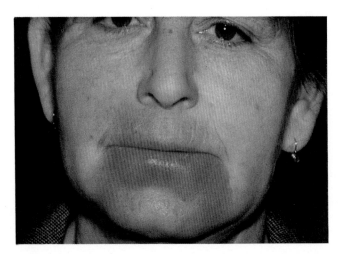

Fig. 57. Plaquelike infiltrate of the lower lip in sarcoidosis.

Fig. 58. Malignant acanthosis nigricans: part of the manifestation on the buccal mucosa.

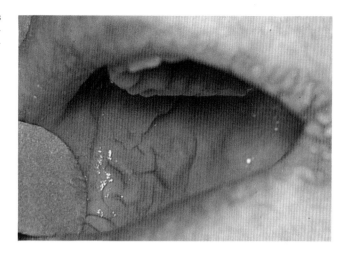

which eventually may result in a post-herpetic elephantiasis of the lips (Fig. 60).[2, 9]

5. Chagas' disease starts typically with a unilateral facial edema. These swellings are caused by the sting of a reduviid bug* harboring *Trypanosoma cruzi*. If the bite, which occurs mostly at night, penetrates the soft skin of the eyelids, the resultant severe itching will cause the unsuspecting person to rub the infected feces of the insect into the bite. Local edema with regional lymphadenopathy and enlargement of the upper external tear gland will follow. Later on an acute phase with attacks of high fever, generalized edema, hepatosplenomegaly, and diffuse meningoencephalitis may develop. Frequently, however, the acute phase will be omitted, and after a prolonged latent period chronic fatal myocarditis will develop.

6. Definitely erythematous and, above all, unilateral edemas of the frontal or eyelid region should direct attention to bacterial **inflammatory conditions** of the nasal sinuses, phlegmonas of the orbit, or osteomyelitis of the maxilla or frontal bone.

7. As the cause of unilateral soft edemas of the hand or forearm appearing as **chronic traumatic edemas of the dorsum of the hand,** artefacts should be suspected (Fig. 61). Such edemas are produced by the patient applying a string or cord, or by beating to cause congestion. The skin within the edematous area is a livid blue. Other diagnostic signs are sharply outlined, circumscribed, and circular borders of the edema, and streaked petechial bleeding or pigmentation at the borders of the cord. The venous flow of the affected part of the

Fig. 59. Cheekbiting (caused by sucking and chewing) of the buccal mucosa.

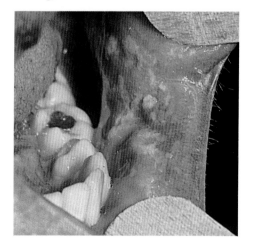

---

* Kissing bug or assassin bug. (Tr.)

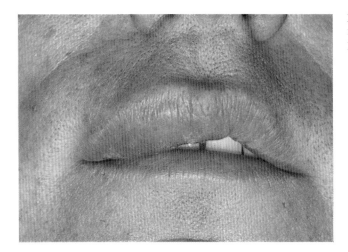

Fig. 60. Snelling of lips following recurrent herpes sim-
plex.

extremity is unobstructed at the time of
the examination, but the edema may
cause a Sudeck-like osteoporosis of the
bone.

Careful application of a plaster cast will
result in disappearance of the edema; the
patient will be unable to produce more
artefacts and the correct diagnosis will be
made.[4, 6, 7, 13]

8. Recurrent edema of the lips and
eyelids is one of the beginning signs of the
Asher syndrome, which is discussed in
Chapter 17, B4 (Fig. 62).

(1) BALABANOW, K., und J. DIMITROWA:
Seltene Lokalisationen und eigentümliche klinische Formen des Melkersson-
Rosenthal-Syndroms (Blepharitis granulomatosa et Hemicheilitis granulomatosa). Derm. Wschr. *151:* 101–107
(1965).

(2) GRABNER, K.: Über ein rezidivierendes
ödematöses Erythem der Lippen. Z.
Haut u. Geschl.-Kr. *43:* 701–710 (1968).

(3) GRANERUS, G., L. HALLBERG, A. B.
LAURELL and H. WETTERQUIST: Studies on the histamine metabolism and
the complement system in hereditary
angioneurotic edema. Acta med. scand.
182: 11–22 (1967).

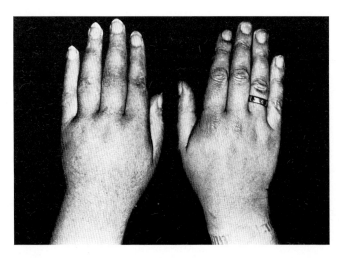

Fig. 61. Traumatic edema of
the dorsum of the left hand.

Fig. 62. "Double lip" in Ascher's syndrome.

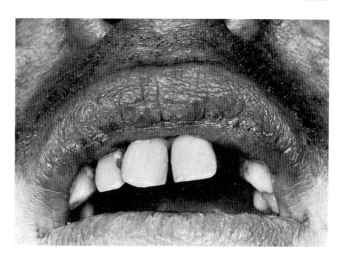

(4) GUMRICH, H.: Begutachtung und Nachweis des Selbststaus. Dtsch. med. Wschr. *83:* 1809–1811; 1821–1822 (1958).

(5) HORNSTEIN, O., und H. SCHUERMANN: Das sogenannte Melkersson-Rosenthal-Syndrom. Ergebn. inn. Med. Kinderheilk. N. F. *17:* 190–263 (1962).

(6) KLOSTERMANN, G. F., und D. MISIC: Artefizielles Oedem mit Haemorrhagien, hervorgerufen durch Schnüren und Klopfen. Z. Haut- u. Geschl.-Kr. *42:* 295–302 (1967).

(7) KUNZE, E.: Artefakt unter dem Bilde eines traumatischen Handrückenödems. Derm. Wschr. *131:* 59–62 (1955).

(8) MISGELD, V., und U. SCHULTZ-EHRENBURG: Zum Quincke-Ödem (hereditäres Angioödem). Med. Klin. *68:* 693–697 (1973).

(9) RATHJENS, B.: Herpes simplex recidivans mit konsekutiver Elephantiasis. Derm. Wschr. *128:* 758–762 (1963).

(10) RAUCH, S.: Neue Gesichtspunkte zum Melkersson - Rosenthal - Syndrom. Schweiz. med. Wschr. *98:* 1743–1750 (1968).

(11) SCHIMPF, A.: Ungewöhnliche Schwellungen beim sog. Melkersson-Rosenthal-Syndrom. Derm. Wschr. *147:* 105–118 (1963).

(12) v. SCHNACKENBURG, K., und K. DÖRNER: Das hereditäre angioneurotische Ödem (Quincke-Ödem) mit bedrohlicher Manifestation im Kindesalter. Med. Welt *22* (N. F.): 1218–1220 (1971).

(13) SCHRÖDER, G.: Röntgenologisch-klinischer Beitrag zur Ätiologie des traumatischen Handödems. Münch. med. Wschr. *101:* 547–549 (1959).

(14) WÜTHRICH, B., und P. GROB: Hereditäres Angioödem: neuere Therapiemöglichkeiten. Schweiz. med. Wschr. *102:* 349–353 (1972).

B. Persistent Swellings

1. Unilateral or bilateral fixed swellings of the temporal or mandibular regions may be due to **hypertrophy of the masseter muscle** caused by simple hyperactivity; younger persons are subject to such swellings resulting from excessive mastication or from faulty position of the teeth or bad chewing habits in the process of eating. Depending on which masseter muscle is more under strain, a slight sensation of tightness or fatigue will be felt on that side; slow diffuse enlargement of the region of the muscle takes place with a definite increase in consistency upon contraction (Fig. 63). As a rule, the opening of the mouth is not impaired; the enlarged muscle remains free from pain on touch or pressure.
[14, 16, 18]

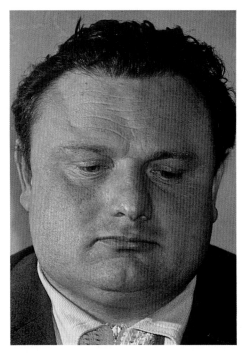

Fig. 63. Hypertrophy of the masseter muscles.

2. In childhood, bulging of the cheeks similar to persistent swelling is a manifestation of the **cherub syndrome.** This condition is caused by osseous dysplasia of the maxilla with upward displacement of the ocular bulbus. The pathologic anatomic basis is a maxillary enlargement due to formation of multiple cysts that are composed of spindle and giant cells; after some time these cells are replaced by collagenous fibers.[9]

3. Tightly elastic swellings in the region of the internal canthus of the eye with displacement of the bulbus are characteristic of the paramedian **mucocele.** The skin covering such a swelling fails to show pathologic changes. The diagnosis is verified by radiography; diagnostic punctures should not be performed.

4. The auricle may show chronic enlargement as part of the **Klippel-Trénaunay syndrome,** together with unilateral hyper-

trophy of the osseous parts of the skull and nevus flammeus. Swellings of the auricle due to hypertrophy of the sebaceous glands with periglandular fibrosis might be called *otophyma* because the appearance resembles rhinophyma of the nose. Elephantiasic enlargement of the auricle due to congenital or acquired *lymphostasis* is extremely rare; this swelling takes decades to develop.[4]

5. Unilateral edema of the arm affects mostly young males with well developed muscles; the edema results from the sudden occlusion of an axillary vein. This **Paget-Schrötter syndrome** is caused by either a sudden or sometimes slowly developing cervicobrachial swelling accompanied by paresthesias and adynamia,* only rarely by cyanosis. Characteristically, the veins of the upper arm become prominent.[23]

6. Surgical elephantiasis of the arm is seen mainly after mastectomy and resection or following excessive radiation of the axillary lymph nodes. Such chronic stasis of the arm quite often results from venous or perivenous circulatory impairment. The **Stewart-Treves syndrome** with elephantiasic stasis of the arm followed by angiosarcomatous changes is reported in Chapter 37, E2.

7. Supraclavicular cushions, i.e., indolent, doughy, soft tissue protuberances of the jugular or supraclavicular fossa, are especially common in older persons with pulmonary emphysema or substernal goiter. However, if such supraclavicular swellings develop relatively rapidly with elevation of the ESR and fever, one should think of *giant cell arteritis.* Such swellings should not be confused with the hump neck after cortisone treatment. Moreover, unilateral supraclavicular swellings should lead to a search for a possible tumor.[30]

_____

* Asthenia. (Tr.)

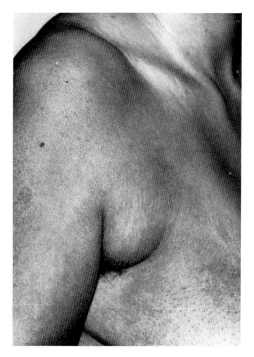

Fig. 64. Fatty pad near the armpit.

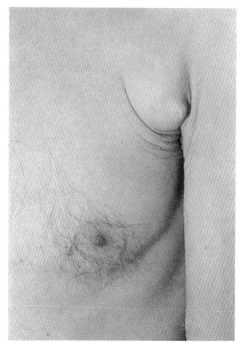

Fig. 65. Accessory breast in the axillary region.

Hibernoma, the rare brown lipoma, is found not only between the scapulae but also in the supraclavicular fossae and in the axillae. Macroscopically, this tumor, covered by normal skin, develops slowly and may reach the size of an apple.[22, 31]

8. Bilateral chronic swellings of the anterior axillary folds (Fig. 64) of soft consistency are not at all rare among obese middle-aged women; they seek medical advice because they are unduly alarmed about having a cancer of the breast. Unilateral **accessory breasts** (Fig. 65) near the axilla can easily be diagnosed by the presence of a nipple.

9. Swellings proximal to the wrists are seen occasionally in climacteric women of pyknic build. In addition, such **cushion-like thickenings** of the extensor side of the forearm are moderately tender with a disposition to dryness of the skin and hypotrichosis. Histologically, one sees displacement of the normal tissue of the upper cutis by fat, especially around the follicles, the sweat glands, and cutaneous muscles.[26]

10. Chronic persistent swellings of one or both dorsal aspects of the hands are the result of paravenous injections of **addictive drugs** such as heroin. In most cases these swellings are firm and cannot be indented by pressure. Other clues to addiction are cutaneous changes such as hyperpigmentations, atrophic or hypertrophic scar formations, and flat ulcerations and abscesses along the veins of the forearms.[32]

11. Genital anal-rectal elephantiasis raises the suspicion of a classic late manifestation of **lymphogranuloma inguinale venereum;** bacterial superinfections today have a greater role in the development of elephantiasis than the original lymphogranuloma infection. The genitoanal region distended by elephantiasis often shows subdivision into lobes and is penetrated by fistulas and ulcerations. An aftereffect of such manifestations is severe stenosis of bodily orifices. In contrast to women, men seldom show urethral stenosis. It is important to remember that malignant tumors can develop on these late manifestations of lymphogranuloma venereum. For verification of the diagnosis, see Chapter 13, A3.

In differential diagnosis of late genital-anal-rectal manifestations, tertiary syphilis should be considered. The possibility of a rectal cancer, common hemorrhoids, or thickenings and fistulization caused by actinomycosis should be considered. Tuberculosis in this region may cause less pronounced swellings. Flat areas of more superficial ulcerations with cobblestone-like granulations covered with purulent

secretions might represent a perianal descending intestinal tuberculosis to be classified as miliary ulcerative tuberculosis of the mucosa and skin.

12. Histologic examination of persistent **edema of vulva and scrotum** shows lymphostasis or lymphectasia as the cause (Figs. 66 and 67). If the history can exclude chronic recurrent erysipelas and if filaria as a cause of elephantiasis of the scrotum is improbable, then in our geographical latitude a careful search for intestinal disorders should be undertaken. Genital elephantiasis not infrequently may be the result of *loss of albumin* due to regional enteritis. Edema of the genitals, usually in conjunction with edema of the lower extremities, has been seen in diseases with primary or secondary *intestinal lymphectasia*. Without exception, the intestinal lymphangiectasia shows lymphocy-

Fig. 66. Lymphangiectatic vulvitis.

Fig. 67. Lymphangiectatic vulvitis: numerous dilated lymph vessels in the corium. HE stain, $63\times$.

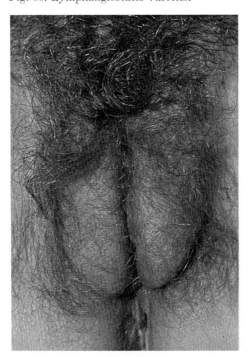

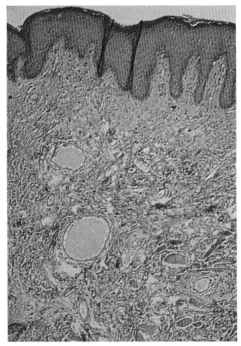

topenia in the peripheral blood smear. Persistent edema of the genitals is observed occasionally in *terminal ileitis*. Chronic swellings of the genitals may be caused by blockage of the lymph vessels or the veins or both together in *retroperitoneal fibrosis*. This disease shows newly formed hard collagenous connective tissue, which constricts not only larger vessels but also the ureters. Such retroperitoneal fibrosis may be observed together with a malignant tumor such as a prostatic cancer or a carcinoid.[3, 10, 12, 15, 17]

13. Chronic edemas of the lower extremities are called elephantiasis simply on inspection; this is a purely descriptive term, unless there is reason to use the more characteristic term lymphedema. A **lymphedema** may be latent for some time until a soft pitting fibrous edema develops, which, however, is still reversible. Finally, an irreversible fibrous sclerosis will result, with a slightly tender, hard, pale swelling; the deformed and thickened lower legs will not return to normal even after prolonged elevation during the night. The surface of the skin is either smooth or, especially on the borders of the lower areas of the legs, shows fine to coarse papillomatous granules. Owing to the mechanics of standing, the soles do not show elephantiasis; neither edema nor verrucous hyperplasia results. However, onychogryphosis often develops. Enlargement of the regional lymph nodes is found only in connection with acute inflammatory conditions (for instance, superimposed attacks of erysipelas) or elephantiasis caused by visceral neoplasias. Uncomplicated lymphedemas do not become especially exacerbated during pregnancy.[8, 11]

Bilateral swellings of the lower extremities require exclusion of **internal causes** such as renal, cardiac, or hepatic diseases. In addition, **static edemas** caused by prolonged standing or sitting, premenstrual edemas due to sodium chloride retention, and the **physiologic edema of pregnancy**

must be considered. This last diagnosis should be made only after a careful search for possible toxemia of pregnancy has been undertaken. **Chronic malnutrition** with resulting albumin deficiency or **exudative enteropathy** is accompanied by a general tendency to edema, especially on the lower extremities. Edema of the legs is observed also after administration of certain drugs such as progesterone, derivatives of guanethidine (ismelin sulfate, Ciba), butazolidin, and corticosteroids.[24]

Unilateral persistent edemas of the lower extremities are not too rarely a late after-effect of a **deep venous thrombosis of the legs.** Inflammatory signs are absent, and the cutaneous temperature is either normal or diminished as compared to that of the unaffected limb. The distal third of the leg very often shows distinct dermatosclerosis, which may form a wide constricting band. Residual deposits of hemosiderin and development of ulcerations may complete the picture of a disease entity best known as post-thrombotic syndrome. Perthes' test and phlebography will determine whether the venae perforantes of the thigh and the deep veins of the lower extremity are patent.

Sometimes, subacute thrombosis of a deep vein of the thigh or leg may be difficult to diagnose. The skin of such a swollen area is not red but there is a certain tenderness of the entire diseased extremity. Characteristic pain is elicited by tapping the sole and by dorsal flexion of the foot, which will cause painful stretching of the calf region. Application of a blood pressure cuff around the thigh, blown up to just above the diastolic blood pressure level, will cause pain in the lower extremity if this disease is present. Unless there is a complicating bacterial infection, fever is absent, although the pulse frequency will be increased independently of the body temperature. The regional lymph nodes will not be affected.

After the fourth decade of life any slowly developing unilateral edema suggests a neoplastic origin (lympho- and reticulosarcomas, cancers of the uterus or prostate, for instance). In such cases it is necessary to perform lymphangiography and phlebography; a biopsy of an inguinal lymph node also may have to be performed.[11]

Erysipelas is of paramount importance in the etiology of the elephantiasis syndrome of the legs. Inconspicuous portals of entry such as mycotic interdigital erosions or ingrown toenails permit the invasion of the organisms. At present, not only do about 80 per cent of all erysipelas cases affect the lower extremities, but they also show a high degree of relapse. Each new additional inflammatory attack with its invasion of streptococci brings about further closures of lymph vessels and an increase in lymphedema. The clinical history allows a diagnosis to be made during an erysipelas-free interval, and additional proof is furnished by an increase in the antistreptolysin titer.[17, 27]

Compared with streptococcic infections other organisms such as *Wuchereria bancrofti* or *Brugia malayi* play no role in the development of elephantiasis in our latitude. In **tropical** or **filarial elephantiasis,** filariae close the lymph ducts and can cause monstrous swellings (Fig. 68). The diagnosis can be established by finding microfilariae in the blood or macrofilariae by puncture of the lymph nodes. **Chromomycosis** (dermatitis verrucosa, "black" blastomycosis) must be considered when verrucous or papillomatous nodular excrescences of the legs with elephantiasic swelling and scar formation are present; these lesions may have a tuberculoid, syphiloid, or psoriasiform aspect. In tropical or subtropical areas this disease may be seen in adults of any age; the causative organism is a fungus belonging to the family Dematiaceae. Clinically, a definite diagnosis cannot be made in an isolated case because one must exclude tuberculosis verrucosa cutis, late syphilis, other mycoses (blastomycosis, sporotrichosis), vege-

tating pyodermias, dermatoses caused by halogens*, and finally, leprosy.

Histologically, there are fairly characteristic findings, with small abscesses in the corium or in the subcutis. These abscesses consist preponderantly of neutrophils; however, they are sometimes tuberculoid structures without central necrosis. Within the abscesses are found numerous giant cells of the Langhans type and fungal spores which are partly extracellular and partly intracellular. These are small, egg-shaped, dark brown, occasionally double-contoured particles (Figs. 69 a and b).

The pathologic-anatomic basis of the various forms of primary lymphedema is a hypoplasia of the subcutaneous lymph vessels. Lymphographic examination of the leg shows only one to two lymphatic ducts per bundle instead of the normal four to five ducts. Another group of primary lymphedemas shows no lymphatic vessels in the subcutis at all except for small separate unconnected cystic spaces. Another malformation consists of dilated and heavily coiled lymphatic vessels, so-called lymphectasia, side by side with normally formed lymphatic ducts. Clinically, several types of primary lymphedema can be differentiated according to their mode of inheritance and time of manifestation. A factor common to all types is the fact that they may be present either unilaterally or bilaterally and that the feet are involved in the formation of the edema.[7]

The **Nonne-Milroy** type is a **hereditary, congenital lymphedema.** The lymphatic stasis often increases during puberty; it affects girls more often than boys. Inheritance is most likely autosomal dominant.[28]

Another kind of hereditary lymphedema is the **Meige type.** In contrast to the Nonne-Milroy type, it starts in late childhood around the time of puberty; the clinical

---

* Such as bromodermas. (Tr.)

course, however, is the same. Sex distribution of females to males is about 1.6 to 1. Concomitant anomalies, also familial, are ptosis of the eyelids and recurrent intrahepatic cholestasis, which becomes evident even before the development of the lymphedema. Patients with the cholestasis syndrome later develop defects and discoloration of the enamel of the teeth. The icteric phase of the disease is accompanied by severe pruritus with diminished excretion of conjungated bilirubin, bile acids, and lipids, with the result that the concentration of these substances in the serum is elevated. 1, 6, 28, 29

Sporadic primary lymphedemas cannot be strictly classified into subgroups like the congenital and noncongenital forms of hereditary primary lymphedema. Because in the vast majority of cases sporadic

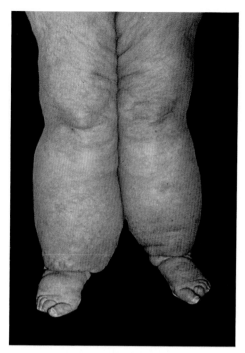

Fig. 68. Tropical elephantiasis.

Fig. 69a. Chromomycosis: cutaneous focus; epidermal hyperplasia, chronic inflammatory infiltrate. Epithelioid cell granulomas with giant cells and central abscess formation. Magnification 65×.

Fig. 69b. Chromomycosis: spores of fungi in an epithelioid cell granuloma. Magnification 400×.

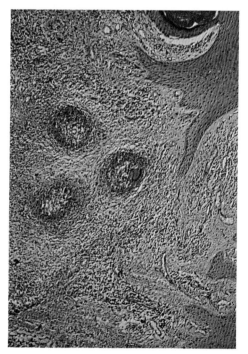

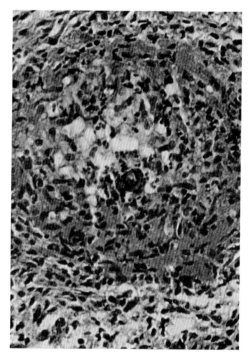

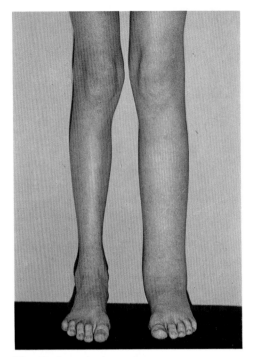

Fig. 70. Lymphedema praecox.

lymphedema occurs before the 35th year of life, it is called **lymphedema praecox** (Fig. 70). Sporadic lymphedema which becomes manifest later is called **lymphedema tarda;** in each case it is necessary to exclude a neoplasm as the cause of the lymph stasis. Lymphedema praecox is the most common form of a primary lymphedema; women are most often affected. The disease begins with a sensation of heaviness in the affected lower extremity, with unilateral, and at first reversible, premenstrual edemas. However, even this early the defects of the lymph vessels mentioned before can be demonstrated in both lower extremities by lymphography. The unilateral start of the disease quickly permits a differentiation from the bilateral edemas resulting from internal causes. Occasionally, lymphedema praecox may start with one attack of erysipelas (locus minoris resistentiae), and this condition may easily be confused with an after-effect of erysipelas. Lymphography will permit

the proper diagnosis. At first the swollen condition is reversible but later hard verrucous hyperplastic swellings of various degrees will appear. The swellings may be restricted to the feet and legs or they may affect the thighs also, and not too infrequently the genital region as well.[7]

14. All primary lymphedemas have an inherent tendency to increase during life, but congenital lymphedemas of the hands and lower extremities in **Turner's syndrome** fail to do so. Such lymphedemas often regress during puberty, and over the age of 17 they are absent as a rule. Practically all patients are of the female phenotype; they have short stature and a webbed neck. The patients are chromatin-negative, and are lacking an X chromosome.[2, 5]

15. In **Klippel-Trénaunay-Weber's syndrome** there is a unilateral hypertrophy of one extremity, starting in childhood with varicosities. The typical diagnostic sign, a nevus flammeus, may be absent in this syndrome, so it is quite possible to confuse the condition with a primary lymphedema (but the latter does not show hypertrophy of connective tissue and bones, and varicosities are absent). Further details will be found in Chapter 18, F4.[21]

16. Progressive lipodystrophy involves irreversible and, after a certain stage of development, stationary enlargement of the circumference of the upper thighs. The increase in volume starts above the knee and reaches its greatest proportions around the buttocks. These disturbances of fat distribution are in pronounced contrast to the emaciated aspect of the upper half of the body, and the thighs may therefore give the impression of elephantiasis.[19]

17. The **cyanotic limb in the shape of a stovepipe** shows a bilateral increase of fatty and connective tissue without lymphostasis. Both lower extremities, beginning at the middle of the legs, resemble stove-pipes. The consistency is hard and does not permit pitting. The color is bluish-red with a changing pattern, while the cutaneous temperature is diminished. In addition, there are similarities between this condition and transitions to perniosis or perniosis follicularis interspersed with vermilion macules. In contrast to most acquired types of swelling of the extremities, uncomplicated cyanotic stove-pipe-shaped limbs in the long run do not develop verrucous hyperplasias.

18. The **anterior tibial syndrome** results from a sudden heavy stress on one leg, which causes an acute unilateral swelling with intense pain. Acute impairment of the circulation of the anterior tibial artery occurs, followed within only a few hours by ischemic necrosis of the musculature of the tibialis compartment. Clinically, a boardlike, extremely painful swelling of the pretibial muscles is observed, with erysipelas-like redness of the overlying skin. The pulse of the dorsal foot artery on the same side is diminished or completely absent. Frequently, subfebrile temperatures and leukocytosis accompany this syndrome, leading to a mistaken diagnosis of erysipelas. The correct diagnosis depends on the extreme pain and the lack of circulation. In the late stage, neuromuscular contractures of the joints of the foot occur. The same signs, but in another location, are found in the acute **ischemic necrosis of the peroneal musculature.**[13, 20, 25]

(1) AAGENAES, O., H. SIGSTAD and R. BJÖRN-HANSEN: Lymphoedema in hereditary recurrent cholestasis from birth. Arch. Dis. Child. 45: 690–695 (1970).

(2) ALVIN, A., J. DIEHL, J. LINDSTEN and A. LODIN: Lymph vessel hypoplasia and chromosome aberrations in six patients with Turner's syndrome. Acta derm.-venereol. (Stockh.) 47: 25–33 (1967).

(3) ANDING, G., C. W. FASSBENDER und J. SÖKELAND: Die retroperitoneale Fibrose. Fortschr. Med. 89: 509–511 (1971).

(4) BECKER, W., und H. THEISEN: Otophym beim Klippel-Trénaunay-Syndrom. Z. Laryng.-Rhinol.-Otol. 41: 487–494 (1962).

(5) BENSON, P. F., M. H. GOUGH and P. E. POLANI: Lymphangiography and chromosome studies in females with lymphoedema and possible ovarian dysgenesis. Arch. Dis. Child. 40: 27–32 (1965).

(6) BLOOM, D.: Hereditary lymphedema (Nonne-Milroy-Meige); report of family with hereditary lymphedema associated with ptosis of eyelid in several generations. N. Y. St. J. Med. 41: 856–863 (1941).

(7) BRUNNER, U.: Das Lymphödem der unteren Extremitäten. Huber, Bern, Stuttgart, Wien 1969.

(8) BUMM, E.: Formenkreis der Extremitäten-Elephantiasis. Dtsch. Gesundh.-Wes. 6: 1149–1153 (1951).

(9) DECHAUME, M., M. GRELLET, J. PAYEN, M. BONNEAU, F. GUILBERT et S. BOCCARA: Le chérubisme. Presse méd. 70: 2763–2766 (1962).

(10) EISSNER, H.: Lymphoedema chronicum penis et scroti bei Enteritis regionalis. Arch. klin. exp. Derm. 210: 558–574 (1960).

(11) FISCHER, H., und W. SCHNEIDER: Die Endstrombahn in der Pathogenese der Elephantiasis. Derm. Wschr. 151: 657–668 (1965).

(12) GAISSMAIER, U., und G. BÜRKLE: Über eine besondere Form der intestinalen Lymphangiektasie. Med.Welt 19 (N.F.): 2292–2298 (1968).

(13) GRUNWALD, A., and Z. SILBERMAN: Anterior tibial syndrome. J. Amer. med. Ass. 171: 2210–2213 (1959).

(14) HARTMANN, W.: Die idiopathische Kaumuskelhypertrophie. Arch. Kinderheilk. 160: 230–235 (1959).

(15) HUNDEIKER, M., und J. PETERS: Zur nosologischen Problematik der Elephantiasis penis et scroti und der retroperitonealen Fibrose. Derm. Wschr. 153: 699–705 (1967).

(16) KERN, A. B.: Masseter muscle hypertrophy. Arch. Derm. Syph. (Chic.) 69: 558–562 (1954).

(17) KONOPIK, J.: Rezidivierendes Erysipel. Med. Klinik *62:* 1162–1164 (1967).

(18) KORTING, G. W., und G. SUNDHAUSSEN: Kaumuskelhypertrophien. Med. Welt *22* (N. F.): 2015–2016 (1971).

(19) LANGHOF, H., und R. ZABEL: Zur Lipodystrophia progressiva. Arch. klin. exp. Derm. *210:* 313–321 (1960).

(20) MEIERS, H. G.: Das Tibialis-anterior-Syndrom und seine Verkennung als entzündliche Unterschenkeldermatose. Dtsch. med. Wschr. *96:* 1357–1359 (1971).

(21) MÜLLER, J. H., K. H. SCHMIDT, M. LÜNING und K. BÜRGER: Doppelseitige Veränderungen beim Klippel-Trénaunay-Weber-Syndrom mit Fehlbildungen im arteriellen, venösen und lymphatischen Gefäßsystem. Radiol. Diagn. *10:* 341–348 (1969).

(22) NOVY, F. G., and J. W. WILSON: Hibernomas, brown fat tumors. Arch. Derm. (Chic.) *73:* 149–157 (1956).

(23) PAPAGEORGIOU, A.: Schlüsselbein-Achselvenensperre (Paget- v. Schroetter-Syndrom). Med. Klin. *55:* 1312–1315 (1960).

(24) v. RECHENBERG, H. K.: Phenylbutazolidin. Unter besonderer Berücksichtigung der Nebenwirkungen. Thieme, Stuttgart 1957.

(25) RESZEL, P. A., J. M. JANES and J. A. SPITTELL: Ischemic necrosis of the peroneal musculature, a lateral compartment syndrome: report of case. Proc. Mayo Clin. *38:* 130–136 (1963).

(26) SCHIMPF, A.: Über polsterartige Verdickungen proximal der Handgelenke. Endokrinologie *32:* 57–66 (1954).

(27) SCHNEIDER, I.: Klinik und Pathogenese des rezidivierenden Erysipels. Hautarzt *24:* 145–149 (1973).

(28) SCHROEDER, E., and H. F. HELWEG-LARSEN: Chronic hereditary lymphedema (Nonne-Milroy-Meige's disease). Acta med. scand. *137:* 198–216 (1950).

(29) SIGSTAD, H., Ø. AAGENAES, R. W. BJÖRN-HANSEN and K. ROOTWELT: Primary lymphoedema combined with hereditary recurrent intrahepatic cholestasis. Acta med. scand. *188:* 213–219 (1970).

(30) WAGNER, A., und U. BRAUN: »Supraclavicularpolster« als Symptom der Riesenzellenarteriitis (Arteriitis temporalis). Schweiz. med. Wschr. *98:* 1720–1722 (1968).

(31) WEGENER, F.: Braunes Lipom und braunes Fettgewebe des Menschen. Beitr. path. Anat. *111:* 252–266 (1951).

(32) WEIDMANN, A. I., and M. J. FELLNER: Cutaneous manifestations of heroin and other addictive drugs. N. Y. St. J. Med. *71:* 2643–2646 (1971).

11. Abnormalities of the Hair

Hypo- and hypertrichoses are discussed in this chapter insofar as they are occasioned by a definite constitution, by changes in the distribution, color, or numbers of the hairs, or by other causes. A description of the pathologic changes in the hairs themselves is not intended.

A. Congenital and Generalized Hypotrichoses

1. Complete lack of all hair (atrichia) may be present at birth and may persist. But even in cases of such **congenital, generalized atrichia** there are areas, especially at the sites of the usual hypertrichosis, such as brows and eyelashes, where a few lanugo hairs still exist. Only those cases of congenital, hereditary, ectodermal dysplasia such as anomalies of the teeth and nails, and disorders in the function of the sweat glands or in keratinization belong to this group of diseases. Occasionally, complete alopecia is preceded by the appearance of normal hair on the scalp. But after the loss of the first hairs no further hair growth ensues. Moreover, these patients develop disseminated papular lesions on the face, the scalp, or other parts of the body. These lesions represent, histologically, follicular horny cysts or hamartias of follicles or sweat and sebaceous glands. This leads to the possibility that this familial picture of *hypotrichia with horny cysts* (Fig.71) represents an incomplete variety of hydrotic, ectodermal dysplasia. Macroscopically, these papular lesions should be distinguished from those of any familial and generalized formation of milia as well as from larger, rather hemispheric syringomas. In such cases of familial miliosis or syringomas hypoplasias of hair and nails are absent.[3, 14, 20, 22]

2. Another "pure" congenital hypotrichia, i.e., lack of hair without associated signs, has been observed in a North German family through seven generations. Clinically characteristic of this **congenital, hereditary, generalized hypotrichosis of the Marie Unna type** are a high degree of congenital lack of hair, delayed growth of bristlelike scalp hair, and alopecia that begins early and leads to complete baldness. In this sibship the hairs were extremely flat and twisted around the long axis. Anomalies of the nails and teeth were not present. Histologically, proliferations of the follicular epithelium occurred at first and at later stages follicular atrophy, foreign body granulomas, and hypertrophy of the sebaceous glands were found.[21, 32]

Besides this type of hypotrichia which followed regular dominant inheritance

Fig. 71. Hidrotic ectodermal dysplasia: hypotrichosis with horny cysts.

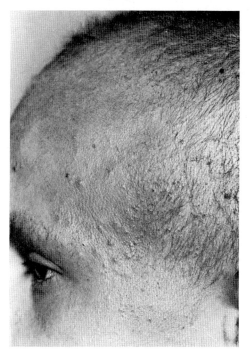

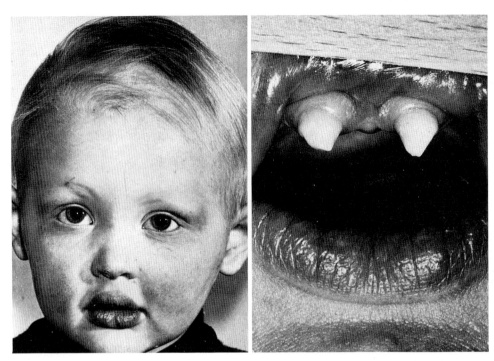

Fig. 72. Anhidrotic ectodermal dysplasia: (a) missing eyebrows and lashes, suggestive saddle nose; (b) peg-shaped teeth.

additional families have been described with congenital hypotrichia but without associated signs and with varying signs in the different families. A few instances of congenital hypotrichia with recessive inheritance have been observed, however.

3. The most important sign of **anhidrotic ectodermal dysplasia** (anhidrosis hypotrichotica), next to hypohidrosis and hypodontia, is hypotrichosis (Fig. 72 a, b). The skin of such patients is extremely thin. In the face, which gives the impression of being "old" or "tired" and simulates congenital syphilis with regard to an olympic forehead, saddle nose, and thick lips, a central paleness is noticeable. Since owing to hypohidrosis, dry skin with a tendency to eczematization soon develops, it is understandable that this biotype of ectodermal dysplasia must be differentiated from endogenous eczema. Occasionally observed in anhidrotic dysplasia are papular elevations caused by rudimentary follicular funnels with solid epithelium and hyperkeratosis. In generalized hypotrichia the lack of hair on the scalp and eyebrows as well as other terminal hair in the axillas and pubic area should be stressed. Lanugo hair seems to be undisturbed in most places. Nonessential signs of anhidrotic hypotrichia are various ocular signs (such as mongoloid lid axis, nystagmus, coloboma, corneal maculae, and cataract) as well as neurolabyrinthine disturbances, ozena, and hypomastias and dysmastias. In many such patients there are, moreover, thin, brittle, and often channelled nails. However, explicit malformations of nails such as are observed in hidrotic ectodermal dysplasia are not present. In the differential diagnosis one should consider, as said before, congenital syphilis and an endogenous eczema. In these two conditions, however, definite disturbances of sweat secretion prevail.[7]

4. A special hereditary type of **anhidrotic ectodermal dysplasia** includes, besides the main signs of hypotrichia, hypodontia, and hypohidrosis, follicular and **palmoplantar keratoses** and centrofacial lentiginosis (Fig. 730).[11]

When **generalized follicular hyperkeratoses** are combined with **universal alopecia** and **deafness,** anhidrosis, which exists simultaneously, points to a relationship with anhidrotic ectodermal dysplasia, although dental changes are not present.[26]

In the **Berlin syndrome,** which has been previously discussed in connection with small macular pigmentations, generalized hair anomalies are also present. Hair of the scalp remains sparse and becomes prematurely gray. A beard, axillary hair, and pubic hair are missing. Lanugo hair is either sparse or absent.[1]

5. In the minor type of ectodermal dysplasia, **hidrotic ectodermal dysplasia,** abnormalities of the sweat glands are lacking, so only hypoplasia of hair and nails is present. Microscopic examination of the hairs does not disclose any changes, but macroscopically they appear thin, short, dry, and brittle. Lanugo, axillary, and pubic hair are sparse or are completely absent. The lateral two-thirds of the eyebrows are sparse and the cilia are poorly developed.

The rarefaction of the lateral eyebrows must be differentiated from **Hertoghe's sign** (Fig. 74) in endogenous eczema, from the loss of the corresponding supercilia in myxedema, and from florid secondary syphilis, intoxication by thallium, Sheehan's syndrome, and trichotillomania.

The nails of the fingers and toes are painfully thickened and streaked, and are often convex on their surface. They are often associated with dental anomalies

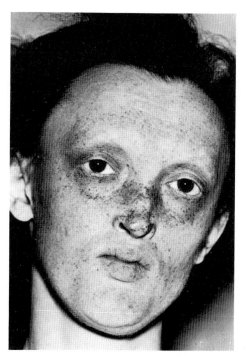

Fig. 73. Anhidrotic ectodermal dysplasia with lentiginosis centrofacialis.

Fig. 74. Hertoghe's sign (rarefaction of the lateral eyebrows) in endogenous eczema.

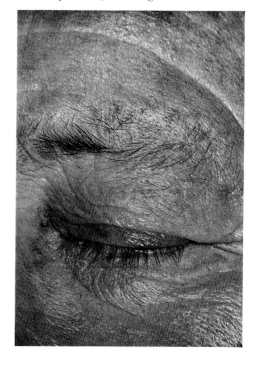

and palmoplantar keratoses, but facial deformities do not occur.

6. The **H. Fischer syndrome** comprises palmoplantar keratoses with hyperhidrosis and onychogryphosis as well as clublike thickening of the distal phalanges of toes and especially fingers. Its association with sparse hair growth but normal sweat secretion permits the classification of this biotype among the hidrotic ectodermal dysplasias.[5]

7. In other special forms of the hypotrichia-hypodontia syndrome dental anomalies are most important. In **Capdepont's disease** small, yellowish caramel-colored teeth with congenital enamel hypoplasia, especially of the chewing surfaces, and palmoplantar keratoses are the cardinal signs. The **Ellis-van Creveld** syndrome, or chondroectodermal dysplasia, shows dental anomalies (hypodontia, conical hypoplastic incisors). More important, however, is the shortening of the extremities (caused by premature epiphyseal closure) combined with the normal size of the trunk. Other signs are congenital cardiac defects and polydactylia; further skeletal malformations complete the features of this syndrome. The nails are thin, short, and brittle, and the hairs are sparse and thin.[10]

8. In the peripheral dysostosis of the **trichorhinophalangeal syndrome,** diffuse hypotrichia (terminal and lanugo hair) is regularly present. All of the hair is sparse, and the individual hairs are thin and easily broken off. Since the hair of the scalp grows only a few centimeters, the patients state that for years they do not need a haircut. Pronounced nail changes are lacking, but occasionally koilonychia is present. In a few cases there are supernumerary teeth. The function of the sweat glands is not impaired. Conspicuous is the broad nose, thickened at the tip – a so-called pear nose. The philtrum is abnormally high and the nasal cartilages

are unusually limp. Some patients are small in every way, but only brachyphalangia, caused by premature epiphyseal closure, is a constant finding. In addition, the fingers are thickened in the area of the middle phalangeal joints and bent to the side. In the radiograph typical phalangeal peg-shaped epiphyses are visualized, which, however, are not pathognomonic.[9, 15]

9. Alopecia areatalike loss of hair, as well as diffuse hypotrichias, constitutes the cardinal sign of the **dyscephaly syndrome of François** (oculomandibulofacial syndrome), which is identical with the Hallermann-Streiff syndrome and the Ullrich-Fremerey-Dohna syndrome. The loss of hair is present on the scalp, eyelashes, eyebrows, beard, and in the axillary and pubic regions. In these hairless areas the skin is often taut, atrophic, dry, and traversed by telangiectases. Other important findings in this congenital malformation syndrome are proportionate dwarfism, bilateral microphthalmia with congenital cataract, dental anomalies, a curved nose, hypoplasia of the mandible, and brachycephaly or scaphocephaly. In the differential diagnosis, Werner's syndrome and progeria might be considered. In Werner's syndrome, however, the cataract is not congenital and no microphthalmia is present. The taut atrophic skin changes are not limited to the hairy body areas, but are located on the extremities also, as in progressive scleroderma. Other distinguishing features are ulcerations of the legs and plantar hyperkeratoses. In progeria the typical ocular changes are absent. In this disorder premature senility affects the entire skin, including the subcutaneous fat tissue. In addition, premature, pronounced arteriosclerosis with all its deleterious sequelae occurs.[6, 28]

10. Familial, congenital hypoplasias of the hair together with cerebral convulsions and oligophrenia characterize **Moynahan's syndrome**.[27]

11. In **pachyonychia congenita**, hypotrichosis caused by follicular hyperkeratoses of the scalp is not of prime importance. The cardinal sign is the congenital pachyonychia of all fingers and toes. For a long time it may present the only manifestation of the disorder. Later, extensive leukoplakias and acneiform follicular keratoses on elbows, knees, and buttocks are additional signs.

12. Men, almost exclusively, develop **dyskeratosis congenita**. The manifestations start around the fifth to the tenth year of life. The first signs are dystrophy or loss of nails accompanying chronic paronychia. At the same time, or only a short time later, the mucous membranes show a transformation of small blisters and erosions to leukoplakias. Within a few years the skin of the face, neck, and chest becomes poikilodermic with pronounced reticular, brown pigmentations. In addition, the skin of the extremities becomes definitely atrophic. The hairs are brittle and sometimes sparse, and tend to become prematurely gray. Occasionally, cicatricial alopecia develops.

13. The **Rothmund-Thomson syndrome**, another congenital poikiloderma, differs from dyskeratosis congenita in that its onset occurs in childhood, a preponderance of the female sex is affected, and there is an absence of leukoplakias and absent or only minor nail changes. From the third month of life on, edematous erythemas leave irregularly formed hyperpigmentations and depigmentations and telangiectases of the skin, which finally becomes atrophic. Patients often suffer from distinct hypersensitivity to light. Between the third and sixth years of life, 40 per cent of patients develop cataracts of both eyes. Hair of the scalp is usually sparse and in a few cases

it is completely absent. The same can be said about the eyebrows, axillary hair, and pubic hair.

14. Progeria of the Hutchinson-Gilford type and Werner's syndrome are characterized by premature senescence and hereditary atrophic features. **Hutchinson-Gilford progeria** is characterized by dwarfism, acromicria, and pronounced senile-looking atrophy and hypoplasia of the skin and subcutaneous layers (Fig. 75). The first cutaneous changes are in general observed between the end of the first and the third year of life. The impression of premature senility is increased by the

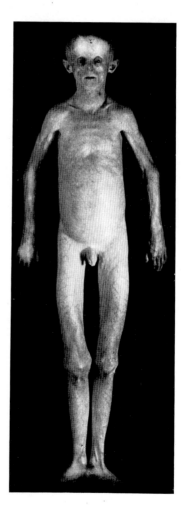

Fig. 75. Progeria (Hutchinson-Gilford type).

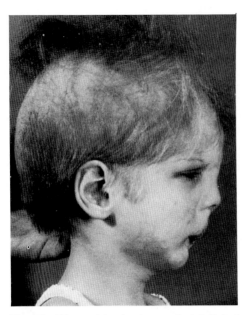

Fig. 76. Hypotrichosis in orofacial-digital syndrome.

deficient development of eyelashes and eyebrows and, last but not least, of the scalp hair. Moreover, the premature loss of hair in the beginning changes into a full picture of a taut atrophic alopecia. Lanugo hair, however, develops without limitation. Radiologically, a short base of the skull and integral coxa valga of both sides are found. The life expectancy of these children is greatly diminished by arteriosclerosis, which begins around the tenth year of life and progresses rapidly.[4, 18, 36]

15. In ulcerative scleratrophy **(Werner's syndrome),** taut atrophy and consequently, a sclerodermic bird-face are characteristic. Peripheral vascular changes, which lead to torpid and trophic ulcerations and juvenile cataracts, are prevalent at an early age. Hyperkeratosis of elbows and soles develops at the same time. The premature senility is underlined by premature graying or even total alopecia. Premature graying usually coincides with the formation of cataracts. Eyebrows,

eyelashes, and beard, and also axillary and pubic hairs are sparse.[16, 17, 36]

16. The syndrome first described as "dysplasia linguofacialis" is today generally called **orofacial-digital syndrome** (Figs. 76 and 77 a, b). It is characterized by atypically placed, hyperplastic, multiple frenula of the oral cavity. In addition, dental aplasias, lobes and fissures of the tongue, fibromas of the tongue, and medial upper lip–palate fissures occur. The impression of a beaked pug nose is caused by the hypoplasia of the cartilage at the tip of the nose and the deep location of the columella of the nose. The extremities show polydactylia, syndactylia, and brachydactylia. On the skin of the face numerous yellowish, epidermal cysts are present. The scalp hair is thin and brittle and several circumscribed areas of alopecia occur. The defective hair growth is caused by numerically diminished hair follicles on the one hand, and by premature breaking of the thin hairs on the other. The number of sebaceous glands is likewise often reduced, and as early as childhood keratinous cysts of the face, scalp, and dorsa of the hands occur. Genetically, the disorder seems to show an X-chromosomal dominant inheritance and a lethal effect in hemizygotes.[8, 29, 30, 33]

17. The designation "chondrodystrophy" includes at present several distinct dysostoses. A special form is **cartilage-hair hypoplasia.** In some cases the disorder, which later leads to distinct dwarfism with a long trunk, bell-shaped thorax, and short extremities, is recognizable even at birth. Moreover, such patients have, in addition, flabbiness of the connective tissue which leads among other signs to hypotonia of the ligaments, and thin, faintly pigmented, brittle, and altogether poorly developed hair on the scalp, brows, lashes, and the rest of the body. The nails may also be short and brittle. It is this hypotrichia

Fig. 77. Orofacial-digital syndrome: (a) multiple frenula of the oral cavity and fissures of the tongue; (b) malformations of the toes.

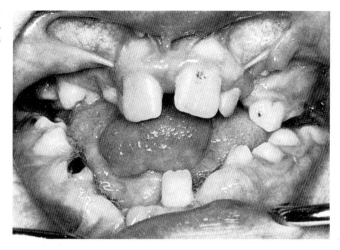

Fig. 77a.

especially that differentiates this disease from other forms of chondrodystrophy.[23, 24]

18. In the **monilethrix syndrome** the scalp hairs are extremely fragile and, therefore, are usually not longer than 1 cm. in length. The individual hair is beaded and thickened. The thicker parts of each hair are formed in a 24- or 48-hour rhythm. Pigment is present only on the thickened parts, and the thin parts remain unpigmented. In addition to the hair of the scalp the eyebrows, eyelashes, axillary hair, and pubic hair can be affected in the same manner. In most cases the hair is normal at birth but is replaced by new beaded hair from the second month of life. In a high percentage of cases koilonychia or keratosis follicularis coexist. The latter is localized especially frequently on the extensor surfaces of the upper arms, but also on the trunk, face, and neck. Accompanying defects in intelligence, as well as dental and ocular anomalies, are rarer. Transitory improvement may occur during pregnancy. Occasionally adults may grow normal hairs again.

In the differential diagnosis pili torti and trichorrhexis nodosa can easily be excluded by microscopic examination. In *argininosuccinuria*, which is associated with congenital imbecility, hairs typical of

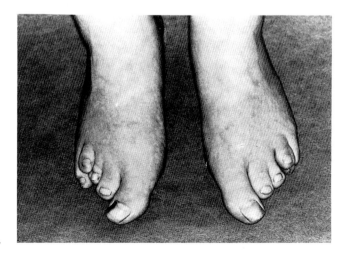

Fig. 77b.

monilethrix occasionally occur. After staining with acridine orange a saturated
green instead of the normal red fluorescence ensues. Due to a diminished or
absent capacity of the enzyme arginino-
succinase, increased argininosuccinic acid is
excreted in the urine. In the hairs argininosuccinic acid can take over the role of
an antimetabolite, since it replaces the
nonexistent arginine in the keratin of the
hair. In the monilethrix syndrome some
mild disturbance of the arginine metabolism
is not infrequent, but it cannot be regularly
proved.[13, 19, 31]

19. Strangely kinky and light hairs,
which simultaneously show microscopically
the picture of pili torti or monilethrix, are
characteristic of the "**kinky hair disease.**"
In this recessively inherited sex-linked
neurocutaneous syndrome, growth is retarded at an early age and in the third to
fourth month of life progressive cerebral
degeneration leads to death.* In the
plasma constantly increased values of
glutamic acid are present.[25]

20. A characteristic sign of **myotonia
atrophicans** is the premature pate, which
may extend to loss of the entire scalp hair.
Other manifestations are a myotonic
cataract and endocrine defects such as
testicular atrophy. The disorder is accompanied by creatinuria. Another dermatologic manifestation of this type of
myotonic dystrophy is acrocyanosis.

21. In children with **hereditary bullous
dystrophy of the macular type** the primarily
sparse scalp hair is lost completely in the
first year of life. About the same time
spontaneous epidermal blisters appear for
the first time. These are followed by
attacks of macular hyperpigmentation and

_____

* In "acquired" progressive kinking of the
hair children or adolescents develop the hair
changes without serious general signs. (Tr.)

depigmentations on the extremities and
the face. Proportionate dwarfism permits
the recognition of a certain microcephaly
with distinct mental retardation. The few
patients known to have suffered from this
X-chromosomal recessive genodermatosis
died before the twenty-fifth year of life.
Important for the differential diagnosis
are (1) epidermolysis bullosa hereditaria,
which, however, lacks the formation of
intraepidermal blisters, pronounced pigmentary changes, and dwarfism, and (2)
incontinentia pigmenti.[35]

22. Another form of alopecia is congenitally present, but becomes manifest
as late as childhood. These **hair follicle
hamartomas** present as universal and
partly cicatricial loss of hair. They begin
with diffuse involvement which becomes
total. This depends on the degree of
development of the individual hamartomas. The tumors can hardly be detected
by the naked eye, so a final diagnosis can
be made only by biopsy. On each root of
the hair benign tumor formations (trichoepitheliomas or trichilemmal cysts) are
present; these probably originate in the
outer sheath of the root. The tumorous
growth, however, always remains benign.
Destructive or infiltrating features do not
occur.[2, 24]

(1) BERLIN, C.: Congenital generalized
melanoleucoderma associated with
hypodontia, hypotrichosis, stunted
growth and mental retardation occurring in two brothers and two sisters.
Dermatologica (Basel) *123:* 227–243
(1961).
(2) BROWN, A. C., R. C. CROUNSE and
R. K. WINKELMANN: Generalized hair-
follicle hamartoma; associated with
alopecia, aminoaciduria and myasthenia
gravis. Arch. Derm. (Chic.) *99:* 478–493
(1969).
(3) DAMSTÉ, TH. J., and J. R. PRAKKEN:
Atrichia with papular lesions: a variant
of congenital ectodermal dysplasia.
Dermatologica (Basel) *108:* 114–121
(1954).

(4) DE BUSK, F. L.: The Hutchinson-Gilford progeria syndrome. Report of 4 cases and review of the literature. J. Pediatr. *80:* 697–724 (1972).

(5) FISCHER, H.: Familiär hereditäres Vorkommen von Keratoma palmare et plantare, Nagelveränderungen, Haaranomalien und Verdickung der Endglieder der Finger und Zehen in 5 Generationen. (Die Beziehungen dieser Veränderungen zur inneren Sekretion.) Derm. Z. (Berl.) *32:* 114–142 (1921).

(6) FRANÇOIS, J.: A new syndrome; dyscephalia with bird face and dental anomalies, nanism, hypotrichosis, cutaneous atrophy, microphthalmia, and congenital cataract. Arch. Ophthal. (Chic.) *60:* 842–862 (1958).

(7) FRIEDERICH, H. C.: Zur Kenntnis der kongenitalen Hypotrichosis (Familiäre Hypotrichosis mit und ohne Nageldystrophie, Anidrosis hypotrichotica, Progerie). Derm. Wschr. *121:* 409–417 (1950).

(8) FUHRMANN, W., und A. STAHL: Zur Differentialdiagnose von Papillon-Léage-Psaume-Syndrom und Mohr-Syndrom. Humangenetik *9:* 54–63 (1970).

(9) GIEDION, A.: Das tricho-rhino-phalangeale Syndrom. Helvet. paediat. Acta *21:* 475–482 (1966).

(10) GOOR, D., Y. ROTEM, A. FRIEDMAN and H. N. NEUFELD: Ellis-van Creveld syndrome in identical twins. Brit. Heart J. *27:* 797–804 (1965).

(11) GREITHER, A.: Über drei Generationen vererbte, auf Frauen beschränkte Keratosis follicularis mit Alopecie, Hypidrose und abortiven Palmar-Plantar-Keratosen in ihren Beziehungen zur Hypotrichosis congenita hereditaria. Arch. klin. exp. Derm. *210:* 123–140 (1960).

(12) GROSFELD, J. C., J. A. MIGHORST and T. M. MOOLHUYSEN: Argininosuccinic aciduria in monilethrix. Lancet *1964/II:* 789–791.

(13) HEYDT, G. E.: Zur Kenntnis des Monilethrix-Syndroms. Arch. klin. exp. Derm. *217:* 15–29 (1963).

(14) HUTCHINSON, J.: Congenital absence of hair and mammary glands with atrophic condition of the skin and its appendages. Med.-Chir. Transact. (London) *69:* 473–477 (1886).

(15) KLINGMÜLLER, G.: Über eigentümliche Konstitutionsanomalien bei 2 Schwestern und ihre Beziehungen zu neueren entwicklungspathologischen Befunden. Hautarzt *7:* 105–113 (1956).

(16) KNOTH, W., R. BAETHKE und L. HOFFMANN: Über das Werner-Syndrom. Hautarzt *14:* 145–152, 193–202 (1963).

(17) KORTING, G. W., und H. HOLZMANN: Die Sklerodermie und ihr nahestehende Bindegewebsprobleme. Thieme, Stuttgart 1967.

(18) LACHMANN, D., und E. ZWEYMÜLLER: Vorzeitiges körperliches Altern bei Kindern. Wien. klin. Wschr. *81:* 499 bis 500 (1969).

(19) LEVIN, B., H. M. MACKAY and V. G. OBERHOLZER: Argininosuccinic aciduria, an inborn error of amino acid metabolism. Arch. Dis. Child. *36:* 622–632 (1961).

(20) LOEWENTHAL, L. J. A., and J. R. PRAKKEN: Atrichia with papular lesions. Dermatologica (Basel) *122:* 85–89 (1961).

(21) LUDWIG, E.: Hypotrichosis congenita hereditaria Typ M. Unna. Arch. Derm. Syph. (Berl.) *196:* 261–278 (1953).

(22) LUNDBÄCK, H.: Total congenital hereditary alopecia. Acta derm.-venereol. (Stockh.) *25:* 189–206 (1945).

(23) McKUSICK, V. A.: Dysostose métaphysaire et modifications des cheveux. Presse méd. *72:* 907–908 (1964).

(24) MEHREGAN, A. H., and I. HARDIN: Generalized follicular hamartoma complicated by multiple proliferating trichilemmal cysts and palmar pits. Arch. Derm. (Chic.) *107:* 435–438 (1973).

(25) MENKES, J. H., M. ALTER, G. K. STEIGLEDER, D. R. WEAKLEY and J. H. SUNG: A sex-linked recessive disorder with retardation of growth, peculiar hair, and focal cerebral and cerebellar degeneration. Pediatrics *29:* 764–779 (1962).

(26) MORRIS, J., A. B. ACKERMAN and P. J. KOBLENZER: Generalized spiny hyperkeratosis, universal alopecia, and deafness. Arch. Derm. (Chic.) *100:* 692–698 (1969).

(27) MOYNAHAN, E. J.: Familial congenital alopecia, epilepsy, mental retardation with unusual electroencephalograms. Proc. roy. Soc. Med. *55:* 411–412 (1962).

(28) PIERARD, J., et J. FRANÇOIS: Le syndrome dyscéphalique de François. Ses

rapports avec le tissu élastique. Arch. belges Derm. *25:* 439–454 (1969).

(29) REINWEIN, H., W. SCHILLI, H. RITTER, H. BREHME und U. WOLF: Untersuchungen an einer Familie mit Oral-Facial-Digital-Syndrom. Humangenetik *2:* 165–177 (1966).

(30) RIMOIN, D. L., and M. T. EDGERTON: Genetic and clinical heterogeneity in the oral-facial-digital syndromes. J. Pediat. (St. Louis) *71:* 94–102 (1967).

(31) SHELLEY, W. B., and H. M. RAWNSLEY: Aminogenic alopecia. Loss of hair associated with argininosuccinic aciduria. Lancet *1965/II:* 1327–1328.

(32) SOLOMON, L. M., N. B. ESTERLY and M. MEDENICA: Hereditary trichodysplasia: Marie Unna's hypotrichosis. J. invest. Dermat. *57:* 389–400 (1971).

(33) STAHL, A., und W. FUHRMANN: Orofacio-digitales Syndrom. Dtsch. med. Wschr. *93:* 1224–1228 (1968).

(34) WIEDEMANN, H. R., J. SPRANGER und W. KOSENOW: Knorpel-Haar-Hypoplasie. Arch. Kinderheilk. *176:* 74–85 (1967).

(35) WOERDEMANN, M. J.: Dystrophia bullosa hereditaria, typus maculatus. Proc. 11. internat. Congr. Dermat. 1957 Bd. III. Acta derm.-venereol. (Stockh.) 678–686 (1967).

(36) ZAUN, H.: Untersuchungen zum Pathomechanismus der Alopecien bei kongenitalen Hautatrophien. Hautarzt *15:* 439–441 (1964).

B. Congenital Circumscribed Hypotrichias

Hairless areas are to be considered circumscribed hypotrichoses in the narrow sense of the word only, if they are not preceded by pathologic conditions or development (such as scars, organic nevi, and others).

1. A special, congenital, circumscribed hypotrichia, the extremely rare **circumscribed congenital alopecia** of the scalp falls under this concept. Typical locations of the affected areas, which are frequently symmetrical, are the frontal hairline, the temporal areas, and along the frontoparietal suture. Atrophic or cicatricial changes of the skin are lacking.[3]

2. Congenital axillary alopecia can occur as a circumscribed familial stigma or can represent part of Unna's congenital hypotrichosis. Compared to such congenital circumscribed hypotrichias or alopecias, alopecia areata is as a rule characterized by reparable and restorable processes, which are absent in congenital hypotrichia.[6, 9]

Unilateral circumscribed absence of axillary hair is also observed in the **Poland syndrome.** Characteristic features are the unilateral syndactylia and brachydactylia as well as a (partial) aplasia of the pectoralis major muscle. Moreover, on the same side hypoplasia or aplasia of the breast may be present.[2, 8]

3. Missing axillary hair is also observed as a main sign in **testicular feminization** ("hairless woman" syndrome). These are completely feminine patients with normal female breast development and female external genitalia. The uterus, however, is always missing, and the vagina ends blindly. The chromosomal and gonadal sex is male XY, with a normal number of chromosomes. In contrast to other gonadal dysgeneses the body growth and the intelligence are not diminished. Pubic hair is not missing as often as the axillary hair. The rest of the body hair corresponds to the female phenotype. The testes very often lie in the inguinal canal or the great labia and simulate inguinal hernias. The high percentage of developing tubular adenomas in these testes is striking.

The diagnosis of testicular feminization is in general not made before puberty, when primary amenorrhea and the lack of sexual hair bring the patient to the physician. Familial cases are frequent since the malformation is transmitted by normal women and always concerns individuals who are males with regard to their chromosomes and gonads. Inheritance is either X-chromosomal recessive or autosomal dominant and is limited to the male sex.[7, 11]

4. Congenital aplasia of the cutis is based on quantitative underdevelopment of cutis and subcutis. Probably it is more a question of a genuine aplasia than of the result of intrauterine pressure necrosis or amniotic adhesions. At birth a round or oval, sharply circumscribed and open area is seen, which after epithelization lies below the level of the surrounding skin. Later, there are scarred and hairless areas, which are usually located near the small fontanelle or paramedianly over the occiput (Fig. 78). Histologically, the typical case of congenital aplasia cutis is characterized by agenesis of the papillary body with hypoplasia or dysplasia of sweat and sebaceous glands and hairs.

5. Circumscribed hypotrichias can be simulated by **pili torti.** This malformation of the hair is preponderantly observed in girls up to the age of puberty and consists of a peculiar twist of the hair around the long axis. There are instances of involvement of the entire scalp, but most fre- quently only the occipital and temporal areas are affected. The hairs, which are thin, dry, and brittle, usually do not reach a length of more than 4 to 6 cm, thus giving the impression of a circumscribed hypotrichia. The peculiar glowing sheen of these twisted hairs is striking. After puberty the malformation of the hair may regress, leaving only a few circumscribed areas, or it may disappear completely. With only a few exceptions persons with pili torti are healthy. There are, however, some reports of the simultaneous occurrence of ectodermal dysplasia or hereditary deafness (see Chapter 9, 2). The diagnosis can be quickly ascertained by microscopic examination of the malformed hairs, which show twists of 90° or 180° around the long axis at distances of between 2 and 10 mm. [1, 4, 5, 10, 12]

(1) BEARE, J. M.: Congenital pilar defect showing features of pili torti. Brit. J. Derm. *64:* 366–372 (1952).

(2) CLARKSON, P.: Poland's syndactyly. Guy's Hosp. Rep. *111:* 335–346 (1962).

(3) FRIEDERICH, H. C.: Zur Kenntnis des angeborenen umschriebenen Haarausfalls. Derm. Wschr. *120:* 712–716 (1949).

(4) FRIEDERICH, H. C., und R. SEITZ: Über eine Form der ektodermalen Dysplasie unter dem Bilde der Pili torti mit

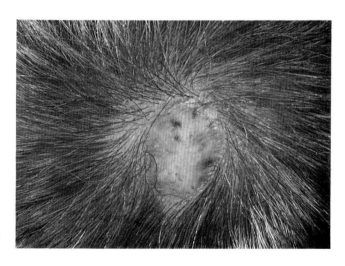

Fig. 78. Congenital aplasia cutis of the scalp.

Augenbeteiligung und Störung der Schweißsekretion. Derm. Wschr. *131:* 277–283 (1955).

(5) GROEGER, H.-W.: Zur Kenntnis der gedrehten Haare (Pili torti). Arch. Derm. Syph. (Berl.) *188:* 521–525 (1949).

(6) LUDWIG, E.: Hypotrichosis congenita hereditaria Typ M. Unna. Arch. Derm. Syph. (Berl.) *196:* 261–278 (1953).

(7) OVERZIER, C.: Die Intersexualität. Thieme, Stuttgart 1961.

(8) PEARL, M., T. F. CHOW and E. FRIEDMAN: Poland's syndrome. Radiology *101:* 619–623 (1971).

(9) TOURAINE, M.: Aplasie pilaire familiale des aisselles. Bull. Soc. franç. Derm. Syph. *47:* 47–48 (1940).

(10) TOURAINE, A., J. HUBER, R. WEISSENBACH, J. A. LIÈVRE et H. BOUR: »Pili torti« familiaux (chez la mère et ses cinq enfants). Bull. Soc. franç. Derm. Syph. *45:* 441–445 (1938).

(11) WILKINS, L.: The diagnosis and treatment of endocrine disorders in childhood and adolescence. Thomas, Springfield, Ill., 1950.

(12) ZAUN, H., und G. BURG: Pili torti veri (Galewsky-Ronchese) mit Beteiligung von Augenbrauen und Lanugines. Aesth. Medizin *18:* 95–100 (1969).

C. Acquired Generalized Hypotrichoses

Paying attention to some fundamental rules will make it easier to classify acquired hypotrichoses and alopecias into proper diagnostic groups. First, the pattern of the loss of hair should be studied, as to whether it is circumscribed, diffuse, or a total shedding of the hair. The next step is to inspect the skin on which the hair grows, deciding whether it shows normal structure or scarring atrophy and whether it presents erythema, bullae, pustules, papules, scales keratoses, or pigmentary changes. Additional diagnostic leads can be gained through evaluation of the condition of the root of the hair (telogen, dystrophic, or mixed effluvium).

1. Generalized acquired losses of hair may have endogenous or exogenous causes. Such endogenous causes are **anomalies of metabolism** (malnutrition, lack of iron [Fig. 79]), **endocrine high points** (pregnancy, lactation, menopause, hyperthyroidism or hypothyroidism), and febrile **infectious diseases** (typhoid, epidemic typhus, grippe, erysipelas, and secondary syphilis).[2, 6]

Rare hypotrichoses are caused by anterior pituitary hypofunction of the **Sheehan's syndrome** type (loss of eyebrows, axillary and pubic hair, with premature graying) and cirrhosis of the liver. The patient with cirrhosis of the liver typically shows loss of axillary hair (Chvostek's sign) and pubic hair ("abdominal pate").[10]

In **hypoparathyroidism** the scalp hair is dry and sparse; the individual hair shafts, however, do not appear thin. Because this type of scalp hair is especially vulnerable to slight traumatic influences, hypotrichosis with small macular, disseminated areas is observed quite often.

At the time of the menopause **androgenic alopecia** (premature alopecia) may be seen, especially as central thinning of the vertex (Fig. 80). Inflammatory changes or atrophic scars of the scalp are always absent. Examination of the hair roots shows a telogenic effluvium confined to about the middle of the vertex and the occiput. This type of hair loss is similar to the male pattern of baldness because it spares the temples and also the lower occipital region. Statistically, these female patients show a higher level of testosterone excretion than normal women, so that etiologically this is probably an equivalent of the male pate. The **chronic diffuse alopecias** of younger women cannot be clinically separated definitely from androgenic alopecia. These women also show thinning of the hair of the scalp around the vertex; however, normal strong hairs are present simultaneously with thin hairs that have a tendency to break off easily. By ascertaining the status of the hair root

Fig. 79. Sparse, thin, and light hairs in iron deficiency.

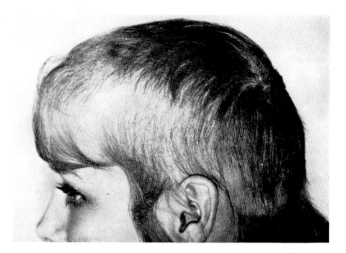

one finds a diffuse dystrophic or mixed type of alopecia. There are no hormonal abnormalities in contrast to androgenic alopecia.[1, 3, 9, 11, 12]

A diagnosis of **neurogenic alopecia** should be made only if there has been a massive psychic trauma and the alopecia started within a few days after the insult or if it took place during the decompensation triggered by the insult.[8]

2. The **exogenous diffuse alopecias** are primarily caused by chemicals or toxic substances such as all *anticoagulants*, cytostatica or thallium. Acute thallium poisoning shows cutaneous manifestations relatively late, with seborrheic erythema of the face (e.g., cheilosis), loss of hair about 14 days from the beginning, and lunulalike areas of the nails another two weeks later, plus symptomatic ichthyosis due to simultaneous damage to the sebaceous glands. An early dermatologic sign is black clumps of melanin within the hair near the root (Fig. 81 a, b).[7]

Rare toxic alopecias caused by drugs are due to lead and to some **thyroid inhibitors** and **antihypertensive preparations** which have now become obsolete. Some of the modern **tranquilizers** (diazepam) have been suspected of causing alopecia. **Cytostatica**

cause a reversible loss of hair after about two to three weeks; this loss starts with the scalp hair and later involves the body also. The metabolic changes due to cytostatica affect the reproduction of the very sensitive matrix cells of the hair bulb

Fig. 80. Androgenic alopecia.

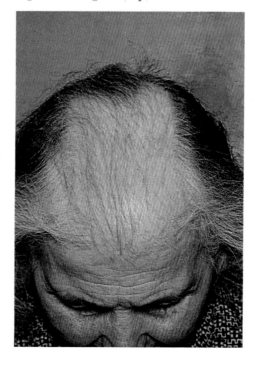

during the anagen phase; duration and dosage of the drugs as well as individual differences are important in this type of effluvium. Such cytostatic alopecia resembles Mieschers' trichomalacia.*[5, 7]

3. The changes of the scalp and the scalp hair caused by **physical** modalities, such as several permanent wave methods using heat and the cold wave process, are well known. Typical of cold wave dermatitis is the irritation of the epithelium, which begins with pruritus at the borders of the scalp especially, and later occurs on the entire hairy scalp; after the exudative reaction subsides, residual pigmentations

may result. Damage to the hairs themselves caused by the cold wave process is demonstrated by a deformation of the hairs resembling twisted fibers or by areas of broken hair shafts.

4. Lipedematous alopecia presents no diminution in the number of scalp hairs but does involve a decrease in the length of their growth. These changes are caused by a marked increase in thickness of the subcutaneous fatty tissue of the scalp without a specific histomorphologic picture. The status of the hair root and the whole hair itself has no diagnostic significance. [4]

* Softening and disintegration of the hair shaft within the follicle. (Tr.)

5. Alopecia totalis has been discussed with alopecia areata (p. 114).

Fig. 81. Thallium poisoning: (a) diffuse alopecia; (b) melanin clumping in the hair.

Fig. 81a

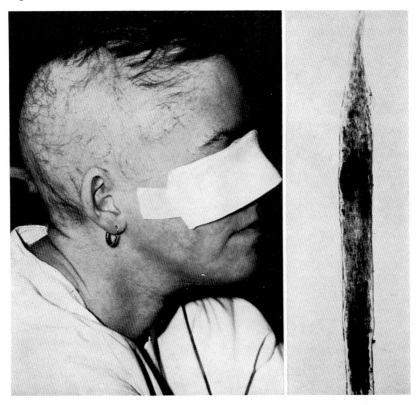

Fig. 81b

(1) Apostolakis, M., E. Ludwig und
    K.-D. Voigt: Testosteron-, Oestrogen-
    und Gonadotropinausscheidung bei dif-
    fuser weiblicher Alopecie. Klin. Wschr.
    43: 9–15 (1965).

(2) Bosse, K.: Haarwachstum und Schwan-
    gerschaft. Schrift. Marchionini-Stiftg. *2:*
    59–68 (1971).

(3) Braun-Falco, O., und H. Zaun: Zum
    Wesen der chronischen diffusen Alo-
    pecie bei Frauen. Arch. klin. exp.
    Derm. *215:* 165–180 (1962).

(4) Coskey, R. J., R. P. Fosnaugh and
    G. Fine: Lipedematous alopecia. Arch.
    Derm. (Chic.) *84:* 619–622 (1961).

(5) Falkson, G.: Endoxan alopecia. Brit.
    J. Derm. *72:* 296–301 (1960).

(6) Freinkel, R. K., and N. Freinkel:
    Hair growth and alopecia in hypothy-
    roidism. Arch. Derm. (Chic.) *106:*
    349–352 (1972).

(7) Herzberg, J. J.: Cytostatische Alo-
    pecien einschließlich Thallium-Alo-
    pecien. Arch. klin. exp. Derm. *227:*
    452–468 (1966).

(8) Kienle, G., und W. Wagner: Haar-
    ausfall und psychische Belastung. Z.
    Psychother. med. Psychol. *6:* 173–184
    (1956).

(9) Ludwig, E.: Über das endokrine Sub-
    strat der diffusen weiblichen (andro-
    genetischen) Alopecie. Arch. klin. exp.
    Derm. *227:* 468–477 (1966).

(10) Lukidis, W.: Über die mangelhafte
    Achsel- und Schambehaarung bei Leber-
    zirrhosen. Z. ges. inn. Med. *10:* 880–882
    (1955).

(11) Sulzberger, M. B., V. H. Witten and
    A. W. Kopf: Diffuse alopecia in women.
    Arch. Derm. (Chic.) *81:* 556–560 (1960).

(12) Zaun, H.: Echte Glatzenbildung (»male
    pattern baldness«) bei Frauen. Z. Haut-
    u. Geschl.-Kr. *35:* 35–41 (1963).

D. Acquired Circumscribed Hypotrichoses

1. Reversible, externally caused hypotrichoses are well known in infants; they
are due to tension affecting the scalp in
connection with the growth of the skull
and involving especially the frontal hairline. As long as the infant remains in a
permanent recumbent position the condition is known as **decubital alopecia** of the
occipital region. Less known is the fact
that during the first months of life parts
of the scalp hair change as if molting.

2. Reversible, nonscarring losses of hair
result from certain fashions of hairdo
(ponytail) and are easily understood as
traction alopecia. Some national fashions
(in Greenland, Schwalm disease; in France,
chignon disease) cause pressure or tension
alopecias. Typically, they are observed as
biparietal macular alopecias above the
ears. The skin of such areas remains
unaffected.

3. Trichotillomania (hair-pulling tic)
consists of frequent habitual plucking of
tufts of hair perhaps as a pleasurable
neurotic tendency (preferred sites are the
crown region, eyelashes, eyebrows, beard,
and pubic hair). Frequently, a circular or
oval, partly alopecic area may reach the
size of a palm (Fig. 82); this condition may
simulate idiopathic alopecia and, if present
on the eyebrows, may suggest Hertoghe's
sign. The close proximity of damaged and
normal hair follicles is typical within these
areas of alopecia. More rarely, this
"alopécie manuelle" is accomplished with
an instrument, for instance, scissors. In
any case, the mania of plucking leaves the
skin itself normal or only slightly scaly.

Symptomatic trichoclasia (such as tinea
capitis, lichen simplex chronicus, and
others) shows pronounced basic changes
of the skin in a circumscribed, partly
alopecic area. Here the hairs appear
broken or knotted, especially when heavy
scaling, itching, or even infiltration is
present.[7]

4. Disseminated neurodermatitis, an
endogenous eczema, sometimes shows
more or less circumscribed, not sharply
limited, and occasionally almost diffuse

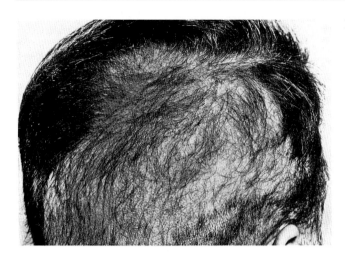

Fig. 82. Trichotillomania.

"alopecia neurodermatitica." Histologically, peculiar inflammatory, strongly eosinophilic infiltrates with a heavy accumulation of eosinophils in the small cutaneous vessels of the scalp are noted. Smaller and more circular areas of neurodermatitis of the scalp differ by their dull grey-reddish color from alopecia areata with its decrease in pigment and its ivory-white, yellowish, shiny sebaceous hyperplasia.

5. The loss of hair seen in **psoriasis vulgaris** has previously received little attention. However, even psoriatic areas without scales show a circumscribed loss of hair; after such psoriatic patches heal, the hair grows back. Also, the density of the hair is definitely diminished within psoriatic areas of the scalp; such hair is much thinner than the surrounding hair. In some cases an inflammatory infiltrate causes destruction of the follicle and results in a scarring alopecia.[8]

6. **Alopecia areata** (pelade, area celsi) is characterized by a reversible, "idiopathic," rapid, and complete loss of hair affecting not only the scalp (Fig. 83) but also the eyebrows, eyelashes, beard, and the axillary and pubic hair. This type of alopecia affects primarily children and adolescents, seldom old people. Spontane-

ous involution is unlikely to occur before puberty and seldom affects lesions of the occipital region in general. **Alopecia areata totalis** describes total loss of scalp hair; such a development is not surprising because alopecia areata is fundamentally a diffuse disease of the entire scalp. **Alopecia areata universalis** describes loss of all hairs of the body (Fig. 84). Hairs can be easily extracted around the circular or oval bald areas, depending on the activity of the attack. These hairs have a small bulb with a thinned-out root and a partially preserved thin follicular portion; they are called "exclamation point hairs." Inflammatory or cicatricial changes of the hairy skin are not characteristic of alopecia areata. The skin of such alopecic areas is smooth and ivory colored, and shows no scaling. In addition, it is remarkable that there may be stippling of all fingernails and toenails (onychosis punctata, Fig. 259 b). However, this stippling is much more superficial than in the psoriatic nail. Occasionally, keratotic changes of the elbows exist also.

The pathologic mechanism consists of a primary mixed effluvium caused by dysfermentation of the matrix of the actively mitotic hair. If there is an especially rapid progression in a case of alopecia areata a determination of the status of the hair

Fig. 83. Alopecia areata.

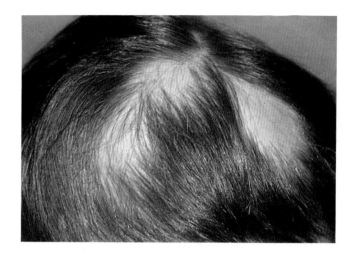

root will show dystrophic hairs; if, on the other hand, progression is especially slow, telogen hairs will prevail. Although again and again familial occurrences seem to indicate a genetic relationship of this circumscribed alopecia, the question of heredity cannot yet be decided definitely.* The syntropy with vitiligo, hyperthyroidism, or intestinal polyposis must be kept in mind. The frequency of alopecia areata-like spots of thinned-out hair in mongolism is striking; ophthalmologically, the condition tends to coincide with pupillary abnormalities, Horner's syndrome, and, possibly, anomalies of refraction, and sporadically with astigmatism, strabismus, cataract, and retinitis pigmentosa. It has been asserted that alopecia areata occurs more frequently in cases of hypertension and also in people with·an atopic constitution, that is, those who have a reactive disposition toward endogenous eczema in its wider sense. In the Vogt-Koyanagi syndrome, which is characterized by uveoencephalitis associated with vitiligo and poliosis, alopecia areata-like loss of hair occurs also. Total alopecia areata with its obviously poor prognosis regarding

regrowth of hair may be caused by a central nervous system disease (for instance, a glioma of the hypothalamic region).[1, 5, 6, 9]

7. The most important small macular type of hair loss, **syphilitic alopecia**

Fig. 84. Alopecia areata totalis.

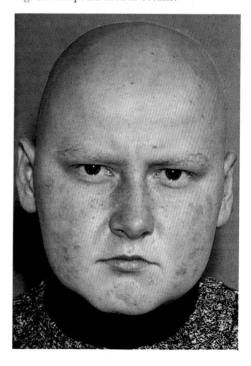

---

* We have observed many members of a family affected with alopecia areata. (Tr.)

areolaris (specific alopecia), starts acutely and frequently at first at the occipital region of the scalp; however, this type of alopecia is irregularly distributed, the numerous hairless areas do not become larger as they would in alopecia areata, and the entire scalp takes on a motheaten appearance. Also, the hairs around a single lesion of alopecia areata are firm. As the hairs grow back in syphilitic alopecia they show mostly normal pigmentation, whereas in alopecia areata they are at first white and become pigmented only slowly.

8. An appearance similar to that of syphilitic alopecia is presented by **alopecia parvimaculata,** * showing atrophic or non-atrophic lesions. It is supposed to occur as an endemic disease in children, probably

---

* Small macular type of alopecia. (Tr.)

Fg. 85. Microsporosis lesion: pale green fluorescence under Wood's light.

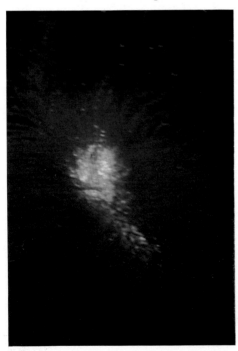

owing to an infection. The etiology of this questionable entity is still unsolved (apathogenic aerobe spore-forming bacilli?). Perhaps one should suspect that such so-called alopecia parvimaculata are microsporum infections which have been overlooked.[4]

9. In any case, a small macular alopecia which occurs as an epidemic with coin-sized and, most important, scaling areas which have hairs broken off shortly above the surface suggests a **microsporum infection (Microsporum audouini, M. canis,** or **M. gypseum)** and requires diagnostic verification. The diseased hairs are put on a slide and covered with a few drops of a 15 per cent solution of sodium hydroxide; microscopic examination will show the hairs densely filled with spores, like "nuts in a sack." Under a Wood's light (quartz lamp with cobalt filter) diseased hairs will show a blue-greenish fluorescence (Fig.85). While microsporum infections may show seborrheic, pityriasiform, and parvimacular variations, it should be emphasized again that seborrheic dermatitis affects more or less the entire scalp in a short time and, when it lasts for some time, it will not be limited to a small macular extension. Also, the seborrheic-eczematous patch is reddish and scaling and the broken-off hairs above the surface are lacking. In seborrheic dermatitis or psoriasis vulgaris, the proximal parts of the hairs are covered with mica or asbestoslike crusts called "tinea amiantacea" (French "teigne amiantacé"). Although a single psoriatic area of the scalp looks like a circular and sharply limited patch of microsporum infection, its base is light or dark red, and the scales are in layers of a thick silvery or yellowish-white color; conversely, microsporum areas lack inflammatory changes and have only a pale red color. In psoriasis the hairs are not clinically changed; they are present within the compact scale but are sometimes not immediately visible.

Fig. 86. Alopecia mucinosa.

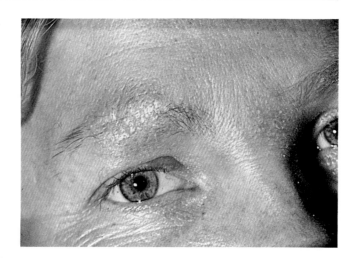

10. Completely different, however, are the findings in **follicular mucinosis** (alopecia mucinosa). The disease is characterized by a mucinous degeneration within the epithelia of the follicle and the sebaceous glands, respectively, or in other words, a follicular mucinosis. As the disease progresses cysts will be formed and metachromic substances will be present in these areas ("mucophanerosis").* Clinically, there is a lichenoid-follicular, and sometimes keratotic focal eruption, which later assumes an orange-peel aspect (Figs. 86, 87). In the beginning alopecia is not always distinctly visible. The differential diagnosis must consider the entire range of cutaneous diseases causing follicular mucinosis, such as keratosis pilaris, follicular eczema, pityriasis rubra pilaris, parapsoriatic plaques, mycosis fungoides, and others. Sometimes such reactions of the hair follicle apparatus, which begin with spongiosis and vesiculation, can be seen in lichen simplex (*"lichénification géante"*) or in cutaneous lupus erythematosus. Without doubt follicular mucinoses are observed frequently in connection with reticulosis and even more often with reticulogranulomatosis. In retrospect one should ask whether the condition formerly called "spinulism" in mycosis fungoides in reality represents follicular mucinosis histologically. In any case, the presence of multiple areas of alopecia mucinosa should lead to a thorough search for premycosis, especially if pruritus is present at the same

Fig. 87. Alopecia mucinosa: edema and mucous degeneration of the outer root sheath. HE stain, 25×.

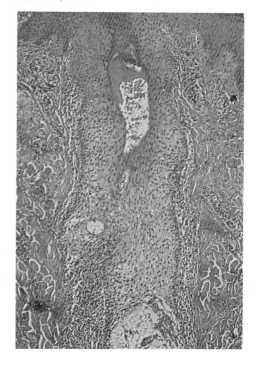

---

* Appearance of acid mucopolysaccharides. (Tr.)

time and if in addition there are faded yellow-brownish, moderately infiltrated or even polycyclically gyrated erythemas.

Besides these symptomatic follicular mucinoses there exist idiopathic forms, which either regress spontaneously after some time or do not show transition to mycosis fungoides even after many years. See also Chapter 29, C.[2, 3]

(1) BRAUN-FALCO, O., und B. RASSNER: Klinik, Pathogenese und Therapie der Alopecia areata. Fortschr. prakt. Derm. u. Ven. Bd. *V*, 227–242, Springer, Berlin, Heidelberg, New York 1965.

(2) CABRÉ, J., und G. W. KORTING: Zum symptomatischen Charakter der »Mucinosis follicularis«: Ihr Vorkommen beim Lupus erythematodes chronicus. Derm. Wschr. *149:* 513–518 (1964).

(3) EMMERSON, R. W.: Follicular mucinosis; a study of 47 patients. Brit. J. Derm. *81:* 395–413 (1969).

(4) HÖFER, W.: Sporadisches Auftreten von Alopecia parvimaculata. Derm. Wschr. *149:* 381–386 (1964).

(5) IKEDA (née MATSUBARA), T.: A new classification of alopecia areata. Dermatologica (Basel) *131:* 421–424 (1965).

(6) KORTING, G. W., und H. HOLZMANN: Hautveränderungen bei mongoloider Abartung. Med. Welt *17* (N.F.): 2801–2802 (1966).

(7) MEHREGAN, A. H.: Trichotillomania. A clinicopathologic study. Arch. Derm. (Chic.) *102:* 129–133 (1970).

(8) SHUSTER, S.: Psoriatic alopecia. Brit. J. Derm. *87:* 73–78 (1972).

(9) WUNDERLICH, CHR., und O. BRAUN-FALCO: Mongolismus und Alopecia areata. Med. Welt *16* (N.F.): 477–481 (1965).

E. Cicatricial Alopecias

The group of circumscribed alopecias, which are irreversible because they are cicatricial, includes those of both endogenous and exogenous cause.

1. The mechanism of the development of **aplasia cutis congenita** ought to be mentioned in this connection (see also Chapter 11, B4). Also, nevoid formations (e.g., nevus sebaceous and others) may cause irreversible circumscribed alopecias.

2. The same can be said for certain forms of the group of follicular or parafollicular keratoses and dyskeratoses, for instance, porokeratosis of Mibelli and **ulerythema ophryogenes** (Fig. 88). In blond people particularly, symmetrical bandlike erythemas with follicular keratoses begin in the region of the eyebrows. In the course of the disorder follicular atrophies with scarring loss of hair develop. The disorder often begins as early as childhood.

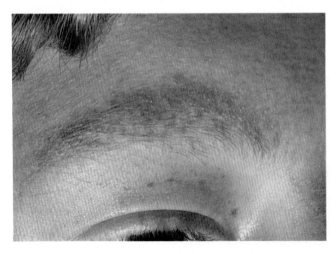

Fig. 88. Ulerythema ophryogenes.

Some patients simultaneously show typical lichen pilaris on the extremities.

3. Follicular spinulous hyperkeratoses of the extensor surface of the upper extremities, face, and neck are also present in **keratosis follicularis spinulosa decalvans.** These keratoses lead to follicular atrophy early, so that on the eyelashes and eyebrows, on the neck, and circumscribed in the middle of the scalp scarring alopecia becomes manifest. At the time of puberty the disorder subsides, and later only atrophic and hairless areas remain. The disturbance of keratinization is a dominant sex-linked hereditary trait with little expressivity in heterozygous women. As early as the first weeks after birth, photophobia and inflammatory changes of the conjunctiva and cornea are present. In female patients the ocular signs are considerably less pronounced and the loss of hair is not as severe as it is in men.[3, 6]

4. Furthermore, scarring alopecias are predominantly the sequelae of preceding dermatoses which also affect other sites. They are mentioned here only briefly since they will be thoroughly discussed in other chapters. Scarring, and sometimes

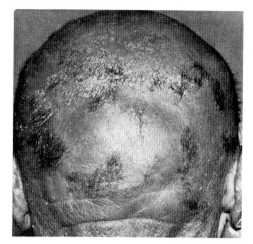

Fig. 89. Cicatricial alopecia in mycosis fungoides.

also nonscarring, alopecias of the axillary, pubic, and scalp hair are observed in *congenital bullous dermatoses*, as for instance in dystrophic, bullous, and hereditary epidermolysis or congenital erythropoietic porphyria.[5, 8] But not every hairless region has preceding eruptions of blisters. Other causes of cicatricial alopecias are *lepromas*, tumors of *mycosis fungoides* (Fig. 89), *carcinomas metastasizing* to the scalp (Fig. 90), syphilitic gummas, *fungous granulomas* (e. g., deep trichophyton infection), *favus* (Fig. 91),

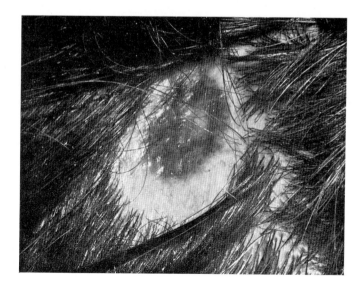

Fig. 90. Circumscribed loss of hair due to a metastasis of a mammary carcinoma to the scalp.

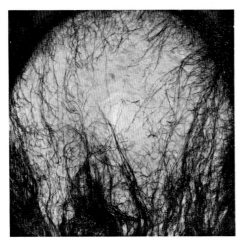

Fig. 91. Scarring alopecia following favus.

and *folliculitis decalvans* (see also atrophic alopecia, p. 122). Not too rare even today are taut, helmetlike alopecias, the end result of *lupus vulgaris*, especially if it has been treated in the previously common aggressive manner (x-rays, ultra-

Fig. 92. Helmetlike, cicatricial alopecia following roentgenologic therapy.

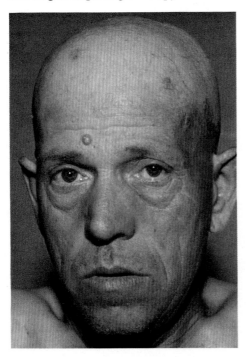

violet light, and salves of pyrogallic acid) (Fig. 92). Scarring and atrophic areas of plaquelike sarcoidosis and necrobiosis lipoidica on the scalp are rarer.

5. Hair losses on the scalp as sequelae of **circumscribed scleroderma** or disseminated **lupus erythematosus** are doubtlessly observed more often. Chronic lupus erythematosus presents in the beginning slowly enlarging peripapillary erythemas, but these affected areas soon assume the highly characteristic follicular atrophic and worm-eaten aspect (Fig. 93). When the stage is reached in which such areas (which are serrated or polycyclically circumscribed, telangiectatic, and tender to palpation) show scarring alopecia with sunken-in skin, restitution of hair is definitely improbable. At the stage of preatrophic follicular erythema, sparse hairs are still present and if treatment comes in time, some hairs may regrow.

6. In the course of **lichen planus** cicatricial alopecia may cause irreversible loss of scalp hair. In so-called lichen planopilaris et acuminatus atrophicus especially, the scalp is involved in about 30 per cent of cases. In lichen ruber follicularis decalvans **(Graham-Little syndrome)**, which favors the third to the sixth decade of life, acuminated lichen papules appear at first on the scalp. These small areas gradually become confluent, forming larger areas with the disappearance of the hair follicles. Large areas have a scarring-atrophic center, but at the periphery they may be surrounded by follicular, millet-sized papules. In comparison with chronic lupus erythematosus, the central scarring and atrophic parts are less extensively characterized by widening and separation of the follicles. Pubic and axillary hair may show the same changes as the scalp hair. A distinct group of papules occurs in

Fig. 93. Chronic cutaneous
lupus erythematosus.

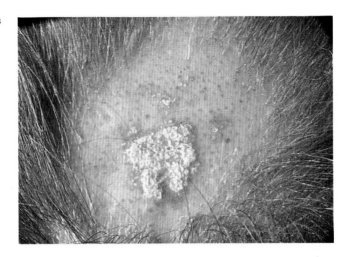

the Graham-Little syndrome, mostly in the lumbosacral region. Here, round, not polygonal, nodules resembling those of lichen nitidus predominate. In *pityriasis rubra pilaris*, which is wrongly identified with lichen ruber acuminatus, the scalp is only moderately erythematous but presents pityriasiform, or plaster-of-paris-like, thick scales. Only exceptionally can isolated, hyperkeratotic nodules or keratotic cones be found in these areas or at the borders. Scarring alopecias do not occur, as a rule.[4,7]

7. Folliculitis decalvans results, in most cases, in small spots of irreversible loss of hair on the scalp. Small papules, limited to the follicles, develop into large pustules centrally penetrated by a hair in a characteristic way. The contents of the pustule often yield cultures of *Staphylococcus aureus*. By confluence, irregularly formed scars develop, which in inflammation-free intervals are differentiated with great difficulty from other scarring alopecias.

8. Sycosiform ulerythema also leaves a cicatricial alopecia. The predominantly exceptional erythematous areas develop into papulopustular infiltrates with characteristic marginal accents. Eventually,

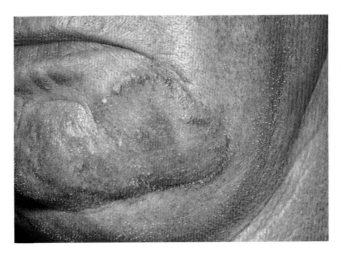

Fig. 94. Sycosiform ulerythema.

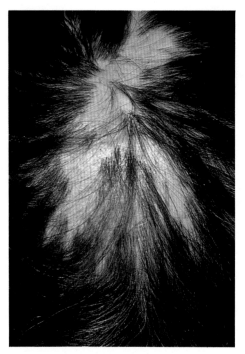

Fig. 95. Brocq's pseudopelade.

serpiginous, slightly sunken scars are present. Histologically, a sheath rich in plasma cells surrounds the sweat and sebaceous glands as well as the hair follicles, which are finally completely destroyed. The beard and the eyebrows are favored sites, but not infrequently, the scalp and the lanugo hairs of the body are also affected (Fig.94). In contrast to nonparasitic sycosis, sycosiform ulerythema does not involve the entire face. It also lacks the abscess-forming nodular aspect. At the present time it is difficult to determine whether these are really two entities.

9. Atrophic alopecia, usually called **pseudopelade,** starts insidiously and causes no symptoms or minimal itching, with no visible signs of inflammation. The loss of hair starts chiefly in the temporal or occipital regions in patients of middle age. Irregularly circumscribed, lentil-sized hair-

less areas develop, which later sink down somewhat. The irregularity in the distribution and borders of the small scarred areas has led to the excellent comparison with "footprints in the snow" (Fig.95). Occasionally, there are periods of great activity, but basically the disorder follows a protracted course.

The preceding remarks on the development of small, cicatricial alopecias in lichen planus, cutaneous lupus erythematosus, favus, folliculitis decalvans, and others have amply shown that *atrophic alopecia* is not a disease entity but a most "anonymous" dermatosis with regard to etiology. It would be advisable, therefore, to speak of a state of pseudopelade rather than of pseudopelade.

10. Incontinentia pigmenti of the Bloch-Sulzberger type almost regularly presents small cicatricial areas of alopecia, which clinically fit in with atrophic alopecia. It is not known whether this alopecia is preceded by inflammatory or bullous changes.[1]

(1) CARNEY, R. G., and R. G. CARNEY JR.: Incontinentia pigmenti. Arch. Derm. (Chic.) *102:* 157–162 (1970).

(2) CARTEAUD, A., et S. BELAÍCH: Tumeurs du cuir chevelu. Presse méd. *74:* 2853–2858 (1966).

(3) FRANCESCHETTI, A., M. JACCOTTET et W. JADASSOHN: Manifestations cornéennes dans la keratosis follicularis spinulosa decalvans (Siemens). Ophthalmologica (Basel) *133:* 259–263 (1957).

(4) GEBHARDT, R.: Little-Lassueur-Syndrom. Med. Welt *18* (N.F.): 2509–2510 (1967).

(5) HEILMEYER, L.: Die erythropoetischen Porphyrien. Med. Welt *16:* 1–8 (1965).

(6) KORTING, G. W.: Zur Kenntnis der multiformen Keratosen. Z. Haut- u. Geschl.-Kr. *11:* 241–244 (1951).

(7) SPIER, H. W., und W. KEILIG: Lichen ruber follicularis decalvans (Graham-

Little-Syndrom) und seine Beziehungen zur Pseudopelade Brocq. Hautarzt *4:* 457–467 (1953).

(8) WAGNER, W.: Alopezie und Nagelver-
änderungen bei Epidermolysis bullosa hereditaria. Z. Haut- u. Geschl.-Kr. *20:* 278–285 (1956).

F. Congenital Generalized Hyper-
   trichoses

1. The name **hypertrichosis lanuginosa** or hypertrichosis universalis congenita was given to an abundance of long, dense, and silklike body hair which remains, as no secondary hairs follow the primary lanugo hair. As a rule, the change from primary to secondary hair takes place about the eighth to ninth month of pregnancy and ends around the first half of the first year of life. Patients with this autosomal dominant persistence of lanugo hair are called apelike human beings because of their furlike surface, which, however, is lacking on palms, soles, and preputium. If they do not resemble apes, they may resemble dogs or lions. These rare anomalies frequently also show deficient dentition.

2. In patients with the **Cornelia de Lange's syndrome** (dwarfism, mental retardation, brachycephaly, hypoplasia of the lower jaw, low-set ears, syndactyly), congenital generalized hypertrichosis of the lanugo-hair type is often present also. Especially dense hair grows on the neck, elbows, and spine. The frontal hairline may extend down almost to the eyebrows. Another frequent finding in this syndrome is generalized cutis marmorata.[2, 3]

3. Occasionally, hypertrichosis of the lanugo-hair type has been observed in **congenital familial acanthosis nigricans**

(Seip-Lawrence syndrome).* These patients also have simultaneous lipoatrophic diabetes mellitus. Moreover, a diabetic is apt to have so-called hirsutism diabeticorum, which is found preponderantly on the face and on the back near the shoulder blades as well as periumbilically.[1]

4. Hereditary **fibromatosis of the gingiva** commonly shows, besides hypertrophy of the gingiva, hypertrichosis of the face, the extremities, and the back. The increased growth of hair starts, however, as late as puberty.[4, 5]

(1) MIESCHER, G.: Zwei Fälle von congenitaler familiärer Akanthosis nigricans kombiniert mit Diabetes mellitus. Derm. Z. *32:* 276–305 (1921).

(2) SALAZAR, F. N.: Dermatological manifestations of the Cornelia de Lange syndrome. Arch. Derm. (Chic.) *94:* 38–43 (1966).

(3) SCHUSTER, D. S., and ST. A. M. JOHNSON: Cutaneous manifestations of the Cornelia de Lange syndrome. Arch. Derm. (Chic.) *93:* 702–707 (1966).

(4) WESKI, H.: Elephantiasis gingivae hereditaria, beobachtet an fünf Generationen in einer Familie. Dtsch. Mschr. Zahnheilk. *33:* 557–584 (1920).

(5) WINKLMAIR, M.: Hereditäre Fibromatosis Gingivae. Dtsch. zahnärztl. Z. *24:* 895–899 (1969).

G. Congenital Circumscribed
   Hypertrichias

1. More abundant growth of hair in circumscribed areas has been observed in constitutional, especially pyknic, body types on the presternum or on the upper parts of the back **(hypertrichosis dorsalis superior).** Conspicuous hypertrichosis may

---

* Acanthosis nigricans at birth is not the characteristic sign in these cases and we would avoid the above name because it leads to confusion with "benign" acanthosis nigricans. (Tr.)

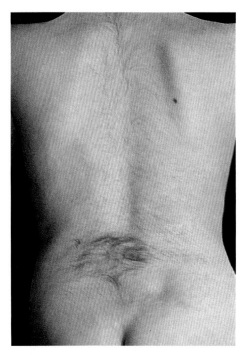 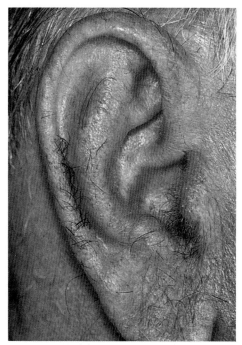

Fig. 96. Spina bifida occulta with hyper-   Fig. 97. Hypertrichosis of the ear.
trichosis.

also exist on the extensor surfaces of the fingers: transitions to the normal amount of hair on the fingers, however, are not sharply delineated.

2. Not too rare also are ponytail-like ("faun-tail") dorsolumbar hypertrichoses **(hypertrichosis dorsolumbalis)** in connection with spina bifida occulta (Fig. 96).[6]

3. Less known are hypertrichoses of the ear (Fig. 97), which have Y-chromosomal heredity. Similar **auricular hypertrichias,** which are acquired and show shorter hair, occur also in patients with porphyria cutanea tarda.*

4. In the **Klein-Waardenburg syndrome** local hypertrichosis occurs in about half

of the cases on the nasal part of the eyebrows.

5. In contrast to the hypertrichoses just mentioned, which present only an increase in the growth of hair, hypertrichias are not infrequently observed on the basis of certain nevoid formations. They show, besides the hypertrichosis, other cutaneous changes. A good example is the papillary and hairy nevus cell nevus, whose maximal variant is the **classic bathing trunk nevus** (nevus pellitus) (Fig. 98).

6. In this connection the **woolly hair nevus** (nevus ulotrichicus) must be mentioned. It is usually found on the scalp and is distinguishable from the surrounding hair by the pronounced woolly hair formation. The scalp itself is in most of these cases unchanged, although a number of linear or verrucous nevi may be present nearby.[2, 5]

---

* These patients also have dark hairs over the cheekbones and eyebrows. (Tr.)

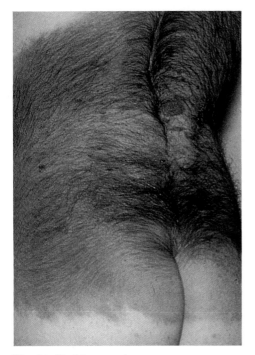

Fig. 98. Bathing trunk nevus.

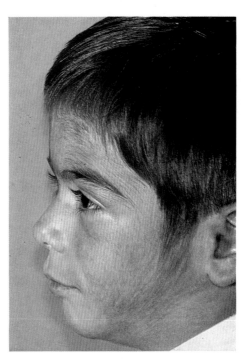

Fig. 99. Acquired hypertrichosis lanuginosa in the healing stage of dermatomyositis.

7. Becker's nevus, which represents a circumscribed hypertrichosis, is identical with **melanosis neviformis**. This milk-coffee-colored, archipelagolike, loose, tardive nevus is often accompanied by hypertrichosis. Its smooth cutaneous surface and homogeneous pigment distribution distinguish it from a bathing trunk nevus. Such a nevus is considerably darker and heterogeneously pigmented. If in doubt, the histologic findings make a sure distinction possible. For more details see Chapter 24, D14.[1, 4]

(1) BECKER, S. W.: Concurrent melanosis and hypertrichosis in distribution of nevus unius lateris. Arch. Derm. Syph. (Chic.) *60:* 155–160 (1949).

(2) BORN, W.: Über umschriebene Kräuselnaevi innerhalb sonst glatten Kopfhaars. Dermatologica (Basel) *115:* 119–121 (1957).

(3) SIEMENS, H. W.: Die naevusähnliche Melanose. Hautarzt *18:* 299–303 (1967).

(4) SOMMER, K.: Untersuchungen zur Genetik der Haardichte auf den Fingern der Menschen. Anthrop. Anz. (Stuttg.) *32:* 46–69 (1970).

(5) STREITMANN, B.: Beitrag zur Kenntnis des Kräuselhaarnaevus. Derm. Wschr. *139:* 185–187 (1959).

(6) THURSFIELD, W. R., and A. A. ROSS: Faun tail (sacral hirsuties) and diastematomyelia. Brit. J. Derm. *73:* 328–336 (1961).

H. Acquired Generalized Hypertrichoses

1. Acute hypertrichoses have been reported after severe **traumas involving the skull** with contusion of the brain and disturbance of the hypothalamic-hypophyseal regulation of hair growth. About two to four months after such severe damage to the brain abnormal growth

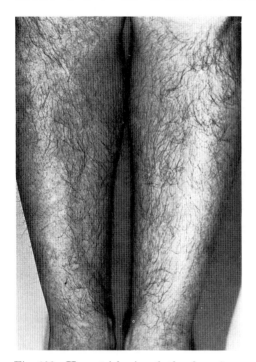

Fig. 100. Hypertrichosis of the legs in a woman who has simultaneous manifestations of progressive scleroderma.

of the hair is said to occur; such growth may last up to one year. In most of the cases the trunk and extremities are covered with lanugolike hair. Occasionally, terminal hairs develop, especially on the lower extremities.[6]

2. Another cause for symptomatic hypertrichosis lanuginosa is **malnutrition,** due either to diminished food intake or to malabsorption in celiac disease or other malabsorption conditions.

3. Dermatomyositis, especially in its healing phase, sometimes presents remarkable hypertrichosis (Fig. 99). Several parts of the body, especially the temples and eyelashes but also the trunk and extremities, are covered with a heavy coat of lanugo hair. This hypertrichosis is more frequent in children but can also be seen

in adults and is independent of corticosteroid medication.[5]

4. Progressive scleroderma may also show increased growth of hair; its characteristic location is on the extremities (Fig. 100).[3]

5. Other causes of diffuse hypertrichoses with a fairly acute beginning are grippe-like diseases or recurrent gastrointestinal ulcerations. Sometimes hypertrichosis can occur in otherwise clinically normal persons.

6. Generalized acquired hypertrichosis lanuginosa (et terminalis) with a sudden onset can occur in combination with visceral neoplasms (bladder, gallbladder, or lung) as part of a paraneoplastic syndrome. Such patients often have a sudden hypertrophy of the papillae of the tongue simultaneously with the hypertrichosis.[1, 2, 4]

(1) HEGEDUS, S. I., and W. F. SCHORR: Acquired hypertrichosis lanuginosa and malignancy. A clinical review and histopathologic evaluation with special attention to the »mantle« hair of Pinkus. Arch. Derm. (Chic.) *106:* 84–88 (1972).

(2) HERZBERG, J. J., K. POTJAN und D. GEBAUER: Hypertrichosis lanuginosa (et terminalis) acquisita als paraneoplastisches Syndrom. Arch. klin. exp. Derm. *232:* 176–186 (1968).

(3) LEINWAND, J., A. W. DURYEE and M. N. RICHTER: Scleroderma (based on a study of over 150 cases). Ann. int. Med. *41:* 1003–1041 (1954).

(4) VAN DER LUGT, L., and C. DUDOK DE WIT: Hypertrichosis lanuginosa acquisita. Dermatologica (Basel) *146:* 46–54 (1973).

(5) SCHUERMANN, H.: Dermatomyositis. Ergebn. inn. Med. Kinderheilk. N. F. *10:* 427–480 (1958).

(6) TARNOW, G., und W. RABE: Zur Frage der zentralen Regulation der Haartrophik (Hypertrichosen und Alopezien nach schweren Schädelhirntraumen). Nervenarzt *40:* 210–215 (1969).

I. Acquired or Symptomatic Circumscribed Hypertrichoses

1. Hereditary hypertrichoses of the auricular region have been discussed previously in connection with a similar condition occurring in combination with **porphyria cutanea tarda;** besides the ears facial hypertrichosis also affects the eyebrows or the beard. Women suffering from porphyria cutanea tarda may also show increased facial hair (Fig. 101).

2. The male patient with **endogenous eczema** has as a peculiar stigma frontal and temporal hypertrichosis extending down the sides of the face and resembling a fur cap.[1]

3. Acquired hypertrichoses may be caused by **external provocation** such as repeated trauma (e. g., carrying heavy loads, irritating ointments or plasters, cupping glasses, or burns). Occasionally, hypertrichoses are observed after fractures or nerve injuries, especially those of the extremities.

4. An increase of hair growth due to drugs is seen occasionally after treatment with vitamin D_2, streptomycin, cortisone, ACTH, and derivatives of hydantoin.

5. Generalized lipodystrophy, which is frequently observed in childhood either as a congenital hereditary condition or as an acquired type, may include hypertrichosis of the face and the extensor surfaces of the extremities. Another dermatologic sign is increased perspiration, and the complete absence of subcutaneous fat (which is absent even inside the abdomen and perirenal region) is striking. Hepatomegaly, muscular hypertrophy, and insulin-resistant diabetes, which appears after several years of the disease, are the main features of generalized lipodystrophy.[3, 5] For the dermatologist the occasional

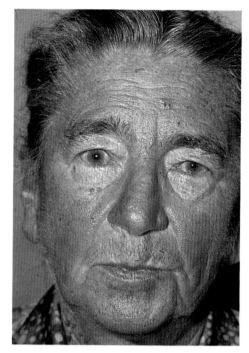

Fig. 101. Hypertrichosis of the cheeks in porphyria cutanea tarda.

finding at birth of acanthosis nigricans, which in its benign form occurs only in very obese individuals, is of special interest.* Most likely there is a close connection to the syndrome described in Section F3 (p. 123).**[2, 4]

6. The **hypothyroid patient** with his doughy, cool, dry skin frequently has increased growth of hair while the hyperthyroid patient presents thin, smooth, warm skin with diminished growth of hair.

7. The **circumscribed, tuberous, or nodular myxedema** of the patient with dysthy-

---

* This condition may also be found in childhood.[2, 4] (Tr.)

** Acanthosis nigricans in very obese individuals is usually pseudoacanthosis nigricans, a phenocopy of "benign" acanthosis nigricans. (Tr.)

roidism is well known to the dermatologist; the areas of myxedema have a distinct increase in hair growth, with especially dark and well-developed hairs sprouting out of funnel-shaped, enlarged follicular openings.

(1) BAUER, L.: Endogenes Ekzem, Konstitution und Behaarung. Aesth. Med. *17:* 95–106 (1968).

(2) BRUBAKER, M. M., N. E. LEVAN and P. J. COLLIPP: Acanthosis nigricans and congenital total lipodystrophy. Arch. Derm. (Chic.) *91:* 320–325 (1965).

(3) LANGSCH, H.-G., D. MICHAELIS und U. FISCHER: Ungewöhnliches Krankheitsbild einer Patientin mit insulinresistentem Diabetes mellitus und hochgradiger Lipoatrophie. Dtsch. Gesundh.-Wes. *24:* 14–18 (1969).

(4) REED, W. B., R. DEXTER, C. CORLEY and C. FISH: Congenital lipodystrophic diabetes with acanthosis nigricans. The Seip-Lawrence syndrome. Arch. Derm. (Chic.) *91:* 326–334 (1965).

Fig. 102. Hirsutism in the Stein-Leventhal syndrome.

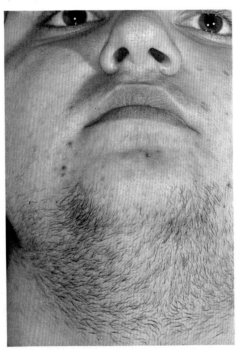

(5) SEIP, M.: Generalized lipodystrophy. Ergebn. inn. Med. Kinderheilk. N.F. *31:* 59–95 (1971).

K. Hirsutism

1. Hirsutism denotes an abnormally excessive growth of hair, especially the hair of the face, genitals, and body in women corresponding to that of men. The most common form of this excessive growth of hair is so-called **idiopathic hirsutism**. Such females have normally functioning ovaries, normal gynecologic findings, and normal 17-ketosteroid values, but the specific testosterone transport protein in the plasma is diminished. Therefore, in such cases the increased amounts of free testosterone in the body act on the target organs – in hirsutism, on the hair follicles. As a rule, hirsutism begins a few years after the menarche and reaches a degree that varies from case to case. In rare cases an increase of 17-ketosteroids can be found in combination with normal ovarian function. Such females show hirsutism usually at the time of the menarche.[3, 4, 6]

2. If hirsutism occurs together with menstrual disturbances, sometimes resulting in long-lasting amenorrhea, **Stein-Leventhal's syndrome** should be considered (Fig. 102). Further signs of virilization such as hypertrophy of the clitoris or huskiness of the voice are quite rare. However, pronounced obesity is not infrequent. Decisive for the diagnosis is the finding of enlarged grey cystic ovaries. Analysis of the hormones may show normal to increased 17-ketosteroid levels. To be on the safe side several hormonal analyses should be performed at different times because the findings in one and the same female may show different values.[1, 4]

3. Hirsutism accompanied by other signs of virilization may in rare instances be due to a **virilizing tumor of the ovary,** i.e., a hilar cell tumor or an arrhenoblastoma. Clinically, the appearance of the patient is very similar to that seen in the Stein-Leventhal syndrome but instead of large ovaries there is in most cases a unilateral ovarian tumor of varying size.[4]

4. Morgagni's syndrome is a combination of hirsutism, obesity, hyperostosis of the frontal bone, and diabetes mellitus. There is some question whether this variable constellation of abnormalities represents a true syndrome.

5. The congenital female adrenogenital syndrome combines virilization with pronounced hypertrophy of the clitoris. Hirsutism becomes evident with the onset of puberty which, however, starts prematurely (pseudopubertas praecox). In child-

hood, growth is increased so that these girls are too tall in comparison with normal children; later however, the epiphyses close prematurely, so as adults they are too short. Helpful in establishing the diagnosis is the pronounced increase of 17-ketosteroids in the urine and an increase in the titer of pregnanetriol in the 24-hour urine due to an absence of C_{21}-hydroxylase in the adrenal cortex. The elimination of the 17-ketosteroids can be suppressed by giving dexamethasone.[3]

6. The so-called **late adrenogenital syndrome** is caused by a tumor (adenoma, carcinoma) of the adrenal cortex or by its diffuse hyperplasia. Such female patients develop pronounced masculinization with hirsutism, huskiness of voice, amenorrhea, and hypertrophy of the clitoris. The elimination of the 17-ketosteroids and espe-

Fig. 103. Late Hurler syndrome: acne, hirsutism and Alder's granulation anomaly of the leukocytes.

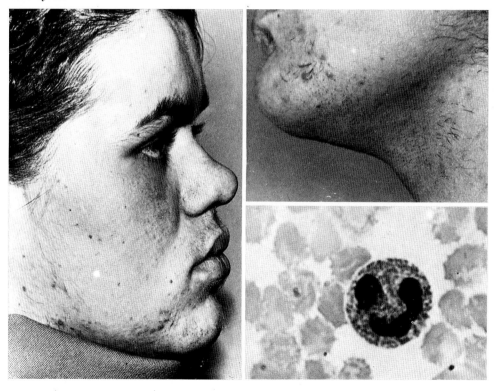

cially their precursor, the dehydroepian-drosterone fraction, is usually increased but it does not present unequivocal dependency on ACTH. The presence of a tumor is diagnostically important.

7. Cushing's syndrome shows hirsutism in about 20 per cent of women in addition to the usual clinical signs such as obesity of the trunk, steroid acne, hypertension, and so on. The urine shows increased excretion of 17-hydroxycorticoids. After ACTH medication this excretion is increased even more. The causes of such increased hormone production may be adenomas, carcinomas, and hyperplasias of the adrenal cortex. Cushing's syndrome may be in rare instances a manifestation of a paraneoplastic syndrome, e. g., a bronchial carcinoma. Cushing's syndrome caused by prolonged cortisone therapy should not be overlooked.[3]

8. Hirsutism due to drugs with signs of virilization can be caused by prolonged or high doses of androgens (e. g., in mammary cancer) or of anabolic drugs; in extremely rare instances it can occur after gestagens.*

---

* Miescher's term for progesterone and allied compounds. (Tr.)

9. The **Hurler-Pfaundler syndrome,** now considered to represent mucopolysac-charidosis storage disease type 1, shows as an associated sign facial hypertrichosis with a lowered hairline of the scalp, excess hair covering the forehead and upper lip, bushy prominent eyebrows, and occasionally, hirsutism of the chin and neck together with disseminated monomorphous acne nodules (Fig. 103).[2]

(1) DECOURT, J., M.-F. JAYLE et P. MAU-VAIS-JARVIS: Syndrome de Stein-Leventhal et virilisme pilaire. Presse méd. *70:* 365–368 (1962).
(2) KORTING, G. W., und I. KORINTHEN-BERG: Hirsutismus als Teilsymptom des abortiven oder tardiven Morbus Pfaundler-Hurler. Z. Haut- u. Geschl.-Kr. *37:* 65–70 (1964).
(3) KUČERA, F., und B. SAREMBE: Zur Differentialdiagnose des Hirsutismus. Dtsch. Gesundh.-Wes. *22:* 60–69 (1967).
(4) STÖCKLI, A., F. KUBLI, M. KELLER und P. KAUFMANN: Zyklusanomalien und Sterilität bei Frauen mit Hirsutismus und polycystischen Ovarien. Schweiz. med. Wschr. *92:* 1687–1697 (1962).
(5) STRAUSS, J. S., and P. E. POCHI: Recent advances in androgen metabolism and their relation to the skin. Arch. Derm. (Chic.) *100:* 621–636 (1969).
(6) TAMM, J., und K. D. VOIGT: Einige klinisch relevante Ergebnisse der neueren Androgenforschung. Schweiz. med. Wschr. *101:* 1078–1083 (1971).

12. Panniculitides

Adipose tissue not only represents a special form of reticular connective tissue but also is equipped with a special form of vascularization of its lobules. This fact presumably also explains the striking disposition of the subcutaneous fat for necrosis. In spite of this the various processes of steatogranulomatosis are included in the concept of panniculitis. This term, then, indicates that at times

only serous or cellular infiltration may be present, although features of adipose tissue necrosis that depend on the intensity of the trigger or the individual disposition may have preceded it.

1. Nodular febrile nonsuppurative panniculitis (Pfeifer-Weber-Christian syndrome) has the greatest clinical significance and is also the most extensive disorder of the subcutaneous and visceral fatty tissue. Predominantly affecting the trunk, the proximal extremities, and the face, subcutaneous pea- to fist-sized inflammatory nodes or palm-sized, plaquelike infiltrates appear, apparently spontaneously. The skin covering these usually tender nodes shows transitory redness or formation of edema. More severe colliquation or spontaneous perforation is rare. A new area of panniculitis may be provoked artificially but this is similarly rare and occurs chiefly only during subactivity. The onset of fresh areas of panniculitis is usually accompanied by episodes of fever. Healing will leave an indented surface and also, infrequently, muscular atrophies, which do not permit any speculation as to the causative disorder. The activity of the disease can be demonstrated in laboratory tests. In the florid stage ESR, SGOT, SGPT, and aldolase activities are increased. Concomitant anemia and leukocytopenia, however, can still be confirmed a long time after the disappearance of the acute manifestations. The prognosis is determined not only by the possibility of a fulminant septic-hyperergic recurrence after many years of afebrile behavior, but also by possible myocardial involvement, granulocytopenia, massive hemorrhagic diathesis following coagulopathy (from too much medication), as well as phlebitides and endangiitides. Histologically, there are usually three stages following each other quite regularly. They are, first, a reticularly arranged grouping of leukocytes, then the formation of a lipophagic granuloma, and finally its replacement by fibrosis. The small arteries, arterioles, and capillaries of the subcutaneous fatty tissue show angiitic changes in many patients. In etiologic-pathogenetic considerations it appears that in spite of a certain preference for young women, various primary diseases such as recurrent polyarthritis, tuberculosis, malignant lymphogranulomatosis, tonsillitis or other streptococcic hyperergies (for example, cholecystitis), or liver cirrho-sis can provoke nodular febrile nonindurative panniculitis.

In the differential diagnosis of nodular febrile panniculitis the following disorders should be mentioned: syphilitic-gummatous lesions deep in the subcutis or muscles; subcutaneous sporotrichosis or fixed abscesses following handling of artefacts (milk or turpentine); and, in fact, all nodose manifestations, especially erythema nodosum and erythema induratum with their similar primary or secondary processes in the fatty tissue. The latter two disorders, however, in contrast to nodular febrile panniculitis, lack the regular previously mentioned sequence of events with regard to tissue reactions, and, above all, the sometimes stormy and threatening course. If the latter is, however, too pronounced, one should consider the presence of a complicating sepsis with consecutive metastases in the subcutaneous fatty tissue (and frequently in the muscles as well). It should be mentioned that panniculitis is observed in typhus and less often also in typhoid or recurrent fever. 3, 4, 9, 10, 14, 16, 17, 19, 21, 24

2. The **syndrome of the metastasizing lipase-forming pancreatic adenoma** differs in its clinical signs from nodular febrile panniculitis in only a few points. The cutaneous changes are identical and do not permit any differentiation. Genuine Weber-Christian disease, however, favors young women; patients with the syndrome under discussion are mostly older men. Other clues are polyarthriticlike joint swellings and evidence of a tumor in the pancreatic region. This can be confirmed by palpation, roentgen rays, or laparoscopic means. Involvement of the joints in nodular febrile panniculitis is limited to arthralgias without swellings. Osseous changes such as necroses of the yellow marrow are considerably rarer. However, pancreatitides of different origin may likewise show these necroses. Important parameters are the increases of serum amylase and lipase

in the serum and urine. Almost always blood eosinophilia is present*.[11, 38]

3. Another important differential diagnosis of nodular febrile panniculitis is represented by the **panniculitis of lupus erythematosus.** Here it is a question of findings which occur in the course of disseminated lupus erythematosus. Firm and only rarely tender nodes of various sizes can be palpated in the subcutaneous fatty tissue. Usually the overlying epidermis is uninvolved; it can, however, be red from inflammation and even ulceration. Predilection sites of such areas of panniculitis are the forehead, chéeks, buttocks, and the proximal parts of the extremities. Some patients note that the areas of panniculitis occur at the site of a mechanical trauma. Healing progresses as in any other deeply located panniculitis process with shallow depressions, which may be circularly arranged. The question arises whether the instances so far described of lipoatrophia anularis were not fatal cases of lupus erythematosus. If the simultaneous and typical cutaneous changes of lupus erythematosus were lacking, the correct diagnosis can only be presumed. It has to be secured by the presence of antinuclear factors and immunofluorescent serologic examinations. [35]

4. In older children, preferentially on the lower extremities, small pea- to cherry-sized nodes, which are multiple but few in number, appear without fever or noticeable impairment of general health.

They are usually caused by **subcutaneous lipogranulomatosis of the Rothmann-Makai type.** Usually, the skin over such nodules remains unaffected or shows perhaps slight edema. Occasionally, however, such lipogranulomas may perforate. In contrast to nodular febrile panniculitis, all general signs and indications of involvement of inner

---

* The histopathologic picture is unique for this disease. (Tr.)

organs are missing. Histologically, subcutaneous lipogranulomatosis in its detailed processes does not differ from the various stages of Weber-Christian panniculitis. It is important that here also the disease process occurs only in the fat lobules, whereas this is not true in erythema nodosum and erythema induratum, in which the involvement of the fatty tissue occurs only contiguously.[2, 18, 24]

5. The **Darier-Roussy sarcoid,** which is etiologically nonhomogeneous, is almost always only a palpable disorder involving small nodules and is hardly ever visible. It occurs not only on the legs but also predominantly on the trunk and occasionally on the arms as well. Such pea-sized or rarely, walnut-sized nontender nodes may represent subcutaneous sarcoidosis, a deeper lying erythema induratum, or even panniculitis of lupus erythematosus. Therefore, a histologic examination is mandatory in all cases. Deep, subcutaneous, circumscribed scleroderma, however, develops in plaques and not in isolated nodules. Infiltrates of the so-called Darier-Roussy sarcoid, which are mostly symmetrical, lack all tendency to softening. Healing occurs as in all panniculitides with shallow depressions.

6. Poststeroid panniculitis is at present one of the most important of the diseases caused by drugs which affect the subcutaneous adipose tissue. It occurs eight to ten days after the end of oral high doses of steroid therapy. The nodes, about 1 to 4 cm in diameter, appear without generalized disturbances. The epidermis covering the nodes remains reaction-free. As in subcutaneous lipogranulomatosis, children are chiefly affected. The histologic examination of these spontaneously involuting nodes shows pathologic changes of the fat lobules exclusively, not of the septa. Besides needle-like holes, many lymphocytes, histiocytes, foam cells, and giant cell reactions to a foreign body are notable in the fat cells.

Multiple subcutaneous abscesses in the fat tissue have also been observed after **potassium iodide** medication. These necroses, however, which in the beginning simulate panniculitis, always lead to perforation and discharge of the necrotic tissue to the outside.[7]

7. In the large fatty cushions of the buttocks and the lower abdomen are found circumscribed, multiple firm tumors, so-called **pingranliquoses,** over which the covering skin is occasionally slightly bluish and delled. These cherry- to chicken egg-sized nodes contain a thin fluid fat in their interior because of an aseptic steatonecrosis. They are surrounded by a firm capsule of connective tissue, inside of which calcium deposits may be found. Spontaneous regression of these "fatty cysts" does not occur.[20, 36]

Cystic **fat necroses of the breast** look similar; the adipose female patients, however, cite trauma as the cause of these nodular formations. Since the skin overlying the nodes is distinctly red and may be folded like an orange peel, a mammary carcinoma is very often suspected. The diagnosis can be ascertained only by excision of a node.*[1, 8]

Following subcutaneous injections of drugs in oily solution or in soft paraffin for cosmetic reasons, the injection site (for example, face or breasts) may show oleomas or **paraffinomas.** If mineral oil has been injected, the histopathologic types predominating are oleogranulomas, oil cysts, and foreign body reactions including epithelioid and giant cells of the Langhans' and foreign body types. If, however, animal or vegetable oils have been injected, necrosis of the fat cells occurs as well as the picture of "sclerosing lipogranuloma" that is similar to the sequelae of fluid silicone

injections. Characteristic of this type of paraffinoma is an appearance resembling that of the cavities of Swiss cheese. This is caused by paraffin leaking out in small channels. Moreover, a striking vascularization with a perivascular grouping of lymphocytes and plasma cells, and to a lesser extent, of neutrophilic leukocytes can be observed, until a slowly developing fibrosis sets in. Because of this histopathologic picture, not to mention the history, it is always possible to differentiate this condition from cutaneous tuberculosis colliquativa or other cutaneous granulomas. If an adequate history is lacking, subcutaneous morphea or sarcoidosis may be considered, which, however, lack the "oil cysts." The significance of such oleomas for the patient lies in the possible sarcomatous degeneration,[5, 23] not to mention the subsequent tremendous disfigurement from the development of sagging and spreading livid swellings.

8. Panniculitis from cold occurs overwhelmingly in adipose women. It develops in two to three days at the site of a strong chilling effect on the fat tissue, as on a double chin, breasts, or buttocks, and forms deep cutaneous, succulent, tender nodes. Experimentally covering the fat tissue on any body site for two to three minutes with pieces of ice will cause the formation of nodes. If further exposure to cold is prevented, this panniculitis will heal without any residua.

Histologically an infiltrate rich in lymphocytes and eosinophils occurs in the fat tissue. Vascular changes and involvement of the cutis, however, are lacking. Similar damage from cold on the cheeks of children has been described as adiponecrosis e frigore. Around the second year of life this disposition, which leads to panniculitis, usually disappears.[6, 26]

9. The deeply located processes of subcutaneous fat tissue heal, as is known, with a boatlike or hollow contraction due to

---

* A histologic examination is also required. (Tr.)

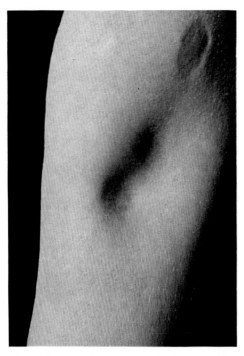

Fig. 104. Atrophy of the subcutaneous fat tissue after the injection of a crystalline cortisone deposit.

lipoatrophy. They have a striking appearance and demand differential diagnostic considerations. In the past, increasingly frequent lipoatrophies have occurred at the site of injection of **crystalline cortisone deposits** (Fig. 104). A stronger concentration of the crystalline suspension and insufficiently deep injections may be responsible for this occurrence. These cortisone lipoatrophies are not accompanied by inflammation and disappear after one or two years. Since the atrophy affects only the fat tissue, the cutaneous surface remains completely uninvolved. The reverse, however, may also happen, and an evidently very superficial cortisone infiltration can lead to thin atrophies of the Pasini-Pierini type of atrophoderma. **Localized panatrophy,** however, is caused by a partial or total loss of the subcutaneous fat layer in conjunction with atrophy of the underlying muscles and bones. Most patients are women between the second

and fourth decades. In these usually distinctly circumscribed places the atrophy of all structures in an area measuring several centimeters develops in a relatively short time (a few months), with no inflammatory phenomena. The affected areas, which almost always occur singly, are located on the back, buttocks, or extremities. In contrast to local cortisone lipoatrophy, reconstitution cannot be expected, even after a long time. It has not yet been decided if localized panatrophy is a disorder sui generis or only the result of other disorders (see also Chapter 16, A9). 15, 28, 31

10. Absence of fat tissue not only may occur in circumscribed areas but also may involve the entire subcutaneous fat tissue. Foremost is **generalized congenital lipodystrophy** (the Seip-Lawrence syndrome), which seems to be inherited as an autosomal recessive trait. In this disorder the extreme diminution of the fat tissue is strikingly apparent as early as birth. Later, often definite muscular hypertrophies develop. The diminution of the fat tissue affects not only the subcutis but also the fat tissue of the intestines and the bone marrow. In contrast, increased fat is stored in the hepatic cells and in the reticuloendothelial system. The fat values of the blood are also increased, so that some patients show eruptive xanthomas. Another manifestation, sometimes to a considerable degree, is hepatosplenomegaly. Many patients have a generalized enlargement of the heart. Mental development is mostly below normal, but somatic maturity exceeds the normal stage of development. The clinical picture is completed by insulin-resistant diabetes with no tendency to ketosis. Diabetes manifests itself usually as late as the tenth year of life; however, prior to that time appropriate tests would show a diabetic predisposition. To the dermatologist, the frequently simultaneous occurrence of acanthosis nigricans (Chapter 24, D20)

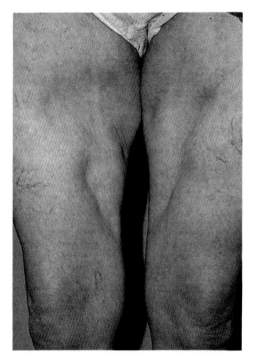

Fig. 105. Acquired generalized lipodystrophy.

and the distinctive hypertrichosis are of interest. [12, 21, 29]

Acquired generalized lipodystrophy occurs in general in children or young adults in the course of infectious diseases (Fig. 105). Here also the associated lipoatrophic insulin-resistant diabetes manifests itself after a few years. Loss of subcutaneous fat progresses step by step and reaches the same dimensions as in the congenital form. The remaining signs depend on the stage of mental development and that of the body at the time the disorder first appears. [29, 30]

Progressive lipodystrophy can probably be considered a partial lipodystrophy. The large majority of patients are girls and young women. Some patients have had a preceding infectious disease, but familial cases have also been observed. Characteristic of progressive lipodystrophy is the limitation of the vanishing fat to the face, arms, and upper parts of the body, whereas the amount of fat from the pelvis and

below is normal. The "skeletal" change of the face owing to the disappearance of the fat over the cheeks and the accentuation of the facial muscles is very conspicuous. Here also the combination with diabetes may occur some time after the disorder begins, but insulin-resistance is considerably less marked. [29, 30, 32, 33, 37]

(1) ADAIR, F. E., and J. T. MUNZER: Fat necrosis of the female breast, report of 110 cases. Amer. J. Surg. *74:* 117–128 (1947).

(2) BAUMANN, R.: Die Panniculitisformen unter besonderer Berücksichtigung der Spontanpanniculitis Rothmann-Makai. Ärztl. Wschr. *8:* 609–613 (1953).

(3) BELLONIAS, E., J. RAFTOPOULOS, F. COSTEAS and C. BARTSOKAS: Myocardial involvement in Weber-Christian disease. Vascular Dis. *2:* 140–148 (1965).

(4) BOSTELMANN, W., und K.-H. STRAUBE: Panniculitis nodularis (Pfeifer-Weber-Christian) mit begleitendem Skeletmuskelschaden. Hautarzt *15:* 235–242 (1964).

(5) COLOMB, D.: L'avenir des paraffinomes. Ann. Derm. Syph. (Paris) *89:* 36–46 (1962).

(6) DUNCAN, W. C., R. G. FREEMAN and CH. L. HEATON: Cold panniculitis. Arch. Derm. (Chic.) *94:* 722–724 (1966).

(7) FARKAS, G., und S. KÖSZEGVARY: Multiple subkutane Abszesse infolge Jodkali-Medikation. Med. Welt *1962:* 1934–1937.

(8) GORINS, A., R. EPFELBAUM, C. HELENON et M. FAVRE: Une observation exemplaire de cytostéatonécrose mammaire. Presse méd. *71:* 2766–2767 (1963).

(9) GOTTRON, H. A.: Krankheitszustände des subkutanen Fettgewebes. Med. Welt *1952:* 1211–1219.

(10) GOTTRON, H. A., und W. NIKOLOWSKI: Pfeifer-Christian-Webersche Krankheit in ihrer Nosologie und Pathogenese. Hautarzt *3:* 530–538 (1952).

(11) GRACIANSKY, P., A. PARAF et E. TIMSIT: Le problème de la maladie de Weber-Christian panniculite aigue fébrile récidivante au cours d'un cancer acineux du pancréas. Ann. Derm. Syph. (Paris) *93:* 503–529 (1966).

(12) GUIHARD, J., R. TESSIER, M. LANIECE, J.-P. FOUCAULT, J.-J. SIBIREFF et J. L'HIRONDEL: Diabète lipoatrophique (syndrome de Lawrence) (nouvelle observation). Ann. Pédiat. *18:* 633–643 (1971).

(13) HAXTHAUSEN, H.: Adiponecrosis e frigore. Brit. J. Derm. *53:* 83–89 (1941).

(14) JUCHEMS, R., und H. KAFFARNIK: Rezidivierende herdförmige Spontanpannikulitis bei Diabetes mellitus. Klin. Wschr. *42:* 574–577 (1964).

(15) KLÜKEN, N., und K.-H. GEIB: Kasuistischer Beitrag zur Panatrophia cutis localisata. Hautarzt *16:* 422–424 (1965).

(16) KORTING, G. W.: Afebrile, suppurative Pfeifer-Weber-Christiansche Erkrankung mit Herdprovozierbarkeit durch Schlag und körpereigene Streptokokkenvakzine. Derm. Wschr. *133:* 521–528 (1956).

(17) KÜNZER, W., H. LOHMANN, W. OEHLERT und M. STRAUCH: Verbrauchscoagulopathie bei Panniculitis nodularis febrilis non-suppurativa (Pfeifer-Weber-Christian). Klin. Wschr. *48:* 193–199 (1970).

(18) LAYMON, C. W., and W. C. PETERSON: Lipogranulomatosis subcutanea (Rothmann-Makai). Arch. Derm. (Chic.) *90:* 288–292 (1964).

(19) MacDONALD, A., and M. FEIWEL: A review of the concept of Weber-Christian panniculitis with a report of five cases. Brit. J. Derm. *80:* 355–361 (1968).

(20) MÜLLER, H., und U. KRAUL: Die Pingranliquose. Derm. Wschr. *153:* 583–589 (1967).

(21) PAMBOR, M., P. KEMNITZ und F. THEURING: Panniculitis nodularis febrilis »non-suppurativa« (Morbus Pfeifer-Weber-Christian) mit foudroyant-letalem Verlauf nach langjährigem, afebrilen Bestehen. Derm. Mschr. *155:* 330–339 (1969).

(22) REED, W. B., R. DEXTER, CH. CORLEY and CH. FISH: Congenital lipodystrophic diabetes with acanthosis nigricans. Arch. Derm. (Chic.) *91:* 326–334 (1965).

(23) REES, H. A.: Sclerosing lipogranuloma. Arch. Derm. (Chic.) *89:* 277–280 (1964).

(24) RÖCKL, H.: Die Bedeutung der Histopathologie für die Diagnostik knotiger Unterschenkel-Dermatosen. Hautarzt *19:* 540–547 (1968).

(25) ROENIGK JR., H. H., J. R. HASERICK and F. D. ARUNDELL: Poststeroid panniculitis. Report of a case and review of the literature. Arch. Derm. (Chic.) *90:* 387–391 (1964).

(26) ROTMAN, H.: Cold panniculitis in children. Arch. Derm. (Chic.) *94:* 720–721 (1966).

(27) SAWICKY, H. H., and N. B. KANOF: Sclerosing lipogranuloma. Arch. Derm. (Chic.) *73:* 264–265 (1956).

(28) SCHULZE, W., und E. KUNZE: Kritische Bemerkungen zur Panatrophia localisata. Derm. Wschr. *138:* 865–878 (1958).

(29) SEIP, M.: Generalized lipodystrophy. Ergebn. inn. Med. Kinderheilk. N.F. *31:* 59–95 (1971).

(30) SENIOR, B., and S. S. GELLIS: The syndromes of total lipodystrophy and of partial lipodystrophy. Pediatrics *33:* 593–612 (1964).

(31) SHELLEY, W. B., and A. K. IZUMI: Annular atrophy of the ankles. A case of partial lipodystrophy. Arch. Derm. (Chic.) *102:* 326–329 (1970).

(32) SIMONS, A.: Eine seltene Trophoneurose (»Lipodystrophia progressiva«). Z. Neurol. Psychiat. *5:* 29–38 (1911).

(33) SIMONS, A.: Lipodystrophia progressiva Z. Neurol. Psychiat. *19:* 377–397 (1913).

(34) SOLOMON, L. M., and H. BEERMAN: Cold panniculitis. Arch. Derm. (Chic.) *88:* 897–900 (1963).

(35) TUFFANELLI, D. L.: Lupus erythematosus panniculitis (profundus). Clinical and immunologic studies. Arch. Derm. (Chic.) *103:* 231–242 (1971).

(36) WASSNER, U. J.: Die Pingranliquose und ihre chirurgische Behandlung. Med. Welt *1962:* 1639–1642.

(37) WEBER, G., und W. G. ROTH: Lipodystrophia progressiva, eine Sklerodermie en coup de sabre simulierend. Arch. klin. exp. Derm. *229:* 194–204 (1967).

(38) WUKETICH, ST., und F. PAVLIK: Syndrom des metastasierenden lipasebildenden Pankreasadenoms. Arch. klin. exp. Derm. *216:* 412–426 (1963).

13. Buboes (Enlargement of Inguinal Lymph Nodes)

A. Venereal Infectious Diseases

1. Enlargement of the inguinal lymph nodes may be due to the presence of a venereal disease. Strongly suspicious for a diagnosis of **primary syphilis** is the finding of indolent, typically hard and movable, tumorous enlargements of the regional lymph nodes (which follow the chancre without fail "as the shadow follows the body"). The characteristic movability of the syphilitic bubo is due to the almost complete lack of periglandular inflammation; the same lack accounts for the typical absence of pain. On the other hand, primary lesions of the finger or mouth due to bacterial superinfection present more readily painful swellings of the cubital, axillary, or submandibular lymph nodes. The enlargement of the regional lymph nodes in primary syphilis develops about three to four weeks after the infection and about one week after the appearance of the chancre. About 15 to 25 days after the chancre becomes manifest, the local lymph nodes attain their largest size; this enlargement continues for several weeks and, therefore, outlasts the primary lesion. The skin overlying such grouped "pleiad-like" lymph nodes is neither red nor adherent, and syphilitic buboes do not form abscesses. Beginning with the superficial inguinal lymph nodes, other iliac or retroperitoneal lymphadenopathies will develop; they usually cannot be perceived clinically. These pelvic lymph nodes are especially significant in women with primary lesions of the cervix or of the neck of the uterus. If the primary lesion is absent, as it is in cases of transfusion syphilis or in congenital lues, generalized swellings of the lymph nodes hardly develop at all; the nodes of the groin cannot be felt (in congenital syphilis it is possible to palpate those of the cubital area or the sides of the thorax). Inguinal lymphadenitis seen in combination with general lymphadenitis and perhaps specific exanthems will permit a diagnosis of secondary syphilis; however, during the last few years such polyadenitis has become much less common than in former decades.

Histologically, the enlarged syphilitic lymph nodes show follicular lymphatic hyperplasia with a high degree of participation of plasma and epithelial cells. Sarcoidlike structures are rare. There may be fibrous thickening of the capsule, and later vascular changes of the periphery of the lymph nodes (endophlebitis and endarteritis). On the other hand, because considerably less characteristic types of lymphadenitis may occur, a definite diagnosis of syphilis requires demonstration of the spirochete (by means of lymph node puncture) or positive serology. This puncture is especially important when the swelling of the inguinal nodes obviously is the first manifestation of syphilis – i.e., when there have been no previous primary lesions.[2, 3, 4]

2. Gonorrhea, as compared to syphilis, shows lymphadenopathy extremely rarely; in such a case a mixed infection with chancroid or lymphogranuloma inguinale venereum must be excluded. Enlargements of lymph nodes in acute gonorrhea are transitory and are only slightly painful.

3. In the early stage of **lymphogranuloma venereum,** a vague, transitory (5 to 15 days duration), painless primary lesion, lymphangitis, and a few small lymph nodes should be kept under observation.

The most prominent sign of the disease occurs from within a few days to a few weeks after the primary lesion with the development of large knobby inguinal-iliac lymph nodes; they are firmly adherent to the epidermis and classically break through with the formation of fistulas, sometimes

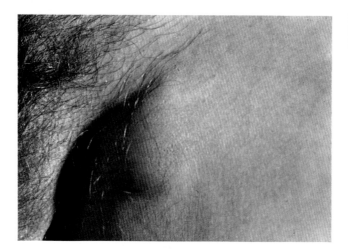

Fig. 106. Enlargement of the inguinal lymph nodes in lymphogranuloma inguinale.

accompanied by chills and fever. The skin overlying the enlarged lymph nodes (which may become as large as hens, eggs) is discolored, the hue varying from reddish-blue to brownish-violet (Fig.106). The enlarged glands soon can no longer be palpated as separate lymph nodes. After the fistulous tracts have dried up, retracted or funnel-shaped scars remain. Occasionally, such pyogenic fistulization will not take place. Characteristic is the spreading of the infection into the iliac group of lymph nodes; they do not suppurate, however. The late manifestations of lymphogranuloma venereum may give rise to malignant tumors similar to those in the genital region caused by sporotrichosis.

The Frei test is diagnostically important during the early period. An antigen derived from the pus of the buboes or from inoculation of the chorioallantoic membranes (Lygranum S.T. [Squibb]) is injected intradermally 0.1 ml; after 48 to 72 hours, if positive, a reddish papule measuring at least 0.6 cm will be seen. Biologic false-positive reactions may be the result of a florid ornithosis or psittacosis (since the virus belongs to the lymphogranuloma psittacosis group). There have been reports of positive Frei tests with plastic induration of the penis (Peyronie's disease). A further

diagnostic aid is the Miyagawanella complement fixation test (titer 1:160 and higher).

Pathologic-anatomic examination of the enlarged lymph nodes of this venereal disease shows them to be fused together with many stellate abscesses, but there is no caseation as in tuberculosis. These findings correspond closely to the clinical picture, which shows the development of many small abscesses and fistulous tracts breaking through the fused epidermis. Histologically, stellate abscesses in conjunction with a considerable increase of plasma cells can be seen within the residuum of the parenchyma. But the more marked reactions of the capsule observed in pasteurellosis or in cat-scratch disease are absent because abscess formation takes place more centrally.[1, 5]

4. Chancroid is characterized by sharply circumscribed, undermined multiple tissue defects (which have an incubation period of two to three days after intercourse); in about 90 per cent of cases these ulcerations are followed by the formation of buboes, first unilaterally and then bilaterally. Shortly after the appearance of the chancroidal ulcerations, griping pains in

Fig. 107. Ulcus molle: regional inflammatory enlargement of the lymph nodes.

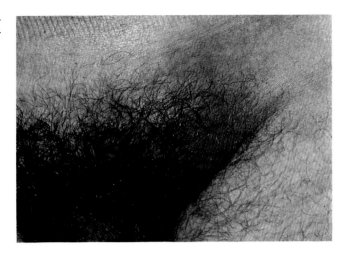

the inguinal region and an increase in temperature precede the enlargement of the inguinal nodes, which will take place some weeks afterwards or even after the ulcerations heal. The initial involvement of the lymph nodes close to the pubic symphysis is typical. The several groups of lymph nodes, which have now been formed, soon become suffused into larger connected conglomerates (periadenitis as opposed to "syphilitic polyadenitis"). The chancroidal bubo is very painful; it is attached to the underlying tissue and also to the slightly red epidermis; it may soon regress by resorption (Fig. 107). On the other hand, surprisingly rapid abscess formation and perforation may occur. The fistulization of chancroidal lymph nodes occurs in only one place with complete liquefaction; in lymphogranuloma venereum, on the other hand, formation of several fistulas occurs almost simultaneously. The chancroid bubo typically may be "strumous", fistulous, or even phlegmonous. As opposed to syphilis, chancroids may be accompanied by cordlike lymphangitis along the shaft of the penis, originating from the sites of the primary ulcerations. Along these lymphangitic cords nodular indurations, which for a long time have been called "bubonoli," may develop.

Histologically, the chancroid bubo shows follicular lymphatic hyperplasia, which soon presents small necroses; they spread in a maplike fashion, thus initiating the final abscess formation. As compared with syphilis, changes of the neighboring vessels are hardly noticeable, and compared with lymphogranuloma venereum with its bee-sting-like abscesses, chancroid shows large abscesses but lacks Langhans' giant cells; in syphilis the formation of abscesses is completely lacking.

(1) DEWALD, W.: Lymphogranuloma inguinale. Hautarzt 3: 337–342 (1952).
(2) GREITHER, A., und H. KLEIN: Syphilis durch Bluttransfusion, Klinik und Pathologie. Arch. Derm. Syph. (Berl.) 187: 569–585 (1949).
(3) HARTSOCK, R. J., L. W. HALLING and F. M. KING: Luetic lymphadenitis: a clinical and histologic study of 20 cases. Amer. J. Clin. Path. 53: 304–314 (1970).
(4) KRESBACH, H.: Zum gegenwärtigen Bild der Frühsyphilis. Z. Haut- u. Geschl.-Kr. 43: 109–118 (1968).
(5) SONCK, C. E.: Lymphogranuloma inguinale. Klinische, epidemiologische und immunologische Aspekte. Hautarzt 23: 280–286 (1972).

B. Nonvenereal Infectious Diseases

1. Analogous to chancroid and lymphogranuloma venereum, inherently pathogenic **pyogenic bacteria,** especially staphylococci, may quickly give rise to abscess-forming inflammations of the lymph nodes. Such a "respectable" bubo is usually caused by erosive ulcerated pyodermas of the legs, occasionally even by hardly noticeable infected fissures of the interdigital spaces of the feet. The same is true of secondarily infected herpes progenitalis, paraphimosis, or condylomata acuminata.

2. Cat-scratch disease is closely related to lymphogranuloma venereum, and both are classified as Miyagawanella. Both diseases can be definitely diagnosed by a papular skin reaction performed with an antigen obtained from the pus of a lymph node (Frei test or Mollaret-Debré antigen). The clinical picture presents an inconspicuous primary lesion at the port of entry of the virus, followed by involvement of the lymph nodes of the regional lymphatic drainage area. If such lymphadenitis is located at the genitals a pseudovenereal character may result, with only a slight, hardly painful swelling of one or two lymph nodes; general signs are very mild with occasional monocytosis in the blood smear. Abscess formation or perforation is rare. Such lymph nodes may reach the size of a small apple or a ping-pong ball (Fig. 108). A cut surface of a node shows a reddish-grey surface with a few yellowish-grey areas near the capsule; histologically, the dominant findings are a "follicular" reticulum cell lymphatic hyperplasia with development of large germinal centers and occasional abscess-forming granulomas.[1, 3]

3. Tularemia, like cat-scratch disease, rarely starts with a primary lesion in the genital area. As a rule the source of the infection is found on the hands, therefore affecting the cubital and axillary groups of lymph nodes. The oculoglandular type and the ulcerogranulomatous conjunctivitides are still more frequent than "lymphadenitis inguinalis tularemica." The clinical history is important for the diagnosis, i. e., contact with rodents* which harbor ectoparasites (deerflies or ticks). Further proof can be furnished through laboratory tests (agglutination, complement fixation, thermoprecipitation) or through the intracutaneous test with tularine (Foshay skin test). Histologically, the tularemic lymph node shows small granulomas with central necrobiosis, an intermediate ring with epithelioid and Langhans' cells, and an external perigranulomatous area. In contrast to tuberculosis and cat-scratch disease, the hemorrhagic component of the tularemic lymph node must be emphasized.[5, 6]

4. Although **leprosy** is of little importance in our latitude, it must be emphasized that regional lymph nodes may be slightly enlarged. In the early stages of leprosy and in association with fever and lepra reaction the inguinal nodes are the first ones to be enlarged.

5. In **plague,** especially bubonic plague, changes in the lymph node system are of first importance. Following an old custom, swellings of the extragenital lymph nodes are also called buboes. This may have originated from the fact that in more than half of the cases the affected lymph nodes show inguinal localization and would therefore be buboes according to present usage. The painful tension caused by the swollen nodes of the groin results in flexion of the lower extremity while the patient is in the recumbent position.[4]

6. A number of **mycoses,** such as American and European blastomycosis, histoplasmosis, or sporotrichosis, may involve the lymph nodes. Sporotrichosis especially shows not only axillary but also inguinal

---

* Such as wild rabbits and muskrats. (Tr.)

Fig. 108. Cat-scratch disease:
swelling of the submental
lymph nodes.

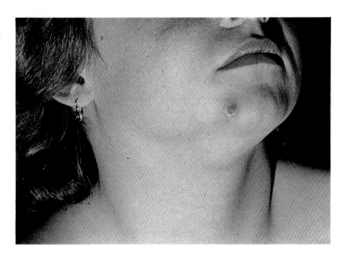

lymphadenitis. This adenitis always starts with an ulcerated chancriform primary lesion from which there is a retrograde lymphatic spread of the infection. Each enlarged lymph node remains indolent and does not tend primarily toward abscess formation. Painful nodes indicate super-infection, and if in doubt, the diagnosis of sporotrichosis should be reevaluated. The patient suffering from sporotrichosis does not feel sick, whereas the patient with tularemia has larger swellings of lymph nodes and shows certain general signs of sickness. Histologically, the PAS reaction is a useful method for demonstrating fungus elements.

7. **Actinomycosis** only rarely involves abscesses of lymph nodes (the pus shows "drusen", or rosettes of granules). This disease basically favors hematogenous spread. However, actinomycosis of the soft tissue with its boardlike, reddish-livid, and polyfistulous infiltrates has a tendency to invade the cutis and subcutis and not infrequently affects bony tissue. From a topographic standpoint the most frequent location is the face and neck, where actinomycosis is frequently observed after trauma (tooth extraction, fractures, or mucous membrane injuries, for example).

8. A "strumous" or fluctuating bubo observed in the temperate zone suggests **tuberculosis,** which may occur as an independent disease of the inguinal lymphatic tissue. As a rule, tuberculosis of the lymph nodes does not appear isolated in the groin only, but in conjunction with scrofuloderma of the lateral neck region or the axillas. One should always look for manifestations in other organs also. Compared to sarcoidosis, in lymphonodular tuberculosis the tuberculin test is strongly positive. Further diagnostic proof can be obtained by finding the tubercle bacillus either in material from a puncture or in surgically obtained tissue.[2, 7]

As long as only enlargement of lymph nodes occurs, with no signs of abscess formation, the differential diagnosis must consider **sarcoidosis.** This disease more frequently involves peripheral lymph nodes than any other organ. In general, nodes of any region may be affected; however, the inguinal region is one of the more rarely involved lymphonodular manifestation sites. The enlarged sarcoidal nodes are painless, firmly elastic, and freely movable without adhering to the tissue above or below. The differential diagnosis in such cases must consider either tuberculosis or malignant lymphogranulomatosis. In addition to biopsy and examination for manifestations in other organs, the Kveim reaction is important. In this connection the differential diagnosis must include either sarcoidlike or, even more frequently, tuberculoid lymphadenopathies that occur within the regional lymph drainage system of the various malignant tumors.[8.]

(1) BREHM, G., und B.-K. JÜNGST: Zur Klinik und Epidemiologie der sog. Katzenkratzkrankheit. Dtsch. med. Wschr. *90:* 1331–1334 (1965).

(2) EISSNER, H.: Skrofulöser Bubo. Med. Welt *1961:* 1310–1315; 1347–1350.

(3) HEDINGER, C.: Die histologischen Veränderungen bei dér sog. Katzenkratzkrankheit, einer benignen Viruslymphadenitis. (»Maladie des griffes de chat, lymphoréticulose benigne d'inoculation«). Arch. path. Anat. *322:* 159–174 (1952).

(4) KRAMPITZ, H. E.: Pest. In: Infektionskrankheiten. Hrsg. O. GSELL und W. MOHR. Bd. II/1, S. 325–344. Springer, Berlin, Heidelberg, New York 1968.

(5) REICH, H.: Zur Kenntnis der Tularämie hautnaher (regionaler) Lymphknoten. Arch. Derm. Syph. (Berl.) *192:* 175–188 (1950).

(6) REICH, H.: Die Tularämie. Hautarzt *3:* 385–390 (1952).

(7) RODER, H., und K. HORN: Zur Differentialdiagnostik des Bubo. Derm. Mschr. *155:* 917–922 (1969).

(8) SCADDING, J. G.: Sarcoidosis. Eyre & Spottiswoode, London 1967.

C. Noninfectious Diseases

1. Malignant lymphogranulomatosis may begin with the enlargement of several groups of lymph nodes close to the skin of the neck or the axillas; they can be grasped like potatoes in a sack. The consistency of these knotty packages is variable. At first the enlarged lymph nodes are rather soft, later they become more firmly fibrous. In any case, it is rare for these enlarged nodes to begin in the groin. If there is any doubt, an early biopsy can provide a definite diagnosis.

2. Mycosis fungoides, the other systemic reticulogranulomatosis, almost always lacks lymph node swelling. Part of the lymph node changes accompanying mycosis fungoides are merely due to the presence of exudative infiltrates or oozing patches in general, or, so to speak, to a neighboring reaction caused by secondary infection. Above all, the possibility of a dermatopathic lymphadenitis (lipomelanotic reticulosis) should be considered as in all other primary or secondary erythrodermas. Although mycosis fungoides seldom shows lymph node enlargement, the inguinal nodes would be affected if any enlargement existed. A histologic examination of such nodes would yield no etiologic information.

3. The **reticuloses,** in the narrow sense, quite frequently show lymphadenopathy but without the groups of enlarged palpable lymph nodes that occur in malignant lymphogranulomatosis. The epidermis covering such enlarged nodes is not especially discolored nor is it attached to them. The lymph nodes of reticuloses are hardly ever as hard as the enlarged nodes accompanying malignant tumors. Histologically, the normal reticulum cells of lymph nodes are slowly displaced by the growth of cell elements of reticulosis, and finally the normal lymph node tissue dis-

appears completely. It can be very difficult to distinguish between real reticulosis
on the one hand, and, on the other, reticular growth within the epidermis and lymph
node region; such growth represents a copy
of reversible responses to external stimuli.
A well-known example of such a stimulus
is the reticular **lymph node hyperplasia**
caused by hydantoin and its derivatives.[2]

4. Lipomelanotic reticulosis, mentioned
before, consists of a nonspecific reaction of
the reticulum cells of the lymph node
caused by deposits of fat, melanin, or
hemosiderin; this happens in a wide
variety of different skin diseases. Cytologically, this elementary reaction involves
foci of increased numbers of reticulum
cells; this proliferation probably is due
mainly to the deposition of melanin. In
addition, admixtures of eosinophils, plasma
cells, and others accompany the development of such lymph node reactions. Clinically, mostly solitary groups of lymph
nodes, plum-sized or larger, are observed,
chiefly in males beyond the fifth decade.
These groups of nodes are hard and firm,
do not coalesce, and have no tendency to
abscess formation or fistulization. Such
enlarged regional lymph nodes have been
known for a long time as inguinal or
axillary *buboes of prurigo*. Today, such
dermatopathic lymphadenitis is observed
primarily in *erythrodermas of the senile
seborrheic type* or as *benign hyperplastic
cutaneous reticulohistiocytosis with melanoderma*. Almost always patients with
erythroderma suffer from intractable pruritus and show marked eosinophilia of the
blood. Such a lipomelanotic reticulosis can
be differentiated without difficulty histologically from a *large follicular lymphoblastoma* and from malignant reticulosis
because the lymph node structures as a
rule remain free of pigment; occasionally
the perinodular space, including the capsule, is infiltrated. A lymph node *metastasis of a melanoma* will frequently show
abundant deposits of melanin, but there
will be other cell proliferations of a
heterogeneous character as well.[1]

(1) KABOTH, W.: Die cutane Reticulohistio-
cytose mit Melanodermie. Z. Haut- u.
Geschl.-Kr. *33:* 69–76 (1962).
(2) KORTING, G. W., und R. DENK: Retikuläre Hyperplasie der Haut durch ein
Hydantoin-Derivat. Derm. Wschr. *152:*
257–262 (1966).

14. Abscesses and Fistulas

A. Abscesses

1. The essential nature of an **abscess**
involves central liquefaction or sequestration of an area of tissue infiltrated with
leukocytes. The accumulation of pus is not
visible because it is located subepidermally or deeper, and ordinarily can be felt
only as a fluctuation of such an inflammatory tumor. The breakthrough of the
abscess through the epidermis by fistulization leads to its evacuation. A *furuncle*
results from the entry of pathogenic
organisms along the funnel of the follicle
into the skin; this is followed by destruction of deeper tissue as in an abscess.

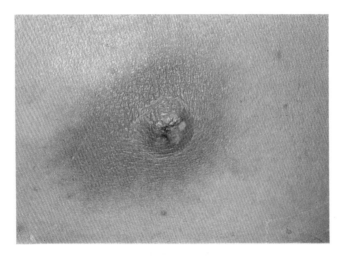

Fig. 109. Furuncle.

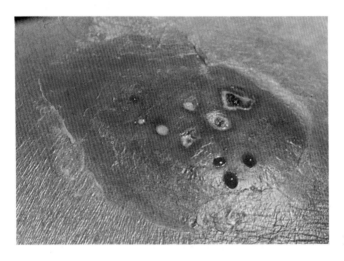

Fig. 110. Carbuncle.

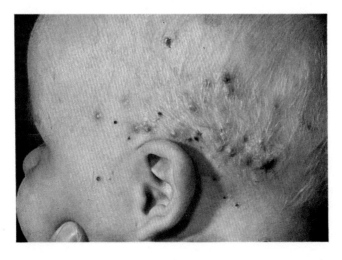

Fig. 111. Multiple abscesses
of the eccrine sweat glands.

The **furuncle** is a special type of folli-cular, mostly staphylococcic pyoderma and can therefore assume various forms (Fig. 109). If several furuncles coalesce into a larger cluster, a **carbuncle** develops (Fig. 110). **Furunculosis** indicates the re-currence of multiple furuncles. Such an event calls for an investigation of consti-tutional factors such as diabetes, granulo-cytopenia, or lack of immunoglobulins. Septic distant metastases from a furuncle, as for instance a subsequent abscess of the lung or osteomyelitis, are rare. On the other hand, some special localizations of a furuncle cause certain complications rela-tively often, i. e., a location on the nose or the upper lip (thrombosis of the cavernous sinus via the vena angularis and ophthal-mica, or thrombosis of the jugular vein via the vena facialis). A beginning furuncle of the nose may be difficult to differentiate from erysipelas. Although there can be superficial redness of the entire nose or the ala nasi, in most cases the beginning furuncle presents a circumscribed painful infiltration, and inspection of the nasal cavity will show follicular redness or formation of a pustule. The patient will not develop fever as long as there are no complications. However, erysipelas will present impressive constitutional signs rather early (chills and high fever). A furuncle of the external ear canal frequent-ly evokes pain when the lobule of the ear is pulled or during chewing. If increased edema of the vicinity occurs, mastoiditis must be ruled out; in this condition pulling the lobule of the ear will not give rise to pain, but the doughy swelling over the mastoid process is tender upon slight palpation.[2]

2. Axillary abscesses develop at the site of the **apocrine glands** as an equivalent, so to speak, of the furuncle. In general, young women develop axillary hidradenitis dur-ing the hot summer months. Apocrine abscesses in adults are seen almost exclu-sively in the axillae and only rarely in the genitoanal or mamillary regions. At first, bluish-red nodules appear, either uni-laterally or bilaterally; they adhere to the epidermis and are freely movable against the epidermis and the subcutis. As opposed to furuncles, which are hardly ever seen in the axillae except perhaps at the edge, abscesses of the sweat glands liquefy or discharge in toto. Therefore, the typical pluglike piece of tissue is lacking. But the infiltration around a single fluctuating or fistulizing sweat gland may develop into phlegmonous infiltration of the entire axillary region; this condition may be accompanied by a great deal of pain and a rise in temperature. In contrast to eccrine sweat gland abscesses, superficial pustules which develop simultaneously are absent. The causes of axillary hidradenitis fre-quently are local traumas (such as dress shields or depilatories). It should be men-tioned that deodorant sticks containing zirconium give rise to papular granulomas (but not abscesses); these growths look histologically extraordinarily like sarcoidal granulomas.

Multiple eccrine sweat gland abscesses of infants are seen mostly in very small, dystrophic babies in body areas subject to pressure from lying (occiput, buttocks) (Fig. 111). Frequently these abscesses are accompanied simultaneously by febrile attacks and the development of typical deep or subcutaneous pea-sized, bluish-red nodules with many pustules surrounded by a red halo ("periporitis").

3. Solitary or multiple abscesses may be the result of self-administered unclean injections by addicts. These abscesses are found within reach of the hand used for the injection. The same is true for inten-tionally caused furunculoid **artefacts,** which can be produced by injections of milk or by pricking the skin with foreign bodies (x-ray examination may be neces-sary) (Fig. 112). In every case such patients should undergo psychiatric examination.[1]

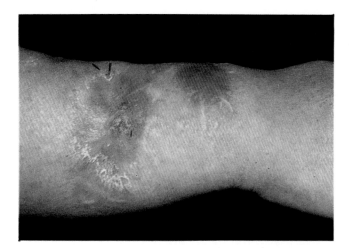

Fig. 112. Abscesses caused by pricks from spines of cacti.

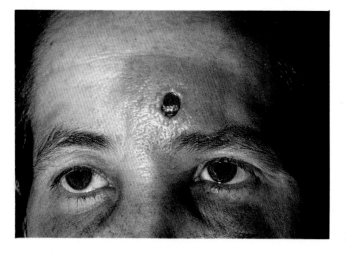

Fig. 113. Anthrax pustule.

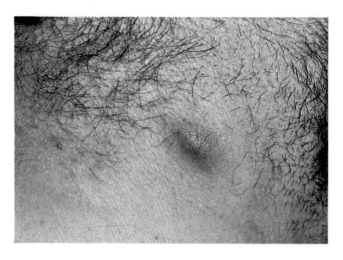

Fig. 114. Tumbu myiasis: furunculoid infiltrate.

4. The carbuncle of **anthrax** and its accompanying edema are observed in 95 per cent of all cases of cutaneous anthrax. Its preferred site is the uncovered skin (hand, forearm, face) where it appears as a slowly growing, papular lesion of bluish-black color (Fig. 113). As a rule, the patient suffering from the carbuncle of anthrax will deny pronounced tenderness, in contrast to the patient with an acute furuncle; on further questioning the patient will state that prior to the now visible blackish eschar there was a rapidly disintegrating pustule. Only on the second day of cutaneous anthrax do septic temperatures and pain in limbs and joints occur; at this time the eschar is surrounded by fresh vesicles and a tight but not especially painful infiltration of the periphery. Most patients suffering from anthrax belong to certain occupations such as butchers, veterinarians, and workers in abattoirs and paint or shaving brush factories.

5. Tumbu myiasis* presents furuncle-like infiltrates. This disease exists all over Africa with the exception of the northern

---

* Caused by the active maggot of the tumbu fly. (Tr.)

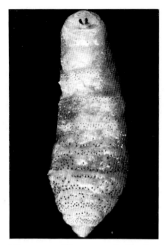

Fig. 115. Maggot of *Cordylobia anthropophaga.*

part; actual cases can be seen in the temperate zone owing to the rapidity of modern intercontinental traffic. The female of the tumbu fly (*Cordylobia anthropophaga* of the Calliphorida family) deposits her eggs in soil that is preferred as a resting place by warm-blooded animals. After only 48 hours the larvae leave the eggs; at first the young maggots remain close under the surface but when stimulated by vibrations or heat they appear in the open. Holding themselves erect, they wave their bodies until they come in

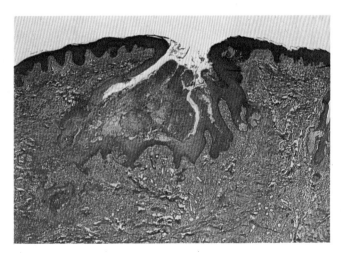

Fig. 116. Tumbu myiasis: fistular duct with pseudo-epitheliomatous hyperplasia. HE stain, 25×.

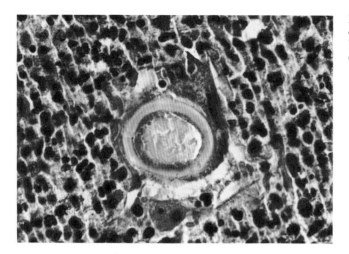

Fig. 117. Tumbu myiasis: exuviae (slough) surrounded by granulocytes in the corium. HE stain, 400×.

contact with an animal host, mainly rats; almost imperceptibly they penetrate the skin of the host. After the second shedding a furunculoid inflammation (Figs. 114, 116, 117) produced by the larva develops around the cavity in the skin; about two weeks later the larva bores itself out in retrograde fashion and forms a pupa in the soil. The larvae of the tumbu fly attack mostly children and nonresidents because local immunity develops after the first infection; the result is that renewed attempts at penetration of a formerly diseased part of the host's skin cause such a pronounced local edema that the tiny larvae quickly die in this edematous tissue.[4, 6]

6. The differential diagnosis of furuncles and carbuncles must include **deep trichophytosis.** The condition starts with superficial areas of trichophytosis, followed by perifollicular inflammation, pustulation, and liquefaction of tissue; with the appearance of flat or semispherical conglomerates, pressure from the side causes discharge of pus through multiple openings. Hairs can easily and painlessly be removed with a pair of forceps from such an area of deep trichophytosis (Fig. 118). On the bearded region of the face furunculoid nodes frequently coalesce into extensive infiltrates with vegetating granulations and multiple fistulous ducts. The diagnosis depends on finding the trichophyton fungus with proper consideration of the secondary bacterial invaders.

Fig. 118. Tinea profunda (deep trichophytosis).

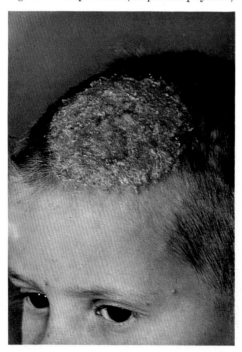

7. Glanders (malleus) is an acute or chronic infectious disease of solid-hoofed animals caused by *Malleomyces mallei*. Encountered in those who handle horses and cattle, it starts with prodromal general signs (fever and headache). Initially, not only is there a primary pustule with consecutive lymphangitis but also furunculoid or acute inflammatory nodular infiltrates are observed as well. The subsequent course of the disease, after the lymphangitis in conjunction with the primary lesion, is characterized by intensive involvement of the lymphatics. The German lay term "Rotz" (mucoid nasal discharge) refers to the pronounced nasal discharge seen in glanders. The nose and upper respiratory pathways show erysipelaslike involvement. The disease becomes generalized with muscular and joint pains and the appearance of boil-like cutaneous manifestations of the skin, which soon begin to ulcerate. The erysipelaslike signs may persist in protracted form for years in the chronic type of glanders, while the involvement of the lymphatics and lymph nodes becomes less conspicuous. The clinical picture by itself may permit a tentative diagnosis of glanders. Erysipelas and gummatous lesions of different origin (syphilis, for example) should be considered. To verify a suspected diagnosis of glanders it is necessary to puncture a closed abscess and to examine the punctate microscopically, as well as by culture and animal inoculations. (Intraperitoneal injection in a male guinea pig results in testicular swelling – Straus' reaction.) In addition, sero-reactions (complement fixation tests, serum agglutination tests) can be performed. However, the intracutaneous mallein test is unreliable.

8. Subacute or chronic **sporotrichosis** takes place almost exclusively in the subcutaneous cellular tissue, appearing as furunculoid or gummalike cutaneous infiltrates, especially on the extremities.

Although in some cases more acneiform or verrucoid lesions (similar to those of tuberculosis cutis verrucosa) have been observed, as well as erythematous desquamating changes, the almost always multiple sporotrichotic granuloma is the more important lesion. Lymphangitic sporotrichosis is especially characteristic, having separate subacute, movable nodes which later adhere to the bluish-red epidermis. Similar to a "gumma," these almost painless nodes, which are arranged along the hard lymph vessels like a string of pearls, present purulent abscesses. As a rule, they extend no further than from the hand to the axilla. This close connection to the lymph vessels in itself shows the difference between sporotrichotic gummas and the softening of nodes in other infectious diseases (e. g., tuberculosis, syphilis); however, ulcerating gummas of sporotrichosis with sharply circumscribed borders may closely resemble crateriform, tertiary syphilitic lesions. But whereas an ulcerated syphilitic gumma will soon heal with scar formation, the postgummatous ulcers of sporotrichosis may show only a covering crust with continued undermining abscess formation. Furthermore, sporotrichosis may also disseminate by metastasizing. In addition to the typical nodes, small papular or pustular lesions may appear, and also ecthymalike or frank furunculoid manifestations; they resemble either common pyodermas or superficial ecthymalike lesions of malignant syphilis. Sporotrichosis may also present as a subcutaneous platelike manifestation that resembles erythema induratum, which, however, is more stationary and rarely shows the tendency to colliquation of sporotrichosis, although it may ulcerate. With regard to involvement of the lymph nodes, lymphadenopathy due to sporotrichosis is extremely rare. The clinical polymorphism of sporotrichosis makes it necessary to verify the diagnosis not only by culture and animal inoculation (peritonitis and orchitis two to three weeks

after injection of the sporotrichotic pus
into the abdominal cavity or the testes of
white rats), but also histologically. On
histologic examination the gumma of
sporotrichosis presents three different
zones, the central one of which shows areas
of leukocytes, bleeding and, less distinctly,
necroses. Then follows a zone of tuberculoid structures with histiocytes, epithelioid cells, and Langhans'-like giant cells.
The peripheral zone consists of proliferation of connective tissue with plasma cells,
fibroblasts, and lymphocytes. However, in
spite of this structural arrangement the
histologic picture of sporotrichosis can
hardly be called specific, because tuberculoid tissue reactions are also definitely
present in tertiary syphilitic nodes. Recently the performance of the PAS-reac-
tion after prior thorough application of
amylase (to facilitate microscopic examination by removing the glycogen present in
leukocytes and necrotic particles) has
appreciably enhanced success in the
search for spores of *Sporothrix schenckii*
and, especially, for asteroid bodies.[3, 5]

(1) BERZEWSKI, H., H. LEONHARDT und V.
    MISGELD: Artefakte unter dem Bild
    einer Furunkulose und haemorrhagi-
    schen Diathese: Aufdeckung und psych-
    iatrische Problematik. Med. Klin. *67:*
    1671–1676 (1972).
(2) DOBERKE, C., und H. ALFF: Lungen-
    abszeß nach Gesichtsfurunkel. Med.
    Welt *18* (N. F.): 2177–2178 (1967).
(3) ITANI, Z.: Die Sporotrichose. Hautarzt
    22: 110–113 (1971).
(4) PETERS, H., und S. KRAMER: Zur
    Differentialdiagnose der Myiasis cutanea
    in der ärztlichen Praxis. Hautarzt *17:*
    195–201 (1966).
(5) STROUD, J. D.: Sporotrichosis presenting
    as pyoderma gangrenosum. Arch. Derm.
    (Chic.) *97:* 667–670 (1968).
(6) SUNDHAUSEN, G., R. DENK und G. W.
    KORTING: Cordylobia anthropophaga.
    Med. Welt *23* (N. F.): 75–76 (1972).

B. Fistulas

1. Fistulas in the maxillary-facial region
always demand a thorough clinical and
roentgenologic investigation. Usually they
are **extraoral dental fistulas,** and develop
via caries, pulpitis, decomposing pulpa,
and involvement of the apex of the root as
chronic granulating inflammations. In
general, the openings of dental fistulas
start in the maxilla at the first molar and
canine tooth; in the mandible, however,
they start at the third molar. In the
maxilla this results in a predilection for the
nasolabial folds and the inner and outer
angles of the eyes, and in the mandible, in
areas medial and lateral to the masseter
muscles, on the chin, and in the floor of the
mouth. Depending on acuity and extent,
there may be fluctuating, slightly painful
red swellings, which may be associated
with enlargement of the regional lymph
nodes. The fresh dental fistula has a slender
opening inside a small wall of granulation.
If this "mouth of the fistula" becomes
clogged, the duct becomes more purulent,
making the connection between the dental
apex and the cutaneous infiltration distinctly palpable. If, however, the fistula
is chronic, the scar is indented like a funnel
and is firmly attached to the underlying
osseous parts (Fig. 119). This firm "attachment" of the dental fistula with its osseous
base is contraindicative of a common
perifolliculitis, an abscess of the soft
tissue, or a purulent atheroma.[17, 19]

2. In contrast to fistulas originating at
the teeth, **congenital cervical fistulas** are
easily recognizable because of their special
location. Median fistulas originating at the
branchial cleft (thyroglossal duct) are rare
and usually represent blindly ending malformations situated at the level of the
thyroid cartilage or jugular fossa (Fig. 20).
The more frequent lateral congenital cervical fistula is always present at birth and
originates because of the persistence of an
intrafetal connection between the second

and third branchial clefts and the corresponding branchial furrows. It ends at the
anterior margin of the sternocleidomastoid
muscle and if "complete," is connected
with the pharynx. The question of whether
a fistula is complete or incomplete can be
solved either by injection of a sugar solution (sweet taste) or by injection of a dye
into the outer opening of the fistula. Occasionally, a mucuslike fluid exudes spontaneously from the cutaneous opening of the
fistula. The lining of such a dysontogenetic
cervical duct consists of several layers of
keratinizing squamous or cylindric ciliated
epithelium. Usually these fistulas and
cysts cause only mild complaints.[11, 20, 23]

3. In contrast to these dental and cervical fistulas, other dysontogenetic fistulas
in this location are less impressive, unless
certain complications draw attention to
them. A good example is the **congenital
auricular fistula,** which in most cases is
hereditary (Fig. 121). It is frequently
associated with other anomalies (auricular
appendages, for instance) or combined
with osseous anomalies. Its opening is
usually above and anterior to the tragus
and is occasionally connected with the
middle ear or pharynx. Its origin is linked

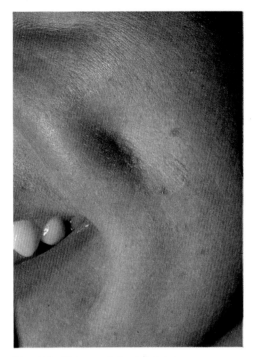

Fig. 119. Extraoral dental fistula.

either to the first branchial arch or to a
faulty coalescence of the auricular protuberances. Such auricular fistulas may
be accompanied by persistent eczemas
of the ear canal and, most important, by

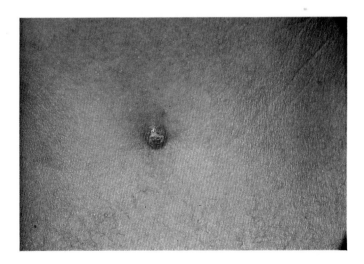

Fig. 120. Fistula of the
middle of the neck.

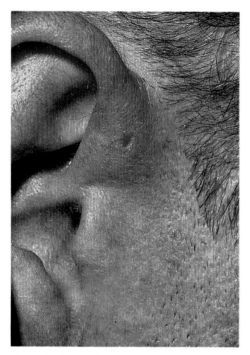

Fig. 121. Congenital fistula of the ear.

lymphocytomas located near such fistulas. Inflammations resembling lupus with a tuberculoid structure as well as those resembling foreign body granulomas may also accompany these fistulas.[3, 21]

4. Considerably rarer are **congenital nasal fistulas,** which superficially resemble common furuncles, sebaceous cysts, or meningoceles or encephaloceles. Occasionally, these dysontogenetic ducts, which are located medianly or paramedianly on the dorsum of the nose, appear only as point-sized indentations.

Labial fistulas on the lower lips appear symmetrically or asymmetrically as slit-like or round retractions. They occur not too rarely in persons with cleft palate or anomalies of the extremities. More frequent are dimples of the labial commissures, which may be explained by the long persistence of a perlèche.[5, 14, 22]

5. Fistulizating **forms of tuberculosis** are not easily confused with the overwhelmingly torpid, median or lateral congenital duct formations but may be mistaken for the above-mentioned dental fistulas. In addition, tuberculous fistulas are slowly progressive and secrete only intermittently. Often such fistulas are diagnosed as tuberculosis of the jaws only by roentgenology. Fistulizating **scrofuloderma** nowadays occurs more often in adults and more often in women than in men. It is a secondary lymphogenous and hematogenous form of tuberculosis. The deep cervical lymph nodes – i.e., the lymph nodes located between the mandibular angle and the anterior side of the sternocleidomastoid muscle in the lateral cervical triangle (Fig. 122) – are the first nodes affected by cervical lymph node tuberculosis. Clinically, the lesions appear as cordlike plaques, or more often, as nodes of a bluish-reddish hue, which are chronic and recurrent, and soften and rupture upon ulceration. Occasionally, however, they form fistulas and granulomas. Because of their tendency to expansion and their continuous development toward the surface, they become the classic "heralds" of lupus vulgaris, ascending step by step. Diagnosis is difficult if for the first weeks and months there is a node in the lateral cervical area that is only cherry-stone-sized, soft or hard, still easily movable, and with no surface change such as erythema or a cutaneous fold. In such instances an excision seems indicated to rule out leukemic lymphomas, which, however, usually occur bilaterally and with corresponding changes in the blood picture. Other possibilities are lymphogranulomatosis or lymphosarcoma or retothelial sarcomas.

In contrast to scrofuloderma, all these nodular formations, which are important in the differential diagnosis, lack to a considerable extent the rapidly developing fluctuation or softening. After the lesions are perforated, the appearance is that of a cold abscess or a serpiginous ulcerating granulating growth. Another characteristic of scrofuloderma is the irregular, partly keloidlike, and generally bulging or pointed forms of scarring.

Cutaneous colliquative tuberculosis usually appears on the chest and back of definitely dysergic older persons. Other sites of predilection of fistulous, tuberculous, softening areas of the skin are the buttocks and the perineum.[1, 4, 6, 8]

6. In contrast to these tuberculous liquefactions the analogous syphilitic lesion moves more rapidly toward fluctuation (2 to 6 weeks) and is firmer in its consistency. It is also less painful. Although the subcutaneous **syphilitic gumma** can develop theoretically anywhere on the body, its location at the usual site of a lymphonodular tuberculous scrofuloderma – i.e., the angle of the jaw – would be extremely rare. The final ulceration of the tertiary syphilitic gumma takes the shape of a hole or a kidney. If the gumma is connected with the bone, it is usually located on the skull or chest, or over the tibia. If there is a connection with a muscle, it is found mostly over the sternocleidomastoid muscle, the biceps, or the gastrocnemius muscles.

7. In contrast, **actinomycosis** favors the skin of the extremities as well as that of the face and neck. From these sites the disease progresses to deeper lying organs, mostly the muscles. On the other hand, actinomycosis may begin deep in the abdomen and involve the skin later. Usually a hard, boardlike, bluish-red infiltration (similar to a carcinomatous induration, among other things) of the soft tissue with several small fistulas and subsequent marked scar formation predominates (Fig. 123).

Human actinomycosis is caused by the anaerobic organism *Actinomyces israelii*. This organism is part of the normal oral flora and is facultatively pathogenic; thus actinomycosis in its cervicofacial as well as

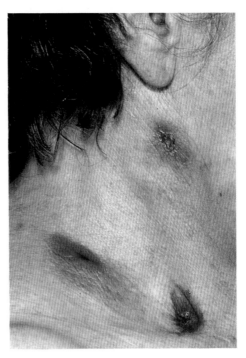

Fig. 122. Cutaneous scrofulodermas.

its thoracic pulmonary forms is an endogenous infectious disease. Of course, concomitant aerobic as well as anaerobic bacteria (among others, *Actinobacillus actinomycetemcomitans*) make actinomycosis a mixed infection basically.

In the acute stage actinomycosis of the jaw region may simulate a dental fistula or a phlegmon of the bottom of the oral cavity. If, however, the development is protracted, it may resemble an osteoma. Primary swellings of the parotid gland are also sometimes imitated. In view of such polymorphism, confirmation of the suspected clinical diagnosis should be sought in each case by proof of the so-called drusen (solid elements of the pus which can be recognized by the crunching noise that occurs when a cover glass is put on a slide with secretion) and by culture (Fortner plate with apathogenic *Serratia marcescens* as oxygen user) in special laboratories.

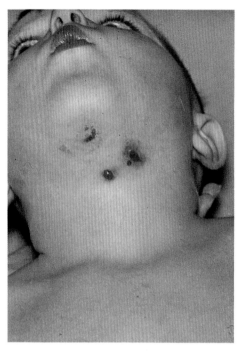

Fig. 123. Actinomycosis.

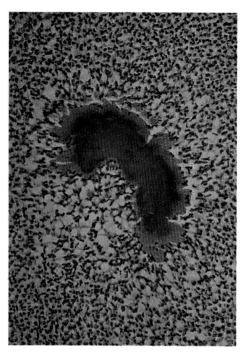

Fig. 124. Actinomyces drusen. HE stain.

Histologically, an unspecific, eosinophilic or plasmacellular, mixed granulation tissue is found. It contains the significant drusen, as mentioned before (mulberrylike, sulfuric- or brownish-yellow bodies, which are homogeneous in the center but have a clublike formation peripherally). Around these drusen a softening necrosis of many leukocytes takes place (Fig. 124).

In the differential diagnosis the clinical picture of boardlike infiltration with multiple fistulous openings, the site (angle of the jaw), and the history (fracture or dental extraction) permit a differentiation from tuberculous or syphilitic gummas. If the infiltration is less pronounced, however, the appearance may simulate ulceroserpiginous syphilis or chronic pyodermia.

8. In the sacral-coccygeal region, furunculoid and centrally fistulous inflammations often originate with the so-called dysontogenetic **pilonidal sinuses.** They occur approximately in the middle of the anal fold over the sacral canal, either as solitary or multiple furuncles or simulating a periproctitic abscess.

Generally, these cavities are lined with multilayered squamous epithelium. Their fistulous ducts become secondarily infected and they grow to the size of nodular protuberant infiltrations. If they remain abortive, they present only small, dimplelike indentations, or pigmented spots with a small central opening, and they can, therefore, be easily overlooked. The secondary infections just mentioned are in general first noticeable after puberty and occur especially after an external mechanical strain ("jeep disease").

Similarly, cystic or fistulous malformations are found in the region of the median raphe of the perineum and scrotum. If they are located deep in the perineum and para-medianly, they may be mistaken for cowperitis, whereas genuine furuncles ("pseudo-cowperitis") usually develop medianly.[7, 9]

The most important differential diagnosis in regard to the sacral or coccygeal fistulas concerns the so-called **anal fistula,** which brings the patient to the physician with complaints of pruritus, secretion, or difficulties with stool. If the buttocks are unfolded in such patients, a fistulous opening may not be seen because it may be covered temporarily by epithelium or because an inconspicuous pigment spot is present. Trans-sphincteral and ischiorectal fistulas are most frequent. The former discharge within a 3-centimeter zone around the anus, whereas the latter are outside this zone. To discover whether a complete fistula is present, methylene blue milk should be injected into the outer fistulous opening with a syringe having a head cannula. In the presence of a complete fistula, a piece of gauze inserted into the rectum would become blue.

9. Fistulization and adjacent perianal ulcerations and granulations demand that **regional enteritis (Crohn's disease)** be ruled out, which is easily done by roentgenologic examination of the small intestines. Before the appearance of fistulas and ulcerations, bluish-red edematous erythemas with condylomalike growths are present (Fig. 125). Occasionally, erythema nodosum accompanies the enteritis. Clinically, patients with Crohn's disease suffer from diarrhea with abdominal pain; they have fever, loss of weight, guarding of the abdomen, and anemia. The microscopic picture of these perianal changes accompanying regional enteritis is very similar to that of tuberculosis or sarcoidosis. Initially, edema and a cellular infiltration which finally destroys the structure of the glandular tissue are present. The focal infiltrates have a tuberculoid aspect, with many giant

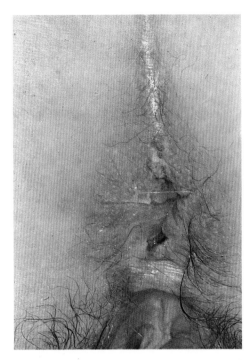

Fig. 125. Perianal fistulization in regional enteritis.

cells of either the foreign body or the Langhans' type. In other cases epithelioid cell granulomas, including Schaumann bodies, predominate. These sarcoidal histologic features differentiate these lesions from common fistulas. If the roentgenologic findings of the intestines are negative, the possibility of tuberculosis or a foreign body granuloma should not be completely overlooked.[13, 16, 24]

10. In the presence of extensive flat miliary or elevated ulcerative, granulating, or purulent-secreting perianal ulcerations **miliary tuberculosis of the mucous membrane and skin** with intestinal tuberculosis (which occurs in 10 per cent of all cases of mucous membrane tuberculosis) should doubtless be considered. It occurs anally or perianally (Fig. 126).

However, **subcutaneous fistulous tuberculosis,** if it occurs at this unusual location,

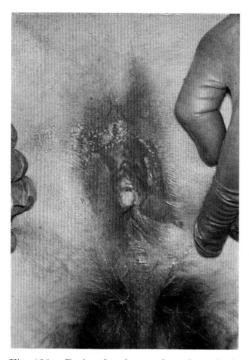

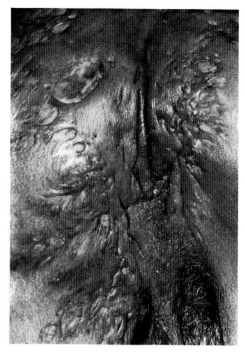

Fig. 126. Perianal ulcerated tuberculosis miliaris of the skin.

Fig. 127. Acne conglobata in the region of the perineum and buttocks.

will appear as an irregular invasion with semispherical protruding formations, in accordance with its scrofulodermatous character. The infiltrates on the buttocks and near the genital area generally do not soften but develop only thin fistulas to the outside. Occasionally, small papillomatous growths develop near the fistulous openings. Larger elephantiasic swellings are rare, and rectal strictures are never observed. Furthermore, **bacterial granulomas,** especially those that are chronic, deeply cutaneous, and enterococcic, may lead to nodular, abscess-forming and fistulizing changes in the perianal-buttock area, which heal with branching, keloid-like scars. For the diagnosis of these enterococcic granulomas, evidence of the causative organism in a pure culture is necessary, since many bacterial granulomas of these areas are caused by a mixed flora as well as by enterococci. These fox-

hole-like, fistulous and pocket-forming disorders of the skin and subcutaneous tissue never transgress the perianal or muscular fascias. The formation of fistulas and pockets stops, therefore, at the anal ring and rectum.[1, 6, 12]

11. If these multilocular, fistulous disorders also contain comedones, **acne conglobata** in the genitoperianal region (Fig. 127) is present. It shows typical, grouped, and giant comedones, bridging and pointed scars, and also "cutis laxa," which leads to the correct diagnosis.[2, 18]

12. Of the late manifestations of **lymphogranuloma venereum** the so-called genitoanorectal syndrome must be mentioned. It may develop many years after the infection as a consequence of the destruction of the inguinal and pararectal lymph nodes. Women are much more often affected than men. The first signs of the genitoanorectal syndrome are chronically persistent edemas of the genital and anal regions. Later, ulcerations, perianal fistulas, and fistulas between urethra, rectum, and vagina develop. Pararectal abscesses and fistulas develop when neighboring lymph node conglomerates become soft and break open. Besides these fistulas, strictures of the terminal intestines and the urethra are common. To confirm the diagnosis a Frei test should be performed, although it does not show a positive reaction in all patients. The chronic ulcerations may years later turn into malignant tumors.[15]

13. Many patients with **dracunculiasis** (guinea or Medina worm) have larvae-containing cysts beneath the skin on the legs and the buttocks; they cause no reactions, however. After the female worm has developed, it migrates through the skin into the open. Shortly before it breaks through the epidermis, the patient develops general signs with fever and lassitude. After the epidermis has opened, a secondary infection of the cysts and ducts, which up to this time had remained sterile, sets in, and deep cutaneous abscesses and furunculoid infiltrates appear. For other cutaneous changes see Chapter 25, B8.[10]

(1) BEUTNAGEL, J.: Tuberculosis subcutanea fistulosa. Tuberkulosearzt 4: 18–28 (1950).

(2) BÖHME, H.: Die Pyodermia fistulans sinifica. Eine seltene fistelnde und taschenbildende Erkrankung des Haut- und Unterhautgewebes. Dtsch. med. Wschr. 89: 1265–1267 (1964).

(3) DONALD, G. F.: Fistula auris congenita. Aust. J. Derm. 1: 253–255 (1952).

(4) EHRING, F.: Wandlungen in der Klinik und Bakteriologie der Halslymphknotentuberkulose. Dtsch. med. Wschr. 92: 62–65 (1967).

(5) EISSNER, H.: »Familiäre Perlèche«, vorgetäuscht durch hereditäre bilaterale Mundwinkelfisteln. Derm. Wschr. 140: 1192–1196 (1959).

(6) EISSNER, H., und G. FUCHS: Zur Klinik und operativen Behandlung der Tuberculosis subcutanea fistulosa. Chirurg 35: 68–70 (1964).

(7) HECTOR, A.: Haarcysten, Fisteln und Abszesse der Steißbeingegend. Med. Klin. 48: 1263–1265 (1953).

(8) JATHO, K.: Zur Pathogenese und Behandlung der Tuberkulose der Halslymphknoten. Dtsch. med. Wschr. 87: 137–143 (1962).

(9) KARCHER, G., W. DEUBZER und A. MEYER: Zur Diagnose, Klinik und Therapie des Pilonidalsinus (Steißbeinfistel). Fortschr. Med. 86: 173–176 (1968).

(10) KATZENELLENBOGEN, I.: Studies on dracontiasis among yemenite immigrants to Israel. Dermatologica (Basel) 108: 129–136 (1954).

(11) KESSLER, L.: Die medianen und lateralen kongenitalen Fisteln und Zysten des Halses. Dtsch. Gesundh.-Wes. 24: 269–273 (1969).

(12) KORTING, G. W.: Chronische tiefkutane Enterokokkengranulome. Derm. Wschr. 126: 999–1005 (1952).

(13) KORTING, G. W.: Zur perianalen Erscheinungsweise der Crohnschen Krankheit. Hautarzt 19: 553–556 (1968).

(14) LEMKE, G.: Über Fisteln der Lippen einschließlich der Mundwinkel. Derm. Wschr. 140: 1085–1089 (1959).

(15) LINSER, K., und A. K. SCHMAUSS: Karzinome bzw. Malignome in Spätformen der Lymphopathia venerea. Derm. Wschr. 135: 337–357 (1957).

(16) McCALLUM, D. I., and P. D. C. KINMONT: Dermatological manifestations of Crohn's disease. Brit. J. Derm. 80: 1–8 (1968).

(17) MEYER, R.: Von den Zähnen ausgehende Hautfisteln und ihre Erkennung. Z. Haut- u. Geschl.-Kr. 13: 1–10 (1952).

(18) NÜRNBERGER, F.: Zur Kenntnis der Akne conglobata im Damm-Gesäßbereich. Z. Haut- u. Geschl.-Kr. 38: 188–197 (1965). ,

(19) PETRES, J., und M. HUNDEIKER: Extraorale Zahnfisteln. Münch. med. Wschr. 110: 1320–1321 (1968).

(20) PETZ, R., und J. MEYER: Zu einigen diagnostischen Irrtümern und therapeutischen Fehlgriffen bei Fisteln im Kiefer-Gesichts-Bereich. Dtsch. Gesundh.-Wes. *22:* 1714–1719 (1967).

(21) SCHACHTER, M.: Recherches sur les fossettes paraauriculaires ou fistules auriculaires congénitales (fist. auris cong.). Schweiz. med. Wschr. *79:* 343–345 (1949).

(22) TAYLOR, W. B., and D. K. LANE: Congenital fistulas of the lower lip. Arch. Derm. (Chic.) *94:* 421–424 (1966).

(23) TSCHESCHMEDJIEV, J., und S. CHLEBAROV: Fistula congenita pharyngocutanea. Derm. Wschr. *142:* 764–766 (1960).

(24) WAGNER, A.: Hauterkrankungen bei Enteritis regionalis (Morbus Crohn). Dtsch. med. Wschr. *96:* 1078–1086 (1971).

15. Gingival Hypertrophies

Tumorlike hypertrophies, fibromatoses, or proliferations of the gingiva are known as macrogingiva when they produce diffuse thickenings. Transient enlargement of the interdental septa combined with a raspberry to dark red color of the dental papillae during pregnancy is called macrogingiva gravidarum; during puberty there may be a trace of such enlargement. More rarely, other endocrine disorders (dysthyroidism, acromegaly) may cause such swellings. Persistent enlargement of the gingiva is seen in acanthosis nigricans, the Melkersson-Rosenthal syndrome, systemic amyloidosis, hyalinosis cutis et mucosae (lipoid proteinosis), leprosy, sarcoid, and mycosis fungoides; however, macrogingivae are rare concomitant signs.[1, 6]

1. In the rare **hereditary gingival fibromatosis,** a high degree of fibromatous hyperplasia of the gingiva is present. Quite suddenly and unpredictably, the gingiva grows to such an extent that it may cover the erupted crowns of teeth either partially or totally. Signs of inflammation are absent. Chewing is not impossible, but macrogingiva may make it impossible to close the mouth. The gingiva itself is not painful, and it has a normal color and shows a fine granular surface. Histologically, hyperplasia of the connective tissue with overgrowth of fibers and small-cell perivascular infiltration is present. As a rule, the bony substance of the alveolar processes remains unaffected. Complete removal of all teeth results in almost full regression of the macrogingiva, but excision of the gingiva itself will not be successful. In many patients, hypertrichosis develops simultaneously (see Chapter 11, F4).[7, 8]

2. In rare instances even small infants may show hypertrophy of the gingiva caused by malformation of the lymphatic

Fig. 128. Pringle's disease: bulging gingival hyperplasia.

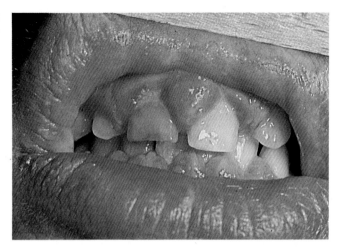

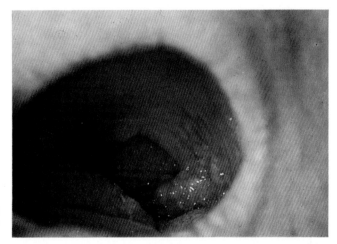

Fig. 129. Pringle's disease: nodular deformity of the tonsil.

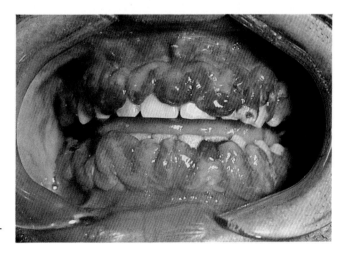

Fig. 130. Gingival hyperplasia in monocytic leukemia.

vascular system. Such primary **intestinal lymphangiectasia** manifests itself by extensive edema, enteral loss of protein, diarrhea, hypocalcemia, and hypoproteinemia.[5]

3. Partial signs of **Pringle's disease** (adenoma sebaceum) are multiple small, regular, protuberant tumors of the gingiva that are mostly closely aggregated and later become confluent (Fig. 128). Similar lesions can be found on the buccal mucosa, tongue, palate, and even on the surface of the tonsils (Fig. 129). The most frequent sites of these whitish-grey to brownish fibromas of the gingiva are the anterior teeth. The diagnosis depends on other manifestations of Pringle's disease, such as periungual lesions, adenoma sebaceum, and lumbosacral connective tissue nevi (shagreen skin). Diagnostic difficulties may arise when dilantin preparations have to be given in the treatment of epileptic fits caused by tuberous sclerosis, a manifestation of Pringle's disease.

4. Dilantin and similar hydantoin compounds cause hyperplasia of the gingiva in about 40 per cent of patients suffering from cerebral epilepsy; such gingival lesions develop mostly in young people within one to three months after the beginning of the medication. The lesions themselves are first soft, later more firm, semispherical to nodular protuberances. Secondary infection may cause increased exudation or hemorrhagic sponginess of the gingiva and loosening of the teeth. If dilantin medication is discontinued, complete involution will take place within a few weeks or months.[2, 3]

5. Leukoses may present diffuse thickening of the gingiva of the anterior alveolar processes. Macrogingiva is an almost pathognomonic sign of monocytic leukemia (Fig. 130), as well as of myeloblastic

leukemia and some reticuloses. Hypertrophies of the gingiva of unknown etiology demand careful hematologic evaluation.[4, 6]

6. Furthermore, hyperplasias of the gingiva with a tendency to light bleeding characterize **scurvy.** These gingival changes affect the dentulous mouth, especially the anterior teeth. Some of the other manifestations of scurvy will help to establish the diagnosis. These include capillary hemorrhages surrounding nutmeg-grater-like follicular papules arranged in a chessboard pattern, petechiae, and subperiostal hemorrhages, especially at sites subject to muscular stress.

7. Polypous tumors are isolated lesions such as an epulis or eosinophilic granuloma of the bone (which presents an ulcerated, necrotic nodular area of granulation tissue of the gingiva), or a rapidly growing carcinoma of the gingiva (which involves 20 to 30 per cent of all cancers of the mouth); a biopsy permits a definite diagnosis. All such isolated tumors differ from the diffuse thickening of the gingiva of macrogingiva.

(1) HORNSTEIN, O., und H. SCHUERMANN: Das sogenannte Melkersson-Rosenthal-Syndrom. Ergebn. inn. Med. Kinderheilk. N. F. *17:* 190–263 (1962).

(2) LIVINGSTON, S., and H. L. LIVINGSTON: Diphenylhydantoin gingival hyperplasia. Amer. J. Dis. Child. *117:* 265–270 (1969).

(3) MATHIS, H.: Zur Frage der Hyperplasie der Gingiva unter Dilantindauerbehandlung. Dtsch. zahnärztl. Z. *9:* 1280–1289 (1954).

(4) OSGOOD, E. E.: Monocytic leukemia; report of 6 cases and review of 127 cases. Arch. Intern. Med. *59:* 931–951 (1937).

(5) PELLER, P., J. SCHAUB, H. ZOBEL und H. J. BREMER: Intestinale Lymphangiektasie. Dtsch. med. Wschr. *95:* 1219–1224 (1970).

(6) SCHUERMANN, H., A. GREITHER und O. HORNSTEIN: Krankheiten der Mundschleimhaut und der Lippen. Urban & Schwarzenberg, München, Berlin, Wien 1966.

(7) WESKI, H.: Elephantiasis gingivae hereditaria. Dtsch. Mschr. Zahnheilk. *3:* 557–584 (1920).

(8) WINKLMAIR, M.: Hereditäre Fibromatosis gingivae. Dtsch. zahnärztl. Z. *24:* 895–899 (1969).

16. Collagenosis Group; Generalized Connective Tissue Diseases

Although doubtless vulnerable in many respects, the practical and useful concept of collagenous diseases applies, at least in dermatology, to a closely related group of clinical entities composed of scleroderma, dermatomyositis, and lupus erythematosus, even though from a phenomenologic standpoint these conditions show very little similarity clinically and microscopically. On the other hand, these collagenoses do present some common factors such as involvement of internal organs, dysproteinemia, occasional fever, chronic progression, and others. Figure 131 shows graphically how each of the three collagenoses prefers certain organs and how a gross differential diagnosis can be arrived at.

Lupus erythematosus involves joints, serous membranes, kidneys, and heart; **dermatomyositis** is characteristically located in the cardiac and skeletal musculature, while **progressive scleroderma** shows a preference for the upper gastrointestinal tract, lungs, kidneys, and also heart. However, each organ is affected differently. In systemic lupus erythematosus the heart shows the Kaposi-Libman-Sacks type of endocarditis, whereas in dermatomyositis

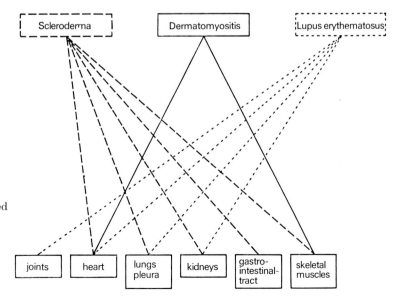

Fig. 131. Preferred involvement of organs in scleroderma, dermatomyositis, and systemic lupus erythematosus.

changes of the myocardium itself occur, and in progressive scleroderma fibrosis of the myocardial tissue takes place. These three rare diseases show a distinctly different distribution according to age and sex. Further differences are based on immunologic phenomena; however, the tendency to the production of abnormal antibodies is principally and definitely restricted to systemic lupus erythematosus. In contrast, dermatomyositis is based on a pathologic enzymatous mechanism and has a higher frequency of association with malignant neoplastic disease than would occur by pure chance. Finally, scleroderma represents primarily a neurovascular problem involving a decisive pathogenetic action on the various collagen fractions.[1-5]

(1) DENK, R.: Elektrokardiographische Untersuchungen bei Hautkranken. Arch. Kreisl.-Forsch. *60:* 33–114 (1969).

(2) KORTING, G. W.: Über einige Wesensunterschiede von Sklerodermie, Dermatomyositis und Lupus erythematodes acutus und die darauf basierende differente Therapie. Dtsch. med. Wschr. *92:* 281–288 (1967).

(3) KORTING, G. W., und H. HOLZMANN: Die Sklerodermie und ihr nahestehende Bindegewebsprobleme. Thieme, Stuttgart 1967.

(4) SCHUERMANN, H.: Dermatomyositis. Ergebn. inn. Med. Kinderheilk. N. F. *10:* 427–480 (1958).

(5) SIEGENTHALER, W., und R. HEGGLIN: Der viscerale Lupus erythematosus (Kaposi-Libman-Sacks-Syndrom). Ergebn. inn. Med. Kinderheilk. N. F. *7:* 373–428 (1956).

A. Circumscribed Scleroses

1. Circumscribed scleroderma (morphea) is a spontaneously involuting disease, whereas the diffuse variety, better called *progressive* scleroderma, is a systemic disease of the vascular connective tissue which has a fatal outcome. However, borderline cases and transitions between these two types do occur. In circumscribed scleroderma several types can be distinguished according to their extension – scleroderma "en plaques," linear morphea ("en bandes," "en coup de sabre"), a small macular variety, a keloidal variety, and a subcutaneous variety. All types of scleroderma occur three times more frequently in women than in men. An area of circumscribed scleroderma develops from a subacute erythematous macule, which fades

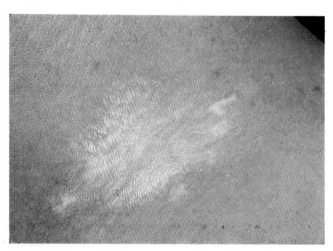

Fig. 132. Circumscribed scleroderma.

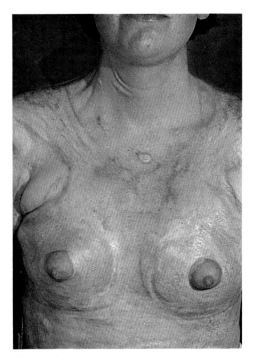

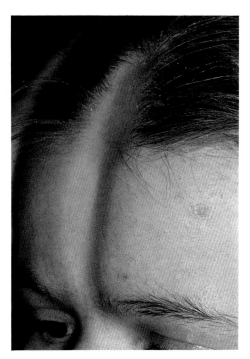

Fig. 133. Generalized circumscribed scleroderma.

Fig. 134. Linear circumscribed scleroderma.

in the center and is surrounded on the periphery by the so-called "lilac ring;" finally, this macule becomes an indurated area with a waxy to boardlike consistency (Fig. 132). Atrophy with or without pigmentation may follow. Similar atrophic areas of a faintly lilac color can be caused by superficial infiltration with cortisone. Subcutaneous circumscribed scleroderma does not involve the epidermis and, as a rule, lacks the peripheral erythematous ring. The same is true for other partly subcutaneous forms such as tuberous, nodular, or keloidal circumscribed sclerodermas.

When induration of an area of scleroderma is minimal or absent and the main feature is pigmentation, the condition is called **idiopathic atrophoderma,** which is identical with "morphea plana atrophicans." Such multiple, oval, slightly depressed, light brown pigmentations of the trunk (occurring mostly in females?) do

not show wrinkles, in contrast to anetoderma, and they lack also hernialike protrusions. Histologically, atrophy of the elastic tissue with no reaction occurs in anetoderma, while idiopathic atrophoderma shows hardly any alteration of the elastica.

Circumscribed areas of scleroderma occasionally form bullae on the legs as a short-lived transitory reaction; sometimes these bullae develop into ulcers.

If a number of different areas of scleroderma occupy almost the total body surface one speaks of generalized circumscribed scleroderma or, preferably, **generalized morphea** (Fig. 133). Even in the generalized stage in which large areas of scleroderma occupy the trunk, typical "lilac rings" persist on the periphery. In contrast to progressive scleroderma, Raynaud's phenomenon on acral areas is absent in generalized morphea. The devel-

Fig. 135. Lichen sclerosus et atrophicus: typical picture with follicular keratoses.

opment of early severe cicatrizing alopecia of the scalp in a helmetlike pattern is characteristic; the breasts show a brassiere-like constriction with a peculiar prolapse of the uninvolved areolae and a tendency of some of the lesions of morphea to form

bullae. The more brownish appearance is striking in contrast to the usual yellowish color tints of scleroderma. Other findings are contractures caused by the diseased skin and constrictions of the connective tissue of the dental alveolar socket (alveolar atrophy). Involvement of inner organs, causing dysphagias, cardiac fibrosis, or pulmonary fibrosis, is, however, seldom seen. The conversion of this generalized morphea into typical progressive scleroderma is extremely rare. More frequent is the combination of generalized morphea and lichen sclerosus et atrophicus.

Linear bandlike circumscribed scleroderma involves the extremities and, when it occurs in children, may endanger the growth of the limbs; in the face, linear lesions may occur in a paramedian location with changes of the underlying bone (Fig. 134).

In **small macular circumscribed scleroderma** there are distinctly yellowish-white, lentil-sized, multiple areas indented below the level of the skin. These lesions are chiefly located on the chest and shoulders and occur like satellites on the periphery of typical circumscribed areas of scleroderma. Intrafocal follicular hyperkeratoses are lacking, but there are "miniature lilac rings" around some of the lesions. Histo-

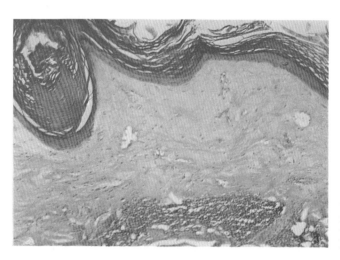

Fig. 136. Lichen sclerosus et atrophicus: follicular hyperkeratosis. Atrophy of the malpighian layer. Homogenization of the upper corium with inflammatory infiltrate lying below. HE stain, 25×.

logically, such firm, hard macules do not show loss of elastic tissue.[3, 5, 11, 18, 20, 26, 32]

2. Lichen sclerosus et atrophicus (Figs. 135, 136) presents porcelain-white, small, macular indurations with intrafocal, follicular hyperkeratoses. A "lilac ring" is not present. Sites of predilection are the neck and clavicular regions. During the course of the disease larger confluent areas of lichen sclerosus may show extensive serous or hemorrhagic subepidermal bullae arising within fissures. Frequently, closely aggregated groups of lichen sclerosus lesions are found in the genitoanal regions. Here the atrophic tendency of the disease is more distinct than in any other location; the surface of the papules is wrinkled and the receding follicular plugs are confluent. The nonspecific term **kraurosis vulvae** describes the manifestation of a number of diseases. Very often kraurosis of the female genital tract is caused by lichen sclerosus; it may occur even in young children. Therefore, in cases of kraurosis with stenosing atrophy of the genitals of otherwise unclear etiology, one should look for single lesions of lichen sclerosus in the vicinity or in other places.

Histologically, elastic fibers are found only in the early stages of lichen sclerosus. Later, they disappear to a large extent, leaving a bandlike area within a subepidermal zone of homogenization; in contrast, the elastica in the small macular type of scleroderma persists permanently. Corresponding to the macroscopic appearance of lichen sclerosus, follicular keratoses are prominent in the histologic picture as well. Under the electron microscope signs of increased newly formed fibrils can be seen in areas of lichen sclerosus et atrophicus. Lichen sclerosus et atrophicus can best be classified as an independent disease entity occupying a place between small macular circumscribed scleroderma and lichen planus. Corroborating this independence is the fact that in

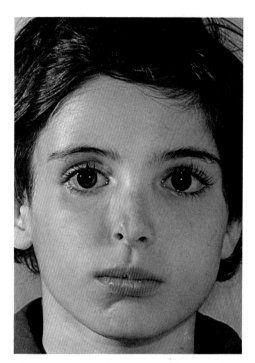

Fig. 137. Progressive hemiatrophy of the face.

the same patient, although not in the same area, there may be simultaneous signs of circumscribed scleroderma, lichen planus, and lichen sclerosus ("lichen-sclérodermie," "sclérolichen").[10, 13, 20]

Because lichen sclerosus and small macular circumscribed scleroderma do not itch, the presence of pruritus and prurigo nodules in other locations, together with similar but more stellar-shaped, retracted, cicatricial, multiple lesions of the shoulder region, point to "**prurigo diathetica leukodystrophica**," which represents a special type of atopic dermatitis. The same considerations apply to postacneiform, whitish, and also cicatricial indurations in similar locations ("Ivanov's spots").[15, 19]

3. Sometimes linear scleroderma is associated with **facial hemiatrophy,** or the scleroderma itself results in the manifestation of a hemiatrophy; the latter occurrence can be substantiated if the

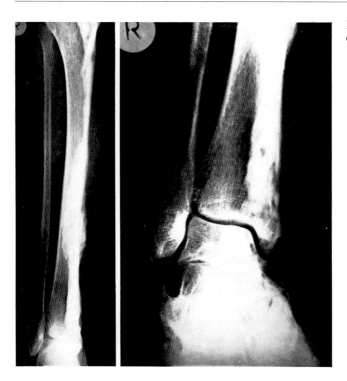

Fig. 138. Melorheostosis in circumscribed scleroderma.

atrophy has been preceded by edematous indurative phases. On the other hand, at least a part of these facial hemiatrophies of Romberg are "idiopathic," especially those which start in early childhood, around puberty, and those occurring in girls; they may be a hereditary degenerative affliction with relatively weak gene penetration. The shrinkage of the skin (which starts with a strikingly pale color), muscles, and bones results in development of an enophthalmus, and also, occasionally, of a complete Horner's syndrome (Fig. 137). Upon inspection, the asymmetry of the face is located paramedianly; at first sight it may suggest facial paralysis.[8]

4. More than a mere coincidence exists between **melorheostosis** and linear circumscribed scleroderma. Roentgenologic examination, often accidental, of the long bones of the extremities of such patients shows hyperostosis extending in a linear

fashion and looking like dripping candle wax (proliferated ivorylike new bone) (Fig. 138). These changes may be restricted to a few bones, but often one or several extremities are affected. Many patients complain of vague pain in bones and joints and of limitation of movement of some joints. Thus, it is possible to confuse the limitation of movement caused by scleroderma itself with melorheostosis. Patients with linear scleroderma and corresponding complaints, therefore, should have a roentgenologic examination of their bones.[16, 22, 30]

5. Acrodermatitis chronica atrophicans with sclerodermalike areas must be considered in the differential diagnosis. Macroscopically, in the vast majority of cases tightly atrophic – i.e., pseudosclerodermic – areas are present. Difficulties will arise only in establishing the proper diagnosis after the typical cutaneous changes of acrodermatitis chronica atrophicans have completely healed; but this can happen only when the therapy is started very early. In such cases histologic examination will offer further possibilities of differentiation, because in acrodermatitis, in contrast to scleroderma, the elastica has become rarefied and may have disappeared completely. The simultaneous occurrence of both diseases in the same patient is quite rare. The therapeutic success of penicillin injections does not permit conclusive evidence of the diagnosis because some sclerodermatic areas will show a spontaneous tendency to regression under such treatment, while, on the other hand, the taut atrophies of acrodermatitis often respond poorly to penicillin.[12, 20]

6. Not all circumscribed areas of scleroderma of the scalp, sometimes with loss of hair, can be associated with scleroderma "en bande." For instance, a sclerodermiform basal cell epithelioma* (Fig. 139) and also **metastases of other malignant tumors** may simulate scleroderma. In contrast to the usually protuberant metastatic tumors of the scalp, which are often discovered when combing the hair, cicatrizing

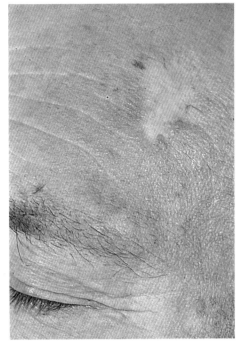

Fig. 139. Sclerodermiform basaloma.

* Cicatricial basal cell epithelioma. (Tr.)

malignant tumors are either at the level of the surrounding skin or sometimes slightly depressed and have a somewhat inflamed border. In such cases only histologic examination will enable one to establish the diagnosis.

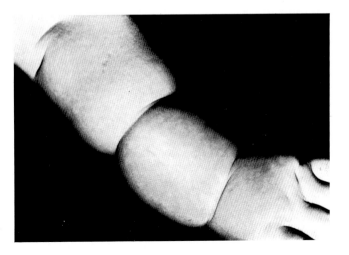

Fig. 140. Constriction by amniotic bands.

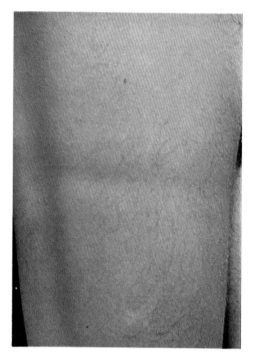

Fig. 141. Annular lipoatrophy.

7. Although linear scleroderma may occasionally be strictly circular, a number of similar diseases showing rings of constriction should be considered also. Prenatal, nonreactive, sometimes deeply marked constrictive rings of the peripheral parts of the extremities are evidence of a congenital malformation called **Simonart's threads**; a band is formed by the stretching of adhesions between the amnion and the fetus. Distal to the constricting sulcus the abdomen shows diffuse thickening similar to a chronic edema (Fig. 140). Histologically, the band of constriction reveals fibrosis and hyperkeratosis.

If constrictions of fingers or toes are observed in newborn or small children as well as signs of local inflammation, the presence of **artefacts** should be considered. Female attendants especially commit such maltreatment by applying long scalp hairs; these hairs can hardly be seen in the deep constricting sulcus.[25, 33]

Circular constrictions of fingers and toes are also found in connection with diffuse keratoses of palms and soles. The furrows of constriction run within the normal folds of the finger and after many years finally bring about mutilation of some digits. The constriction itself is probably the result of the retraction phenomena of the hyperkeratoses. The hyperkeratoses themselves are distributed diffusely on the palms and soles and, occasionally, may spread to the dorsal surfaces. In addition, linear and islandlike keratoses are found on the extensor aspects of the knee and elbow joints. The disease is called **mutilating palmar and plantar keratosis** or keratoma hereditaria mutilans (pseudo-ainhumlike dermatosis) and may in some families be associated with deafness.[23, 24, 28, 29]

Marked local vascular changes of the subcutaneous fatty tissue may result in circular constrictions called **annular lipoatrophy**. The furrows usually begin at the proximal parts of the extremities and are most often arranged symmetrically (Fig. 144). Palpation of the skin within these furrows does not give the impression of infiltration or induration, but the bottom of the furrow feels like bone. Except for a moderate amount of atrophy the epidermis shows no changes; clinical signs of inflammation are absent.[3, 9]

8. **Necrobiosis lipoidica** is observed almost always on the legs and in women; clinically and microscopically, it differs only slightly from granulomatosis disciformis. Almost always, there are lentil- to palm-sized, brownish-yellow to reddish-blue indurations of tissue on the extensor aspects of the legs. These later fade into a whitish-yellow color; as in morphea, the border may be surrounded for a long time by a hyperemic zone. Later, the central portion becomes slightly depressed and, in contrast to circumscribed scleroderma, the entire lesion is conspicuously crisscrossed by telangiectases. Frequently, such necrobioses of the legs are interspersed with

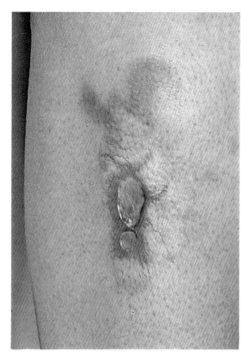

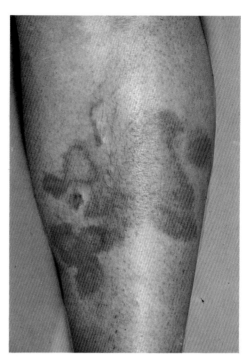

Fig. 142. Necrobiosis lipoidica with ulcerations.

Fig. 143. Granulomatosis disciformis.

ecthymatous or punched-out ulcers (Fig. 142). The diagnosis is often facilitated by the finding of outright diabetes or by an abnormal glucose tolerance curve; necrobiosis lipoidica is sometimes present before diabetes mellitus is diagnosed.

Histologically, necrobiosis lipoidica is completely different from the homogenized sclerosis of the corium that is found in circumscribed scleroderma. The usual findings are conspicuous thickenings of the vascular walls with sometimes obliterative proliferations of the intima or productive arteriopathies, and necrobiosis (rarely advancing to necrosis) with peripheral cellular screening and areas of deposition of PAS-positive material stained by Hale's iron stain – specifically, alcian blue. Additional findings are deposition of some sudanophil lipids, mostly in droplet form, not only within the necrobiotic zones themselves, but also between bundles of collagen.[6, 7]

Granulomatosis disciformis should be considered when the extensor aspects of the legs in particular show areas of necrobiosis that become progressively worse over the years and have a marked proclivity for confluence and bizarre configuration but no tendency toward ulceration (Fig. 143). Microscopically, this is understandable because the trend toward necrosis recedes as the prevalence of granulomatous signs increases. Epithelioid cells, giant foreign body cells, and also Langhans' type cells are more numerous than in typical necrobiosis lipoidica; the combined result is one of sarcoidlike or, to a lesser extent, of tuberculoid structures. In addition, there are deposits of lipids which are more extracellular than intracellular, and also circumscribed areas with a positive PAS stain; mucin, however, is absent. In general, the histochemical findings are similar to those in necrobiosis lipoidica.

9. Localized panatrophy, in contrast to the subcutaneous circumscribed scleroderma mentioned earlier, usually presents a single lesion a few centimeters in diameter with a wide depression as well as atrophy of the epidermis. Such atrophies, when located in the gluteal region, are seen nowadays after the injection of repository cortisone suspensions. Soon after the injection, panatrophy of all layers of tissue from the epidermis to the muscles develops with no definite inflammatory signs. In some cases it is not clear whether the panatrophy has started from **scleroderma** or **panniculitis.** However, in cases of panniculitis, a clinically obvious inflammatory reaction precedes the atrophy. The final result will be more or less a lipoatrophy but not an atrophy of all layers of tissue. The circumscribed atrophies of tissue observed after injections of insulin are almost always lipoatrophies; they are due to the contamination of proteins present in insulin and to the acid pH of the insulin solution. Lipoatrophies are much less common if a neutral insulin solution is chosen; the injection of mono-component insulin will cause no side effects at all. 17, 27, 30

10. Cutaneous fibroses following x-ray radiation usually are confined to the field of exposure and are reversible late reactions to radiation. In contrast to these milder sequelae, intensive telecobalt radiation will cause indurative reactions of the subcutis; starting within a few weeks after the termination of the radiation these reactions develop successively as erythemas with platelike, hypertrophic infiltrations and livid pigmentation. Although the fibrosis is confined to the field of radiation, there are occasionally reactions that go beyond that field or even become generalized. Such indurations of the subcutis are frequently quite painful and favor the adipose abdominal, lumbar, and paravertebral regions of the body (Fig. 144). Histologically, an increase in alcian blue positive material is present only in the beginning, while interstitial proliferation of cells remains longer; this fact permits some differentiation from scleroderma. Otherwise, the histologic differentiation is difficult because diffuse sclerosis of the corium is present in morphea as well as in radiation sclerosis. However, radiation sclerosis sometimes extends as deep as the subcutaneous septae of the adipose tissue, while the main sclerotic development in morphea occurs in the middle of the corium. 2, 14

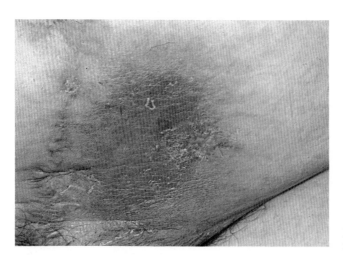

Fig. 144. So-called x-ray fibrosis.

(1) BARAN, R.: Les métastases alopéciantes scléroatrophiques des cancers mammaires. Dermatologica (Basel) *138:* 169–181 (1969).

(2) BIRKNER, R., und B. HOFFMANN: Unterhautindurationen nach Telekobalttherapie. Strahlentherapie *116:* 463–477 (1961).

(3) BRUINSMA, W.: Lipo-atrophia annularis, an abnormal vulnerability of the fatty tissue. Dermatologica (Basel) *134:* 107–112 (1967).

(4) CANIZARES, O., P. M. SACHS, L. JAIMOVICH and V. M. TORRES: Idiopathic atrophoderma of Pasini and Pierini. Arch. Derm. Syph. (Chic.) *77:* 42–60 (1958).

(5) CHRISTIANSON, H. B., CL. S. DORSEY, P. A. O'LEARY and R. R. KIERLAND: Localized scleroderma. Arch. Derm. Syph. (Chic.) *74:* 629–639 (1956).

(6) DEGOS, R.: Nekrobiosis lipoidica diabeticorum (Oppenheim-Urbach). Münch. med. Wschr. *109:* 1518–1523 (1967).

(7) DENK, R.: Insulinantikörper bei einem Diabetiker mit Nekrobiosis lipoidica. Arch. klin. exp. Derm. *220:* 329–333 (1964).

(8) ERLER, D.: Ungewöhnliche Form einer Sclérodermie faciale en bande mit Mundschleimhautveränderungen und Alveolaratrophie. Z. Haut- u. Geschl.-Kr. *35:* 342–347 (1963).

(9) FERREIRA-MARQUES, J.: Lipoatrophia annularis. Arch. Derm. Syph. (Berl.) *195:* 479–491 (1953).

(10) FORSSMANN, W. G., H. HOLZMANN und J. CABRÉ: Elektronenmikroskopische Untersuchungen der Haut beim Lichen sclerosus et atrophicans. Arch. klin. exp. Derm. *220:* 584–599 (1964).

(11) GARB, J., and CH. F. SIMS: Scleroderma with bullous lesions. Dermatologica (Basel) *119:* 341–359 (1959).

(12) HAUSER, W.: Akrodermatitis chronica atrophicans. Ergebn. inn. Med. Kinderheilk. N. F. *22:* 58–89 (1965).

(13) HERZBERG, J. J., J. MEYER-ROHN und P. J. UNNA: Sclérolichen Gougerot. Arch. klin. exp. Derm. *216:* 246–259 (1963).

(14) ISHIKAWA, H., W. THIES, W. SCHUMACHER und F. KLASCHKA: Vergleichende Untersuchungen über das Verhalten der sauren Mucopolysaccharide bei Sklerose der Haut nach Betatron-Bestrahlung, bei Sklerodermie und einigen sklerosierenden Dermatosen. Hautarzt *18:* 174–180 (1967).

(15) IWANOW, W. W.: Über weiße atrophische und narbenähnliche perifollikuläre Flecke der Rumpfhaut. Arch. Derm. Syph. (Wien, Leipzig) *64:* 369–380 (1903).

(16) KELLER, H. L., R. KUNZE und H.-J. VOGT: Melorheostose Léri-Joanny mit bandförmiger Sklerodermie. Münch. med. Wschr. *113:* 1081–1084 (1971).

(17) KLÜKEN, N., und K.-H. GEIB: Kasuistischer Beitrag zur Panatrophia cutis localisata. Hautarzt *16:* 422–424 (1965).

(18) KORTING, G. W.: Über keloidartige Sklerodermie nebst Bemerkungen über das etagenmäßig differente Verhalten von einigen sklerodermischen Krankheitszuständen. Arch. Derm. Syph. (Berl.) *198:* 306–318 (1954).

(19) KORTING, G. W.: Zur Pathogenese des endogenen Ekzems. S. 20–21. Thieme, Stuttgart 1954.

(20) KORTING, G. W., N. HOEDE und H. HOLZMANN: Zur Frage des Elasticaverhaltens bei einigen sklerosierenden und atrophisierenden Hautkrankheiten. Hautarzt *20:* 351–361 (1969).

(21) KORTING, G. W., und F. NÜRNBERGER: Ungewöhnliches Basalzellepitheliom unter dem Bilde einer »Sclérodermie en bande« im Bereich des behaarten Kopfes (Basaliom en Coup de sabre). Med. Welt *20* (N. F.): 479–480 (1969).

(22) MULLER, S. A., and E. D. HENDERSON: Melorheostosis with linear scleroderma. Arch. Derm. (Chic.) *88:* 142–145 (1963).

(23) NEUMANN, A.: Pseudoainhum. Arch. Derm. Syph. (Chic.) *68:* 421–427 (1953).

(24) NOCKEMANN, P. F.: Erbliche Hornhautverdickung mit Schnürfurchen an den Fingern und Zehen und Innenohrschwerhörigkeit. Med. Welt (Stuttg.) *1961/II:* 1894–1900.

(25) PETERSEN, D.: Entstehung angeborener Gliedmaßenabschnürµngen. Med. Klin. *66:* 45–50 (1971).

(26) POIARES BAPTISTA, A., A. BASTOS ARAUJO et J. CORTESAO: Sclérodermie bulleuse en plaques. Ann. Derm. Syph. (Paris) *95:* 29–38 (1968).

(27) SCHULZE, W., und E. KUNZE: Kritische
     Bemerkungen zur Panatrophia locali-
     sata. Derm. Wschr. *138:* 865–878 (1958).

(28) SPENCER, G. A.: Ainhum associated
     with hyperkeratosis palmaris et plan-
     taris. Arch. Derm. Syph. (Chic.) *45:*
     574–577 (1942).

(29) VOHWINKEL, K. H.: Keratoma here-
     ditarium mutilans. Arch. Derm. Syph.
     (Berlin) *158:* 354–364 (1929).

(30) WAGERS, L. T., A. W. JOUNG JR. and
     S. F. RYAN: Linear melorheostotic
     scleroderma. Brit. J. Derm. *86:* 297–301
     (1972).

(31) WATSON, B. M., and J. S. CALDER: A
     treatment for insulin-induced fat atro-
     phy. Diabetes *20:* 628–632 (1971).

(32) WEIDNER, F., und O. BRAUN-FALCO:
     Gleichzeitiges Vorkommen von Sympto-
     men der circumscripten und progressi-
     ven Sklerodermie. Hautarzt *19:* 345–350
     (1968).

(33) WERTHEMANN, A.: Allgemeine Ein-
     führung und Mißbildungen aus placen-
     tarer Beeinträchtigung, insonderheit
     sog. amniogene Schnürungen und Schä-
     digungen durch die Nabelschnur. Bull.
     Schweiz. Akad. med. Wiss. *20:* 313–335
     (1964).

B. Diffuse Scleroses

1. Progressive scleroderma starts with the same signs as Raynaud's syndrome – i. e., an interchange between syncope and acroasphyxia of the fingers except the thumbs. After this comes the indurative stage with a waxy to boardlike consistency of the upper layers of the skin and firm adherence to the bone. Acrosclerosis, sclerodactylia, and microstomia develop, and at the same time, the inner organs become involved. Progressive scleroderma is, therefore, a systemic disorder of the vascular and connective tissue structures whose significance lies in the fact that it is a fatal general disease.

Prominent signs of this progressive systemic sclerosis are vasomotoric distur-bances (Fig. 145), which in the beginning are felt by the patient as increased sensitivity to cold and later as a symmetrical painful deadening, mostly of the second and fourth fingers. At the onset these **Raynaud's symptoms** should arouse the suspicion, especially if they are unilateral, of an occupational cause (such as contact with vibrating tools) or of pathologic anatomic conditions (such as a cervical rib). If at the same time bluish erythemas develop as the effect of cold temperatures, the presence of cold agglutinins, cryoglobulins, or paroxysmal hemoglobinuria should be investigated. Raynaud's signs, although much rarer than acroparesthesias, occur in chronic intoxication with heavy metals and in ergotism. Although much less frequently observed than in progressive scleroderma, these Raynaud's phenomena are also seen in other collagenoses such as dermatomyositis or systemic lupus ery-thematosus (see also Chapter 5, B2).

Similar to these Raynaud's phenomena is **sclerodactylia,** the characteristic fixation of the fingers in flexion, which occurs occasionally in mild form or somewhat changed in other diseases. The initial Raynaud's symptoms, however, have long disappeared by the time sclerodactylia develops. The sclerodermatous claw forma-tion shows conspicuous upward thinning of the terminal phalanges ("fingers of the madonna") before the characteristic wooden, stiff stumps develop. The nails also contribute to this bird-clawlike deformity as a consequence of extreme curvature and transverse streaks. In addition, the cuticle becomes thick and hardened (Fig. 146). However, these sclero-dermatous contractures of the connective tissue, which occasionally are difficult to differentiate from arthropathias in rheumatoid arthritis, always lack rheumat-ic features such as swellings and mutila-tions of the joints as well as ulnar finger deviations. In arthropathic psoriasis,

Fig. 145. Raynaud's phenomenon.

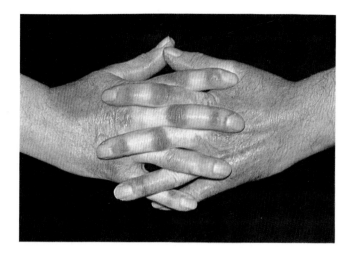

which has negative results on serologic tests for rheumatoid arthritis, the appearance is never that of a sclerodermalike hand deformity, since apart from all other psoriatic skin changes, the nail changes alone (pits, yellowish discoloration, and crumbling) are characteristic of psoriasis. It is important for the differential diagnosis, therefore, when dealing with an "isolated" sclerodactylia and not with complete acrosclerosis (of hands and face), to consider the trophoneuroses of the "acropathie ulcéromutilante familiale" type, the sclerodermalike cutaneous changes in parathyroid diseases, and the carpal tunnel syndrome in women (which is characterized by nightly paresthesias that always spare the little finger and almost always the thumb). Sclerodermatous hands caused by trauma develop from paresis of the arm plexus, as for instance after a gunshot wound. Occupationally, workers with pneumatic tools may experience necroses of the fingertips (Fig. 147); such changes were previously seen in shoe workers, who used hammers. In the generalized stage of Wegener's granulomatosis, extensive necroses of the fingertips may occur.[8, 23, 24]

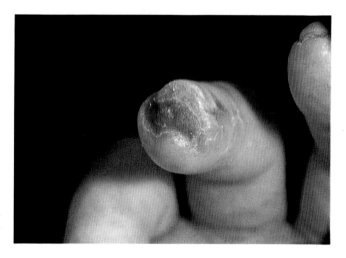

Fig. 146. Progressive scleroderma: necrosis of the fingertip.

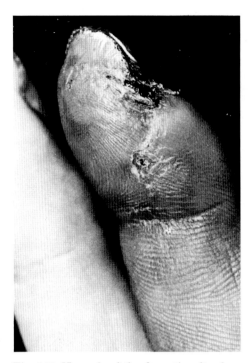

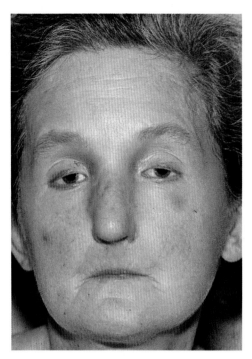

Fig. 147. Necrosis of the fingertip after long use of a hydraulic press.

Fig. 148. Progressive scleroderma: "mummy face."

Conspicuous upward thinning of the terminal phalanges is caused by a diminution of the adipose layer of the fingertip. It is also found in the syndrome of **apical dysplasia of the fingers,** which is inherited as an autosomal dominant trait. In addition to the hypoplasia of the end phalanges, dysplasia of the skin markings and transverse furrows of the nail plate are also present, but the typical firm cutaneous changes that are characteristic of scleroderma are missing.[10]

The mutilating processes of the terminal finger phalanges in progressive scleroderma are not confined to the connective tissue of the skin but also involve the deeper lying osseous tissue. Such **acroosteolyses** begin at the palmar side at the top of the terminal phalanges and are, therefore, demonstrable only in a lateral radiograph. In the differential diagnosis similar osteolytic conditions in neurosyphilis, leprosy,

syringomyelia, and diabetes mellitus must be ruled out.

Most cases of familial acroosteolyses (Thévenard syndrome) develop in young people on the feet and hands (see Chapter 5, A3). In all such cases the presence of neuropathic familial amyloidosis must be excluded (by rectal biopsy), especially since here also sclerodermiform cutaneous changes of the hands may occur. Acroosteolyses may also indicate acrodermatitis chronica atrophicans and also late damage of the fingers caused by x-rays.[3, 7, 13, 21, 34, 36]

Associated with sclerodermiform cutaneous changes on the arms and hands, **acroosteolyses** of the fingers have been observed in workers who have had a long-continued contact with **vinyl chloride polymers.** As in progressive scleroderma, the patients in the beginning experience such subjective sensations as pronounced sensitivity to cold, paresthesia, and

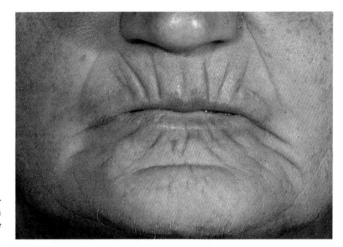

Fig. 149. Progressive scleroderma: microstomia with
radial folds around the
mouth.

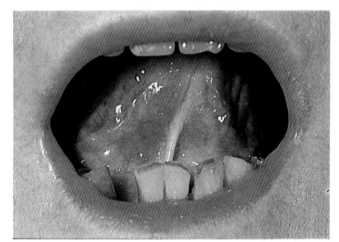

Fig. 150. Progressive scleroderma: microstomia and
wardened and shortened frenulum.

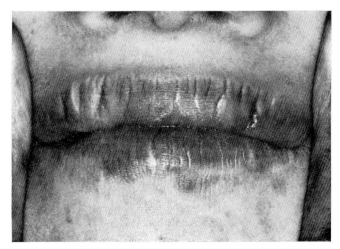

Fig. 151. Transverse folds of
the lips in Down's syndrome.

hypesthesia. At the same time, these patients have symptoms typical of Raynaud's disease. The affected skin is pasty, pale, and edematous and becomes gradually hard, resulting in the disappearance of skin markings and a limited mobility of the joints. In some patients, closely aggregated papules develop, whitish-yellow to skin-colored, and about the size of rice grains. Characteristic roentgenologic findings, which are typical and determine the diagnosis, show bandlike osteolysis and shortening of the terminal phalanges.[27, 28, 38]

Just as sclerodactylia characteristically afflicts the hands of the patient with scleroderma, the face is also affected (Fig. 148), especially by **microstomia** (Fig. 149). The frenum of the tongue becomes hard and short (scleroglosson) (Fig. 150). With increasing limitations the facial features develop a masklike rigidity, and the mouth is surrounded by a ring of folds similar to those of a tobacco pouch. Somewhat similar microstomias are occasionally observed in extensive atrophies of the facial area caused by x-rays and in the syndrome of craniocarpotarsal dystrophy. Microstomias and poikiloderma in x-ray atrophies (for instance, as the result of roentgenologic treatment of lupus vulgaris) are limited to the size of the field. In **craniocarpotarsal dystrophy** (Freeman-Sheldon syndrome, the whistling face syndrome), microstomia, a distinctly masklike facies, a receding chin, protruding lips, and, above all, a tower skull are conspicuous. The muscles of the arms are thin and extremely slack, and the hands and fingers show flexion contractures and ulnar deviation.[16, 31, 37]

If, however, only radial perioral folds are present, but no microstomia or scleroglosson, Parrot's rhagades of congenital syphilis may have to be considered. These are caused by specific preceding infiltrative processes around the lips. Similar radial perioral rhagades may be present in endogenous eczema (disseminated neurodermatitis); however, they extend within the borders of the lips, which occurs in Parrot's rhagades only at the inflammatory stage. Fissures of the mouth are also found in erythropoietic protoporphyria and in Down's syndrome (Fig. 151). In no case, however, are the perioral radial fissures diagnostically decisive. This is one stigma to be considered within the framework of many other signs.[5] For microstomia in oral submucous fibrosis see Chapter 34, A12.

Rather frequently, progressive scleroderma will show calcium deposits, in which case it is usually called the **Thibierge-Weissenbach syndrome.** Such calcinoses are, of course, detectable by x-rays but they may become evident clinically by the discharge of crumbling material. In progressive scleroderma calcinosis usually occurs in circumscribed areas, which, however, sometimes become rather large, whereas in dermatomyositis these calcifications of soft tissue, especially in the healing stage in children, are larger and more widespread. If the calcifications are associated with signs of Raynaud's disease, sclerodactylia, and telangiectases, a clinical picture evolves which has recently been called the CRST syndrome. Telangiectases, however, are regularly seen in every stage of progressive scleroderma. Only very infrequently will the intensity and extension of such dilatations of end vessels suggest Osler's disease. Therefore, it can be said that in progressive scleroderma teleangiectases are mainly present on the face and upper chest and in association with interlacing ("guilloche") pigmentations (Figs. 152, 153, and 154).

The extracutaneous components of progressive scleroderma are generally not important to the dermatologist interested in differential diagnosis. Scleroderma of the esophagus (Fig. 155), however, will occasionally demand exclusion of other esophageal spasms or esophageal carcinoma, and the rigidity of the gastric mucosa must be differentiated from that of "linitis plastica." One should keep in mind that malabsorption or late ileus may be due to scleroderma. Pulmonary involvement in progressive scleroderma, however, demands special differential diagnostic considerations. If the clinical picture is typical, it will clearly indicate that it belongs to a disorder of the pulmonary supportive tissue, since fibrosis of the lungs occurs rather frequently in collagenoses, among them, progressive scleroderma. Increased fibrosis, however, which causes shortness of breath and chronic cough and may lead to a cor pulmonale, is also observed in sarcoidosis. Interstitial pulmonary fibrosis of the Hamman-Rich syndrome presents a uniform pulmonary picture clinically and anatomically, which, however, may also be caused by pneumoconioses (silicosis), organic dust, x-rays, some drugs (hydralazine and hexamethonium), and, very rarely, may occur also in rheumatic polyarthritis. In all these presumably exogenous pulmonary fibroses, which do not occur in connection with systemic skin manifestations, the history is invaluable. Reports on frequent and simultaneous occurrence of silicosis and progressive scleroderma in miners or workers exposed to inhalation of dust are suggestive. On the other hand, interstitial fibroses resulting from pulmonary mycoses, pulmonary amyloidoses, or neoplastic reticuloses are only rarely observed.[4, 9, 14, 15, 17, 39]

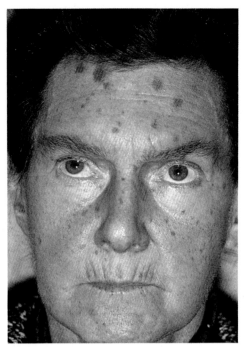

Fig. 152. Progressive scleroderma: so-called CRST syndrome.

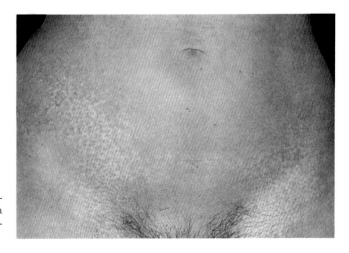

Fig. 153. Progressive scleroderma: pigmentations in "guilloche" (intertwined ornamentation).

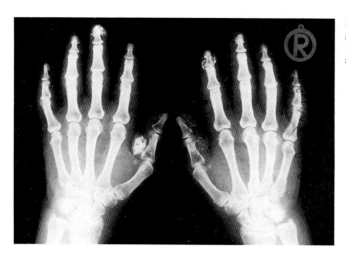

Fig. 154. Calcinosis in progressive scleroderma (Thibierge-Weissenbach syndrome).

2. Different conditions that resemble progressive scleroderma include, first of all, "edematous" scleroderma, **scleredema adultorum.** It is a transitory mucopolysaccharide thesaurismosis which has no preference for age or sex. When the disease is fully developed, the skin has a waxy or hard-as-paraffin consistency, which is more apparent palpably than visibly and which on the surface may look somewhat nodular

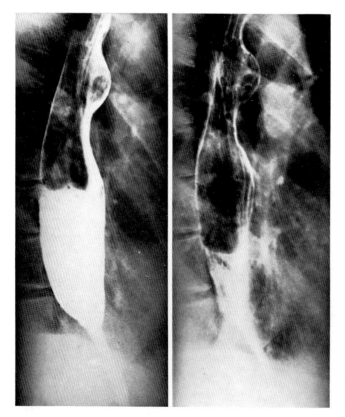

Fig. 155. Progressive scleroderma: sclerosis of the esophagus with pronounced prestenotic dilatation.

Fig. 156. Scleredema adultorum: Trabecular surface
of the indurated cutaneous
areas.

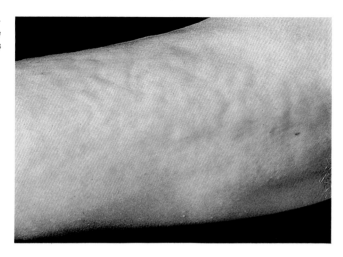

or wavily trabecular (Fig. 156). Except in rare cases, the inner organs are not affected. Occasionally, myocarditis is discovered in the EKG and electromyographic changes occur in the skeletal muscles. In the differential diagnosis against progressive scleroderma, it is significant that scler-edema almost always follows an infection, has a rapid onset and a tendency to spontaneous involution, and does not involve the inner organs. Furthermore, Raynaud's phenomenon is missing and hands, feet, and nipples are rarely involved. If the ability to open the mouth is restricted, it is due to the hard consistency of the surrounding facial skin and not to a genuine diminution in the opening of the mouth.[9, 12, 28]

3. In **scleromyxedema,** papular and diffuse myxodermas lead to a thickening of the skin and bulging folds (Fig. 157a, b). In contrast to progressive scleroderma, the primary cause of scleromyxedema is mucinous storage, which leads secondarily to sclerofibrosis. In progressive sclero-derma the patient is endangered by possible visceral involvement, whereas in sclero-myxedema the danger lies in the vascular changes or in a possible cerebral mucinous infiltration. Furthermore, most cases of scleromyxedema are complicated by para-proteinemia, but other indications of a plasmacytoma need not be present (see also Chapter 31, B1).[33]

4. Deposits of amyloid may resemble scleroderma. **Scleroderma amyloidosum,** part of a "primary" systemic amyloidosis, can be determined by the presence of Bence Jones proteinuria, histologic evidence of amyloid in the skin, and most important, the result of a rectal biopsy.[25, 30, 35]

Edematous-indurative hardening of the skin can also accompany **multiple myelomas.** In most cases these sclerodermiform changes are caused by amyloidosis. There are, however, patients with myeloma with diffuse cutaneous scleroses, in whom no deposits of amyloid can be found. In these patients the sudden onset of induration and the lack of involvement of inner organs rule out progressive scleroderma. The similarity with scleredema adultorum is, however, greater, since both cutaneous indurations favor the shoulder girdle and the upper arms.[19]

5. A sclerodermalike picture is also seen in **porphyria cutanea tarda.** Based on our

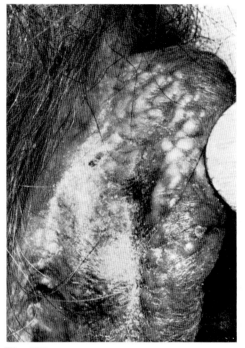

Fig. 157a.

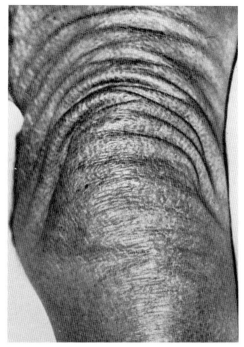

Fig. 157b.

Fig. 157. Scleromyxedema: (a) isolated lichen myxedematous nodules behind the ear; (b) gross folds of the thickened skin near a joint.

present knowledge, previously reported cases of progressive scleroderma with porphyrinuria were apparently those of porphyria cutanea tarda with sclero-vitiliginous features. Signs favoring a diagnosis of sclerodermiform porphyria are any lesions on skin exposed to light, and, above all, the associated postbullous excoriations and crusts. Histologically, a differentiation between sclerodermiform porphyria and progressive scleroderma is difficult; sclerodermiform features in chronic porphyria are rare, however.[32]

6. Even rarer than these manifestations in porphyria cutanea tarda are the sclerodermalike fibroses and indurations in the **carcinoid syndrome.** But here it is strictly a question of cutaneous scleroses, which lack any progressive tendency toward generalization, and, therefore, the character of a systemic disorder.[1, 40]

Sclerodermiform cutaneous changes on the distal portions of the extremities may be associated with muscular hardening in children with untreated **phenylketonuria.** [2, 18]

7. In sclerodermalike diseases of childhood – genuine progressive scleroderma with involvement of the inner organs is rare in children – unusual, flat, circumscribed areas of induration of the cutaneous and subcutaneous cellular tissues constitute **sclerema** of the newborn. In sclerema adiposum, in contrast to sclerema edematosum, finger pressure will not result in pitting. In spite of this alleged difference in the character of the edemas, both disorders show a similar alabaster to whitish-yellow hue, which is occasionally marble-like and may be cyanotic at the periphery. The first cutaneous changes occur on the surface of the lower body but soon cover the entire skin. Typically, body areas that are prone to edema (genitals, eyelids, and ankle region) are spared. The surface of the affected skin is smooth; its deeper portions are sometimes interspersed with palpable nodules or cystic formations. The skin cannot be lifted in folds and cannot be moved from its base, or only to a small degree. It is important to differentiate this condition from other forms of hydrops (Rh incompatibility, hypoproteinemia in pancreatic fibrosis, and others) in the newborn. The prognosis for these usually hypothermic infants, whose muscular mobility (and respiration) is restricted, is extremely unfavorable, and about two-thirds of the cases will end fatally.[26, 28]

8. Subcutaneous fat necrosis of the newborn is mainly located as a frequently symmetrical fat sclerosis in the shoulder region, buttocks, cheeks, and proximal parts of the extremities. It is characterized by plaquelike subcutaneous infiltrates in infants who are in good general condition but overweight, and therefore, have been born under hard labor. The induration can be moved only a little from its base and is demarcated like an epaulet. The overlying skin is often brownish or bluish-red (Fig. 158). Sometimes septic softening intervenes; otherwise involution ensues after months with no significant residual lipoatrophy. In this disorder, caused by trauma to the subcutaneous adipose tissue, the fats liberated in the necrosis undergo enzymatic influences and the resulting products cause granulomatous proliferation. The prognosis for such children is somewhat unfavorable if the internal fat tissue is also affected.[26,28]

9. In **Werner's syndrome,** which is an inherited dermatosis classed with progeria, sclerodactylia and a sclerodermalike face that resembles that of a bird are especially important for the differential diagnosis.

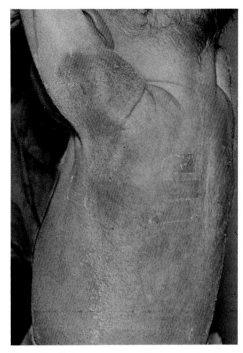

Fig. 158. Subcutaneous adiponecrosis of the newborn.

This disorder is observed mostly in men and usually begins after the twentieth year of life. It is characterized by fluctuations in pigment as well as by a taut atrophy that begins on the extremities and later makes the limbs spindly owing to loss of subcutaneous tissue and wasting of muscles. Special features of this scleratrophy are trophic (mostly plantar) ulcerations, warty hyperkeratoses, hypofunction of the gonads, or arrest of development on an infantile level. Patients with this disorder look alike: they are small in stature, and have birdlike faces; their hair is prematurely gray or is brittle and total alopecia follows. The nails are frequently dystrophic. Another characteristic is the rasping voice (leukoplakia of the vocal cords). A cardinal sign is a juvenile cataract, which begins about the third decade of life and eventually occurs in both eyes. Roentgenologically, Werner's syndrome is characterized by osteoporoses, "metastatic" calcifications in the connective tissue, peripheral arteries, cardiac valves, and coronary arteries, as well as trophic disturbances of the bones of the feet. The prognosis of patients with Werner's syndrome is dim, not only because of their tendency to juvenile arteriosclerosis but also because of their increased disposition to malignant tumors.[9, 11, 20, 22]

10. It is difficult to distinguish progressive scleroderma from **rheumatoid arthritis** because in the former there are arthritic rheumatoid manifestations which affect the proximal parts of the extremities rather than the distal ones and are accompanied by severe general signs. If, however, a definite ulnar, fish-finlike finger abnormality is present, and the affected hands – not so much the feet – are enlarged rather than reduced in size, possible sclerodermiform changes that are otherwise impressive are not considered progressive scleroderma. Some help can be derived from the determination of the rheumatoid factors, which, however, are positive in 15 per cent of patients with scleroderma. On the other hand, sclerodermalike visceral involvement (e. g., esophageal stenosis) is not expected in rheumatoid arthritis. Roentgenologically, polyarthritis in progressive scleroderma can be differentiated from rheumatoid arthritis by the lack of cystlike clear spaces and proliferative osseous changes.[23,36]

(1) ASBOE-HANSEN, G.: Scleroderma in carcinoid syndrome. Acta derm.-venereol. (Stockh.) *39:* 270–273 (1959).
(2) BATTIN, J., P. CHAVOIX, J. ALBERTY et J.-P. HEHUNSTRE:Phénylcétonurie avec infiltration de type sclérodermique. Pédiatrie *25:* 777–784 (1970).
(3) BISCHOFF, A.: Zur diabetischen Amyotrophie (Neuromyopathie). Schweiz. med. Wschr. *89:* 519–525 (1959).
(4) BREDNOW, W.: Zur klinisch-röntgenologischen Differentialdiagnose seltener Lungengerüsterkrankungen. Internist: *3* 339–346 (1962).

(5) BUTTERWORTH, T., E. P. LEONI, H. BEERMAN, M. GRAY WOOD and L. P. STREAN: Cheilitis of mongolism. J. Invest. Dermat. *35:* 347–351 (1960).
(6) CLARK, J. A., R. K. WINKELMANN and L. E. WARD: Serologic alterations in scleroderma and sclerodermatomyositis. Mayo Clin. Proc. *46:* 14–107 (1971).
(7) DELANK, H.-W., G. KOCH, G. KÖNN, H.-P. MISSMAHL und K. SUWELACK: Familiäre Amyloid-Polyneuropathie Typus Wohlwill-Corino-Andrade. Ärztl. Forsch. *19:* 401–416 (1965).
(8) DENK, R.: Fingerkuppennekrose bei einem Preßluftwerkzeugarbeiter. Med. Welt *17* (N. F.): 1595–1596 (1966).
(9) DENK, R.: Elektrokardiographische Untersuchungen bei Hautkranken. Arch. Kreisl.-Forsch. *60:* 33–114 (1969).
(10) DODINVAL, P.: A propos de la dysplasie des crêtes épidermiques. Mise en évidence d'une dysplasie apicale des doigts. Humangenetik *15:* 20–24 (1972).
(11) EPSTEIN, CH. J., G. M. MARTIN, A. L. SCHULTZ and A. G. MOTULSKY: Werner's syndrome. Medicine (Baltimore) *45:* 177–221 (1966).
(12) FLEISCHMAJER, R., and J. V. LARA: Scleredema. Arch. Derm. (Chic.) *92:* 643–652 (1965).
(13) GNÄDIGER, A., und E. LANDES: Fingergangrän als Röntgenspätschädigung. Arch. klin. exp. Derm. *231:* 170–186 (1968).
(14) GÜNTHER, G., und E. SCHUCHARDT: Silikose und progressive Sklerodermie. Dtsch. med. Wschr. *95:* 467–468 (1970).
(15) HOLZMANN, H., und W. FRISCH: Über die Beziehungen zwischen progressiver Sklerodermie und malignen Tumoren. Ärztl. Forsch. *24:* 129–140 (1970).
(16) HORNSTEIN, O. P., und G. GERDES: Klinische und röntgenologische Symptome der progressiven Sklerodermie in der Mundhöhle. Hautarzt *22:* 471–476 (1971).
(17) JABLONSKA, S.: Pseudosklerodermien. Med. Klin. *62:* 1151–1154 (1967).
(18) JABLONSKA, S., et A. STACHOW: Pseudosclérodermie ou sclérodermie coexistant avec la phénylcétonurie. Ann. Derm. Syph. (Paris) *99:* 257–262 (1972).
(19) JABLOŃSKA, S., and A. STACHOW: Scleroderma-like lesions in multiple myeloma. Dermatologica (Basel) *144:* 257–269 (1972).

(20) JACOBSON, H. G., H. RIFKIN and D. ZUCKER-FRANKLIN: Werner's syndrome: a clinical-roentgen entity. Radiology *74*: 373–385 (1960).

(21) JÄNNER, M., B. ROHDE und G. JANNASCH: Zum Krankheitsbild der familiären Akroosteolyse. Z. Haut- u. Geschl.-Kr. *34*: 65–73 (1963).

(22) KNOTH, W., R. BAETHKE und L. HOFFMANN: Über das Werner-Syndrom. Hautarzt *14*: 145–152, 193–202 (1963).

(23) KORTING, G. W., und H. HOLZMANN: Das Erscheinungsbild der Hand bei den sogenannten Kollagenosen. Med. Welt *20* (N. F.): 603–605 (1969).

(24) KÜSTNER, W., P. LÜBBERS, H. UTHGENANNT und F. WEGENER: Die Wegenersche Granulomatose. Diagnostische Probleme und klinischer Verlauf unter immunsuppresiver Therapie. Schweiz. med. Wschr. *101*: 1137–1142 (1971).

(25) LEACH, W. B., PH. S. VASSAR and CH. F. CULLING: Primary systemic amyloidosis presenting as scleroderma. Canad. Med. Ass. J. *83*: 263–265 (1960).

(26) LINDLAR, F., und V. MISGELD: Die Adiponecrosis subcutanea neonatorum unter lipoidchemischem Aspekt. Hautarzt *18*: 115–118 (1967).

(27) MEYERSON, L. B., and G. C. MEIER: Cutaneous lesions in acroosteolysis. Arch. Derm. (Chic.) *106*: 224–227 (1972).

(28) MISGELD, V.: Adiponecrosis subcutanea neonatorum – Sclerema neonatorum – Sclerödem Buschke. Nosographie unter Berücksichtigung der Literatur ab 1950. Arch. Kinderheilk. *183*: 5–22 (1971).

(29) MISGELD, V., H.-J. STOLPMANN und S. SCHULTE: Zur Intoxikation durch Vinylchlorid-Polymerisate und/oder deren Begleitstoffe. Z. Haut- u. Geschl.-Kr. *48*: 425–436 (1973).

(30) MISSMAHL, H.-P.: Erbbedingte generalisierte Amyloidosen. Dtsch. med. Wschr. *89*: 709–712 (1964).

(31) OTTO, F. M. G.: Die »Cranio-carpo-tarsal Dystrophie« (Freeman und Sheldon); ein kasuistischer Beitrag. Z. Kinderheilk. *73*: 240–250 (1953).

(32) PERROT, H., J. THIVOLET et G. CARDIN: Les aspects sclérodermiformes de la porphyrie cutanée tardive. J. Méd. Lyon *51*: 159–165 (1970).

(33) PROPPE, A., V. BECKER und TH. HARDMEIER: Skleromyxödem Arndt-Gottron und Plasmocytom. Hautarzt *20*: 53–59 (1969).

(34) RASCHKE, G.: Über den Zusammenhang der Akrodermatitis chronica atrophicans Pick-Herxheimer und der Akroosteolyse. Derm. Wschr. *137*: 21 7–221 (1958).

(35) RUKAVINA, J. G., W. D. BLOCK, CH. E. JACKSON, G. F. FALLS, J. H. CAREY and A. C. CURTIS: Primary systemic amyloidosis; a review and an experimental, genetic, and clinical study of 29 cases with particular emphasis on familial form. Medicine (Baltimore) *35*: 239–334 (1956).

(36) SCHACHERL, M., und H. HOLZMANN: Zur Polyarthritis bei progressiver Sklerodermie. Fortschr. Röntgenstr. *107*: 485–493 (1967).

(37) WEINSTEIN, S., and R. J. GORLIN: Cranio-carpo-tarsal dysplasia or the whistling face syndrome. I. Clinical considerations. Amer. J. Dis. Child. *117*: 427–433 (1969).

(38) WILSON, R. H., W. E. MCCORMICK, C. F. TATUM and J. L. CREECH: Occupational acroosteolysis. J. Amer. Med. Ass. *201*: 577–581 (1967).

(39) WINTERBAUER, R. H.: Multiple telangiectasia, Raynaud's phenomenon, sclerodactyly and subcutaneous calcinosis: a syndrome mimicking hereditary hemorrhagic telangiectasia. Bull. Johns Hopk. Hosp. *114*: 361–383 (1964).

(40) ZARAFONETIS, C. J., S. H. LORBER and S. M. HANSON: Association of functioning carcinoid syndrome and scleroderma. Amer. J. Med. Sci. *236*: 1–14 (1958).

C. Dermatomyositis

1. Dermatomyositis is a systemic disease of both skin and muscles; the role of each, however, changes in each case and in the course of the disorder. Cutaneous manifestations may precede myositis by months; in the acute stage, they are characterized by a saturated wine-red color, and later also by telangiectatic or porcelain-white spots, especially on the osseous prominences of the hands (Fig. 159) and knees. Additional signs are closely agminated, slightly glassy nodules on the neck (Fig. 160) and a painful thickened cuticle (Fig. 161). However, after healing or extraneous to the eruptions themselves a unique, checkered, cutaneous appearance sometimes remains (see Chapter 23, B2, dealing with poikiloderma). Especially in the burnt-out final stage, extensive hypertrichoses (Chapter 11, H3) and massive calcifications (Figs.

163, 164, 165) may be present. The patient with dermatomyositis has a strange, sad, and suffering expression, and his movements (lifting arms, bending knees, fastening an apron, or trying to reach a back pocket) are diminished. This is a valuable diagnostic sign. Men and women in their first to fifth decades are affected about equally. It is always important to search for a malignant tumor, including thymoma. In about twenty per cent of dermatomyositis patients over the age of 40 such an association can be found. Often repeated investigations are necessary since in the beginning the tumor may be too small for detection. Figure 166 shows which organs are involved.

Associated involvement of inner organs occurs least in dermatomyositis among all the "collagenoses." But foremost among these is the involvement of the heart,

Fig. 159. Dermatomyositis.

Fig. 160. Dermatomyositis: nuchal erythemas interspersed with small papules.

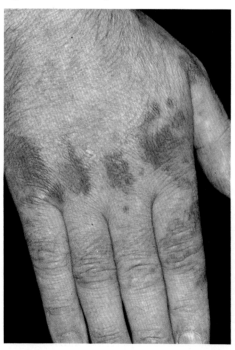

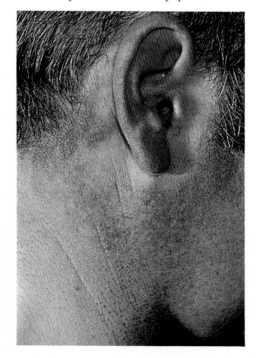

which in acute cases is often responsible for a fatal outcome. Pulmonary fibroses and degeneration and fibrosis of the smooth muscles of the esophagus and urinary bladder are rare.[3, 6, 8, 9, 12 15, 17, 19]

Histologically, one finds, especially when a muscle biopsy has been taken following an electromyogram, circumscribed and discontinuous edematization of muscle fibers leading to myolysis (empty sarcolemma tubes) (Fig. 167). In an acutely diseased area, swollen cutaneous nerves and involvement of the arrector muscles are remarkable. Of greater importance, however, are the interstitial cell proliferations situated between the muscle fibers. The number of eosinophilic leukocytes in these proliferations is not particularly great. It should be noted however, that the histologic findings differ with the different phases. In the acute stage, edema and vacuolar degeneration are notable, and in

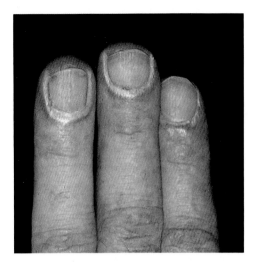

Fig. 161. Dermatomyositis: sclerosis of the cuticle.

the subacute or chronic stages lymphocytic infiltrates predominate, especially interstitially between the muscular fibrils.

Fig. 162. Dermatomyositis: wine-red facial erythemas.

Fig. 163. Calcinosis cutis after healed dermatomyositis.

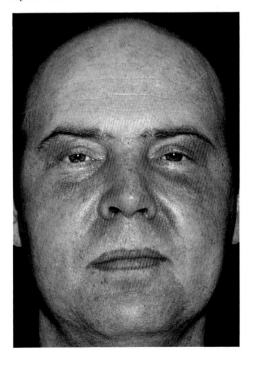

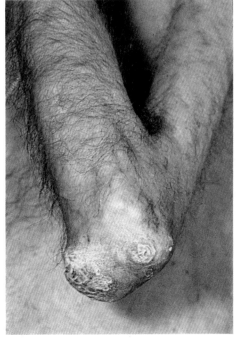

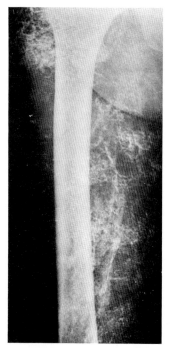

Fig. 164. Dermatomyositis: radiologic picture of calcifications in the soft tissues of the thigh.

Moreover, in muscles, skin, and the gastrointestinal tract distinct scleroses of smaller arteries and arterioles can be observed; these must be distinguished from similar vascular artefacts produced by cortisone.

Fig. 165. Dermatomyositis: massive calcium deposits in the corium. Von Kossa stain.

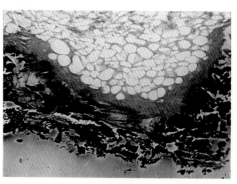

It is difficult to diagnose dermatomyositis from the histologic findings. Quite often, the changes correspond to those of acute lupus erythematosus. No correlation exists between the degree of myositis and the intensity of the changes in the corium. The essential change in the corium in dermatomyositis is mucoid edema without simultaneous accumulation of cells. Usually, loose perivascular infiltrations of lymphocytes or granulocytes are present. The mucinous deposit, however, is at times so extreme that the histologic appearance may resemble that of exquisitely mucinous states such as the circumscribed mucinoses (pretibial tuberous myxedema, lichen myxedematosus, and scleromyxedema). This severe mucoid infiltration may be responsible for the vacuolar degeneration of the basal cell line, a characteristic histologic finding in dermatomyositis. This degeneration of basal cells is obviously noninflammatory, because it appears without connection with cellular infiltration; it is, therefore, distinctly different from similar changes in lichen planus or some forms of parapsoriasis, in which liquefaction of the basal cells is apparently connected with the adjacent dense cellular infiltrate.[1, 2, 10]

In addition to the muscle biopsy and the determination of increased creatinine excretion in 24-hour urine (normal values are 0.1–0.4 g per 24 hours), the diagnosis of dermatomyositis has been facilitated by the use of an electromyogram. The electromyogram shows characteristic features only in the acute and subacute stages (brief duration of the action potentials, strongly increased polyphasia, diminution of the tension of the potentials of the motoric unity, and a dense interference pattern in spite of distinct pareses). On the other hand, in chronic cases the electromyographic findings permit only the diagnosis of myogenic dystrophy without additional classification. It must be said that the decisive value of electromyography lies in its ability to distinguish

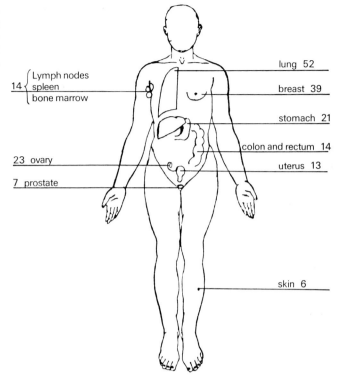

Fig. 166. Frequency of localization of malignant tumors
in 233 patients with der-
matomyositis and tumor
(from Holzmann and Herz,
1969).

Lymph nodes
14 { spleen
bone marrow

lung 52

breast 39

stomach 21

colon and rectum 14

uterus 13

23 ovary

7 prostate

skin 6

between primary myogenous disorders and central or peripheral neurogenic muscular damage, but a differentiation among the myopathies using the electromyogram is rather limited. But electromyography is valuable in determining the site of a muscle biopsy, since with its help areas of myositis can be verified.[23]

In the serum the enzymes GOT, GPT, aldolase, creatine-phosphokinase, and myo-kinase change with the activity of the disease. On the other hand, the so-called seroreactions, such as the Wassermann reaction, Coombs test, rheumatoid factors, lupus induction test, and antistreptolysin titer, are negative or uncharacteristic. If the muscle fibers deteriorate excessively, the urine may show a red-brown color indicating myoglobinuria.

The concept of **carcinomatous neuro-myopathy** covers those cases of dermato-myositis which show neuropathy and a malignant tumor. If these are polymyo-

sitides with typical cutaneous changes, the establishment of a special entity different from dermatomyositis appears unneces-sary.[6, 13]

2. The differentiation of dermatomyosi-tis from infectious or parasitic myositis is generally easy (bacterial, e. g., staphy-

Fig. 167. Dermatomyositis: muscle fibers with loss of transverse streaks and interstitial cell proliferation. HE stain.

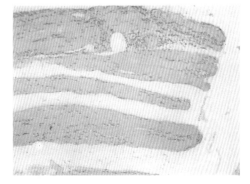

logenous **suppurative myositis,** syphilitic myositis, also circumscribed myositides in leptospirosis, salmonellosis, toxoplasmosis, trypanosomiasis, and so on. Especially important in this connection is the differential diagnosis from **trichinosis,** which simulates dermatomyositis so closely that the latter has sometimes been called "pseudotrichinosis." In the beginning trichinosis shows severe general signs (hyperhidrosis, fever, nausea, vomiting, diarrhea, and insomnia) and occasionally edema of the lids. The patients suffer violent muscular pain, so that they anxiously avoid any body movements. Additional signs are hypoglycemia, involvement of the myocardium and creatinuria. Dermatomyositis as well as trichinosis may be accompanied by eosinophilia. Important signs in trichinosis are its epidemic character and the regression of the acute manifestations, beginning usually with the second month. The diagnosis of trichinosis can be secured by proof of trichinellas, at the earliest, on the tenth day of the disease. (A biopsy should be obtained from the deltoid muscle.) The specimen is put between two slides and squeezed; glycerin is then added (Fig. 168). In trichinosis calcification phenomena similar to those in dermatomyo-

Fig. 168. *Trichinella spiralis* in a squeezed muscle preparation.

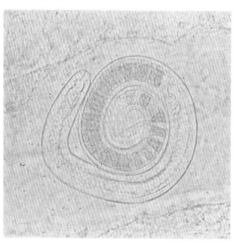

sitis also occur; however, they affect only the capsules of the trichinellas. After about six months they can be detected roentgenologically as small lancet-shaped shadows in the muscles. Since trichinosis also shows increased serum ferments (GOT, GPT, myokinase, LDH [lactic dehydrogenase]), the outcome of the precipitation test from the fifth week of illness on is decisive.[4, 16]

3. Another "epidemic" **myositis,** especially in children, is caused by the coxsackievirus **(Bornholm disease** or myalgia epidemica). The characteristic signs are pleurodynia, peracute pericarditis and, occasionally, dry pleuritis, myocarditis, and encephalitis. Genuine pareses are rare. Evidence of the causative organism is found in the stool or by the outcome of the complement fixation test.

4. In **sarcoidosis (Boeck**'s **disease)** muscular granulomatous infiltrates of epithelioid cells may appear but do not cause any symptoms. Only in a few cases of acute sarcoidosis are painless nodes in the muscles of the extremities or on the head and neck palpable. Rare cases of muscular sarcoidosis have signs similar to those of progressive muscular dystrophy or polymyositis. Occasionally, an additional association with polyneuritis occurs so that at first confusing overlapping signs may develop (see also Chapter 7, E1).[18]

5. Involvement of the muscles is observed in endocrinopathies, especially in **hyperthyroidism** (paresis of the ocular muscles in thyrotoxic crisis is frequent in contrast to its rare occurrence in dermatomyositis). But also **hypothyroidism,** disturbances of the **parathyroid** function, and **Cushing**'s **disease** are known to show muscular involvement. Moreover, **hyperkalemia** (e.g., in severe renal insufficiency) and **hypokalemia** can produce abnormal tiredness and muscular cramps and pareses. The latter may show ascending flaccid paresis with a tetraplegic picture.[22]

6. Apart from the **myopathies caused by drugs or toxins** following corticosteroids, chloroquine, and vincristine, myasthenias have been observed following certain antibiotics such as neomycin, streptomycin, kanamycin, colistin, polymyxin-B, and viomycin. The occurrence of myasthenia caused by antibiotics depends heavily on the dosage and is caused by competitive inhibition at the end plate. Since some anesthetic and muscle-relaxing drugs have the same effect, a combination of their actions may cause dangerous incidents during anesthesia.[11, 14]

7. In a dermatologic work it is necessary to discuss the manifestations of the various dermatoses among the collagenoses. In **systemic lupus erythematosus** (SLE) facial erythema, comparable to that in dermatomyositis, may exist. Cutaneous changes in SLE include spotty palmar erythema, intrafollicular bleeding points and those on the mucous membranes, and follicular hyperkeratoses, whereas in dermatomyositis lichenoid eruptions of the neck are of special diagnostic significance. Polyserositis is an indication in favor of SLE; involvement of the myocardium, of dermatomyositis. Finally, SLE is characterized by the LE-cell, the results of immunofluorescence, distinct leukopenia with lymphocytosis, higher values of ESR, and marked dysproteinemia.

8. Chronic dermatomyositides may show mild sclerodermalike features. The course of typical **progressive scleroderma,** however, differs from that of common dermatomyositis; it is not violent but slowly progressive, starting with distinct Raynaud's phenomena. Its later course is characterized by widespread involvement of inner organs (lungs, gastrointestinal tract, kidneys, and heart). Poikilodermalike changes characterize much more frequently the end stages of dermatomyositis than those of progressive scleroderma, in which scleratrophy, hyperpigmentation,

and depigmentation, and occasionally, secondary wasting of muscles dominate the whole final process of mummification. The enzymes mentioned earlier in the serum and creatine in the urine are not present unless the muscles are distinctly affected. On the other hand, electromyography can, in many cases, also show an involvement of the muscles in progressive scleroderma.[20, 21]

9. The concept of **generalized fibrous myositis** covers those chronic progressive muscular diseases in which conspicuous hardening and shortening of the muscles predominate, with resulting stiffening and contracture. Etiologically, no uniform cause is responsible. In a considerable number of such patients the existing disease is chronic dermatomyositis or its end stage, as the accompanying cutaneous manifestations will indicate. Clinically, there is also some similarity with the *"stiff man syndrome"* which, however, lacks any morphologic or biochemically proven muscular damage. The occasionally extremely painful bracing of the skeletal muscles develops progressively over a period of months and may be increased by external stimuli. Mimic expression remains unaffected. Electromyographically, permanent fixed activity cannot be distinguished from voluntary activity. Doses of diazepam* lead to conspicuous diminution of the muscular stiffness.[5, 7, 15]

---

*Librium. (Tr.)

(1) BOLCK, F.: Zur Morphologie des Lupus erythematodes, der Dermatomyositis und der Sklerodermie. Derm. Mschr. *155:* 3–35 (1969).

(2) BOYLAN, R. C., and L. SOKOLOFF: Vascular lesions in dermatomyositis. Arthritis, Rheum. *3:* 379–386 (1960).

(3) DENK, R.: Elektrokardiographische Untersuchungen bei Hautkranken. Arch. Kreisl.-Forsch. *60:* 33–114 (1969).

(4) HENNEKEUSER, H. H., K. PABST, W. POEPLAU und W. GEROK: Zur Klinik und Therapie der Trichinose. Dtsch. med. Wschr. *93:* 867–873 (1968).

(5) HEYCK, H., und C.-J. LÜDERS: Myositis fibrosa generalisata – ein uneinheitliches Krankheitsbild. Mit kasuistischen Beiträgen und Schilderung einer ungewöhnlichen Myopathieform. In: Rheuma und Nervensystem. Ein Arbeitsgespräch in Wiesbaden vom 28./29. XI. 1969. S.105–129. Hoffmann-La Roche AG., Grenzach, Baden, 1970.

(6) HOLZMANN, H., und E. HERZ: Über die Beziehungen zwischen Dermatomyositis und malignen Tumoren. Ärztl. Forsch. *23:* 335–348 (1969).

(7) HUHNSTOCK, K., R. BROCK und E. KUHN: Über das Stiff-man-Syndrom. Dtsch.med.Wschr. *87:* 1388–1394 (1962).

(8) ILLIG, L.: Zur Begriffsbestimmung der sogenannten pseudomuskeldystrophischen Form der Polymyositis. Arch. klin. exp. Derm. *227:* 317–322 (1966).

(9) IRMSCHER, J., und S. ENGEL: Beteiligung der glatten Muskulatur bei Dermatomyositis. II. Arch. klin. exp. Derm. *228:* 364–371 (1967).

(10) JANIS, J. F., and R. K. WINKELMANN: Histopathology of the skin in dermatomyositis. Arch. Derm. (Chic.) *97:* 640–650 (1968).

(11) KAESER, H. E., und R. KOCHER: Iatrogene Muskelsymptome und Myopathien. Therapeut. Umschau *27:* 387–393 (1970).

(12) KLEINE-NATROP, H.-E., und S. ENGEL: Beteiligung der glatten Muskulatur bei Dermatomyositis. I. Arch. klin. exp. Derm. *228:* 353–363 (1967).

(13) KORTING, G. W.: Zur sog. karzinomatösen Neuromyopathie. Med. Welt (Stuttg.) *1963:* 1053–1057.

(14) McQUILLEN, M. P., H. E. CANTOR and J. R. O'ROURKE: Myasthenic syndrome associated with antibiotics. Arch. Neurol. (Chic.) *18:* 402–415 (1968).

(15) MERTENS, H. G., und K. RICKER: Übererregbarkeit der γ-Motoneurone beim »Stiff-man«-Syndrom. Klin. Wschr. *46:* 33–42 (1968).

(16) NITSCHE, W.: Trichinose unter besonderer Berücksichtigung ihrer Verbreitung und Bekämpfung. Münch. med. Wschr. *115:* 141–146 (1973).

(17) PUFF, K. H., und ST. ZSCHOCKE: Differentialdiagnose und Therapie der »Polymyositis«. Internist *7:* 170–175 (1966).

(18) SANDBANK, M., M. GRUNEBAUM and I. KATZENELLENBOGEN: Dermatomyositis associated with subacute pulmonary fibrosis. Arch. Derm. (Chic.) *94:* 432–435 (1966).

(19) SCADDING, J. G.: Sarcoidosis. Eyre & Spottiswoode, London 1967.

(20) SCHUERMANN, H.: Dermatomyositis. Erg. inn. Med. Kinderheilk. N. F. *10:* 427–480 (1958).

(21) SOLLBERG, G., R. DENK und H. HOLZMANN: Neurologische und elektrophysiologische Untersuchungen bei progressiver Sklerodermie und Morphaea. Arch. klin. exp. Derm. *229:* 20–32 (1967).

(22) SPIESS, H.: Myopathien und Muskelsymptome bei internen Krankheiten. Schweiz. med. Wschr. *99:* 1471–1477 (1969).

(23) STEINBRECHER, W.: Elektromyographie in Klinik und Praxis. Thieme, Stuttgart 1965.

D. Lupus Erythematosus Syndrome

Today the two forms of lupus erythematosus, the chronic discoid or cutaneous type and the acute systemic type which affects many organs, are considered varieties of the same disease.

1. Chronic cutaneous lupus erythematosus (discoid lupus erythematosus, discoid LE) of the face is usually characterized by a butterfly-shaped erythema with follicular hyperkeratoses; at first, only follicular atrophy is present, but later a larger, superficial area becomes atrophic. The diagnosis is much more easily ascertained when follicular hyperkeratoses become visible or when some of the atrophic areas show the well-known worm-eaten appearance (Fig. 169 a, b), which can be made more distinct by rubbing or by degreasing with ether. The same procedure is impor-tant in diagnosing cicatricial alopecia of the scalp.[4, 11, 31]

Histologically, chronic discoid LE does not offer, as a rule, any diagnostic difficulty, although other dermatoses also show hyperkeratosis or degenerative liquefaction of the basal cell line. The subepidermal basal membrane of the upper portion of the follicles, including the sebaceous glands, is distinctly widened (PAS positive) (Fig. 170 a, b, c). Especially characteristic are nodular circumscribed infiltrations of the middle of the follicle ("mediofollicular") within the corium and the formation of considerable edema within the subepidermis. In contrast to this perifollicular type of infiltration of discoid LE, some other diseases present such infiltrations in a more perivascular arrangement, such as secondary syphilis or toxic allergic exanthems, or in a different

Fig. 169. (a) Chronic discoid lupus erythematosus of the face. (b) Chronic discoid lupus erythematosus with central atrophy.

Fig. 169a.

Fig. 169b.

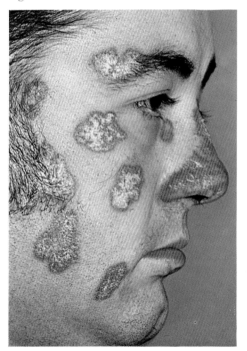
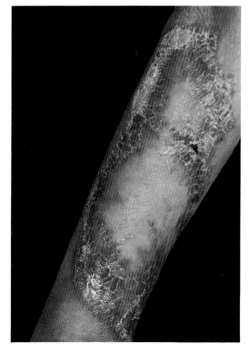

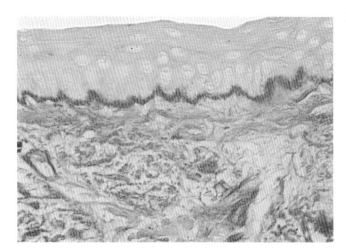

Fig. 170a.

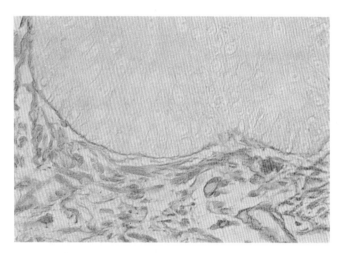

Fig. 170b.

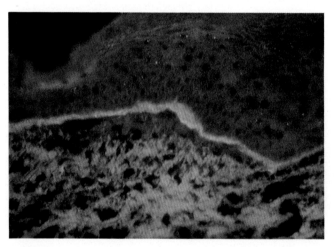

Fig. 170c.

Fig. 170. (a) Chronic discoid lupus erythematosus: widened basal membrane zone. PAS stain, 400×. (b) Normal skin in comparison. PAS stain, 400×. (c) Band of continuous fluorescence of the basal cell membrane.

cellular arrangement (plasma cells in syphilis, lymphocytes in lymphocytoma). Besides, there are very few other cutaneous diseases with such massive changes in the corium and corresponding characteristic alterations of the epidermis (vacuolization of the basal cell layer, hyperkeratoses) as in discoid LE. Lichen planus also shows epidermal changes (flat but not follicular hyperkeratoses; circumscribed widening of the granular layer; suggestive sub-epidermal formation of vacuoles with closely adjoining, dense, bandlike round cell infiltrates without perivascular or adnexal arrangement). Another differential diagnostic criterion is the immunohisto-logic detection of a wide, ill-defined band of fluorescence below the basal membrane of the epidermis (Fig. 170c).[3, 6, 7]

During the course of this disease a number of manifestations are observed, ranging from congestive seborrhea to occasionally mutilating "ulerythema cen-trifugum." The auricles and parts of the extremities are sometimes affected; how-ever, if there is further rapid dissemination (especially over the back), the condition is called **cutaneous discoid LE with acute exacerbation.** This disease has a wide spectrum of manifestations, consisting of erythematous, infiltrated, and hyperkera-totic lesions, as well as atrophy, telangiec-tasia, and pigmentary changes. In each case there can be several manifestations depending on the prevalence of each component; in some patients such com-ponents may remain unchanged during the entire course of the disease.

Simple, ill-defined erythematous patches that are conspicuous by their stubborn persistence **(erythema perstans)** are diffi-cult to diagnose, especially when firmly adherent scales and increased hyper-esthesia to touch are absent. However, the diagnosis is facilitated if early equilateral butterfly distribution of the lesion is present; discoid LE shares this clinical appearance with a number of dermatoses

(allergic dermatitis, rosacea, the exan-thems of scarlet fever, the constitutional vegetative facial mask also known as the rustic type of persistent chronic vaso-motoric erythema, and others). Compared with seborrheic dermatitis chronic discoid LE has firmly adherent scales, especially when attached to follicular openings (so-called thumbtack scales); also, sebor-rheic dermatitis, while it shows the same marginal peripheral exudative component as LE, has a faded brownish-yellow color. Characteristically, the margins of the lesions of this superficial type of discoid LE change relatively rapidly, and they are obviously exacerbated by exposure to light and weather; in principle, these influences are characteristic of all varieties of LE.

Such lesions approximate the appear-ance of **lymphocytic infiltration.** In spite of its character as an abortive type of LE,* this disease occupies an undisputed special phenomenologic position, especially because lymphocytic infiltration lacks hyperkeratosis and heals without atrophy. The flat infiltrates of lymphocytic infiltra-tion, pink to red-brown in color, start as small papules; histologically, sharply cir-cumscribed, perivascular and peri-appen-dicular infiltrates with a preponderance of small lymphocytes and only a few plasma and reticulum cells are present. Other attributes of lupus erythematosus are absent (such as follicular hyperkeratoses, atrophy of the epidermis, degeneration of the basal cell layer, and dilatations of blood vessels with red cell extravasations). The differential diagnosis of the **Sweet syndrome** (acute febrile neutrophilic dermatosis) is discussed in Chapter 1, B7.[9]

The solitary character of the lymphocytic infiltration may occasionally make it diffi-cult to separate it from **lymphadenosis benigna cutis** (LABC, lymphocytoma cutis)

---

* This opinion is shared by some, but not all, dermatologists. (Tr.)

because germinal centers surrounded by small mature lymphocytes are not regularly present. Clinically, LABC lacks the evanescence and the tendency to rapid recurrences of lymphocytic infiltration.[2]

Eosinophilic granuloma of the skin (granuloma faciale) is usually seen in middle-aged persons as a circumscribed, long-lasting reticulogranulomatosis of the skin. These reddish-brown to greyish-red, orange peel-like infiltrates of the face show a typical histologic picture: at first a polymorphic, perifollicularly arranged infiltrate with many eosinophils, which is later transformed into a lymphoreticular granulomatous infiltrate. Traces of such polymorphic cellular infiltrates mixed with many eosinophils can be seen in some pyodermas, hyperergic vasculitis, or leukoses with as yet unspecific cutaneous manifestations.[22]

A certain counterpart to the lymphocytic infiltration of the skin are the **angular atrophic plaques of the face;** running an eminently chronic course, they show sclerosis and fibrosis of the upper and middle corium, as well as lymphocytic inflammation and epidermal and follicular atrophy. Other characteristics arguing for a certain special position for such "annular atrophic facial plaques" are the lack of light sensitivity and the absence of therapeutic response to cortisone and antimalarial drugs.[8]

It remains an open question whether one is justified in establishing a special category of **erythematosuslike actinic dermatosis** in addition to the erythematous kind of polymorphous light eruptions. (Such an erythematosuslike actinic dermatosis has a required response to light and is correspondingly limited to exposed areas of skin, with sharply outlined areas of fine, lamellar scaling. Histologically, the appearance is that of hyperkeratosis.) However, healing takes place without atrophy.[37]

Sarcoidosis may show butterflylike, delicate erythemas of the cheeks, sometimes combined with a distinctly saturated, blue color of the nose **(lupus pernio)** or as annular centrifugal areas with accentuated edges. Such annular lesions of sarcoidosis fail to show follicular hyperkeratoses or other epidermal involvement. In addition, these lesions are located near the frontal hairline or in front of the auricles. Atrophy does not occur, and sensitivity to light is absent. When in doubt, histologic examination will be necessary.

The lupus erythematosuslike cutaneous changes of **Bloom's syndrome** will be discussed separately (Chapter 23, A4).

A variant of discoid LE with increased infiltrates consists of nodular special lesions located in various different layers. In **hypertrophic discoid** LE, a characteristic lesion with marked hyperkeratosis is present; the infiltrates are platelike, protruding, and resemble specific leukemic cutaneous infiltrates or platelike reticuloses, especially in the absence of a typical butterfly distribution. However, the two malignant neoplasms never show hyperkeratoses or marked atrophic regression.[12]

In **lupus erythematosus profundus,** the counterpart of hypertrophic discoid LE, deep subcutaneous nodules occur, completely isolated from other typical cutaneous lesions; they heal either spontaneously or with treatment, forming depressions of the skin (Fig. 171a, b). Histologically, LE profundus produces in the subcutis a combination of granulomatous infiltrates with massive, extensive, proliferative or degenerative vascular changes; however, these criteria by themselves do not permit a diagnosis without knowledge of additional facts about the disease process.[27,36]

Additional rare varieties of **chronic discoid** lupus erythematosus include **bullous types;** they resemble erythema multiforme and probably occur more often in connection with systemic LE. Bullous exacerbations are sometimes seen in **chilblain lupus** (Fig.172). This is a special type with large, dark wine-red, chilblain-like erythemas of the hands and face; however, in contrast to the "lupus pernio" of sarcoidosis, they do not involve in particular the lower two-thirds of the nose.[21, 38]

Discoid LE with acute exacerbation differs from the acute systemic type of LE in that it is a mostly transitory new development of numerous additional lesions in formerly healthy skin, especially of the back and the extensor aspects of the upper arms, without a simultaneous stormy exacerbation of the existing chronic discoid lesions of the face.[31]

A cicatrizing circumscribed loss of hair requires a differential diagnosis between chronic discoid LE and lichen planus decalvans (also known as **Graham-Little [Lassueur's] syndrome**), together with other lichen planuslike lesions (see also Chapter 11, E5 and E6). However, these lesions are not the usual flat, polygonal papules but more circular, acuminate nodules located in the lumbosacral region.

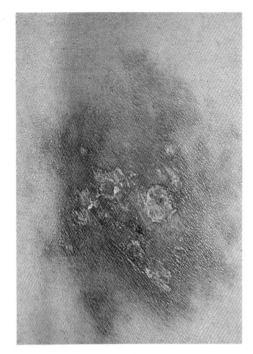

Fig. 171a.

As far as mucous membrane involvement is concerned, the genital region remains almost always free from chronic discoid LE, in contrast to lichen planus. The main mucous membrane lesion of LE is located on the lower lip; here short striae are

Fig. 171. Discoid lupus erythematosus profundus: (a) sunken-in area on the right side of the back, paravertebrally; (b) simultaneous hypertrophic facial areas.

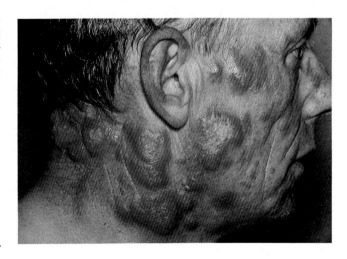

Fig. 171b.

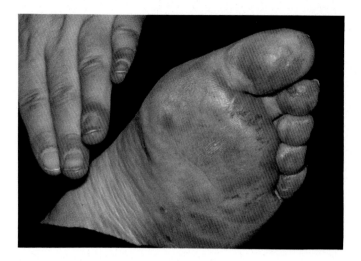

Fig. 172. Discoid lupus erythematosus: so-called chilblain lupus.

arranged in radial polycyclic fashion. Sometimes painful erosive and later atrophic depressed areas with crisscrossing telangiectases are present; they differ distinctly from the more uniform, flat, homogeneous lesions of leukoplakia.

In contrast, lichen planus of the lips and buccal mucosa has a lacy and cloudy network suggesting a fine spider web. The presence of atrophic areas with enlarged follicles around the periphery favors the diagnosis of lichen planus, in contrast to *lupus vulgaris* which is located in the midface region. Mild pressure with a blunt probe penetrates the skin easily; pressure with a diascope (i. e., a glass slide) will show a lack of blanching.* Recurrence within a scarred lesion favors a diagnosis of lupus vulgaris rather than of LE.[14]

2. Systemic lupus erythematosus, abbreviated SLE, is one of the few human diseases with definite autoimmune phenomena; it affects mainly middle-aged or young women between the ages of 20 to 40, who suffer from a triad of fever, arthralgia, and loss

of weight. The disease has a chronic intermittent course with many spontaneous remissions and exacerbations.

Cutaneous lesions of SLE are inconspicuous, such as intrafocal bleeding points or isolated petechiae of the mucous membranes together with other systemic manifestations. Light sensitivity exists to a high degree and results in delicately red, butterfly-type erythemas; in addition, uncharacteristic maculopapular eruptions, alopecia (of the frontal region), and various vascular phenomena are also present (among others, Raynaud's lesions with gangrene of the digits, livedo reticularis, and leg ulcers) (Figs.173, 174). Simultaneous facial lesions of chronic discoid LE are seldom seen. Although palmoplantar changes compared with other locations are less frequently observed in discoid LE, they are even rarer in SLE, and are observed only when there is extensive spreading. In contrast to other areas of the body, palmoplantar lesions show more hyperkeratosis and atrophy. Special sites of involvement are the prominent parts of the volar aspect of the tips of the fingers, toes, and the thenar eminence of the thumb, while palms and soles show only faint erythemas, similar to hepatic palmar erythema.[1, 11, 16, 18, 30, 33]

* As well as the presence of apple-jelly nodules. (Tr.)

Fig. 173. Systemic lupus erythematosus.

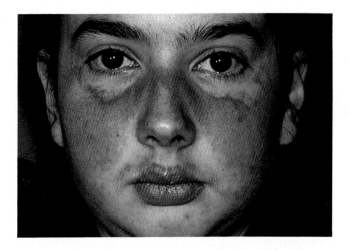

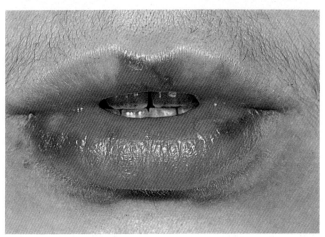

Fig. 174. Systemic lupus erythematosus: erosions of the
vermilion border.

Clinical signs of SLE, in addition
to the cutaneous changes and various
febrile episodes characteristic of the
disease, are caused not only by hyperergic
disease but also by intercurrent infections
(sinusitis, otitis, and others) and by
involvement of a number of internal
organs. Atypical verrucous endocarditis
(Kaposi-Libman-Sacks disease) is one of
the cardinal signs of SLE. The differential
diagnosis must include other cardiac
diseases, such as **Löffler's parietal fibro-
plastic eosinophilic endocarditis,** a rare
febrile disease which can seldom be
diagnosed except at autopsy, and subacute bacterial endocarditis **(endocarditis
lenta)** which is usually superimposed on
an organic cardiac defect. Characteristic
of subacute bacterial endocarditis are
microemboli of fingers and toes, known as
Janeway's spots, and, much more rarely,
exudative necrotizing arteriitis. In addition to endocarditis, cardiac involvement
of SLE may manifest itself as myocarditis
and, especially, as pericarditis. Complicating hypertension usually is of renal
origin. One of five patients with severe
SLE dies of cardiac insufficiency due to
this disease.[10,11,30,34]

Pulmonary changes have both specific
and unspecific manifestations; among the
latter are pneumonias of the lobes or

lobuli, abscesses, and empyemas. SLE of the lungs may show itself either intra-alveolarly or interstitially; diminution of the exudation finally results in pulmonary fibrosis. The extent of respiratory insufficiency due to SLE can frequently not be detected by roentgenologic examination but only by appropriate determination of the respiratory capacity. The straw-yellow effusion of pleurisy due to SLE is usually not massive, but even in the early phase LE cells can be found or the LE phenomenon can be induced.

The tendency to polyserositis manifests itself in the gastrointestinal tract by subjective and objective signs (meteorism, diarrhea, and colitis). Occasionally, severe edema of the gut or inflammation of the esophagus takes place. Enlargement of the spleen, lymph nodes, and also of the liver is found, and the histologic picture resembles rather unspecific reactive mild hepatitis. So-called *"lupoid hepatitis"* is a serious chronic-aggressive liver disease that progresses to cirrhosis with SLE-like general signs; it is, however, not a special type of LE but an independent primary disease of the liver.

Neurologically, SLE may start mono-symptomatically with chorea, epilepsy, apoplexy, polyneuritis, transverse paralysis, or Wallenberg's syndrome; only when other signs of SLE appear, such as typical light-provoked cutaneous changes, will the correct diagnosis be made. On the other hand, clinically suspicious of a supervening central nervous involvement in connection with already existing SLE symptoms are headaches and increasing lethargy. Psychoses and epileptic fits after the start of treatment with antimalarial drugs should be considered as possible therapeutic side-effects, while convulsive disorders should be investigated as the effect of corticosteroids.[32]

Renal involvement of SLE practically always manifests itself as glomerulone-phritis; this may be present for some time as a focal nephritis, but in other cases nephrotic conditions develop with a poor prognosis. In any case, albuminuria, microhematuria, cylindruria, and limited renal function point to renal involvement in the disease process. However, a biopsy is the best way to prove early involvement of the kidney. During remission lupoid nephritis may be the only recognizable manifestation.

The fate of the patient depends to a large extent on the degree of kidney involvement. Histologically important are changes of the capillaries of the glomeruli, which sometimes show massive thickening of the basal membrane; a special feature is the (rare) renal wire-loop lesions of this membrane. Immunofluorescent tests show the arrangement of small particles of aggregates of immunoglobulins at the glomeruli; electron-microscopy shows bundles consisting of a density of electrons at the glomeruli.[19, 26]

Examination of the fundus of the eye in cases of chronic LE shows fairly typical pigmented areas in the periphery of the choroid, whereas in acute LE papillary edema, hemorrhages, frequently vascular changes, cotton-wool exudates, or circumscribed whitish lesions ("cytoid bodies") are present.[23]

Histologically, SLE shows basic changes similar to those in discoid LE. However, inflammatory changes (development of infiltrations) and keratinization (follicular hyperkeratosis) distinctly subside, while flattening of the epidermal band and, above all, mucoid edematization of the corium with PAS-positive sweat phenomena become especially evident. The liquefaction degeneration of the basal cell layer is also distinct. Histochemically, PAS-positive accentuation of the basal membrane, inclusive of the cranial and medial sections of the follicles, is noteworthy. As in discoid LE, immunofluorescent methods show a wide subepidermal band of fluorescence; in addition, spotty fibrinoid swellings within the dermal collagen or in the arterial walls can be conspicuous. Hematoxylin bodies found occasionally in the upper corium are of even greater diagnostic significance; however, in exceptional instances, these bodies can be found in diseases of different etiology, even in the nevus cell nevus. In later phases of SLE, penetration of fibroblasts through the lesions or hyaline transformation of precipitates occurs; less frequently, there is moderate collagenous production of new fibrils so that, in contrast to scleroderma, the clinical sign of fibrosis is usually lacking. As a general principle, SLE fails to show the acute and massive inflammatory intensity of dermatomyositis. Also in contrast to dermatomyositis, in SLE there are areas of degeneration, mainly in the connective tissue between the muscle bundles, therefore, chiefly interstitially and less in areas of inflammation within the muscle and less parenchymatously. Finally, in rare instances SLE may show vacuolar myopathies; within these vacuoles the myofibrils have disappeared and fine eosinophilic precipitates may be found.[6, 7, 13, 24]

SLE localizes in a great number of different places. Serologically, it can be diagnosed by the antinuclear factor or the nuclear autoantibody test; the autoantibody causes lysis of the nuclei of the granulocytes, and they in turn undergo phagocytosis by leukocytes and monocytes. This phenomenon results in the appearance of the so-called LE cell: a homogeneous, somewhat eosinophilic, nuclear inclusion mass that attaches itself to the semilunar nucleus of the phagocytized cell (Fig. 175).

Quite exceptionally, such LE cells have been found in cases of strong hypersensitivity to penicillin, hydantoin (Dilantin), or other drugs (INH, hydralazine), and also in autonomous diseases such as

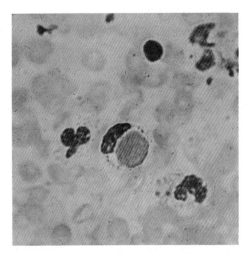

Fig. 175. Lupus erythematosus cell.

pernicious or hemolytic anemia, multiple myeloma, or miliary tuberculosis. LE cells can be found in SLE in other body fluids (pleural effusions and urine). Tart cells (monocyte or granulocyte with phagocytosed cell nucleus) should not be confused with the LE cell phenomenon. If the chromatin structure of the cell nucleus remains intact it is a type-A cell. After the cell nucleus becomes disintegrated and homogenized, a type-B cell results. In any case, the cellular nucleus shows a basophilic border, which helps to avoid confusion with LE cells. As a supplement to the morphologic qualities of LE cells, a number of antinuclear seroreactions (serologic fluorescent antiglobulin-consumption test, indirect immunofluorescent antibody technique) that permit the demonstration of nuclear autoantibodies are available. Probably the autoaggression of SLE is produced, not by a certain altered antigen, but by a multiplicity of antibodies. A decisive factor in the serologic diagnosis is the demonstration of antinuclear factors by the indirect immunofluorescent technique; the degree of the titer permits a differentiation between SLE and positive findings in other diseases, for instance, rheumatoid arthritis.[5, 7, 25]

SLE patients with a positive reaction to the serologic test for syphilis (biologically false ?) due to antilipoid antibodies always require control tests with the *Treponema pallidum* immobilization (TPI) or the fluorescent treponemal antibody absorption (FTA) tests. Less characteristic are serologic findings of considerably increased ESR and the presence of hypergammaglobulinemia. However, the blood picture is especially remarkable because it shows cytopenia. Pathognomonic for the patient with SLE are leukocytopenias from under 4000 WBC to agranulocytosis with a relative lymphocytosis. This constellation of reactions can be found also among clinically healthy family members ("LE-diathesis"). In addition, SLE patients have different anemias such as the aplastic and hemolytic types, often at the same time as a positive Coombs test. SLE with thrombocytopenia is not rare and occasionally is of clinical importance because the disease may start with the monomorphic manifestation of a thrombocytopenic purpura. Splenectomy is sometimes performed for monosymptomatic hemolytic anemia; in such cases manifestations of SLE may follow later. Coagulation defects can be observed in connection with thrombocytopenic purpura.[20]

Lesions masquerading as or **precipitating SLE** occur after initial sensitization by streptococci and subsequent allergy to drugs such as Dilantin, griseofulvin, tetracyclines, penicillin, sulfonamides, hydantoin, chlorpromazine, procainamide, PAS, and gold.[15]

In considering the various aspects of SLE for a diagnosis, one must start with the fact that most patients first develop one or two lingering, not acute, basic signs (fever, increased ESR, joint pains, pleurisy, and others). Frequently, only the appearance of cutaneous lesions leads to diagnostic steps such as examination for LE cells and immunoglobulins. Treatment with corticosteroids or immunosuppressive drugs should not lead to neglect of the possibility of an exacerbation of SLE or of overlooking bacterial or septic complications, or the flare-up of pulmonary tuberculosis. Also, there are reports of a disturbance of the immunologic balance so that SLE regresses, through the association with lymphogranulomatosis.[11, 29, 30, 31]

(1) ALEXANDER, M., und W. ROTHENBERGER: Zur Diagnostik des Erythematodes disseminatus. Med. Klin. *59:* 205–209 (1964).

(2) BÄFVERSTEDT, B.: Über Lymphadenosis benigna cutis. Acta derm.-venereol. (Stockh.) *24:* Suppl. 11 (1943).

(3) BARTHELMES, H., und N. SÖNNICHSEN: Die Bedeutung der Immunofluoreszenzverfahren für die Dermatologie. Derm. Mschr. *156:* 184–211 (1970).

(4) BIELICKÝ, T., und VL. VOLEK: Morphologische und biochemische Veränderungen der Leber bei chronischem Erythematodes. Hautarzt *15:* 171–174 (1964).

(5) BITTER, TH.: Systemic lupus erythematosus: antinuclear serology and cell-mediated immunity in the light of clinicohematologic diagnostic criteria. Schweiz. med. Wschr. *101:* 181–186 (1971).

(6) BOLCK, F.: Zur Morphologie des Lupus erythematodes, der Dermatomyositis und der Sklerodermie. Derm. Mschr. *155:* 3–35 (1969).

(7) BURNHAM, T. K., G. FINE and T. R. NEBLETT: Immunofluorescent »band« test for lupus erythematosus. II. Employing skin lesions. Arch. Derm. (Chic.) *102:* 42–50 (1970).

(8) CHRISTIANSON, H. B., and W. T. MITCHELL: Annular atrophic plaques of the face. Arch. Derm. (Chic.) *100:* 703–716 (1969).

(9) CRAMER, H.-J.: Beitrag zum Krankheitsbild der lymphocytären Infiltration (Jessner-Kanof). Hautarzt *13:* 543–547 (1962).

(10) DENK, R.: Elektrokardiographische Untersuchungen bei Hautkranken. Arch. Kreisl.-Forsch. *60:* 33–114 (1969).

(11) DUBOIS, E. L.: Lupus erythematosus. McGraw Hill, Toronto, London, Sydney 1966.

(12) v. EICKSTEDT, U. M., und K. H. HASSENPFLUG: Zur Kenntnis des Lupus erythematodes hypertrophicus (et profundus) Bechet. Arch. klin. exp. Derm. *214:* 471–481 (1962).

(13) ERBSLÖH, F., und W. D. BAEDEKER: Lupusmyopathie. Dtsch. med. Wschr. *87:* 2464–2470 (1962).

(14) GEBHARDT, R.: Little-Lassueur-Syndrom. Med. Welt *18:* (N. F.): 2509–2510 (1967).

(15) GOERZ, G.: Erythematodes-Provokation durch Goldtherapie wegen primärchronischer Polyarthritis. Dtsch. med. Wschr. *94:* 2040–2045 (1969).

(16) GOLDEN, R. L.: Livedo reticularis in systemic lupus erythematosus. Arch. Derm. (Chic.) *87:* 299–301 (1963).

(17) GRIMMER, H.: Beitrag zur Morphologie der L. E. Zelle. Z. Haut- u. Geschl.-Kr. *24:* 62–76 (1958).

(18) HAFERKAMP, O.: Morphologie und Pathogenese der Autoaggressionskrankheiten. Med. Welt *21* (N. F.): 999–1003 (1970).

(19) HARTL, W., R. Roos und E. GENTH: Zur Klinik und Prognose der Nierenmanifestation bei Lupus erythematodes. Klin. Wschr. *48:* 711–723 (1970).

(20) HASERICK, J. R., and R. LONG: Systemic lupus erythematosus preceded by false positive serologic tests for syphilis: presentation of five cases. Ann. Int. Med. *37:* 559–565 (1952).

(21) KOGOJ, FR.: Über eine blasige Abart des Erythematodes discoides. Dermatologica (Basel) *117:* 325–335 (1958).

22) KORTING, G. W.: Granuloma eosinophilicum faciale. Med. Welt *17* (N. F.): 397–398 (1966).

(23) KORTING, G. W.: Haut und Auge. Eine Korrelationsdermatologie der Periorbitalregion. Thieme, Stuttgart 1969.

(24) KORTING, G. W., und K. H. HASSENPFLUG: Über das Vorkommen von »Hämatoxylin-Körpern« bei einem Naevuszellnaevus und einer Melanosis Dubreuilh. Arch. klin. exp. Derm. *224:* 81–89 (1966).

(25) PERCY, J. S., and CH. J. SMYTH: The immunofluorescent skin test in systemic lupus erythematosus. J. Amer. Med. Ass. *208:* 485–488 (1969).

(26) ROTHER, K.: Autoaggression gegen Niere. Med. Welt *21:* (N. F.): 1029–1035 (1970).

(27) SCHIRREN, C. G., und D. EGGERT: Beitrag zum Erythematodes profundus (Kaposi-Irgang). Arch. klin. exp. Derm. *216:* 541–555 (1963).

(28) SCHMID, M.: Zum Begriff der lupoiden Hepatitis. Dtsch. med. Wschr. *95:* 783–784 (1970).

(29) SCHMIDT, W., und R. GEBHARDT: Zur Assoziation von Autoimmunerkrankungen und Lymphogranulomatose. Med. Welt *20* (N. F.): 567–570 (1969).

(30) SIEGENTHALER, W., und R. HEGGLIN: Der viscerale Lupus erythematosus (Kaposi-Libman-Sacks-Syndrom). Ergebn. inn. Med. Kinderheilk. N. F. *7:* 373–428 (1956).

(31) SÖNNICHSEN, N.: Diagnostische Kriterien des Lupus erythematodes unter besonderer Berücksichtigung der Hautveränderungen. Derm. Mschr. *157:* 14–26 (1971).

(32) STUTZER, G.: Lupus erythematodes acutus mit Wallenberg-Syndrom. Z. Haut- u. Geschl.-Kr. *42:* 329–334 (1967).

(33) TUFFANELLI, D. L., and E. L. DUBOIS: Cutaneous manifestations of systemic lupus erythematosus. Arch. Derm. (Chic.) *90:* 377–386 (1964).

(34) UEHLINGER, E.: Zur pathologischen Anatomie der Myokarditis und Myokardose. Regensburg. Jb. ärztl. Fortbild. *14:* 175–183 (1966).

(35) VACHTENHEIM, J.: Livedo reticularis bei akutem Erythematodes. Z. Haut- u. Geschl.-Kr. *39:* 331–335 (1965).

(36) WALTHER, D.: Über den Lupus erythematodes profundus (Lupus erythematodes mit subcutanen Knotenbildungen). Arch. klin. exp. Derm. *204:* 182–204 (1957).

(37) WEBER, G.: Zur Klinik und Differentialdiagnose der erythematodes-ähnlichen Lichtdermatose. Hautarzt *9:* 400–406 (1958).

(38) WEISSER, H.: Chilblain-Lupus als Form des Lupus erythematodes chronicus. Z. Haut- u. Geschl.-Kr. *26:* 9–16 (1959).

17. Atrophies

The concept of "atrophy" includes the universal or circumscribed reduction of an organ, and takes place through the dwindling of previously present substances. The various tissues show different modes of atrophy. Atrophying epidermis undergoes loss of cellular numbers and a wasting of volume, although the stratum corneum may show increased volume; the characteristic saw-toothlike rete profile is flattened and the epithelial band is distinctly thinner.

A. Plane Atrophies

1. The substrate of **senile atrophy** is mainly transformed collagen, especially in the light-exposed areas, such as the face, neck, and dorsum of the hands. Histologically and biochemically, it occurs in the elastica and the collagen. The main macroscopic features of senile skin are somewhat firmly thickened, yellow-white to yellow-brown, structural transforma-

tions. In addition, senile atrophic skin tends to the formation of folds or wrinkles. Because of reduction of the sebaceous and sweat glands such areas not only show pityriasiform scaling but are often transformed into gross rhombic areas (Fig. 176).

On the back of the neck these changes are called *"cutis rhomboidalis nuchae"* (Fig. 177). Such forms of senile elastosis usually occur after the third decade of life only in men who have been exposed to wind, weather, and sun. This is part of the appearance of *"farmer's"* or *"sailor's skin."* Histologically, senile elastosis is hardly distinguishable from actinic elastosis. In pseudoxanthoma elasticum, however, elastorrhexis with calcium incrustations immediately permits differentiation (histologically!) Senile atrophies show often remarkable pigmentary changes in addition to the already mentioned furrows (see also Chapter 24, E4). Together with leukomelanoderma, streaklike or bizarrely indented pseudoscar formations ("pseudo-cicatrices stellaires spontanées") occur (see also Chapter 24, A9) as well as bizarre jagged suggillations (purpura senilis). The main cause of these "flores cimeterii," aside from senile elastosis, is the rigidity of aged vessels.[3, 17]

The diagnosis of senile atrophy is facilitated if additional signs are present besides the cardinal signs of pale yellow, flabby, and wrinkled skin; for instance, the combination of skin atrophy and "old age comedones" on light-exposed areas, sometimes together with cystic elements. Such a picture is called "elastoïdose cutanée-nodulaire avec kystes et comédons" (Fig. 178). It is found mainly on the forehead and cheeks of older people or in skin areas that have been strongly traumatized. Quite often the sides of the face are unequally affected since they have been unequally exposed to the weather. The deeper lying follicular cysts appear as white-yellowish nodules, while those situated more shallowly have comedones at their follicular openings, which, however, cannot be expressed like the usual comedones but instead show whitish, crumbly, and friable formations. However, if "chafing comedones" are conspicuous in adolescents and in patients with no cystic translucent nodular lesions at

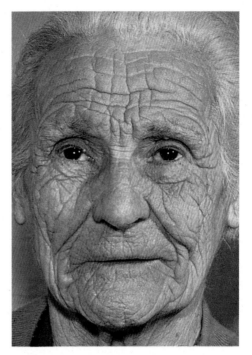

Fig. 176. Severe colloidal degeneration of the skin.

sites of common traumatization (such as straps of brassieres), a diagnosis of folliculitis ulerythematosus or acneiform ulerythema should be considered.[7, 14, 16]

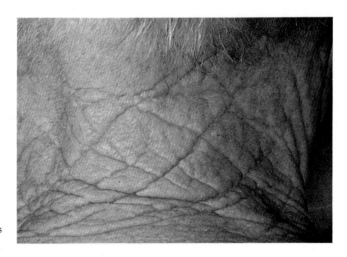

Fig. 177. Cutis rhomboidalis nuchae.

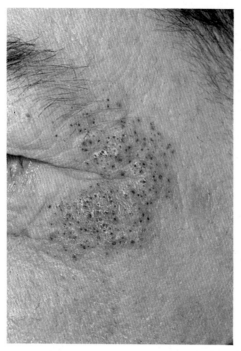

Fig. 178. Nodular and cystic cutaneous elastoidosis.

The differential diagnosis between senile atrophy and acrodermatitis chronica atrophicans is easy because the latter has a characteristic predilection for sites at the ends of one or all extremities. In the atrophic areas sclerodermiform changes develop. Because of their atrophying character, both senile atrophy and acrodermatitis chronica atrophicans involve histologic rarefaction to complete disappearance of the elastica in the final stages of development. Senile atrophy, however, develops acellularly and without infiltrates of the connective tissue during the whole process, while acrodermatitis chronica atrophicans shows its true atrophying character following an edematous infiltrative cellular phase.

Similarly, hereditary, atrophic, premature senescence of the skin (i. e., manifestations of the progeria group) are easily distinguishable from true senile skin because of their additional stigmata (dwarfism and acromicria).

Like pseudoxanthoma elasticum, senile atrophy may show white-yellow to lemon-colored nodules on the skin. They are, however, limited to the areas exposed to light. If the lemon color is associated chiefly with distinct depression points, the condition is called "peau citreine." If, however, the color is pale yellowish – with no essential changes – it is called *elastoma diffusum*.[6]

Similar white to white-yellow streaklike or reticularly grouped "deposits" also characterize the cutaneous changes of pseudoxanthoma elasticum. In this disorder, however, the changes are already present in the first or second decade of life, do not depend on light, and are located on the axillas and inguinal fold and inner surface of the thighs, locations which are unusual in senile atrophy.[19]

2. But **colloid milium** (pseudomilium colloidale or hyaloma), a special form of senile elastosis, can also be lemon-colored. In contrast to pseudoxanthoma elasticum, it occurs only on light-exposed sites (especially on the middle of the forehead) in the form of pinhead-sized and somewhat transparent, grouped nodules, which give the affected skin the quality of soft leather (Fig. 179a). In exceptional cases colloid milia may assume a more yellow-brownish color, and they may appear even in adolescents who, however, have a familial history of this disorder. Histologically, homogeneous and circumscribed colloidal conglomerates, fused into clumps, are present; wherever they occur, distinct changes and rarefactions of the elastica can be found. The substrate of colloid stains slightly less eosinophilic with HE than does normal collagen; in rare cases, however, it stains mildly basophilic. The colloid degeneration of the colloid milium differs from the usual

Fig. 179. Colloidal pseudomilium: (a) Multiple yellowish papules on the cheek
and temporal area; (b) circumscribed masses of colloid
in the upper corium. Van
Gieson stain, 25×.

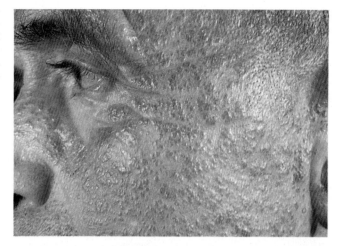

Fig. 179a.

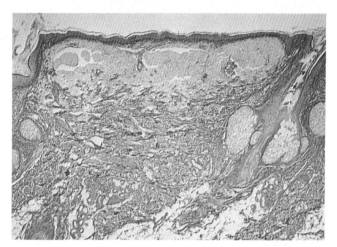

Fig. 179b.

colloid degeneration of the skin by not
forming diffuse subepidermal bands, but
rather areas or clefts of degenerated
collagen (Fig. 179b). Excessive colloid milia may require differentiation from nodular amyloidosis (Congo red, methyl violet)
and hyalinosis cutis et mucosae. Finally,
colloid milium may be imitated by erythropoietic, familial protoporphyria (see
also Chapter 25, A10).[11, 15]

3. In senile atrophy, because turgor or
elasticity is diminished, loose and permanent folds of the skin develop. In the
differential diagnosis the **cutis laxa syn-**
drome (dermatochalasis, "loose skin")
must be considered. The entire skin
appears to be "too wide," and hangs in
large folds (Fig. 180). Correlated with the
systemic degeneration of the elastica of
the skin is the decrease of elasticity in
the pulmonary supporting system. This
appears clinically as chronic substantial
pulmonary emphysema, and may also
affect the heart and gastrointestinal tract.
One should distinguish between a congenital and an acquired cutis laxa syndrome. The former is either present at
birth or develops in earliest childhood. No
other cutaneous changes exist at any time.

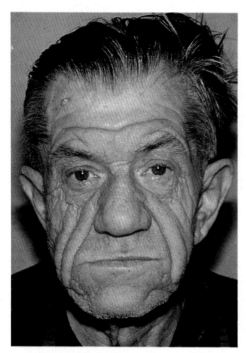

Fig. 180. Cutis laxa syndrome.

A hooked nose and a long, overhanging upper lip are rather typical and are not present in the acquired form of cutis laxa, which manifests itself in late childhood or adulthood. Usually, the development of "too wide" skin is preceded by uncharacteristic, inflamed erythematous or urticarial cutaneous changes. Histologically, there is no difference between the two forms of cutis laxa. In both types the whole elastica is rarefied and fragmented but, in contrast to the Ehlers-Danlos syndrome, it is never incrusted with calcium salts. Another differential diagnostic point in regard to the Ehlers-Danlos syndrome is the lack of hyperextensibility of the joints. The skin of the patient with the Ehlers-Danlos syndrome is hyperextensible (cutis hyperelastica) but returns to its original form without folds after the cessation of tensile stress, whereas in the cutis laxa patient it is always hanging ʾ in large folds. Likewise, the symptomatic slackness of the skin of a patient with acne conglobata is not cutis laxa but cutis hyperelastica, without, however, additional signs of the Ehlers-Danlos syndrome. Further pseudosenile atrophic formations of slackened skin, which in a certain sense represent premature senility of the skin, occur in granulomatous angiitides.[4, 10, 22–25]

4. Periocular loose skin, called **blepharochalasis** (Fig. 181), perhaps represents

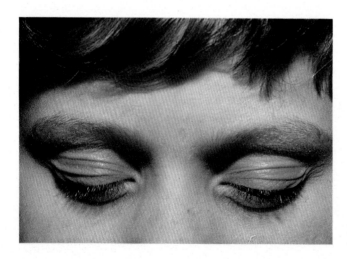

Fig. 181. Blepharochalasis (dermatolysis palpebrarum).

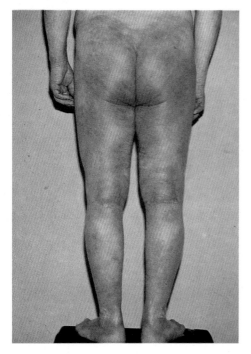 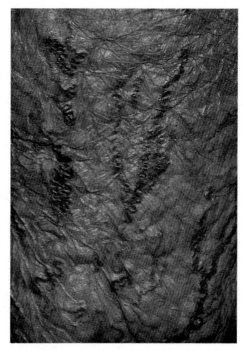

Fig. 182a.   Fig. 182b.

Fig. 182. Acrodermatitis chronica atrophicans: (a) stage of erythromelia, and (b) atrophy with thin folds and transparency of veins.

a heterogeneous developmental stage similar to kraurosis. In most cases, as in acrodermatitis chronica atrophicans, the tendency toward atrophy ends with folds of the lids and transparency of the vessels. There is an edematous preceding stage. Moreover, blepharochalasis is a definite sign of the **Ascher syndrome,** which includes changes in the upper lip (double lip) and struma with various endocrine disturbances. The disorder begins in most cases with recurrent edema of the upper lids, whereas the lower lids are rarely involved. The development of the double lip (upper lip) likewise begins with changing stages of swelling, until gradually a persistent enlargement remains with a double fold in the transitional zone between the skin and mucous membrane of the lip.[1, 8, 26]

5. In **acrodermatitis chronica atrophicans** fine, shallow erythemas develop, which then acquire more pasty infiltrations and finally end in slack atrophy. At the onset, they are unnoticed and affect only one extremity; later, they appear more or less symmetrically on the other extremities as well. The condition of the skin in the atrophic stage has been compared with the folds of Russian cigarette paper or those of a baked apple. A characteristic feature is the transparency of the veins (Fig. 182a, b). In the beginning, wide erythematous streaks along the ulna (ulnar streaks) and tibia are typical. Additional frequent manifestations are "fibroid" juxta-articular nodes, which occasionally may be plaquelike (see Chapter 8, A2). Sometimes, sclerodermiform, taut, pathological changes de-

velop in this way (see Chapter 16, A5). Acrodermatitis chronica atrophicans may begin at any age, but the incidence of disease peaks distinctly in the fifth to sixth decade of life. General signs such as fever, lassitude, or a feeling of weakness are always absent. Nevertheless, a high ESR and an increase of plasma cells in the bone marrow and lymph nodes are present. Lately, accompanying paraproteinemia has been reported. For accompanying acroosteolyses see Chapter 16, B1, and for joint involvement see Chapter 7, E2. Histologically, in acrodermatitis chronica atrophicans far-reaching rarefaction of the elastica which extends to areas of complete disappearance is observed early and synchronously with "inflammatory"-cellular infiltrations. Areas of disappearing elastica occur also in the accompanying fibroid nodes, ulnar streaks, and sclerodermalike areas. Within the sclerodermiform cutaneous changes there are, however, also areas without diminishing elastica. These areas react to aldehyde-fuchsin stain in the same way as typical scleroderma. Therefore, after the stain for elastica has been applied, a safe distinction between circumscribed scleroderma and acrodermatitis chronica atrophicans cannot always be made.

Most probably, acrodermatitis chronica atrophicans does not represent a treponematosis, although evidence of spirochetes in the tissue and a positive pallida reaction in the serum have been reported in isolated cases. Changes in the regional lymph nodes and bone marrow and an increase in ESR suggest a generalized disease, which may have been caused by an infectious agent (transmission by ticks?). This theory has been confirmed by recent transplantation experiments. At the present time, acrodermatitis chronica atrophicans, erythema chronicum migrans, and lymphadenosis benigna cutis, in which the transmission of ticks is discussed, are considered to be "probable infectious diseases of the skin."

In practice, acrodermatitis chronica atrophicans most often is mistaken for "frostbite," which is understandable because the patients interpret the paresthetic subjective pain sensations as increased feelings of cold from cold damage. We should recall the fact that frostbite mostly occurs symmetrically and bilaterally and, above all, at distal sites, whereas acrodermatitis chronica atrophicans begins usually on one extremity with definite sparing of the distal phalanges of fingers or toes. Against a diagnosis of Raynaud's syndrome or beginning progressive scleroderma is their symmetrical onset and, above all, the rhythmic changes between more syncope at first (digitus mortuus) and later, a relatively greater acroasphyxia. Erythromelalgia, which is found mostly in juveniles or young adults, can be differentiated by its tormenting, burning pain, a simultaneous diffuse, reddish, nonlivid hue, and swelling. Pain in the affected areas becomes intolerable with the application of heat. Furthermore, in erythromelalgia atrophies do not remain permanently. Palms and soles are the favorite sites of occurrence of erythromelalgia (see also Chapter 5, B4) in contrast to acrodermatitis chronica atrophicans. Acrocyanosis, the chronic peripheral blood stasis, in which the skin is distinctly cooler and moist, affects far younger persons than does acrodermatitis chronica atrophicans. Light, anemic, or cinnabar-red spots are interspersed on the skin. By pressing with a finger (iris diaphragm phenomenon) the skin can be made excessively anemic, and its character as a purely functional angiopathy without any cellular infiltrative aspects becomes evident. Other characteristic manifestations are the follicular marks ("perniosis follicularis") on the lower legs. Further, the reticular or dendritic, bluish marbleizing of cutis marmorata or livedo reticularis is not to be confused with the transparent large veins of acrodermatitis chronica atrophicans, considering the widespread

Fig. 183. Pseudoacrodermatitis in chronic lymphadenosis of the skin.

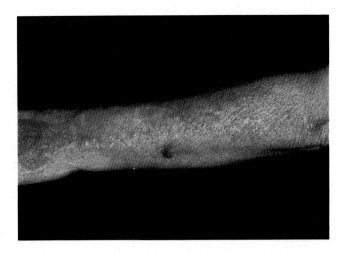

thin condition of the skin. Erysipeloid, although it also has articular changes and responds promptly to doses of penicillin, is not difficult to distinguish from acrodermatitis chronica atrophicans because it is unilateral, has a predilection for the fingers, starts conspicuously with burning and itching (within a few hours after infection), and presents a light red, inflammatory erythema, which slowly covers the fingers and occasionally the dorsum of the hands. Likewise, a fixed drug eruption with its smaller round lesions, which occur on other sites as well as the extremities, offers no difficulties to a differential diagnosis from acrodermatitis chronica atrophicans. However, in subsiding, the infiltrate of a drug eruption leaves a transient dirty greyish-brown erythema.

Early stages of acrodermatitis chronica atrophicans can in rare cases develop from erythema migrans, which, however, differs from the fully developed picture of the former by its vast central involution and its migratory character. It occasionally happens that erythema migrans and confirmed acrodermatitis chronica atrophicans exist coincidentally.

Worth mentioning in the differential diagnosis against acrodermatitis chronica atrophicans are cutaneous manifestations following chronic *intoxication with arsenic.* In recognizing the character of these lesions the simultaneous presence of arsenical keratoses, epitheliomas on the trunk, and epitheliomas of the Bowen type is of great help. The history would show that the edematous early stages and consequently the tendency to atrophy that is typical of acrodermatitis chronica atrophicans did not occur. Cutaneous manifestations resembling those of acrodermatitis chronica atrophicans have been observed in *chronic lymphatic leukemia* (Fig. 183). The specific character of such lesions is evident in the histologic findings.[2, 5, 9]

(1) ASCHER, K. W.: Blepharochalasis mit Struma und Doppellippe. Klin. Mbl. Augenheilk. *65:* 86–96 (1920).

(2) BREUCKMANN, H.: Über ein der Akrodermatitis chronica atrophicans ähnliches Krankheitsbild bei Winzern mit Arsenschädigungen. Arch. Derm. Syph. (Berl.) *179:* 695–702 (1939).

(3) COLOMB, D., J.-A. PINÇON et J. LARTAUD: Individualisation anatomo-clinique d'une forme méconnue de la peau sénile: Les pseudo-cicatrices stellaires spontanées. Ann. Derm. Syph. (Paris) *94:* 273–286 (1967).

(4) Denk, R.: Elektrokardiographische Untersuchungen bei Hautkranken. Arch. Kreisl.-Forsch. *60:* 33–114 (1969).

(5) Denk, R., und H. Holzmann: Acrodermatitis chronica atrophicans-ähnliches Hauterscheinungsbild nach chronischer Arsen-Intoxikation. Med. Welt *17* (N. F.): 2027–2028 (1966).

(6) Dubreuilh, W.: Elastome diffus de la face. Bull. Soc. franç. Derm. Syph. *1921:* 247–248.

(7) Favre, M., et J. Racouchot: L'élastidose cutanée nodulaire a kystes et a comédons. Ann. Derm. Syph. (Paris) *78:* 681–702 (1951).

(8) Findlay, G. H.: Idiopathic enlargements of the lips: Cheilitis granulomatosa, Ascher's syndrome and double lip. Brit. J. Derm. *66:* 129–138 (1954).

(9) Gebhardt, R.: Acrodermatitis chronica atrophicansähnliche Hautmanifestation einer chronisch lymphatischen Leukämie. Med. Welt *19* (N. F.): 1651–1652 (1968).

(10) Goltz, R. W., A. M. Hult, M. Goldfarb and R. J. Gorlin: Cutis laxa. Arch. Derm. *92:* 373–386 (1965).

(11) Guin, J. D., and E. R. Seale: Colloid degeneration of the skin (colloid milium). Arch. Derm. Syph. (Chic.) *80:* 533–537 (1959).

(12) Hauser, W.: Akrodermatitis chronica atrophicans. Ergebn. inn. Med. Kinderheilk. N. F. *22:* 58–89 (1965).

(13) Hopf, H. Ch.: Acrodermatitis chronica atrophicans (Herxheimer) und Nervensystem. Springer, Berlin, Heidelberg, New York 1966.

(14) Kleine-Natrop, E.: Seltenere Varianten der Elastoidose cutanée nodulaire avec kystes et comédons (Favre-Racouchot). Z. Haut- u. Geschl.-Kr. *39:* 250 bis 255 (1965).

(15) Klingmüller, G., und O. Hornstein: Protoporphyrinämische Lichtdermatose mit eigentümlicher Hyalinosis cutis. Hautarzt *16:* 115–122 (1965).

(16) Korting, G. W.: Folliculitis ulerythematosa. Derm. Wschr. *149:* 91–93 (1964).

(17) Korting, G. W., und R. Gebhardt: Zur hepatischen Co-Genese der Purpura senilis. Derm. Mschr. *155:* 124–128 (1969).

(18) Korting, G. W., N. Hoede und H. Holzmann: Zur Frage des Elasticaverhaltens bei einigen sklerosierenden und atrophisierenden Hautkrankheiten. Hautarzt *20:* 351–361 (1969).

(19) Korting, G. W., und H. Holzmann: Zur Frage humoraler Kollagen-Begleitkomponenten beim Pseudoxanthoma elasticum. Arch. klin. exp. Derm. *231:* 408–414 (1968).

(20) Krebs, A., und H. U. Andres: Zum Krankheitsbild der Erythromelalgie. Schweiz. med. Wschr. *99:* 344–349 (1969).

(21) Ludwig, E.: Erythema chronicum migrans im Frühstadium der Acrodermatitis chronica atrophicans Herxheimer. Hautarzt *7:* 41–42 (1956).

(22) Maxwell, E., and N. B. Esterly: Cutis laxa. Amer. J. Dis. Child. *117:* 479–482 (1969).

(23) Obermayer, M. E., and T. Winsor: Angiitis with nodule formation, vasomotor instability and secondary cutis laxa. J. Invest. Derm. *32:* 529–537 (1959).

(24) Reed, W. B., R. E. Horowitz and P. Beighton: Acquired cutis laxa. Primary generalized elastolysis. Arch. Derm. (Chic.) *103:* 661–669 (1971).

(25) Robinson, H. M., and F. A. Ellis: Cutis laxa. Arch. Derm. (Chic.) *77:* 656–664 (1958).

(26) Stehr, K., K. Werb und H. J. Löblich: Pathogenese und Therapie des Ascher-Syndroms. Dtsch. med. Wschr. *87:* 1148–1155 (1962).

B. Striae

Atrophic striae of the skin are linear atrophies due to weakening of the elastic tissue of the cutis, especially in areas subject to great distention. These cutaneous changes are frequently observed during *pregnancy* or in *obese adolescents*. Accordingly, striae are found two to three times more frequently in women than in men, and for a long time the only other causes of this condition were thought to be *infectious disease* or long-endured hunger.

Recently the atrophic striae of the skin after extended *systemic* or even *local cortisone therapy* have been recognized (Fig. 184). This explains the great importance of the hormones of the hypophysis and the adrenal cortex in regard to the slackness of the elastic tissue in general and the etiology of the striae in particular; striae also occur with tumors of the adrenals and the anterior lobe of the hypophysis *(Cushing's syndrome)*. There is no histologic difference between atrophic striae occurring after either local or systemic cortisone therapy and those following other causes. Moreover, observations on the evolution of such atrophic striae in *Marfan's syndrome* indicate that next to the disintegration of elastic tissue probably a pathogenic basic defect in the ground substance plays a role.

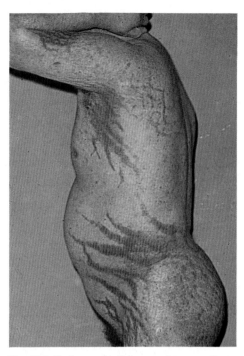

Fig. 184. Striae cutis distensae from cortisone treatment.

Local inflammatory factors may be responsible for the development of striae in patients suffering from inguinal intertriginous dermatitis. There is no doubt that individual factors are important because not every pregnant woman and not every patient treated with corticosteroids develops this cushingoid sign.

In the differential diagnosis striae can hardly be confused with other atrophic lesions (linear scars; anetoderma, including linear scleroderma). The same is true for the molluscoid and mostly protruding scar formations of the Ehlers-Danlos syndrome. Pronounced keloidal but nonatrophic striae that suggest linear atrophic striae in appearance can be observed in the gluteal region in progressive scleroderma.[1, 8]

(1) BISMARK, H. D.: Zur konstitutionellen Bedeutung der Striae cutis atrophicae. Med. Klin. *62:* 51–53 (1967).

(2) DENK, R.: Ungewöhnlich hochgradiger Steroid-Cushing bei Psoriasis vulgaris. Med. Welt *16* (N.F.): 2115–2116 (1965).

(3) EPSTEIN, N. N., W. L. EPSTEIN and J. H. EPSTEIN: Atrophic striae in patients with inguinal intertrigo. Arch. Derm. (Chic.) *87:* 450–457 (1963).

(4) GSCHWANDTNER, W. R.: Striae cutis atrophicae nach Lokalbehandlung mit Corticosteroiden. Hautarzt *24:* 70–73 (1973).

(5) PINKUS, H., M. K. KEECH and A. H. MEHREGAN: Histopathology of striae distensae with special reference to striae and wound healing in the Marfan syndrome. J. Invest. Derm. *46:* 283–292 (1966).

(6) ROSENTHAL, O.: Striae distensae et keloideae. In: Ikonographia Dermatologica. Hrsg. A. NEISSER u. E. JACOBI. S. 295–296. Urban & Schwarzenberg, Berlin, Wien 1906.

(7) STREITMANN, B.: Eigenartige Elasticaveränderung nach lokaler Cortison-Infiltration. Z. Haut- u. Geschl.-Kr. *42:* I–IV (1967).

(8) THIERS, H., G. MOULIN et M. LARIVE:
Les vergetures de la corticothérapie lo-
cale. Ann. Derm. Syph. (Paris) *96:* 29–36
(1969).

C. Isolated and Disseminated Circumscribed Atrophies

1. Macular atrophy of the skin (anetoderma) occurs in adolescents and adults; it is more common in females. The lesions consist of single or irregularly multiple, circular, sharply circumscribed and frequently wrinkled areas with thinning of the skin (Fig. 185). Anetoderma of the Pellizari type develops from an urticarial lesion, the Alexander type starts from an initially bullous stage, and, finally, the Schweninger-Buzzi type presents saccular or hernialike atrophic lesions elevated above the level of the surrounding skin. Sometimes the same patient has different areas at various stages of development – for instance, erythematous macules, soft atrophic lesions with peripheral erythema, and old involuted areas without an erythematous border.

Histologically, this kind of atrophy shows in the beginning a peculiar acellular swelling, an increase in the volume of the collagenous connective tissue, with early and at times simultaneous rarefaction of the elastic fibers; eventually, these fibers disappear completely. The early elastolysis resulting in complete disappearance of the elastica is completely different from the sclerosing skin diseases and accordingly becomes an important landmark of the (atrophying) course of this disease. Occasionally, an early lesion may give the appearance of leukocytoclastic vasculitis. Another possibility is the combination with other mesenchymal diseases (for instance, osteogenesis imperfecta or Blegvad-Haxthausen syndrome), or histioreticulocytotic conditions (for instance, lymphocytoma). Involvement of the lymph nodes (primarily those of the dermatopathic lymphadenitis type) very rarely develops in anetoderma.

The differential diagnosis of the anetodermas revolves around the question of whether it is a primary or a secondary cutaneous macular atrophy. The secondary type can be easily diagnosed as such by its tendency to pigmentation (as for instance after pyodermas), which is lacking in primary anetodermas, or by the nature of its arrangement (for instance, after herpes zoster). Other atrophic skin diseases, for instance, discoid LE or circumscribed scleroderma, cause no differential diagnostic difficulties in their final stages because of accompanying signs or history. However, morphea and anetoderma may both show annular bluish-red, peripheral borders, but circumscribed scleroderma almost always heals without residual signs and only rarely with pigmentation or pitting, while anetoderma does not regress. Generalized neurofibromatosis may in rare instances produce flaccid, soft, molluscalike fibromas, which at first suggest herniating, protuberant, atrophic cutaneous sacculi. But palpation of a tumor, in addition to other findings, will leave no doubt.*

Anetoderma may also look like nodular amyloidosis because it already has a partial tendency to anetodermalike atrophic transformation (nodular atrophic cutaneous amyloidosis), even when the original primary nodes are quite hard (Fig. 186). Histologically, the deposition of amyloid in this large nodular form takes place throughout the skin with the exception of the dermal papillae.[4, 5, 7, 13]

2. Not too rarely heterotopic fat lobules within atrophic lesions are found moving upward as a result of shrinking tissue. It

---

* Pressure with the finger will permit invagination of the tumor through a ring in the skin. (Tr.)

is understandable that anetodermic pro-
lapsing areas consisting of high-lying
aggregates of fatty cells produce a macroscopic phenocopy. The clinical representative of such a condition is the mostly
multilocular and closely aggregated **nevus
lipomatosus cutaneus superficialis;** it is in
most cases located on buttocks, hips, and
thighs but, in contrast to the connective
tissue nevus, not in the lumbosacral
region. Because this lipoid nevus definitely
shows less compactness than dermatofibroma protuberans, it may very well
resemble anetoderma of the Schweninger-
Buzzi type owing to its only moderately
taut swelling. Rarely is this lipoid nevus
already present at birth; it consists almost
always of several closely adjacent tumors.
Associated malformations have never been
seen. Similar congenital heterotopias of
lipoid tissue are an integral component
of the Goltz-Gorlin syndrome **(focal dermal hypoplasia);** in this condition the
subepidermal connective tissue is completely replaced by fatty tissue so that
such an area macroscopically resembles
anetoderma and the superficial cutaneous
lipomatous nevus. However, other signs
of this malformation syndrome (bandlike
atrophy of the skin with telangiectases,
papillomas of the oral and anal regions,
and syndactyly, among others) will quickly

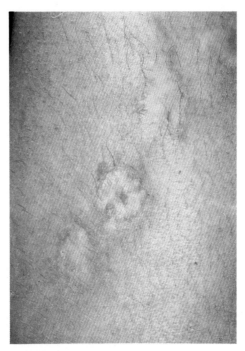

Fig. 185. Dermatitis maculosa atrophicans:
affected round areas on the leg.

permit the correct diagnostic classification
(see Chapter 23, A7).[14]

3. Folliculitis ulerythematosa reticulata
is characteristically limited according to
site (cheeks) and time of life (children and

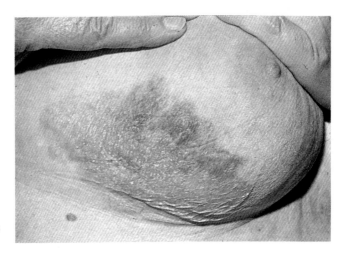

Fig. 186. Amyloidosis cutis
nodularis et atrophicans.

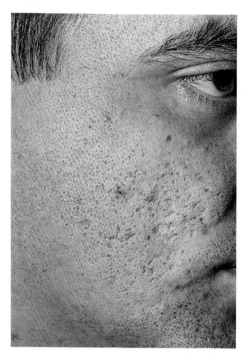

Fig. 187. Atrophoderma vermiculare.

4. Ulerythema ophryogenes, however, also produces upon involution a fine granular worm-eaten aspect, but it starts with a persistent reticular erythema favoring the eyebrow region. In addition, ulerythema ophryogenes is frequently associated with lichenoid follicular keratoses of the extensor aspects of the upper extremities. Histologically, ulerythema ophryogenes typically lacks comedo plugs and, on the whole, keratinization of the sebaceous glands.

5. Polygonal-to-longish, "punched out" scar formations of at first unclear etiology that involve the zygoma, forehead, cheeks, and also the nose should lead to a tentative diagnosis of **erythropoietic protoporphyria;** erythrocytes of such patients show coral-red fluorescence (see Chapter 5, B4).[1, 8, 9]

6. Congenital ectodermal facial dysplasia (hereditary symmetrical aplastic nevus) also shows circular or bandlike atrophic scarlike lesions. These congenital cutaneous changes favor the temporal or supraorbital regions; they are as a rule symmetrically arranged and affect the face only. Preceding inflammatory or ulcerous changes have not been observed. The atrophic areas are slightly depressed and, occasionally show a yellow or light-brown tinge; such areas of the scalp lack hairs. Additional concomitant findings are an unusually low frontal hairline and a very wide and flat nasal bridge; the eyebrows are scanty, the outer two-thirds being absent. According to observations so far available it is suggestive of an autosomal dominant mode of inheritance with extremely variable penetration and expression.[2, 12]

7. Follicular atrophies and cicatrizing alopecias are present in **chondrodystrophia calcificans congenita** (Conradi's syndrome) as inconstant cutaneous accompaniments. Follicular atrophies are observed only on the distal parts of the extremities and not on the face as in folliculitis ulery-

adolescents); it results in a cutaneous atrophy with peculiar netlike lesions having dilated follicles and in the formation of pseudocomedones that give the skin a worm-eaten appearance (Fig. 187). Varieties with "active" folliculitis, comedones, or pseudocomedones are rather rarely seen in this type of atrophy. Only exceptionally do these lesions occur in the region of the zygoma; thus in the differential diagnosis in such cases diseases of different etiology accompanied by dimpling must be considered (for example, vermicular scars after the small macular type of discoid LE, the results of acne vulgaris or acne necroticans, and, to a lesser extent scars after smallpox). Nevus comedonicus has a tendency to smouldering suppuration and extraction of groups of comedones is easy. In contrast to folliculitis ulerythematosa reticulata, nevus comedonicus is usually a strictly unilateral disorder of wide extension.[11]

thematosa reticulata. On the scalp the cicatrizing alopecia looks like pseudopelade but is not progressive. For ichthyosiform cutaneous lesions see Chapter 22, A1.[3, 6, 10]

8. Atrophia alba (atrophie blanche) occurs in two varieties ("en plaques" and "segmentaire") with circumscribed areas due to venous insufficiency or combined arterial and venous circulatory disorders. Characteristically, small circular or somewhat bizarrely frayed, slightly depressed cicatrized areas are observed; they favor the perimalleolar region (Fig. 188). Ten per cent of such cases of "atrophie blanche" develop nonhealing painful ulcers with limited extension. Perifocally, atrophie blanche in most cases has a washed-out brown pigmentation (see also Chapter 33, D2).

The same perimalleolar location as atrophie blanche is favored at first by *progressive pigmented purpura*; it can be recognized by somewhat spotted, reddish-brown areas, which later may spread to the legs and thighs (also observed after continued use of carbromal [German, "adalin"] and other sedatives and hypnotics). Secondary depigmented scars following leg ulcers are to be differentiated; however, these ulcerations usually fill up to the level of the surrounding skin, do not appear indented, and are not interspersed with knobs of angiomalike growths. Lesions of necrobiosis lipoidica and similar granulomatoses of the legs are not located in the malleolar region but favor either the edge of the tibia or its vicinity.

(1) ANTON-LAMPRECHT, I., und A. BERSCH: Histopathologie und Ultrastruktur der Haut bei Protoporphyrinämie. Virchows Arch. path. Anat. Abt. A *352:* 75–89 (1971).

(2) BRAUER, A.: Hereditärer symmetrischer systematisierter Naevus aplasticus bei 38 Personen. Derm. Wschr. *89:* 1163–1168 (1929).

(3) COMINGS, D. E., C. PAPAZIAN and H. R. SCHOENE: Conradi's disease, chondrodystrophia calcificans congenita, congenital stippled epiphyses. J. Pediat. *72:* 63–69 (1968).

(4) GOTTRON, H. A.: Amyloidosis cutis nodularis atrophicans diabetica. Dtsch. med. Wschr. *75:* 19–24 (1950).

(5) GRIMALT, FR., und G. W. KORTING: Anetodermie und Osteopsathyrose (Syndrom von Blegvad-Haxthausen). Z. Haut- u. Geschl.-Kr. *22:* 361–365 (1957).

(6) JENSEN, N. E.: Congenital actodermal dysplasia of the face. Brit. J. Derm. *84:* 410–416 (1971).

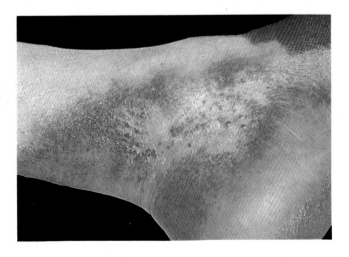

Fig. 188. Capillaritis alba.

(7) KORTING, G. W., J. CABRÉ und H. HOLZMANN: Zur Kenntnis der Kollagenveränderungen bei der Anetodermie vom Typus Schweninger-Buzzi. Arch. klin. exp. Derm. *218:* 274–297 (1964).

(8) LANGHOF, H., H. MÜLLER und L. RIETSCHEL: Untersuchungen zur familiären, protoporphyrinämischen Lichturticaria. Arch. klin. exp. Derm. *212:* 506–518 (1961).

(9) LYNCH, P. J., and L. J. MIEDLER: Erythropoietic protoporphyria. Arch. Derm. (Chic.) *92:* 351–356 (1965).

(10) OLLENDORF CURTH, H.: Follicular atrophoderma and pseudopelade associated with chondrodystrophia calcificans congenita. J. Invest. Derm. *13:* 233–247 (1949).

(11) SCHULZ, T., E. BOTEZAN und N. GANEA: Bemerkungen zu einem Fall von Atrophodermia vermiculata. Derm. Wschr. *140:* 1346–1351 (1959).

(12) SETLEIS, H., B. KRAMER, M. VALCARCEL and A. H. EINHORN: Congenital ectodermal dysplasia of the face. Pediatrics *32:* 540–548 (1963).

(13) STREITMANN, B.: Amyloidosis cutis nodularis atrophicans. Z. Haut- u. Geschl.-Kr. *38:* 115–123 (1965).

(14) SUNDHAUSSEN, G.: Die Klinik der fokalen dermalen Hypoplasie. Inaug.-Diss. Mainz 1971.

D. Kraurosis

Originally, the concept of kraurosis was established for a disease consisting of sclerosis, atrophy, and flattening of the genital profile, followed by shrinkage and stenosis of the vaginal introitus; later, the same expression of kraurosis was applied to a similar condition of the male genitals (Fig. 189). Today we more and more recognize that kraurosis represents a characteristic final stage of shrinkage of the genitals but that this condition obviously can be the result of a number of different diseases. This means that kraurosis, etiologically and pathologically, in spite of its morphologic distinctive character, represents an "anonymous" disease entity.

However, one cannot completely overlook the extremely rare occurrence of **primary kraurosis** without preceding pruritus or leukoplakia. Widespread **acrodermatitis chronica atrophicans** may be accompanied by atrophy of the vulva; lichen sclerosus et atrophicus as a cause of kraurosis in men and women (thoroughly discussed in Chapter 16, A2) plays a role that is still underestimated.

Terminal kraurotic conditions of the genitals will hardly permit differential diagnostic conclusions as to the underlying disease which led to the kraurosis. The definitions of a purely senile involution of the genitals are fluid. Pronounced lichenified areas or **giant lichenification** (Pautrier's "lichénification géante") do not belong to the picture of kraurosis in the strict sense and should be classified differently (lichen simplex hypertrophicus, lichen planus verrucosus et atrophicus). In such cases a finding of other chronic areas of circumscribed neurodermatitis or lichen planus lesions (inspection of the mouth is necessary) will often aid in the diagnosis. Solitary or a few plaquelike circumscribed areas with whitish and definitely infiltrated lichenification should be called leukoplakia or **leukoplakic vulvitis** only if simultaneous shrinkage is lacking. However, one should consider that markedly pruritic areas of leukoplakia within the framework of a diffuse genital kraurosis but also independent of such a kraurosis could be the result of chronic irritation (not at all always obvious). The significance of this finding is that it is considered precancerous.

Lichen sclerosus et atrophicus is doubtless the most frequent cause of kraurosis (Fig. 190). From the point of view of classification it occupies a place between small circumscribed scleroderma on the one hand and lichen planus on the other hand, but it cannot be completely identified with either of these two disease entities. Lichen sclerosus favors the exten-

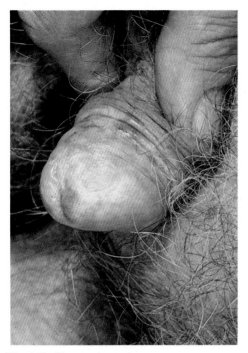

Fig. 189. Kraurosis penis.

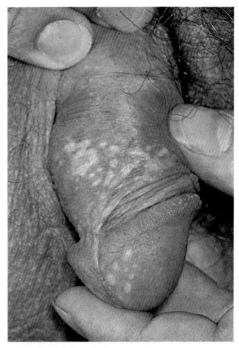

Fig. 190. Lichen sclerosus et atrophicus of the penis.

sor aspects of the large labia but may spread also to the anal region and the thighs.

The hard, white, sometimes slightly dimpled papules, typically with small horny plugs, measure 2 to 5 mm in diameter; histologically, one sees subepidermal areas with few nuclei within homogeneous and sclerotic connective tissue; the elastica disappears quite early, Such

homogeneous areas of connective tissue sometimes are surrounded by a wall of round cells; this appearance results in a lichen planuslike aspect. After a transitory phase of hyperkeratosis and parakeratosis with acanthosis, the epidermal band soon begins to become rather narrow, while the follicular hyperkeratoses that were observed macroscopically earlier persist much longer.

18. Erythemas and Exanthems

An erythema is the simplest reaction of the skin to various irritants and is caused by arteriolar or capillary hyperemia. Red areas of varying intensities usually lie at the level of the surrounding skin and are therefore macular. Occasionally, however, they are slightly raised, i. e., moderately

urticarial, because of fluid excreted from the vessels. We are dealing with an exanthem, and in an analogous way an enanthem, only if a multitude of small single endogenous elements are present simultaneously (i. e., in the blood stream, or less frequently, the lymphatics or nerve

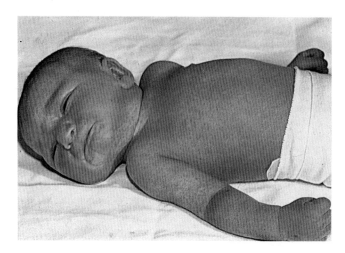

Fig. 191. Toxic erythema of the newborn.

impulses) and with distinctly increased intensity (stadium floritionis). Occasionally recurrences develop, and then the eruption subsides. In previous chapters the differential diagnosis of erythrodermas (see Chapter 22) and poikilodermas (see Chapter 23) was discussed and these entities need not be described again.

A. Noninfectious Erythemas of Childhood

1. Toxic erythema of the newborn appears on the second or third day of life. For the most part the lesions are urticarial (erythema papulatum) but may also be morbilliform or lichenoid. In later stages the confluent erythemas of the trunk or extremities (Fig. 191) disappear after a few days, usually without complications from involvement of other organs. Occasionally, vesicular lesions develop. Most pediatricians consider this form of erythema a postnatal reaction to the change of environment of the newborn. If minimal exanthems are considered representative, this eruption of the newborn occurs in up to 50 per cent of newborn children.[3, 8, 9]

Erythema of the newborn should be separated from the toxic erythema of the newborn. It develops more or less immediately during the transition from the inside of the uterus to the completely new environment. In premature infants the erythema lasts somewhat longer. In this practically physiologic postnatal erythema urticarial, papular, and vesicular lesions as well as considerable blood and tissue eosinophilias or leukocytopenias are absent, although they occur in the toxic erythema of the newborn. (A diaper rash has a different localization [see the following paragraph]. It develops, by the way, not before the fifth or sixth day of life.) If vesicles and pustules are present, they do not show eosinophilia, whereas neutrophils or bacteria are predominant. If the vesicular-pustular component is more pronounced, miliaria may be present. Toxic erythema of the newborn differs from miliaria by its rapid return to normal. Toxic miliaria of the newborn, on the other hand, which favors intertriginous, flexural, or similar locations, can persist for weeks as long as a warm environment increases the retention of sweat. The gyrated erythemas of beginning incontinentia pigmenti can be recognized by their speedy change to vesicles with high

Fig. 192. Erythema papulosum posterosivum.

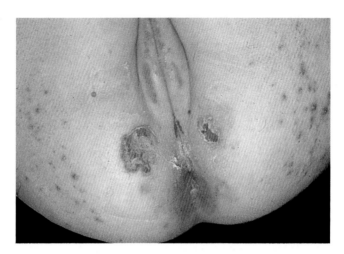

eosinophilia in blisters and blood (see also Chapter 1, A3 and Chapter 24, E9).

2. The most common dermatosis of the infant is **erythema of the gluteal region** (seu papulosum posterosivum) (Fig. 192).

Its other names are dermatitis pseudo-syphilitica papulosa and dermatitis ammoniacalis, among others. It represents a very common erythematous diaper rash. It may, however, become aggravated by blisters, erosions, and firm vegetating

Fig. 193. Acanthoma from irritation by dripping urine in patient with epispadias.

Fig. 194. Acanthoma from irritation around fistula of the ureter.

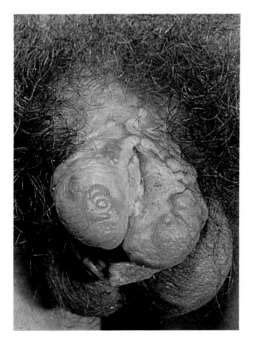

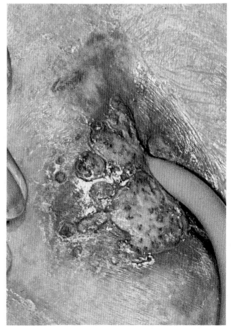

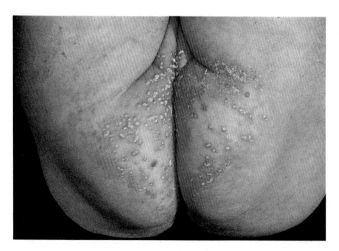

Fig. 195. Intertriginous candidiasis.

papules, and is identical with *papular pseudosyphilis* of the adult (for instance, urine and stool incontinence or urinary fistulas, Figs. 193, 194). "Ammonia", liberated in an alkaline milieu, is the harmful agent. Whereas a diaper rash in an acutely dyspeptic infant is character-

Fig. 196. Istizin dermatitis.

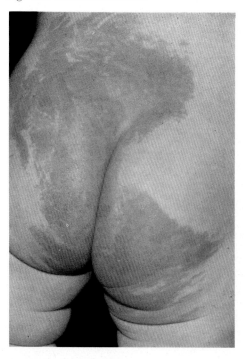

ized by flat, well circumscribed erythema immediately around the anus, gluteal erythema, also in contrast to syphilitic papules, leaves the region around the anus free. It is, however, wise to pay attention to the possibility of congenital syphilis (search for spirochetes and serum reactions) and not only when palms and soles are also involved. Swollen inguinal glands may also occur in confirmed gluteal erythema on account of superimposed unspecific secondary infections. On rare occasions gluteal erythema can become diffusely macerated, especially in intertrigenous eczematized areas. Then the differential diagnosis against moniliasis (Fig. 195) becomes important. Seborrheic eczema usually manifests itself simultaneously at the so-called intertriginous areas, i. e., face and most of all, behind the ears. Even if it is strongly macerated, it will lack nodular and papuloerosive lesions. Also confluent and erythematous is dermatitis venenata in this region (from rubber sheets or pants, salves, or remnants of salves). Another erythematous dermatitis venenata is caused by the excretion of the cathartic Istizin (Fig. 196), which is transformed in the colon to Cignolin. Intertriginous psoriasis vulgaris of the gluteal region, often with superimposed moniliasis, appears for the first time as "diaper psoriasis" after the second month of life. It appears rapidly in a few days with a few scales and sharply circumscribed areas of light or saturated red color, which, obviously, do not itch. Dermatitis herpetiformis with large bullae and a pemphigoid appearance, but always with a relatively grouped arrangement of single lesions, may be limited for weeks to the genitoanal area. Finally, as the original rash develops on additional sites the diagnosis of staphylogenic impetigo or a vesiculobullous diaper rash will be ruled out. In hereditary epidermolysis the pressure points of the gluteal region may limit the eruption for a while, but as in acrodermatitis enteropathica (see also Chapter 26E) the involvement of other body regions makes a diagnosis of a common gluteal erythema improbable.[6, 7]

3. Erythema annulare rheumaticum is today only rarely found as a cutaneous manifestation in rheumatic patients. It affects the upper abdomen almost exclusively, forming marginated and polycyclic, slightly saturated, reddish erythematous rings. It is without sequelae and disappears after a few days. A longer duration is exceptional. Recurrences have been observed. The presence of erythema annulare rheumaticum indicates a florid cardiac complication of acute rheumatic fever.

Histologically, a hardly characteristic vascular and cutaneous inflammation is present, which by dilatation of lymph spaces and edema of papillary bodies might suggest urticaria, but discrete perivascular masses of lymphocytes, histiocytes, and monocytoid elements are also present. In any case, the histologic picture does not show rheumatic tissue substrates.[5]

In the differential diagnosis of this extremely evanescent and, by its location, typical exanthem, one should consider urticaria, which, however, would itch, or

a toxic-allergic eczema which has a tendency to polymorphism. In fifth disease (infectious erythema) garlandlike "Ringelröteln" (round erythemas) with their jumping way of spreading are preceded by slight redness described as "papillon" of the lateral face. Annular erythemas of adults (see erythema annulare centrifugum or gyratum repens, discussed elsewhere) show larger arches or networks and last much longer. Furthermore, they are not limited to the upper abdomen and show in their round shapes greater infiltration, succulent induration (and therefore elevation), and, occasionally, fine lamellar scaling. Allergic subacute sepsis (see also Chapter 1, B7) may have a passing similarity with erythema annulare rheumaticum. The presence of septic intermittent bouts of fever may cause a false diagnosis, but the variability of its cutaneous manifestations (scarlatiniform, morbilloid, petechial), its location, and recurrences which last for weeks and months but hardly affect the general well-being, will point to the correct diagnosis. Allergic subacute sepsis, furthermore, has no cardiac complications. In Still's disease evanescent, mostly morbilliform or scarlatiniform eruptions appear on the extremities, trunk, and face. Moreover, in addition to its evanescent nature, the high rate of recurrences is typical. Finally, cutis marmorata, representing a vasoneurotic sign in more or less healthy individuals, favors the lower extremities. It is occasionally observed on the lower abdomen, but the favorite site of erythema annulare rheumaticum, the epigastric angle, is hardly ever involved.[10]

4. Acrodynia (Feer's disease) is a vegetative neurosis of infants. It is characterized by pronounced acral cyanosis and large lamellar palmoplantar desquamation with often considerable maceration (Fig. 197). Not infrequently, evanescent exanthems of the trunk and extremities are present. The rather impressive picture

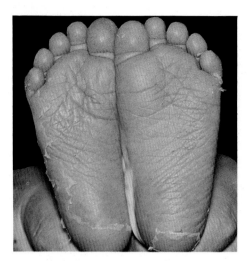

Fig. 197. Acrodynia.

is initiated by profuse sweats and tormenting insomnia. There usually is no fever but
considerable tachycardia is present. Generalized muscular weakness and hypertonia are most characteristic. In severe
cases hair, nails, and teeth may be lost.
Feer's disease is considered a late neuro-
allergic reaction to mercury.

In the differential diagnosis of miliaria-
like exanthems, miliaria rubra must be
ruled out, and in the differential diagnosis
of scarlatiniform rashes, especially if
palmoplantar desquamations develop subsequently, a recurrent scarlatiniform erythema should be considered. If one takes
notice of the accompanying general signs,
Feer's disease can hardly be missed.[1, 2, 4]

(1) BODE, H.-G.: Die Feersche Krankheit
    im Lichte der Dermatologie. Arch.
    Derm. Syph. (Berl.) *167:* 15–46 (1933).

(2) BODE, H.-G., und A. SCHEUFFLER:
    Feersche Krankheit. Zbl. Haut- u.
    Geschl.-Kr. *43:* 241–252 (1933).

(3) FREEMANN, R. G., R. SPILLER and
    J. M. KNOX: Histopathology of ery-
    thema toxicum neonatorum. Arch.
    Derm. (Chic.) *82:* 586–589 (1960).

(4) GÄDEKE, R., und E. HEUVER: Intra-
    familiäre, subakute Quecksilbervergif-
    tung bei Kindern. Med. Welt (Stuttg.)
    1962: 1768–1771.

(5) GREITHER, A.: Über das Erythema
    anulare rheumaticum. Arch. klin. exp.
    Derm. *204:* 205–212 (1957).

(6) IPPEN, H.: Ätiologie und Pathogenese
    des sogenannten Istizin-Exanthems.
    Dtsch. med. Wschr. *84:* 1062–1063
    (1959).

(7) LIPSCHÜTZ, B.: Untersuchungen über
    nicht venerische Gewebsveränderungen
    am äußeren Genitale des Weibes. III.
    Das Bild der Pseudosyphilis am äußeren
    Genitale des Weibes. Arch. Derm.
    Syph. (Berl.) *131:* 104–113 (1921).

(8) MAYERHOFER, E., und M. KRAJNOVIĆ-
    LYPOLT: Erythema neonatorum toxi-
    cum (Leiner) und allgemeine Allergie
    der Neugeborenen. Wien. klin. Wschr.
    40: 991–995 (1927).

(9) TAYLOR, W. B., and C. P. BONDURANT:
    Erythema neonatorum allergicum. Arch.
    Derm. Syph. (Chic.) *76:* 591–594 (1957).

(10) WISSLER, H.: Subsepsis allergica. Er-
    gebn. inn. Med. Kinderheilk. N. F. *23:*
    202–220 (1965).

B. Exanthems in Infectious Diseases

1. Measles (rubeola). The causative
organism of this childhood disease belongs
to the myxovirus group and enters the
body through the respiratory tract and
the conjunctivae. After a constant incubation time of 9 to 11 days a complex of
prodromal signs (biphasic elevations of
temperature, blepharoconjunctivitis, photophobia, rhinitis, and bronchitis) sets in.
On the thirteenth or fourteenth day a
characteristic but not specific exanthem
(Fig. 198) develops very rapidly. It consists of small, faintly red spots, which
later enlarge and become dark red and
confluent. The initial lesions behind the
ears, as in rubella, are characteristic. If
"vesicular measles" (the so-called pemphi-

goid measles) appear, this is a pronounced morbilloid-bullous Lyell's syndrome.* A hemorrhagic variant of the exanthem does not seem to indicate an unfavorable prognosis, in contrast to the situation in other infectious exanthems. Because of the morbilliform character of some other exanthems, the appearance of Koplik's spots around the parotid duct, opposite the molars, is of great diagnostic significance, as they are exclusive in measles. They are chalky-white spots and represent aggregated, superficial epithelial necroses, which may simulate elements in thrush. The latter, however, can be wiped off, leaving easily bleeding erosions. An important diagnostic point is the fact that measles never occur in the first months of life in infants whose mothers had measles themselves. The hemogram initially shows leukocytosis; later there is leukopenia with a shift to the left and an eosinophilia. The urine becomes diazopositive. Typical sequelae or complications of measles are otitis media, croup, bronchiolitis, pneumonia, and encephalitis.

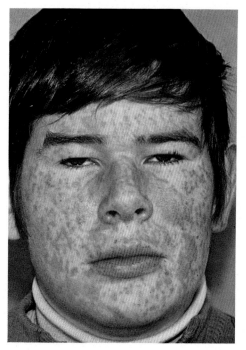

Fig. 198. Measles.

Histologically, an impressive vascular dilatation of the upper corium with moderate perivascular and also perifollicular infiltration with lymphocytes and granulocytes predominates in the exanthem of rubeola. Occasionally, analogous to the exudation in the papillary body, epidermal changes occur (edema, vesicles, and microabscesses), but these histologic findings are of little diagnostic aid.

If the exanthem of measles is at first follicular or mainly follicular, it may simulate scarlet fever. If sore throat and perioral paleness do not indicate the correct diagnosis, then the subsequent scaling in the form of membranous, glovelike desquamation will confirm the diagnosis of scarlet fever, since in measles

the disappearing exanthem eventually shows fine, small, branlike scales. A differentiation between weak measles and strongly developed rubella can become difficult in some cases, but the latter will show striking lymph node swellings and increased plasma cells in the hemogram. In a toxic-allergic exanthem of morbilliform character, the extremities and the gluteal region are usually especially affected, while catarrhal involvement of the conjunctivae and respiratory tract are absent. It may happen, however, that the eruption is caused by a drug given to combat the existing catarrhal viral infection.[10]

2. In **rubella** (German measles) swelling of the lymph nodes – chiefly the occipital-nuchal nodes – occurs five to seven days before the exanthem. This is followed by a faint enanthem (macules or petechiae on the soft palate), and finally the exanthem

---

* According to Korting, who observed such cases. (Tr.)

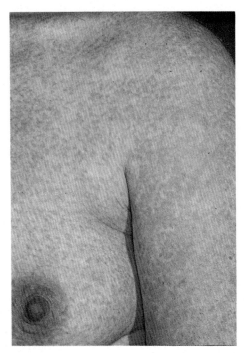

Fig. 199. Rubella.

glutination inhibiting test. Although the eruption of infectious mononucleosis may imitate that of German measles to a high degree, it starts with diphtheroid or Plaut-Vincent-like tonsillitis, is more febrile, and, in addition, shows generalized lymph node enlargement, as well as swellings of spleen and liver. In the hemogram, after a short leukocytopenic beginning phase, a pronounced leukocytosis occurs with up to 80 per cent mononuclear cells. The diagnosis is proved by the heterophilic antibody reaction (Hanganatziu-Deicher or Paul-Bunnell) test. Rubella-like exanthems of secondary syphilis would show a positive seroreaction. Moreover, enlarged lymph nodes of secondary syphilis are generalized, if present at all, and are not especially located in the nuchal region. In dengue the eruption remains morbilliform. After the initial facial congestion the characteristic secondary exanthem is present for only a few days and heals with a few scales. Furthermore, the general picture is one of catarrhal signs, characterized by muscular and joint pains, sudden high fever, and bradycardia. Rubella-like drug eruptions have apparently been observed, especially following administration of hydantoin; they may be accompanied by enlarged lymph nodes. Hemogram and serologic investigations must, therefore, be undertaken in doubtful cases in order to arrive at the correct diagnosis.[14]

becomes visible. As in measles, it starts retroauricularly or on the face and then spreads craniocaudally within a total span of three to four days. The rubella eruption is similar to that of rudimentary measles but lighter, and the individual lesions are smaller and have less tendency to confluence (Fig. 199). Postexanthematic scaling is almost always lacking. In epidemics of German measles about 30 to 40 per cent of cases show no exanthem. If it is present, it varies so much from case to case that it may have to be differentiated from either measles, scarlet fever, or infectious mononucleosis.

The state of health of the patient with rubella is only slightly affected. In the beginning the hemogram shows leukopenia which is soon followed by a relative lymphocytosis. An increase (5 to 20 per cent) of plasma cells is characteristic. A diagnosis of German measles is confirmed if antibodies increase in the cold hemag-

3. Scarlet fever (scarlatina) is caused by beta-hemolytic streptococci of group A (and perhaps an additional virus) and begins in the upper respiratory tract. Within a few hours to days a flaming dusky redness of the pharynx develops, with dirty grayish tonsillar membranes; this is accompanied by high fever, rapid pulse, and vomiting. The exanthem, which soon follows, is observed initially on the inner aspects of the thighs, arms, and anterior axillary folds. Circumorally, the

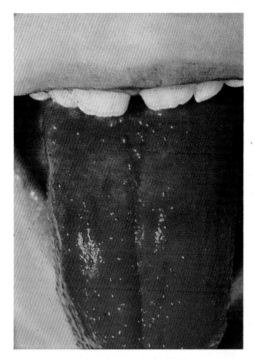

Fig. 200. Scarlet fever: so-called raspberry tongue.

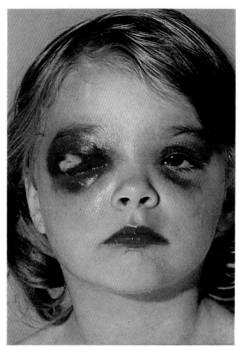

Fig. 201. Bacterial gangrene of the upper lid as complication of scarlet fever.

skin remains pale in contrast to the flaming redness of the body. The tongue reveals swollen papillae at the tip and the sides ("raspberry tongue") (Fig. 200). The exanthem itself appears at first glance to be a solid erythema, known as a concomitant of high fever. On closer inspection, however, it is seen to consist of many closely aggregated, tiny to pinhead-sized, light red or flaming red, erythematous spots, which may become temporarily succulent, while the skin between the lesions assumes a slightly yellowish hue. As early as one to two days later the eruption loses its characteristic appearance, and after one week has usually disappeared completely. Occasionally, however, the rash is followed, after two or three weeks, by characteristic branlike scales, located on the hands, feet, and auricular pinnae; these scales peel off in large lamellae or in a glove-like manner. There is no relationship between the intensity of the exanthem and the mem-branous desquamation. Also, in scarlet fever the exanthem varies with regard to intensity and extension, so that occasionally petechiae and small watery blisters (scarlatina miliaris) occur. It is important to realize that in scarlet fever the eruption intensifies in expression by the appearance of new single elements and not by enlargement of the single lesions as in measles. Occasionally, small petechiae are located only in larger body folds and in linear order. If the circulation is greatly impaired, star-shaped capillary hyperemia appears on the palms and soles or the whole eruption assumes a bluish hue ("blue scarlet"). In rare instances, as in mild cases or in scarlet fever resulting from wounds, there is no exanthem and only the subsequent membranous desquamation indicates the past infection. In doubtful cases the outcome of the Rumpel-Leede phenomenon will confirm the diagnosis; it is negative in cases of scarlatina. Other convincing data are the presence of hemo-lytic streptococci in a nasal or pharyngeal smear, numerous Döhle bodies in neutro-phil leukocytes, and a positive blanching phenomenon 12 to 20 hours after intra-cutaneous injection of scarlet fever con-valescent serum or 0.3 ml of antistrepto-coccic serum. Scarlatiniform exanthems can appear in the course of *viral hepatitis* (increased transaminase), as an eruption of smallpox, and as drug or hypersensitivity reactions (see Table 2).[19]

4. Erythema infectiosum (fifth disease) is observed in children under 14 years of age with initial varying catarrhal signs. The eruption begins on the cheeks with a mild erythema in butterfly distribution ("papillon"). This is followed by a dis-continuous eruption on the extensor sur-face of the upper arms, later on the flexor sides of the forearms, and finally on the

Table 2. Drugs Causing Morbilliform and Scarlatiniform Eruptions.

Allopurinol	Novobiocin
Barbiturates	Penicillin
Chlorothiazide	Phenacetin
Diazepam	Phenazone
Flufenisal	Phenothiazine derivatives
Gold salts	Phenylbutazone derivatives
Griseofulvin	Pyrazolone derivatives
Hydantoin	Salicylates
Indomethacin	Streptomycin
Insulin	Sulfonamides
Mepacrine	Sulfones
Mephenamine	Thiouracil
Meprobamate	

buttocks in reticular or maplike erythema-tous forms (Fig. 202a, b). The palms and soles remain uninvolved. The duration of the disease is about seven days.

Fig. 202. Erythema infectiosum: (a) beginning exanthem of the shoulder region; (b) poly-cyclic rings on the forearm.

Fig. 202a.

Fig. 202b.

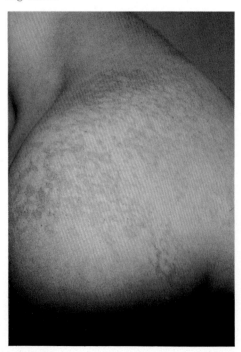
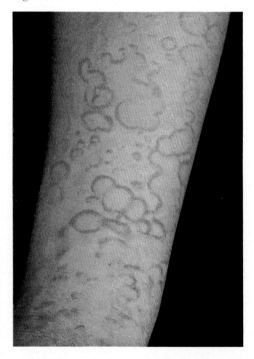

Histologically, one observes uncharacteristic, exudative, inflammatory changes which highly resemble the histologic appearance of measles, since there are also distinct perifollicular infiltrations. But in contrast to measles, there are swollen connective tissue fibers. Whereas in erythema infectiosum no remarkable endothelial alterations occur, such changes in pronounced form characterize the histologic substrate of the roseola of typhus.

In the differential diagnosis there are no difficulties in classic erythema infectiosum, certainly not if this exanthem in epidemic form is seen together with epidemics of measles and rubella. But if one is confronted only by the initial facial erythema in butterfly distribution, other infectious diseases (scarlet fever) and dermatoses (lupus erythematosus, erythematous rosacea) have to be considered. If the facial erythema lasts longer, a constitutional facial erythema of the "rustic type" may be present. Erysipelas in the facial region hardly ever has a symmetrical butterfly shape but remains more pronounced on the side of the portal of entry of the infection. Above all, it is initiated by acute general signs (chills and high fever) and, in contrast to erythema infectiosum, there are no lesions on other body areas even if it lasts a long time. Erysipelas moves continuously, erythema infectiosum jumps. Different from measles are the absence of high fever, Koplik's spots, and catarrhal manifestations. Discontinuous spreading and sparing of the trunk also argue against measles, which always involves the trunk. The feverless course of erythema infectiosum permits its differentiation from exanthema subitum, which affects infants almost exclusively. Infections caused by the ECHO virus may sometimes simulate erythema infectiosum, but they show higher prodromal temperatures and ulcerating mucous membrane changes. Erythema multiforme, which may occur in epidemics, has an eruption of typical target lesions; it favors the extensor surface of the upper extremities, or else a so-called inverse localization on the flexor sides with simultaneous pluriorificial involvement of the mucous membranes.[11]

In the epidemic of *erythema infectiosum variabile** in 1958 the eruption resembled classic erythema infectiosum or erythema multiforme in spite of its pronounced urticarial, vesicular, and partly petechial character. In this epidemic the palms were quite regularly affected.[13]

5. Exanthema subitum (roseola infantum), with an eruption lasting three days, occurs in children up to two years of age. After the sudden and high fever has dropped, a fleeting pink rash appears and spreads centrifugally from the trunk to the extremities, leaving the face unaffected. The eruption, which is rubella-like or morbilliform, heralds the beginning of recovery. The hemogram shows leukopenia and lymphomonocytosis. Although the eruption does not itch, there are mild accompanying neurologic signs, such as hypersensitivity to touch, increased tension of the fontanelles, and convulsions.**

Without discussing otitis media, rhinopharyngitis, and other signs at the outset of the disease, an eruption will make us consider measles first. However, measles show leukocytosis first and only later leukopenia. The exanthem of measles, moreover, in contrast to that of exanthema subitum, is accompanied by another elevation of temperature. In infectious mononucleosis the enlargement of lymph nodes and spleen and the atypical lymphonuclear cells in the hemogram together with a positive Paul-Bunnell reaction will confirm the diagnosis. Viral influenza as

---

* Margarine disease. (Tr.)
** The convulsions are related to the high fever, not the infection. (Tr.)

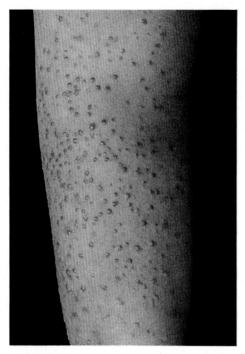

Fig. 203. Acrodermatitis papulosa eruptiva infantum (Gianotti-Crosti syndrome).

well as measles has an initial catarrhal stage, which does not occur in exanthema subitum. Besides, influenza shows biphasic temperature curves.[16]

6. Acrodermatitis papulosa eruptiva infantilis (Gianotti-Crosti syndrome) is a typical children's disease which presents a lichenoid-papular eruption (Fig. 203) starting on hands and feet and is accompanied by moderate fever. It quickly spreads symmetrically in a caudocranial direction. The face and neck are in general affected last and the trunk is not affected at all. Occasionally, one sees a discrete purpuric sign. Almost always the lymph nodes are enlarged, but liver and spleen are not always palpably larger. In the hemogram increased monocytes are found. The involvement of the liver is suggested by the increased serum transaminase values. The single elements of the disorder may

last a long time; nevertheless, the lesions disappear with no tendency to recur.

Considering the age of the patient and the absence of itching, it is the involvement of the lymph nodes and the monocytosis in the blood that demand differential diagnostic considerations. Infectious mononucleosis, acute or subacute lymphoreticuloses, and chronic malignant reticulohistiocytoses, including Letterer-Siwe's disease, must be considered. Lichen planus in children is rare; it is diagnosed by the presence of pruritus, possible mucous membrane involvement, its site of predilection on the forearms, and finally, its histology. Papular or lichenoid drug eruptions can always be ruled out by their history.[2, 4, 21]

7. Typhoid fever, paratyphoid, and exanthematous typhus. Typhoid fever starts slowly with general signs such as cough, sore throat, headaches, diarrhea or constipation, bradycardia (pulse rate less than 60), leukopenia, splenomegaly; in addition, there are a few typical cutaneous signs such as typhoid facies with a flushed face and a dusky, leaden hue frequently associated with distinct acrocyanosis of fingers and auricles, as well as the greyish-yellow tongue of typhoid with its uncoated tip. Other characteristic accompanying signs are an erythematous, spotty, later perhaps ulcerated enanthema, which soon changes into moniliasis of the oral cavity, marked dermographism, and miliaria crystallina caused by heavy perspiration. Late dermatologic complications are diffuse post-typhoid alopecias, onychopathias (transverse dystrophy and fragility of nails), and venous thromboses. Similar characteristic signs of the late stage of typhoid are succulent infiltrates together with specific ostitis and a lack of resistance of the patient toward infection with pathogenic organisms such as pyogenic cocci (ecthymas, furuncles, abscesses caused by injections or a parotid abscess due to an ascending infection of Stensen's duct); larger ulcerated pyodermas comparable to noma have become rare owing to the use of antibiotics. The diagnosis of typhoid is substantiated by evidence of the causative organism (in stool, urine, or blood) and by agglutination tests (Gruber-Widal reaction); typical cutaneous signs are the typhoid roseola (rose spots) of the abdominal skin. They appear between the seventh and tenth days, usually on the lower abdomen, less often on the trunk and extremities. These lesions are pale red and macular at first, later almost always distinctly papular and lenticular. Ordinarily, they appear as a few single lesions only, seldom in profusion, and occurring in several attacks. Very often the exanthem appears in one sudden outbreak but spares the neck and face; however, the face shows deep red erythema and marked conjunctivitis (rabbit eyes). The rose spots begin to fade out after a few days, their color turning to a greenish-yellow. Interspersion of the rose spots with petechiae is rare in typhoid, but it is almost typical in typhus.

A histologic distinction between the cutaneous lesions of typhoid and typhus is not possible and is of no practical importance. One sees predominantly perivascular infiltrates with masses of typhoid bacilli. In contrast to the roseola of typhus the vascular walls in typhoid and paratyphoid remain intact.

It seems desirable to differentiate between the exanthemas of typhoid mentioned earlier and those of **paratyphoid A and B**. Although the final decision can only be made bacteriologically, it can be said that the rose spots are rather more scarce in paratyphoid than in typhoid fever. When present they are larger and more numerous, but spare the hands and feet. In addition to rose spots, paratyphoid shows bluish-red, sometimes deeply located spotty changes. In contrast to typhoid, paratyphoid very often starts with herpes simplex labialis.

Exanthematic typhus, which is one of the rickettsiae, is at first characterized by severe headache and an exanthem. According to Wunderlich's curve, there is a remission of the fever between the third and fourth day, followed by its renewed elevation and a simultaneous change from bradycardia to tachycardia as a result of severe impairment of the CNS. After six to seven days, an exanthem presenting many closely adjacent, separate lesions becomes evident (Fig. 204). The lesion frequently appears somewhat jagged; it is found in abundance on palms and soles. In contrast to typhoid, the exanthem of typhus is more macular than papular; the macules tend to be interspersed with petechiae. Accordingly, the Rumpel-Leede phenomenon as a sign of marked vascular fragility is usually distinctly positive. Like the initial roseolar exanthems of secondary syphilis, the first and chief locations of the exanthems of typhus are the sides of the trunk and the flexor aspects of the forearms. After the twelfth day the exanthem begins to fade, leaving a conspicuous tendency to scaling; it can be compared to the effect of a rubber eraser on paper. Sometimes an additional sign is the interspersion of the rose spots of typhus with dark erythematous lesions that look like areas of cutis marmorata (Murchinson's spots). These phenomena, combined with the tendency to white dermographism, which otherwise occurs in such characteristic fashion almost exclusively in atopic eczema, are difficult to recognize because the entire skin may show excoriations and pyodermas, the effect of infestation with lice.

8. Trench fever (five-day fever, febris quintana, or Wolhynia fever) is due to *Rickettsia quintana* transmitted by body, head, and crab lice; they act as hosts for the organisms. After an incubation period of up to two months, the disease lasts from one to several months with periodic febrile attacks repeating themselves about every

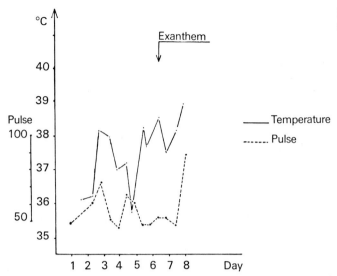

Fig. 204. Wunderlich's remission in exanthematic typhus.

five days, accompanied by chills and profuse sweating. Another important sign, as observed by the author himself, are painful paresthesias of the tibial regions, which are more frequent than the pain in the calves that accompanies leptospiral jaundice (Weil's disease). In a few cases, during the first few febrile attacks, a scarlatiniform eruption appears for a short time; it is roseolalike as well as macular or petechial in nature and is not of much importance in the diagnosis. A definite diagnosis can be achieved by letting healthy lice, enclosed in a capsule applied to the arm, feed on the patient.*

The differential diagnosis must consider other pyrexias, such as intermittent and recurrent fevers and malaria; however, erythema and hemorrhagic diathesis are not among the more prominent signs. Drug eruptions, for instance those due to quinine, have to be considered in malaria. Rarely does malaria show morbilliform or petechial exanthems or infiltrative after-effects, such as erythema nodosumlike

or vasomotoric phenomena of Raynaud's character.

9. Benign **Q**(ueensland) **fever,** described in Australia but worldwide in distribution, (also known as Balkan grippe or Cretan pneumonia), produces no cutaneous changes of any importance, whereas the clinical signs such as primary atypical pneumonias and bradycardia, in spite of periods of high fever with chills, are to be stressed. Late sequelae are orchitis and epididymitis, which can be identified by the complement fixation test for *Coxiella burnetii (Rickettsia diaporica)* with negative cold agglutination of the erythrocytes.[7, 12]

10. The harmless **pappataci fever** (phlebotomus fever) starts with headaches, retrobulbar pain, and conjunctivitis. The skin is hot and dry and in most cases shows no exanthem. A few cases, however, have shown morbilliform, roseolar, scarlatiniform, urticarial, and purpuric eruptions. More characteristic, according to the author's own observations, are spotty or bandlike, dark red enanthemas, especially of the soft palate. Because some cases of

_____

* The infected lice then die. (Tr.)

pappataci fever also produce mucous enteropathies, it may be necessary to consider typhoid or paratyphoid, while dengue fever has a prolonged febrile course and an increased tendency to exanthems.[15]

11. Infection with cytomegalovirus (cytomegalic inclusion disease; CID or salivary gland viral disease) occurs mostly in very young infants in correlation with interstitial plasma cell pneumonia. Jaundice and hemorrhagic diathesis are the most important signs; however, both are absent in the localized form which affects only the parotid gland. In addition, CID may present maculopapular eruptions, desquamative or eczematous erythrodermas, and petechial exanthems. CID in the adult does not involve the salivary glands; it occurs in combination with severe systemic signs. Dermatologically, the most important differential diagnosis is against congenital syphilis, toxoplasmosis, and listeriosis (intracranial calcifications, hydrocephalus, chorioretinitis).[3, 23]

12. Tularemia is caused by *Francisella tularensis (Pasteurella tularensis).* * Depending on the place of entry, the disease may develop into an ulceroglandular type or a grippe-typhoidlike form. More rarely, its course may be pulmonary (infiltrates of the lungs) or abdominal (diarrhea or constipation, swellings of mesenteric lymph nodes). The diagnosis can be verified by subcutaneous or intraperitoneal injections of animals with material obtained from the primary lesion, from blood, or from lymph node punctures, and also by an agglutination reaction (beginning with the second week of the disease). Tularemia can be suspected when there is a history of contact with rodents harboring biting ectoparasites such as deerflies, ticks, mites,

or animal lice.* The possibility of laboratory infections should be kept in mind.

The ulceroglandular type begins with one lesion or multiple primary lesions; it should be differentiated, depending on site and number of lesions, from a syphilitic primary chancre and from a perforated broken-down lymph node, as well as from mildly infiltrated actinomycosis, scrofuloderma, and especially, cat-scratch disease. If the portal of entry is located in the groin, lymphogranuloma inguinale venereum must be considered because its primary lesion, as well as that of tularemia, is an inconspicuous circumscribed lesion with a subsequent clinical picture of regional lymphadenopathy. Should nut-sized, subcutaneous infiltrated nodes develop successively along the lymph paths, one should consider sporotrichosis; however, such nodes in tularemia would break down less readily than those of sporotrichosis. Only the oculoglandular type is really definitely diagnostic. The primary lesion produces severe conjunctivitis accompanied by unilateral enlargement of the preauricular, submaxillary, and cervical lymph nodes together with unilateral edema of the lids. Also, the eyelids and folds of the lids show villous growths and yellow nodules. Ulcerogranulomatous conjunctivitis usually heals without scar formation after several months.

In addition to the cutaneous lesions of tularemia, already mentioned, there are further secondary manifestations of the skin, the so-called tularemides. They may appear as scarlatiniform, papulopustular, or pustular exanthems, and also as erythema multiforme or erythema nodosumlike cutaneous lesions.

Histologically, the structure of tularemic lymph nodes located near the skin resembles the already discussed possibili-

---

* In Germany, this disease is reportable on suspicion. (Tr.)

* Handling the products of contaminated animals, such as raw hides, can also transmit the disease. (Tr.)

ties in the macroscopic differential diagnosis, in which the tularemic lymph node
necrobioses can look especially like the
wasp-stinglike necroses in lymphogranuloma inguinale venereum. Compared to
the lymph nodes of tuberculosis with
caseation, the tularemic nodes are more
polymorphic and irregular.

Also, the granuloma of the tularemic
lymph nodes corresponds to the cutaneous
granuloma of the primary lesion of
tularemia; in the early stage such a
primary lesion shows necroses, and later a
sarcoidlike structure prevails. In contrast,
lymph nodes in cat-scratch disease show
hyperplasia composed of reticulum cells
with occasional formation of abscesses.[1,9,
17,20,22]

13. Bang's disease (which causes abortion in cattle) may cause local infections
owing to contact of the skin with the
vagina of a diseased cow.* These infections produce either fleeting erythematous
or persistent folliculopapular, pruritic but
not pustular, lesions. Only later will
pustules and necroses occasionally occur.
Such cutaneous lesions of Bang's disease –
apparently allergic reactions – are not
accompanied by fever.[6]

14. Smallpox in the initial stage shows
variable, mostly fleeting exanthems. After
an incubation period of from 8 to 18 days
with steep elevation of temperature
accompanied by severe headaches and
pains of the lumbar region, joints, and
testes, an exanthem of morbilliform,
rubeolalike, or scarlatiniform character
appears. The eruption, present on the
flexor aspects of the large joints, shows a
few petechiae. Extensive petechial bleedings are a bad prognostic sign. If a drop
in temperature occurs, such unspecific
exanthems may change occasionally

directly into the specific smallpox eruption. It is impossible to make a diagnosis
of smallpox during the phase of the
initial exanthem (see paragraph C2,
page 234, and Chapter 1, E3).[8]

15. Influenza (grippe). Some epidemics
of influenza show an increased incidence
of exanthems, which can be distinguished
only with difficulty from measles or scarlet
fever. Sites of predilection are the chest,
neck, abdomen, and neck, while the extremities remain relatively free. Such a
maculopapular exanthem is extremely
evanescent and can be observed only for
a few hours. There is no definite connection with the course of the disease as in
smallpox. After the disappearance of the
rash, diffuse facial redness with perioral
blanching and a macular enanthema
remain. The buccal mucosa and also the
mucosa of the mouth may show so-called
influenza dots. These are solitary, pinhead-
sized lesions of yellowish-white color
arranged in groups which lie completely
within the level of the mucous membrane.
In contrast, Koplik's spots of measles are
elevated and have a different size and
arrangement than the influenza dots.
Near these whitish dots, as in many
infectious diseases, are petechial areas of
bleeding located on the mucous membranes of the oral cavity.[5,18,24]

(1) ARZT, L.: Die Tularämie im Gebiet von
    Niederdonau im Herbst und Winter
    1936/37 mit besonderer Berücksichti-
    gung der Haut- und Drüsenveränderun-
    gen. Arch. Derm. Syph. (Berl.) *178:*
    294–317 (1939).

(2) BOLOGA, E. I.: Sur la participation
    hépatique dans l'acrodermatite papu-
    leuse infantile (syndrome Gianotti-
    Crosti). G. ital. Derm. *107:* 1385–1402
    (1966).

(3) BRODKIN, R. H., M. WEINBERG and M.
    LEIDER: Generalized cytomegalic in-
    clusion disease. Arch. Derm. (Chic.) *84:*
    650–653 (1961).

---

* The disease is usually seen in veterinarians. (Tr.)

(4) CROSTI, A., et F. GIANOTTI: Dermatose éruptive acro-située d'origine probablement virosique. Dermatologica (Basel) *115:* 671–677 (1957).

(5) EHM, O. F.: Beobachtungen über Schleimhautveränderungen bei Grippe. Münch. med. Wschr. *99:* 1904–1905 (1957).

(6) HAXTHAUSEN, H., und A. THOMSEN: Brucella-Ausschlag bei Tierärzten. Arch. Derm. Syph. (Berl.) *163:* 477–491 (1931).

(7) HENGEL, R., G. A. KAUSCHE, A. LAUR und K. RABENSCHLAG: Das Q-Fieber. Ergebn. inn. Med. Kinderheilk. N. F. *5:* 219–305 (1954).

(8) HERRLICH, A.: Die Pocken. Erreger, Epidemiologie und klinisches Bild. Thieme, Stuttgart 1967.

(9) JUNG, H.-D.: Die Tularämie als neue differentialdiagnostisch wichtige Erkrankung gegenüber den Geschlechtskrankheiten und der Hauttuberkulose. Derm. Wschr. *123:* 73–76 und 274–275 (1951).

(10) KÖTTGEN, U., und G. W. KORTING: Zur Frage des Masernpemphigoids. Dtsch. med. Wschr. *89:* 2318–2321 (1964).

(11) KORTING, G. W.: Megalerythema epidemicum. Derm. Wschr. *124:* 785–796 (1951).

(12) KORTING, G. W.: Orchitis und Epididymitis als Erscheinungsformen von Q-Fieber. Hautarzt *2:* 168–170 (1951).

(13) KORTING, G. W.: Das bisher bekannte Bild des Erythema infectiosum und die jetzige exanthematische Pandemie. Med. Welt (Stuttg.) *1958:* 2064–2068.

(14) LENNARTZ, H.: Virusdiagnostik der Rubeolen. Dtsch. med. Wschr. *95:* 2439–2440 (1970).

(15) MARCHIONINI, A.: Zur Klimatophysiologie und -pathologie der Haut. Arch. Derm. Syph. (Berl.) *182:* 613–651 (1942).

(16) MÖBUS, L.: Das Exanthema subitum und seine Differentialdiagnose. Dtsch. Gesundh.-Wes. *11:* 392–404 (1956).

(17) NETHERTON, E. W.: Tularemia with reference to its cutaneous manifestations. Arch. Derm. Syph. (Chic.) *16:* 170–184 (1927).

(18) NEUMANN, D., und CHR. LENGSFELD: Exanthematischer Verlauf der Influenza-B-Virus-Grippe bei Kindern. Dtsch. med. Wschr. *97:* 263–265 (1972).

(19) PRESTIA, A. E., and Y. L. LYNFIELD: Scarlatiniform eruption in viral hepatitis. Arch. Derm. (Chic.) *101:* 352–355 (1970).

(20) REICH, H.: Zur Kenntnis der Tularämie hautnaher (regionaler) Lymphknoten. Arch. Derm. Syph. (Berl.) *192:* 175–188 (1950).

(21) REICH, H.: Das Gianotti-Crosti-Syndrom. Hautarzt *14:* 315–318 (1963).

(22) SCHUERMANN, H., und H. REICH: Zur Klinik und Histologie des cutan lokalisierten tularämischen Primäraffekts. Arch. Derm. Syph. (Berl.) *190:* 579–604 (1950).

(23) SEIFERT, G., und J. OEHME: Pathologie und Klinik der Cytomegalie. Thieme, Stuttgart 1957.

(24) YUNG TSÜ, T.: Weitere Erfahrungen über die sogenannten Grippepünktchen bei 1070 beobachteten Grippefällen. Münch. med. Wschr. *101:* 1904–1905 (1959).

C. Varioliform and Pustular Exanthems in Infectious Diseases

1. Varicella (chickenpox), a highly contagious, worldwide, and occasionally epidemically or endemically spreading disorder, is a typical infectious disease of children, mostly of those up to the tenth year of life. Newborns and adults are infrequently affected. Two to three weeks after the infection, initially mild general signs such as fatigue, headaches, and subfebrile temperatures set in. Rarely, an evanescent preexanthem of morbilloid or scarlatiniform character appears. Subsequently, mildly saturated and distinct erythemas develop over the thorax. Within these erythemas nodules and thin-walled transparent blisters, which later become cloudy, appear. Subsequent eruptions are the rule, so that different developmental stages exist next to each other, causing a relatively polymorphous

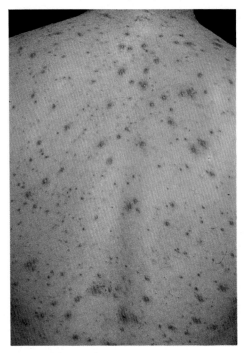

Fig. 205. Chickenpox.

picture (Fig. 205). The single, chickenpox pustules, which are sometimes umbilicated, last only a short while and heal in two to three days, sometimes leaving scars or depigmentations. Until the loss of the crusts the patient is contagious (the portal of entry is a droplet infection of the nasopharynx). Most of the lesions are on the trunk, although the head and face are favored initially. Not at all rare is the involvement of the oral cavity, but that of the genital mucous membranes is less frequent. These areas show a lentil-sized erythema with central vesiculation. Although this is usually a mild disorder, hemorrhagic or gangrenous changes may occur (caution should be exercised with corticosteroids). Other rare complications are pneumonia or involvement of the cornea and the CNS.

2. In **variola vera** (smallpox) there is a symptom-free incubation period of 12 to 18

days (isolation is, therefore, 18 days). Then a fulminant, peracute rise of fever with pain in the sacrum, extremities, and testes, an uncharacteristic scarlatiniform preexanthem, and catarrhal manifestations reveal the generalization of the causative organism. Three days of prodromal signs are followed by lytic temperatures and the eruption of the smallpox exanthems. The first lesions are millet-sized papules. They erupt on the forehead, nose, upper lip, and scalp; then the trunk and extremities, including the palms and soles, are affected. Renewed attacks increase the number of lesions; after a vesicular stage all lesions change synchronously on the eighth day to umbilicated pustules (Figs. 206a, b). Typically, the face is affected very early but small areas in the groin or armpits may be spared. Around the fifteenth day of the eruption acute septic changes (pyarthrosis, phlegmons, and pulmonary abscesses, among others) are possible. The smallpox exanthem heals with multiple small, flat, sunken-in scars (Fig. 207).

The laboratory diagnosis is performed by placing a thin smear of the contents of a pustule on a slide; this is covered by a second slide. (In Germany these slides are carefully wrapped and sent off to the examining place together with another thick, air-dried smear of the contents of a pustule and 5 to 10 ml of venous blood). The diagnosis is made with the help of an electron microscope, animal experiments, and serologic tests.

Judging from the experience gained from previous smallpox epidemics, a definite diagnosis of smallpox from the appearance of the skin alone is impossible – at least at the stage of the high initial fever or the initial rash. At that phase we must consider the possibility of endemic infections such as pappataci, dengue, or yellow fever, as well as typhoid, and even scarlet fever, measles, and rubella. Hemorrhagic scarlet fever may

Fig. 206. Smallpox: (a) monomorphic pustular eruption in the suppurative stage; (b) prepustular, intraepidermal virus blister with ballooning cell degeneration. HE stain, 100×.

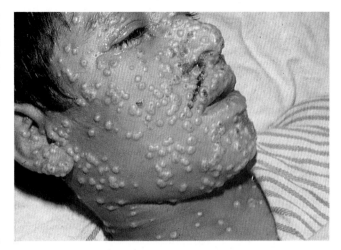

Fig. 206a.

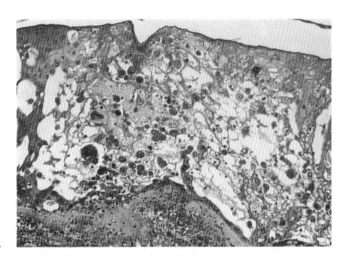

Fig. 206b.

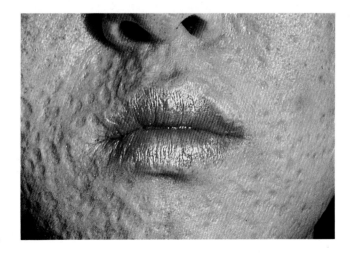

Fig. 207. Scars of smallpox.

imitate purpura variolosa closely. In scarlet fever, however, the eruption often favors the triangle between the thighs and the areas near the axillas. Chickenpox can become hemorrhagic under the influence of cortisone. Also, the cutaneous manifestions in meningococcic sepsis, when associated with acute high temperature, chills, and so on, may simulate purpura variolosa.

It is most important, however, to differentiate the smallpox exanthem, which occurs accompanied by lysis, from varicella. In smallpox, spots, papules, and blisters develop in eruptions and at the first pustular stage the lesions achieve the same level of development. In chickenpox, water-droplike blisters develop from macular, not papular, lesions and are often surrounded by a red border. Also in chickenpox, there is the different "star map," with lesions constantly different at the various stages. The differentiation, however, becomes difficult if we are dealing with "mild" smallpox and "severe" chickenpox. A diagnosis of varicella is favored, in principle, by a more colorful and therefore more polymorphous early exanthem with less clearly umbilicated, single lesions, although occasionally also in smallpox umbilication may be absent or only suggestive. The eruption of chickenpox, furthermore, is characterized by a denser distribution of lesions on the trunk. The lesions are more superficial and, therefore, more vulnerable or frail compared to the firm and tense lesions of smallpox. The lesions of chickenpox burst much more easily on pressure and their base is less red than that of smallpox lesions. Smallpox, on the other hand, is abundant on light-exposed or irritated areas. Often, but not without exception, smallpox eruptions spare the palms, axillas, back of the knee, and the neck. The differential diagnosis of chickenpox from varioloid, the smallpox infection of patients who have been vaccinated, may be especially difficult. The presence of

even one superficial water-clear blister with a red halo, dripping fluid if pricked, argues in favor of varicella. In varioloid, by the way, as in smallpox, the fever occurs before the eruption. In any case, the study of varioloid in its differentiation from varicella shows the great significance of obtaining a precise epidemiologic history when confronted with any varioliform eruption.*

Even less often than in smallpox are the palms and soles affected in pustular drug eruptions. Pustular iodide and bromide acne have afebrile courses. Iodide acne, moreover, is accompanied at the beginning of the eruption by conjunctivitis, rhinitis, and laryngitis. During a smallpox epidemic even acne vulgaris may have to be considered in the differential diagnosis since acne patients who are well protected by vaccination may conceal a few smallpox lesions between acne lesions.[2, 4, 7]

3. Like smallpox lesions, **vaccinia (eczema vaccinatum)** lesions favor light-exposed areas; multilocular, persistent, umbilicated, thickly covered vesicles appear after an incubation period of from 5 to 12 days. Frequently, lesions of the oral mucosa are present.

Eczema herpeticum is caused by rapid dissemination of the herpes simplex virus, practically always in eczematous patches (infantile eczema, disseminated neurodermatitis). The vesicles may be smaller than those of vaccinia and are unilocular. The changes of the oral mucosa closely resemble those in aphthae. Herpetic dendritic keratitis may occur. The incubation period of eczema herpeticum, 75 per cent of which occurs in children, is two to five days; it is definitely shorter than the incubation period of vaccinia. The mortality rate in adults is 10 per cent and

---

* The Tzanck smear is confirmatory in varicella. (Tr.)

in very young infants it is 20 per cent. The differential diagnosis must consider a common impetiginous eruption of a type known as **varioliform pyoderma** versus the eruptions of vaccinia and eczema herpeticum (Fig. 208). Dermatitis venenata caused by iodine, menthol, eucalyptol, and similar products may show secondary staphylococcic pyoderma, in which some of the single lesions resemble smallpox or vaccinia.[6]

Staphylococcic pyodermas showing umbilicated vesicles are seen very rarely.

4. In the **large pustular syphilid** lentil-sized, firm pustules are seen. Rarely is there a suggestion of umbilication, as they soon dry up or change into thinly crusted or rupioid lesions followed by intense pigmentation. Such pustular syphilids apparently develop after intense sun exposure and run an irregularly remittent, highly febrile course. Vomiting, lumbar pain, and constant fever as in smallpox are absent. The monomorphous pustule of smallpox shows a light red halo, whereas the more polymorphous syphilitic pustule with its tendency to rapid change is surrounded by a brown-red halo; it resembles rather the lesion of chickenpox.

The exanthem of **glanders** starts with a roseolar and papular stage, which turns into an acute pustular eruption. The semispherical, prominent, yellow to copper-colored pustules, however, are not umbilicated and almost always become ulcerated.

During its second week, septicemic and usually lethal *melioidosis** may show on the face lentil-sized pustules that also resemble smallpox. In addition, petechial exanthems and deeper subcutaneous abscess formation have been observed.[3]

_____
* A disease of rodents; it is transmissible to man, and is caused by *Malleomyces pseudomallei* which are endemic in Southeast Asia. (Tr.)

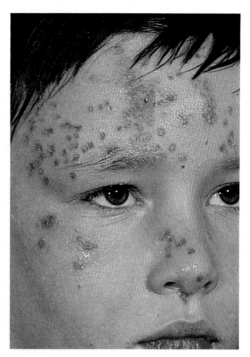

Fig. 208. Varioliform pyoderma.

5. Orf (ecthyma contagiosum) is caused by a virus which produces a contagious pustular dermatitis in sheep and goats. It is transmissible to man; after an incubation period of 3 to 11 days, pustules develop. The fingers and hands show circumscribed, nodular, elevated, and pustular lesions which are of semisolid consistency. They occur in the same location as milker's paravaccinial nodules and must be differentiated from anthrax pustules, pyogenic granuloma, chronic papillomatous pyoderma, accidental vaccinia, and such primary lesions as tularemia and sporotrichosis.[1, 8]

6. Listeria. *Listeria monocytogenes*, a genus of the family Corynebacteriaceae, causes miliary granulomas in newborn infants and develops into granulomatosis infantum septica. The following types can be distinguished in humans:

(a) tonsillar, septic form with mononucleosis;

(b) oculoglandular form with conjunctivitis;

(c) cervicoglandular form;

(d) central nervous form with meningitis, meningoencephalitis, and psychoses;

(e) granulomatosis septica and typhoid-pneumonia form;

(f) granulomatosis infantum septica (of the newborn without meningitis);

(g) listeriosis of pregnancy; and

(h) other forms (exanthematous, venereal, and so on).

Pathognomonic are approximately millet-sized, cutaneous granulomas appearing clinically as roseola or minute pustules. The posterior pharyngeal wall shows minute whitish clots. In 'the adult (especially veterinarians or agricultural workers) inoculation with the gram-positive coccoid rods takes place through pre-existing – for instance, eczematous – changes. The eruption starts with papulovesicular, papulopustular lesions, some surrounded by a hyperemic wall; such infections are especially common after manual evacuation of the bovine uterus following abortions, an occurrence which is similar to the direct cutaneous infection by Bang's bacillus.

In the differential diagnosis pustulosis of listeria must be compared mainly with folliculitis due to staphylococci; such staphylococcic infections develop either as pure ostiofolliculitides or, more frequently, as primary pustules.[5]

7. Hand-foot-mouth disease produces separate palmar and plantar pustules and aphthoid erosions of the anal mucosa. Aphthoid lesions of the oral mucosa exist at the same time. Further details are in Chapter 35, A3.

(1) BLAKEMORE, F., M. ABDUSSALAM and W. N. GOLDSMITH: A case of Orf (contagious pustular dermatitis): Identification of the virus. Brit. J. Derm. 60: 404–409 (1948).

(2) DIXON, C. W.: Small pox. Churchill, London 1962.

(3) FLEMMA, R. J., F. C. DiVINCENTI, M. L. N. DOTIN and B. A. PRUITT: Returning servicemen carry unfamiliar, fatal organisms. J. Amer. Med. Ass. 207: 1275 (1969).

(4) HERRLICH, A., A. MAYR und E. MUNZ: Die Pocken. Thieme, Stuttgart 1967.

(5) KALKOFF, K. W., und W. SCHIFF: Listeriose der Haut durch Kontaktinfektion. Hautarzt 11: 201–204 (1960).

(6) STREITMANN, B.: Über varioliforme Pyodermien. Arch. Derm. Syph. (Berl.) 178: 99–105 (1939).

(7) STÜTTGEN, G.: Die Rolle der Dermatologen bei der Pockenbekämpfung. Fortschr. prakt. Derm. Venerol. 5: 45–59 (1965).

(8) WHEELER, C. E., E. P. CAWLEY and J. H. JOHNSON: Ecthyma contagiosum (Orf). Arch. Derm. Syph. (Chic.) 71: 481–485 (1955).

D. Exanthems of Generalized Syphilis

Syphilis is still known as the "great imitator" because it simulates many different dermatoses, although toxic-allergic exanthems seem to do this to an even greater extent. The generalized syphilitic eruptions of the early and late periods do not offer any differential diagnostic difficulties. A typical sign of this chronic infectious disease, which occurs in stages, is the fact that the lesions of the early (secondary) period are quite small and numerous, whereas later attacks from successive relapses show fewer but larger lesions. Together with the appearance of the early lesions impressive constitutional signs will become evident, including fever, chills, early changes of the cerebrospinal fluid, and nocturnal sweats; upon questioning, the patient will admit severe nocturnal periosteal, bone, and joint pains.

Secondary syphilis occasionally may present **hilar adenopathy.** "Specific" treatment can cause similar anaphylactoid

Fig. 209. Secondary syphilis:
(a) macular recurrent exanthems; (b) maculopapular
recurrent exanthems.

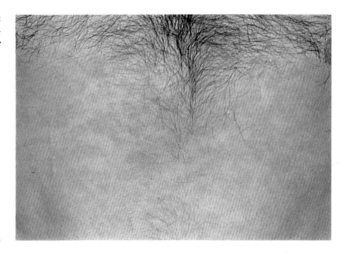

Fig. 209a.

changes of the lungs and kidneys; such changes should be separated from those caused by syphilis proper. In cases with a slow course, characterized by coughing and positive seroreactions, a Wassermann-positive pseudosyphilitic bronchopneumonia with involvement of the hilar region should be considered. Other possibilities are tuberculous infiltration, psittacosis, or adenoviral infections of the upper respiratory tract. Such infections can now easily be classified as pseudosyphilitic by the negative Nelson reaction;* it is not

_____

* Or FTA-ABS test. (Tr.)

necessary any longer to wait for the spontaneous drop in the titer of the Wassermann reaction.[1, 2]

Macular syphilids as a rule are typical for the beginning of the **secondary stage of syphilis,** but basically they can – although mostly with the larger macular lesions – occur as a recurrent exanthem ("roseole en retour"); sometimes such lesions have to be separated from a circinated "érythème tertiaire" (Fig. 209a, b). Whenever such lesions show fine scaling in addition (Fig. 210), study of a single lesion will require exclusion of dermatomycosis and to a lesser extent,

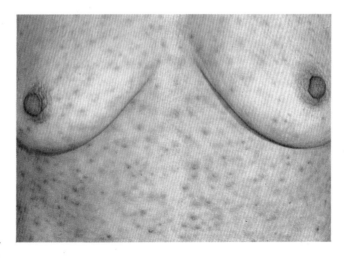

Fig. 209 b.

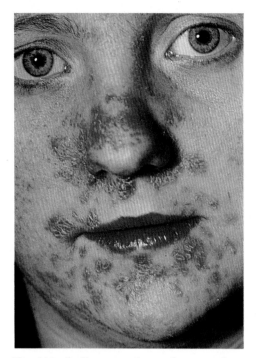

Fig. 210. Scaling maculopapular secondary syphilis of the face.

of a toxic-allergic exanthem, especially after ingestion of cubeb and balsam of copaiba; such allergic reactions would show pruritus but no adenopathy. Even less difficult is a differentiation from pityriasis rosea with its herald spot, peripheral scaling of the subsequently appearing lesions, and arrangement along the lines of cleavage. In contrast to the discretely beginning roseolas, the bluish marks (maculae caeruleae) caused by crab lice have a lead grey color; in addition, the lesions are slightly depressed.

Papular syphilids, as mentioned before, should be considered as recurrent exanthems (Figs. 211, 212). Among these syphilids the miliary small nodular type, in particular the syphilitic lichen, may resemble lichenoid tuberculids and sarcoids. The differential diagnosis of psoriasiform and pustular syphilitic exanthems will be discussed more extensively with the erythematosquamous dermatoses (see Chapter 19, A), and that of the varioliform syphilitic lesions will be discussed with the varioliform exanthems (see Chapter 18, C4). In addition to the large pustular varioliform syphilid a small pustular type called "syphilitic acne" occurs occasionally; when close to the scalp, temples, or similar locations, it can be confused with acne necroticans; the latter is characterized by a dark red infiltrated edge and tends to form a firmly attached brownish scab instead of a pustule.[3]

Syphilitic leukodermas have been discussed in the chapter dealing with pigmentary disturbances (Chapter 24, A11);

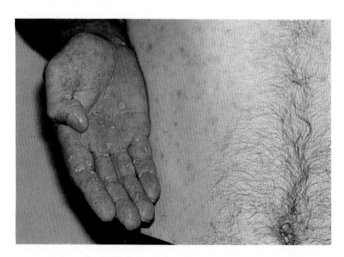

Fig. 211. Secondary syphilis: maculopapular exanthems.

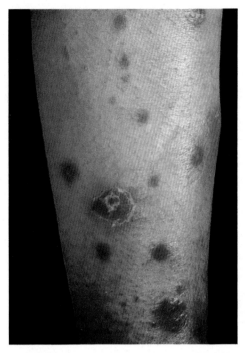

Fig. 212. Secondary syphilis: papulonodose exanthems.

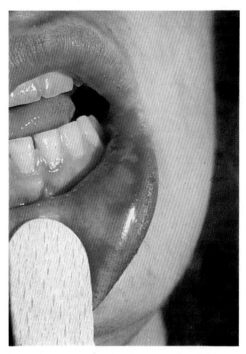

Fig. 213. Secondary syphilis: white plaques ("plaques opalines") of the oral mucosa.

here, attention is called to the rare, atrophic, final syphilitic manifestations resembling macular atrophy or anetoderma of an "idiopathic" character. Typical of **syphilitic shiny macular atrophy** ("lei-odermia syphilitica"), a distinctive manifestation of late syphilis, is the fact that recurrent eruptions do not arise out of such atrophic lesions, in contrast to post-tubercular cutaneous atrophy.

Syphilitic mucous membrane erythemas are, analogous to roseola, early manifestations of the disease; on the mucosa such lesions appear as dark red spots. Other manifestations, such as specific catarrhal sore throat, perhaps associated with an aphonic specific laryngitis, are also striking, not least by their tendency to recur. Slightly elevated and papular infiltrates have an opalescent or erosive, sometimes luxuriant aspect; on the tongue, one sees circumscribed – diphtheroid or papillary – atrophic lesions (Fig. 213).

The hypertrophic character of some of these changes is doubtless aided by corresponding original anomalies, such as a fissured tongue (lingua plicata), while hypertrophic papules on the posterior margin of the tongue may look like a heterotopic lingual tonsil. However, such pinkish-reddish almond-sized swellings frequently have a cerebriform surface and, above all, occur symmetrically bilaterally. For these reasons, the differentiation of syphilitic mucous membrane lesions against other diseases during the period of recurrences and especially when the lesions are exanthematous, is difficult. Not infrequently, the history, other specific cutaneous manifestations, and the serologic tests have to be taken into consideration, even though the finding of spirochetes in the oral cavity is not conclusive evidence because nonpathogenic oral spirochetes closely resemble *Spirocheta pallida*. Whereas formerly, stomatitis due to

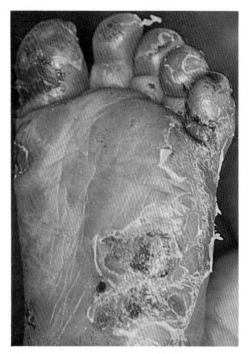

Fig. 214. Congenital syphilis: bullous plantar syphilid of the newborn.

Fig. 215. Saddle nose of congenital syphilis.

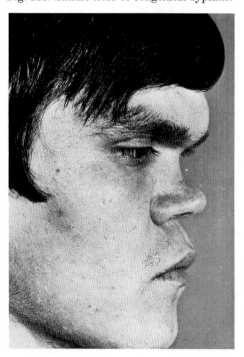

injections of mercury could be confused with a syphilitic enanthem despite profuse salivation and spongiosis of the interdental papillae (as in scurvy), among other signs, today the differential diagnosis must consider erythema multiforme (diphtheroid, easily bleeding mucous membranes, especially those close to the lips, and hemorrhagic crusting of the vermilion border of the lips, simultaneously with irislike cutaneous erythema), bullous drug eruptions of the mucous membranes (antipyrine, iodine), chronic pemphigus vegetans (erosions, fungoid vegetations), and, finally, habitual recurrent aphthae (very painful lesions located on tongue or gingival papillae).

There are only a few differential diagnostic possibilities in regard to the exanthematic eruptions of **congenital syphilis.** The bullous syphilid appears exclusively on the palms and soles (Fig. 214); the lesions contain an enormous amount of spirochetes, and simultaneously, a specific macular eruption is often present, which may resemble toxoplasmosis or listeriosis with enlargement of the liver, spleen, and pseudosyphilitic osseous changes. In contrast, **pemphigus neonatorum** (dermatitis exfoliativa neonatorum), also known as bullous impetigo, is not confined to palms and soles. Quite characteristic, if not actually confirmatory, are the **diffuse syphilids** favoring the palms and soles with large lamellar scaling ("shiny soles"), the buttocks, and especially the midface region; the differential diagnosis of congenital syphilis at the present time lacks specific characteristic stigmas. The well-known stigma of Parott's perioral rhagades deserves special mention, however; an adult may have similar formations of folds in progressive scleroderma or if there is an actually lichenified allergic eczema in this region. Similar superficial infiltrates are the basis for the frequently observed mucous membrane sign of congenital syphilis, the syphilitic coryza; its clinical appearance is such that today it can hardly be separated from the rarely

Fig. 216. Barrel-shaped and notched teeth.

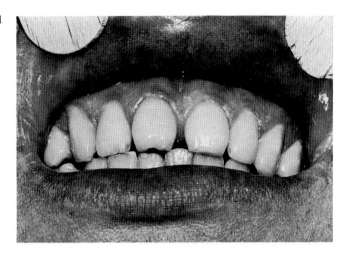

observed diphtheric coryza. Saddle nose and Hutchinson's teeth are seen only in older children after secondary dentition (Figs. 215, 216).[4]

(1) HERZOG, H., und W. PULVER: Die pseudoluische (Wassermann-positive) Viruspneumonie. Schweiz. med. Wschr. *83:* 227–234 (1953).

(2) HORNBERGER, W.: Hilusdrüsenbeteiligung bei Lues II. Fortschr. Röntgenstr. *73:* 553–558 (1950).

3) KORTING, G. W.: Zur Differentialdiagnose und Spezifität einiger luischer Krankheitszeichen. Med. Welt (Stuttg.) *1954:* 704–709.

(4) WECHSELBERG, K., und J. D. SCHNEIDER: Morbidität und klinische Symptomatik der konnatalen Lues im Säuglingsalter. Dtsch. med. Wschr. *95:* 1976 bis 1981 (1970).

E. Palmoplantar Erythemas

1. Palmar erythemas are seen most often with chronic **insufficiency of the liver** ("red liver palms") and are supposedly an expression of general peripheral hypervolemia. Over elevated plantar areas the same erythemas that occur on thenar and hypothenar eminences appear also on the soles as hyperemic spots, in combination with an increase in local temperature. Moreover, fine arterial dilations may be observed as erythematous plaques **(diffuse hepatic erythema);** ordinarily, such dilations are an expression of acute decompensation of the liver. In rare instances such erythematous patches may be present in other locations, for instance, on the forehead. Depending on the stage of liver function, hepatic erythemas of the thenar and hypothenar eminences may have distinct variations.

The watch-glass nails that are associated with palmar erythema are not always an expression of liver disease because isolated "hippocratic nails" are found also in other diseases, for instance, pulmonary disorders, nephroses, and others. However, the fingernails of "red liver palms" are either whitish or like an opaque frosted glass. Palmar erythemas due to other underlying diseases are quite rare. Occasionally, such an erythema can be observed with hyperthyroidism, cardiac insufficiency, ulcerative colitis, malnutrition, or rheumatoid arthritis. In contrast to the warm hand of the patient with cirrhosis of the liver, the palmar region of the arthritic is sweaty cold, cyanotic in places and also sclerodermic, tightly atrophic, or shiny, with the result that an erythema may be concealed among a multitude of other signs. Palmar erythema can occur with diabetes mellitus correlated to "rubeosis

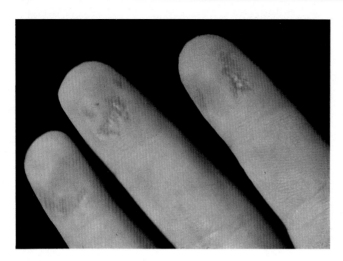

Fig. 217. Systemic lupus erythematosus.

diabeticorum." Conspicuous red palms are seen also in vegetative dystonia; however, dystonic erythemas look like cutis marmorata, are reticular, and have a slightly bluish undertone.[3,9]

2. Intensive light red, plaquelike pigmentation of the volar aspect of the hands, favoring the thenar and hypothenar areas, the fingertips, and the soles, occurs as **hereditary palmoplantar erythema,** a constitutional sign of genetic transmission. This erythema, transmitted as an irregular dominant trait and favoring the male sex, is more marked on the palms than on the soles. If it becomes established in childhood, it usually lasts throughout life. Hereditary palmoplantar erythema can be classified as a special abortive form within the groups of diffuse hereditary palmoplantar keratoses. It can occur not only alternately as erythema but also as a residual, distinctly red peripheral zone in palmoplantar keratoses.[5, 6, 8, 10]

3. Systemic lupus erythematosus (SLE) may sometimes produce bilateral macular erythema of the vola manus (Fig. 217), together with other acral or livedo reticularislike erythemas. However, not every patient with SLE develops palmar erythema, suggesting that special constitu-

tional preconditions for the appearance of such lesions must exist.[1, 2, 7] In contrast, the lesions of dermatomyositis, the "white-spot lilac" disease, occur mainly on the dorsal bony prominences of the hand; in addition, there are pathognomonic scleroses of the cuticle.[1, 2, 7]

4. Palmar and plantar erythemas accompanied by painful sensations due to changes of temperature may be due to **erythromelalgia.** This disease has already been thoroughly discussed (see Chapter 5, B4).

5. In contrast to these symptomatic palmar erythemas, **artificial discolorations of the palms,** for instance, in industrial workers, will have to be excluded in the differential diagnosis. It is understandable that such impregnations will hardly ever occur on the soles.[3]

(1) BERRY, TH. J.: The hand as a mirror of systemic disease. Davis, Philadelphia 1963.

(2) BRAVERMAN, I. M.: Skin signs of systemic disease. Saunders, Philadelphia, London, Toronto 1970.

(3) BUCKLEY, W. R., and W. WEST: Persistent dye staining of the skin. Arch. Derm. (Chic.) *102:* 71–77 (1970).

(4) BÜRGER, M., und H. KNOBLOCH: Die Hand des Kranken. Lehmann, München 1956.

(5) GAHLEN, W.: Erythema palmoplantare als genetisches Äquivalent zur Keratodermia palmoplantaris eines scheinbaren Solitärfalles. Hautarzt 15: 242–245 (1964).

(6) GEISER, J. D.: L'érythéme palmoplantaire héréditaire ou maladie de Lane. Rev. méd. Suisse rom. 79: 564–571 (1959).

(7) KORTING, G. W., und H. HOLZMANN: Das Erscheinungsbild der Hand bei den sogenannten Kollagenosen. Med. Welt 20 (N. F.): 603–605 (1969).

(8) LANE, J. E.: Erythema palmare hereditarium (red palms). Arch. Derm. Syph. (Chic.) 20: 445–448 (1929).

(9) LÖFGREN, R. C.: Erythema of the palms associated with pregnancy. Arch. Derm. Syph. (Chic.) 46: 502–511 (1942).

(10) PERNET, G.: Symmetrical lividities of the soles of the feet. Brit. J. Derm. 37: 123–125 (1925).

F. Facial Erythemas

1. Fleeting facial erythemas, especially **emotional erythemas** in women, frequently spread to the upper chest. The same may happen after swallowing or breathing dilators such as alcohol or trichloroethylene. The redness disappears quickly after the stimulating effect has ceased, and does not leave persistent cutaneous changes in spite of many repetitions. Differential diagnostic considerations are superfluous.

2. Persistent erythemas of the face may be interspersed with or consist of closely agminated telangiectases. Such redness of the cheeks is called a **constitutional facial mask** (rustic type). It exists from childhood on, involves the dorsum of the nose as well, and may occur as a familial disorder. The chin and the vicinity of the mouth, however, remain free (Fig. 218). The number of **acquired facial masks** is probably even greater. Such groups of telangiectases, if they exist even in early childhood, especially over the cheeks and nose but sparing the mouth and chin, may be the sequelae of a difficult delivery

(e.g., a twisted umbilical cord). Persistent erythemas that develop later as vasomotoric redness are less telangiectatic and are limited in their extension by the Lähr-Sölder lines. These erythemas may suggest a central bulbar trigeminal projection and have been observed in the terminal stages of brain tumors (strangulated cerebellar tonsil). The appearance of unilateral, flat red "spots," which end at the periphery with fine branches, depends on the size of the vascularization and may show different saturated colors (and occasionally complete blanching in death). They can be caused by trauma of the cervical or thoracic spine and a disturbance in the vasomotoric equilibrium (so-called *post-traumatic nevus flammeus*). In any case, if a chronic vasomotoric persistent facial redness exists, the question of a neural cause should be investigated. Frequently, however, these permanent erythemas or the more or less generalized, essential telangiectases offer no clue to the cause. [2, 3, 5, 17, 19, 24]

Fig. 218. Chronic vasomotoric and permanent redness (rustic type).

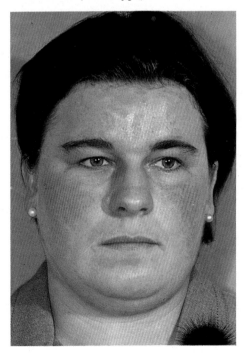

3. Dilations of the face which are diffuse, congenital, telangiectatic, and vascular belong to four different disorders. These are the familial telangiectases of the cheeks, ataxia telangiectatica, hereditary hemorrhagic telangiectasia, and Bloom's syndrome. The latter two are discussed in the chapters on angiomas (Chapter 36) and poikilodermas (Chapter 23, A4).

Familial telangiectases of the cheeks are present as early as infancy and do not favor one sex over the other. The closely agminated telangiectases of the cheeks make the cheeks look intensely red, but the nose and ears always remain unaffected. This makes them distinctly different from constitutional facial masks. Accompanying malformations, as for instance those in Sturge-Weber syndrome, are absent. In other cases, the telangiectases are not limited to the face but are distributed over the entire body as **generalized telangiectases.**[25, 27]

Ataxia telangiectasia, the Louis-Bar syndrome, shows the combination of cerebellar ataxia (abasia, astasia, and dysarthria) and progressive dilations of the end vessels of the face. It can be assumed that the atrophying cerebellar changes are caused by analogous telangiectases. The arrangement of the dilated vessels is rather typical – they are located on the head, nose, neighboring parts of the cheeks, concha of the auricle, and on the back of the neck. Moreover, there may be involvement of the antecubital and popliteal surfaces, as well as the dorsa of the

Fig. 219. The Louis-Bar syndrome: telangiectases of the bulbar conjunctiva.

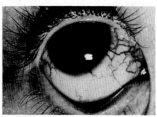

hands and feet. Associated with the facial telangiectases are frecklelike hyperpigmentations and varioliform atrophies. Before the onset of the cutaneous changes, telangiectases of the conjunctivae bulbi are detectable (Fig. 219). The life expectancy of these patients is distinctly shortened by accompanying infections (bronchitis, pneumonia, and sinusitis) or a tendency to malignant tumors (leukemia and gastric cancer). This pronounced susceptibility to infections is, in general, based on a diminution of the serum immune globulins, especially IgA.[1, 8, 9, 18]

4. Facial nevi telangiectatici look like erythemas. **Nevi telangiectatici mediales** are predominantly present on the back of the neck and on the middle of the forehead. Occasionally, the eruption of the midline extends symmetrically to the eyelids, nostrils, upper lips, and lower lips. These faint, pale to light red spots often assume a V-form on the middle of the forehead, and barely impinge on the anterior hairline. They are usually present at birth but almost completely disappear before the third year of life. In contrast to lateral hemangiomas, associated malformations* are lacking.

Lateral telangiectatic nevi are often associated with other malformations. On the face, angiomatosis encephalo-oculocutanea, the **Sturge-Weber syndrome,** is most important. It is mainly localized in the region of the first or second trigeminal branch, or both (Fig. 220). In exceptional cases the nevus is present on both sides. In the first years of life this lateral telangiectatic nevus remains relatively pale but tends later to develop an intense wine-red color; after the fourth decade of life it

---

* H. O. Curth and E. Goldensohn (Hautarzt **10**:366, 1959), reported on six out of seven patients with at least one important neurologic manifestation of the Sturge-Weber syndrome. They also showed pale and inconspicuous vascular nevi of the facial midline.

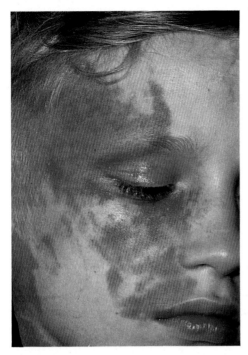 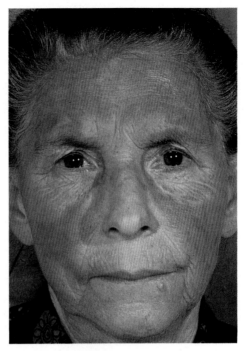

Fig. 220. Lateral nevus telangiectaticus (Sturge-Weber syndrome).

Fig. 221. Erythema perstans: early stage of discoid lupus erythematosus.

often shows numerous tuberous angiomas. As a consequence of this systematized angiomatosis of the cutis, deep ocular sheaths, and leptomeninx, some of the patients develop glaucoma, jacksonian epilepsy or migrainelike equivalents. The various combinations of manifestations have been considered different syndromes. The trisymptomatic forms of the Sturge-Weber syndrome are less frequently observed than the bisymptomatic forms. They include *encephalocutaneous angiomatosis* (Krabbe syndrome) and *oculocutaneous angiomatosis*. The latter should be subdivided according to the ophthalmologic findings into: *Schirmer's syndrome* with glaucoma in early childhood and with bulbar enlargement; *Lawford's syndrome* with late glaucoma but without bulbar enlargement; and *Milles syndrome* with angioma of the choroid but without glaucoma. *Oculoencephalic angiomatosis* is

not accompanied by cutaneous changes and, therefore, plays no role in dermatologic practice. Changes in the roentgenologic picture of the skull are diagnostically important: doubly contoured, mostly occipital, winding calcium shadows corresponding to calcifications of cerebral gyri.[7, 14, 16]

5. The concept of **erythema perstans of the face** (Fig. 221) requires special discussion. Under no circumstances should every persistent erythema of the face be called erythema perstans since the signs of erythema perstans faciei may mask the monotonous initial form of *lupus erythematosus*. This is a distinctly congestive erythema, which shows a butterfly distribution and is accompanied by few subjective complaints; it may remain unchanged for weeks at the same intensity. More rarely, it varies in its expression or recurs

at the same strength after it had seemingly completely disappeared. Follicular hyperkeratoses or a squamous component, which are characteristic of typical discoid lupus erythematosus, are lacking. Only if either is present can one speak of "congestive seborrhea." If, finally, infiltrations develop subsequently one cannot – in contrast to real erythema perstans of the face – hope for complete restitution but must expect the usual at first follicular and later confluent atrophic sequelae of lupus erythematosus. In general, in discoid lupus erythematosus the facial erythemas are exudative-papular, whereas in SLE they are more discrete and macular.[26]

In the differential diagnosis one must consider phenocopies of different toxicodermas and of flat but more annular appearing types of sarcoidosis, which, however, develop nearer the hairline. The diagnostic differentiation of erythematous rosacea with a butterfly distribution can be difficult in the beginning, especially if telangiectases and signs of "acne" are missing. In rosacea, however, erythemas which are not sharply demarcated toward normal skin and tend to confluence of nodular spots do not show any firmly attached follicular hyperkeratoses. The presence of pustules is an unequivocal sign

in favor of rosacea. Injected conjunctivae or even keratitis are frequently present in distinct rosacea, but absent in lupus erythematosus. In rosacea, in contrast to lupus erythematosus, the border of the auricle of the ear and the scalp remain free, whereas spreading of the cutaneous changes to the V of the neck occurs in both diseases. If yellowish-brownish squamous components are present, one should also consider, besides "congestive seborrhea," microbial seborrheic eczema. Apart from additional sites of localization, as on the chest or middle of the back, a certain accumulation of lesions should occur in the nasolabial folds. The coloring of the face is yellow-red in psoriasis vulgaris, with few scales and wide distribution, as for instance following light or heat exposure, but in pellagra a mahogany brown hue prevails following a transient erythema of an Indian brown color. In pemphigus erythematosus butterflylike erythemas are distributed on the face; these are scaly, oozing, and crusted, and even show follicular hyperkeratoses for a long time. There is, however, no atrophy. In all these differential diagnostic possibilities consideration must be given to additional localizations. Only then will the true nature of such an "anonymous" erythema perstans faciei be recognizable.

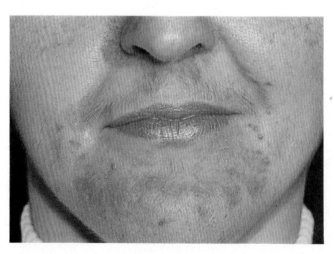

Fig. 222. Perioral rosacealike dermatitis.

6. A position between rosacea and seborrheic dermatitis is occupied by the so-called **perioral rosacealike dermatitis.** This disease entity has been observed with a few exceptions only in women. In the beginning it appears periorally, but with a small strip of skin around the lips remaining uninvolved; symmetrical dissemination of the very small papulopustular elements on primarily normal skin appears on the cheeks, with accentuation of the nasolabial folds, the lower lids, and the forehead (Fig. 222). Later, a vaguely circumscribed, yellowish-red, moderately scaling basic erythema (iatrogenic?) develops. The patients, who are mostly women, experience only a disagreeable tension.

For the differential diagnosis, according to stage of the disease, seborrheic dermatitis (with affected areas also on other sites but no pustules), candidiasis (presence of yeast), or rosacea has to be considered (see also Chapter 30, B1 and B2). [11, 23]

7. In acrodermatitis chronica atrophicans the face may occasionally be affected with an erythema perstans-like eruption of the forehead, nose, and cheeks. According to the stage of the disorder, we observe superficial or deeper, edematous and infiltrated or mildly atrophic lesions. In contrast to erythema perstans faciei as initial expression of lupus erythematosus, acrodermatitis chronica atrophicans of the face starts unequally on both sides. If one agrees with the etiology of ticks, the eruption is dependent on the portal of entry of the suspected causative organism. Less difficult is the differentiation of erythema perstans faciei from erysipelas (fever) or preeruptive herpes zoster beginning as an edematous erythema. In both disorders, however, the subsequent course discloses the cause. [15]

8. Redness of the face is an important sign of **dermatomyositis.** Simultaneously, edematous erythemas are present, which in the beginning are light red, later becoming livid red, mainly on the eyelids or the whole periorbital region (Fig. 162). The erythema then spreads cape-like over the shoulders and upper chest and is accompanied on the back of the neck by small and succulent papules. Occasionally, the facial erythemas spread in butterfly fashion like lupus erythematosus. In dermatomyositis the initial edematous erythema soon shows telangiectases or sunken-in alabaster-white spots. Moreover, the subsequent development of dermatomyositis tends more than lupus erythematosus to a complete picture of poikiloderma. Scattered pinhead-sized bleedings, which are sometimes observed only by applied pressure (with a glass slide), occur in both disorders either intrafocally on the skin or isolated on the mucous membranes of the cheeks. The final decision between the two would then depend on the subsequent course and the result of laboratory examinations (see also Chapter 16, C and D). [20]

Certain similarities with the facial appearance of dermatomyositis are found in the beginning stages of **trichinosis.** For instance, recurrent edemas of the lids are always present, the entire face often being involved in the process of swelling. These edemas are rarely preceded by macular or extensive erythemas. They are, however, without the wine-red component as well as the white spots in between (see also Chapter 16, C2). [22]

9. Attacks of erythema (called the flush phenomenon) characterize, above all, the **carcinoid syndrome** (with signs of ileus, diarrhea, tachycardia, right-sided cardiac valve defect, voracious appetite, and bronchial asthma). In the beginning, the attacks of macular or confluent blue-red erythema of the face and the upper part of the trunk last only a few minutes (Fig. 223). Gradually, persistent vascular dilatations develop. There are also pella-

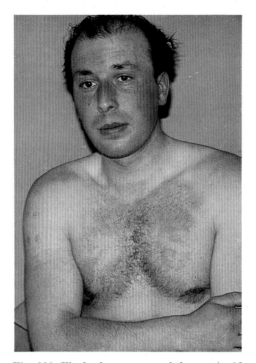

Fig. 223. Flush phenomenon of the carcinoid syndrome.

groid features, which may be caused by increasing depletion of nicotinamide, caused by misdirected tryptophan metabolism. The typical flush of the carcinoid syndrome is a pronounced vaso-motoric attack with accompanying spastic signs in the intestines and bronchi. These attacks are triggered by excitement, alcohol, or certain foods and may occur several times a day. Of diagnostic value is the determination of 5-hydroxyindole-acetic acid as an end-product of serotonin metabolism (add 10 per cent ferrous chloride solution in a ratio of 1 : 1; if positive, the urine assumes a dark-violet color). In progressive stages, apparently from the influence of serotonin, fibrosis of the endocardium of the right ventricle and sclerodermalike skin areas occur. On the tongue nodose thickening is present which, histologically, proves to have neuroid cell growth with hyperplasia of the connective tissue.[4, 21]

Little cause for confusion in the differential diagnosis will arise with *Quincke's edema,* with its suggestive pale reddish hue and, most important, its characteristic distended swellings, or with recurrent erysipelas. In essential pellagra, following sun exposure, there are from the beginning distinctly symmetrical, sharply circumscribed, and macular areas, whereas sun erythema at first manifests itself in tiny follicular spots. After a certain time pellagra assumes a mahogany-brown tone. Later, flour-dustlike or small lamellar scaling becomes visible.

10. Carcinoidlike flushes are also observed in well-developed **urticaria pigmentosa,** most probably due to histamine released from mast cell infiltrates. The trigger of such episodes, which last distinctly longer (15 to 30 minutes) than the flush phenomena of the carcinoid syndrome and do not leave any permanent signs, may be abrupt thermic changes, rubbing of the skin, or certain drugs such as aspirin, codeine, or polymyxin B. During a glowing red mast cell flush the histamine content in the urine is definitely increased, but the amount of 5-hydroxyindoleacetic acid is normal (see also Chapter 24, E12).

Occasionally, distinct flush attacks are observed in **pheochromocytoma.** Moreover, flush phenomena occur most of all in association with heat sensations in the **periclimacterium** or subsequent to **ovariectomy.** Such episodes may occur during sleep, causing the patient to awake. They are often associated with outbreaks of sweat (heat sensations), and depressive moods.

11. One-sided, acutely beginning swellings, alternating with erythemas and associated with simultaneous paroxysmal rhinitis, epiphora, and neuralgia, occur in the **pterygo-**(spheno-)**palatinum syndrome.** In contrast to the Melkersson-Rosenthal syndrome episodic facial paresis and lingua plicata are missing.[6]

Also, in the parotid disturbance of sweat secretion **(auriculotemporal syndrome),** distinct red hyperemia may precede limited preauricular hyperhidrosis (see also Chapter 3, A1).

12. In **erythroprosopalgia** pain in the temporal region is followed by distinct redness with feelings of warmth in the facial area (see also Chapter 5, B12).

(1) AMMAN, P., V. LÒPEZ, R. BÜTLER und E. ROSSI: Das Ataxie-Teleangiektasie-Syndrom (Louis-Bar-Syndrom) aus immunologischer Sicht. Helv. paed. Acta *20:* 137–146 (1965).

(2) BLAICH, W., und H. ENGELHARDT: Intermittierende Erythembildung als Ausdruck syndromatischer Verknüpfung bestimmter Hautveränderungen mit einer Polyneuroradikulitis (Guillain-Barré) Derm. Wschr. *123:* 289–297 (1951).

(3) BLAICH, W., und H. ENGELHARDT: Zur Frage der Entstehung der essentiellen Teleangiektasien, der »vasomotorischen Dauerrötung« und ähnlicher Gefäßveränderungen. Hautarzt *5:* 357–362 (1954).

(4) DEGOS, R., R. TOURAINE, P. GODEAU et PH. BLANCHET: Les manifestations cutanées du syndrome carcinoïdien. Ann. Derm. Syph. *99:* 243–255 (1972).

(5) FEGELER, F.: Naevus flammeus im Trigeminusgebiet nach Trauma im Rahmen eines posttraumatisch-vegetativen Syndroms. Arch. Derm. Syph. (Berl.) *188:* 416–422 (1949).

(6) FEGELER, F.: Halbseitige chronisch-intermittierende Gesichtsschwellung als parasympathische Funktionsstörung im Ganglion pterygopalatinum. Hautarzt *4:* 315–317 (1953).

(7) FRANÇOIS, J.: Angiomatose oculo-cutanée de Lawford. Ophthalmologica (Basel) *122:* 215–227 (1951).

(8) GRÜTZNER, P.: Augensymptome bei Ataxia teleangiectatica (Louis-Bar-Syndrom). Klin. Mbl. Augenheilk. *135:* 712–717 (1959).

(9) HAERER, A. F., J. F. JACKSON and C. G. EVERS: Ataxia teleangiectasia with gastric adenocarcinoma. J. Amer. Med. Ass. *210:* 1884–1887 (1969).

(10) HEYCK, H.: Über das Bingsche Kopfschmerzsyndrom (Erythroprosopalgie). Dtsch. med. Wschr. *87:* 1942–1947 (1962).

(11) HJORTH, N., P. OSMUNDSEN, A. J. ROOK, D. S. WILKINSON and R. MARKS: Perioral dermatitis. Brit. J. Derm. *80:* 307–313 (1968).

(12) KAMMER, G.: Beitrag zur Erbbiologie und Klinik der Sturge-Weberschen Erkrankung. Z. menschl. Vererb.- u. Konstit.-Lehre *33:* 203–220 (1955).

(13) KREIBICH, C.: Sklerodermieartige Lichtdermatose. Arch. Derm. Syph. (Berl.) *144:* 454–457 (1923).

(14) LAMPERT, F.: Akute lymphoblastische Leukämie bei Geschwistern mit progressiver Kleinhirnataxie (Louis-Bar-Syndrom). Dtsch. med. Wschr. *94:* 217–220 (1969).

(15) MIESCHER, G.: Akrodermatitis atrophicans des Gesichtes und der rechten oberen Extremität mit Knotenbildung. Dermatologica (Basel) *86:* 233–235 (1942).

(16) NONNENMACHER, A.: Augenärztliche Betrachtungen zum Symptomkomplex Morbus Sturge-Weber, Klippel-Trénaunay und Parkes-Weber. Klin. Mbl. Augenheilk. *126:* 154–164 (1955).

(17) OHNSORGE, K.: Über einen vasomotorisch-psychischen Symptomenkomplex. Z. ges. Neurol. Psychiat. *167:* 180–186 (1939).

(18) RUITER, M.: Die oculo-cutanen Erscheinungen bei Ataxia teleangiectasia. Hautarzt *15:* 667–670 (1964).

(19) SCHNYDER, U. W.: Zur Klinik und Histologie der Angiome 2. Mitt.: Die Feuermäler (Naevi teleangiectatici). Arch. Derm. Syph. (Berl.) *198:* 51–74 (1954).

(20) SCHUERMANN, H.: Dermatomyositis. Erg. inn. Med. Kinderheilk. N. F. *10:* 427–480 (1958).

(21) SCHUERMANN, H., und O. Hornstein: Über Mundschleimhautveränderungen bei maligner intestinaler Karzinoidose. Dermatologica (Basel) *115:* 641–648 (1957).

(22) SEMPLE, A. B., J. B. M. DAVIES, W. E.
     KERSHAW and C. A. St. HILL: An out-
     break of trichinosis in Liverpool in 1953.
     Brit. Med. J. *1954:* 1002–1006.

(23) STEIGLEDER, G. K.: Die rosacea-artige
     Dermatitis: ein neuartiges Krankheits-
     bild. Dtsch. med. Wschr. *94:* 1393–1398
     (1969).

(24) TUPATH-BARNISKE, R.: Zur Frage des
     posttraumatischen Naevus flammeus.
     Z. Haut- u. Geschl.-Kr. *33:* 379–384
     (1962).

(25) WEBER, G., und W. G. ROTH: Generali-
     sierte essentielle Teleangiektasien an
     Haut und Conjunctiven. Z. Haut- u.
     Geschl.-Kr. *42:* 855–858 (1967).

(26) WHITE, J. W., and H. O. PERRY: Ery-
     thema perstans. Brit. J. Derm. *81:* 641–
     651 (1969).

(27) WORINGER, F.: Téleangiectasies de la
     face chez la mère et le fils. Bull. Soc.
     franç. Derm. Syph. *59:* 493 (1952).

G. Nodular Erythemas

1. Typical **erythema nodosum** is a disease that can hardly be mistaken. These "red nodules" affect the deep vascular regions, i.e., the deep cutis, and the septa of the subcutaneous fat, favoring the extensor aspects of the lower extremities. The disease starts with a succession of up to walnut-sized, partly superficial, partly subcutaneous, nodular and occasionally also plaquelike infiltrates (Figs. 224, 225), which upon pressure are very tender. Exceptionally, children may show lesions on the extensor aspects of the upper arms and even on the face. Erythema nodosum as a classical "réaction cutanée" may have many etiologic factors, making it difficult to find the cause in every case. The decision is easy when an acute febrile sore throat and arthralgias point to *streptococci* as the cause. The far-reaching importance of

Fig. 224. Contusiform erythema nodosum.

Fig. 225. Erythema nodosum.

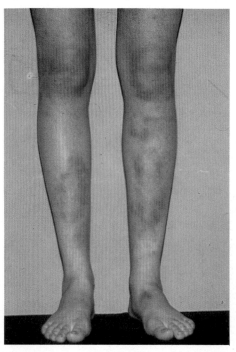

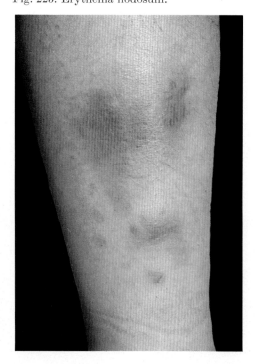

streptococci in the pathogenesis of erythema nodosum becomes evident by the not infrequent occurrence of the lesions after scarlet fever. In addition, erythema nodosum often occurs together with *erythema multiforme* on the upper extremities; in such cases the proper classification can be made without difficulty. In childhood, erythema nodosum represents a hyperergic reaction to an infection with tuberculosis; however, in adults this will happen only exceptionally, for instance, after an inoculation with BCG vaccine. Such "tuberculous" erythema nodosum usually lasts only a short time and as a rule heals quickly. Small endemics of erythema nodosum may have a tuberculous origin, but doubtless there are other possibilities for an apparently "contagious" outbreak of erythema nodosum, for instance, gastrointestinal infections. In any case, at present, the former dependence of infantile erythema nodosum on tuberculosis does not play the same role as before. Today, *rheumatic fever* occupies first place as cause of erythema nodosum in childhood. The usual former course of rheumatic fever has undergone a change insofar as severe rheumatic carditis has decreased while the frequency of nodose erythemas has increased (see also Chapter 1, B6).[22] During the last few years there has been an increase of erythema nodosum in cases of sarcoidosis; this has been described, especially in young females between the ages of 15 and 35, under the name of *Löfgren's syndrome*. The pulmonary changes in such an acutely starting sarcoidosis (which has a good prognosis) are so transitory that the bilateral hilar lymphadenopathy hardly reaches a fully developed sarcoidal stage. The transition of Löfgren's syndrome to chronic sarcoidosis rarely takes place. Hilar lymphomas of more than six months, duration with a negative Kveim test require exclusion of malignant lymphogranulomatosis, even more so because they also may be accompanied by nodular erythemas. Löfgren's

syndrome may be confused with rheumatic fever. It will be difficult to decide whether lepromas are present in a case of leprosy or whether a *lepra* reaction produces febrile erythema nodosum. This reaction can be mitigated by antihyperergic therapeutic measures (cortisone, thalidomide), but these drugs are ineffective against *Mycobacterium leprae*. Perhaps in some of these cases of erythema nodosum leprosum a similar acute panniculitis is more likely. [19, 25]

Nodular erythema may occur in all venereal diseases but also in some nonvenereal infections of the genitals as well, for instance, in *ulcus vulvae acutum* (as a manifestation of Behçet's syndrome). *Nodular syphilids* develop during the first year of syphilis in connection with other manifestations of this infection. Usually these nodular lesions either begin from the subcutaneous veins as a specific syphilitic manifestation with prompt response to antisyphilitic treatment, or they develop like a Herxheimer reaction only during treatment.

Exceptionally, *gonorrhea* may present inflammatory nodules on the extremities. Similar lesions have been observed with *chancroid* infections and this argues against the assumption that the streptobacillus causes only a strictly localized infection. Erythema nodosum is of greater importance in the early stages of *lymphogranuloma inguinale venereum*, but it may occur also during the late manifestations of this disease. *Behçet's syndrome*, one of the nonvenereal disorders of the genitals, also produces nodular erythemas; pathologically, these lesions show thromboses and hemorrhagic vasculitis, together with intensive fibrinoid degeneration and necrosis of the collagen fibers within the cutis and also within the septae of the subcutis. One to two days later, such areas show cellular penetration with mononuclear cells and granulocytes. Sometimes, these pathologic anatomic changes give the impression of severe panniculitis. Lately, erythema nodosum exanthems have been discussed in connection with *trichomonas infections*. [16]

Mycotic infections may show erythema nodosum; for instance, in connection with *Coccidioides immitis* infections.

Drug-induced nodular erythemas are observed on either a toxic or an allergic basis after the administration of bromides, iodides, salicylic acid, salvarsan, and especially sulfonamides. Recently, oral contraceptives have to be mentioned also.[1]

Erythema nodosum due to gastrointestinal infections is seen, not too rarely, in ulcerative colitis; sometimes a reaction to sulfathalidine therapy for colitis may be responsible. Nodular erythemas occur also with the extremely rare infection of the human mesenteric lymph nodes due to Yersinia pseudotuberculosis.* The list of rare causes of isolated cases of erythema nodosum includes typhoid, typhus, trypanosomiasis, helminthiasis, smallpox, chickenpox, diphtheria, whooping cough, leptospiroses of the types L. grippotyphosa (Schlammfieber in western Europe) and L. australis (cane field fever in Australia and Indonesia), and finally, cat-scratch disease.[10, 17, 23]

As mentioned before, erythema nodosum represents a uniform response to different stimuli. Therefore, the histology of the reaction does not permit conclusions as to the cause that has triggered it; the histology can only confirm the diagnosis of erythema nodosum. The subcutaneous tissue shows infiltrates of varying thickness, consisting of lymphocytes and a few neutrophils within the septa of fatty tissue and also between the fatty tissue cells themselves. Eosinophils and giant cells of the Touton type are seen rarely, and plasma cells are absent. The infiltrate can be so scanty that only a few scattered accumulations of cells are seen. Formation of

---

* A common pathogen in rodents and birds. (Tr.)

abscesses, necroses of fatty tissue, and tuberculoid structures do not belong to the histology of erythema nodosum. However, there are vascular changes affecting smaller blood vessels and the medium-sized veins; these vessels present cellular infiltrations of the walls and proliferations of the endothelium. In contrast, erythema induratum presents many giant cells and, especially, caseating necroses. The cellular infiltrate is also much more marked than in erythema nodosum and the vascular changes of erythema induratum affect the arterial segments also.

Differential diagnostic difficulties arise with atypical, acute, or subchronic superficial erysipeloid or contusiform types as well as with migrating types (*erythema nodosum migrans*). All these varieties, and also *chronic erythema nodosum*, have the same histopathologic changes; however, when the lesions are more deeply situated, early "inflammatory" infiltrations with palisading granulomalike structures will lead eventually to fibrosis.[2, 3, 7]

In contrast to all such variations of the typical appearance of erythema nodosum this diagnosis can be excluded when an ulcerative breakthrough occurs; for instance, in erythema induratum, papulonecrotic (ulcerated) tuberculids, or chronic deep pyodermas. A nodular, less painful, and only slightly discolored appearance at the surface may suggest panniculitis caused exogenously (trauma or injection), or by drugs (halogens), or by the course of an infectious disease. To be considered clinically and histologically is spontaneous panniculitis (especially Weber-Christian disease). More cordlike nodules of the legs suggest the presence of "nodular vasculitis;" it differs histologically from typical erythema nodosum as well as by its longer duration, smaller nodules, and tendency to recur. Extensive granulomatous vasculitis is usually seen with thrombophlebitis migrans; it differs from erythema nodosum by its multiple discontinuous mode of spreading.[4, 12, 13]

2. Granulomatous follicular and nodular tinea of the legs has multiple nodules that are almost always subacute "inflammatory," erythematous, and pea-sized; they appear in a follicular pattern (lichen pilaris, perniosis). These usually indolent nodes with superficial scales occur mainly on the legs of younger females. The diagnosis is facilitated by the presence of other mycotic changes (tinea of the feet, onychomycosis). Histologically, the granulation tissue may show a tuberculoid structure and may undergo central necrosis either with or without secondary infection. This process by itself is contraindicative of erythema nodosum, aside from its follicular inflammatory character and its marked chronicity. Scaly material obtained from the surface of the nodes shows fungi; tineae can also be found histologically in a PAS preparation.[9]

3. Circumscribed myxedema develops in patients after treatment for hyperthyroidism as pretibial, plaquelike, or tuberous swellings (Fig. 226). Exceptionally, myxedema may also show multiple, semispherical, elevated, reddish-yellow nodes; however, in contrast to erythema nodosum they are not bluish-red. The plaquelike and tuberous myxedemas may show a sugges-tion of peau d'orange surface. A strikingly high percentage of patients with circumscribed myxedema have a long-acting thyroid stimulator (LATS) in their serum. The correlation between circumscribed myxedema and LATS-activity is closer than that between LATS-activity and hypothyroid exophthalmos (see also Chapter 11, 17).[5, 8, 15, 20]

4. Erythema induratum has a clinical picture of inflammatory, nodular, and sometimes definitely plaquelike changes of the calf of the legs. Quite frequently, central necrotic softening can be observed, terminating in circular ulcerations without undermined edges. Erythema induratum occurs usually in young or middle-aged women of pyknic build and increased susceptibility to cold. Histologically, common inflammatory changes prevail. In contrast to erythema nodosum, erythema induratum presents deeply localized infiltrations in the fatty tissue. At the present time the histologic picture does not permit an association with tuberculosis such as the former concept of "tuberculosis cutis indurativa." In addition, there is doubt whether erythema induratum represents an entity sui generis and whether it should belong to the same

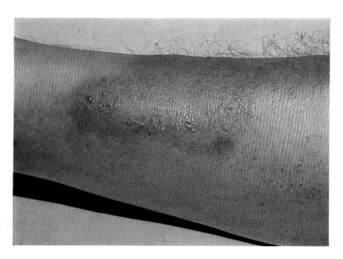

Fig. 226. Tuberous myxedema of the anterior aspect of the tibia.

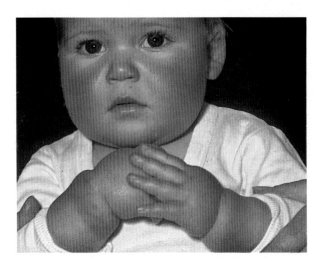

Fig. 227. Frostbites in an infant.

group as chronic erythema nodosum, subcutaneous lipogranulomatosis, nodular vasculitis, and others.[6, 11, 12, 18, 21, 24]

5. The different types of **panniculitis** start out during their early inflammatory stage as nodular erythemas. They are discussed in a separate chapter (see page 130).

6. Necrobiosis lipoidica may start at the extensor aspects of the legs as a reddish-brown, distinctly elevated infiltration. These areas may be single or multiple, are not painful, and fail to show any other inflammatory phenomena. During the later course of the disease the typical aspect of necrobiosis lipoidica (Fig. 142) appears as yellow-white, slightly depressed lesions crisscrossed by telangiectases. Necrobiosis lipoidica has the same tendency to central ulceration as does erythema induratum (see also Chapter 16, A8).

From a differential diagnostic point of view one should mention in this connection the distinction from sarcoidal granulomas, which may sometimes be caused by, among other things, penetrating foreign bodies.

7. Typically, **chilblains** appear during cold and wet weather, and favor somewhat adipose girls and women. Sites of predilection of chilblain lesions are the hands, feet, and legs, and also an adipose chin or the breasts (Figs. 227, 228). Clinically, the lesions appear as bluish-red, almost semispherical, doughy nodes occasionally progressing to blisters. The lesions may develop into chronic, torpid ulcerations with a special tendency to secondary infection. Chilblains cause relatively little pain and present characteristic findings on palpation. All other acute inflammatory nodular erythemas differ completely. Patients with chilblains often show **perniosis follicularis** (Fig. 229) as another sign of a cold effect. Arms and lower extremities show bluish-red, pinhead-sized follicular swellings on a cool skin. There are no subjective complaints except occasional pruritus and cold sensations. The differential diagnosis of facial perniosis has to consider the diffuse infiltrated form of facial sarcoid known as *lupus pernio* (Fig. 230). Lack of dependence on cold, involvement of internal organs, point-sized brown infiltrates visualized under diascopy, a positive Kveim test, and the characteristic histology will permit the

Fig. 228. Frostbites on the lower abdomen.

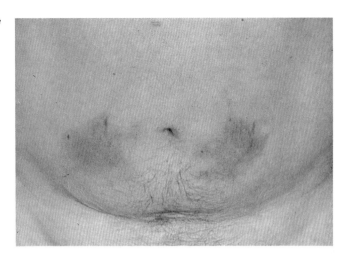

correct diagnosis. Nodular erythemas resembling frostbite of hands and feet are part of systemic lupus erythematosus (see also Chapter 16, D1).

8. Sweet's syndrome may present nodular or plaquelike erythemas on the extensor aspects of the extremities. It is not possible to make this diagnosis from the

Fig. 229. Perniosis follicularis.

Fig. 230. Cutaneous sarcoidosis: so-called lupus pernio.

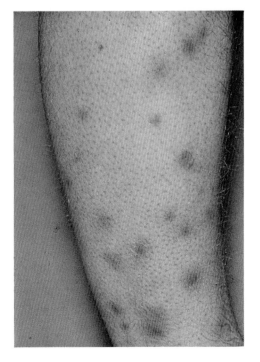

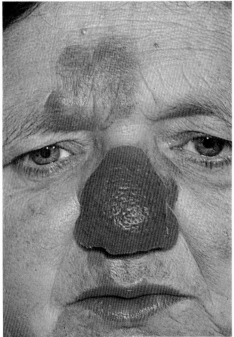

clinical picture alone. A thorough description of this disorder was given in Chapter 1, B7.

(1) BADEN, H. P., and F. D. HOLCOMB: Erythema nodosum from oral contraceptives. Arch. Derm. (Chic.) *98:* 634–635 (1968).

(2) BÄFVERSTEDT, B.: Zur Kenntnis des atypischen Erythema nodosum. Arch. klin. exp. Derm. *208:* 291–300 (1959).

(3) BÄFVERSTEDT, B.: Erythema nodosum migrans. Acta derm.-venereol. (Stockh.) *48:* 381–384 (1968).

(4) BEHREND, H., T. BEHREND und M. WILCKENS: Zur Differentialdiagnose des Erythema nodosum. Z. Rheumaforsch. *26:* 65–73 (1967).

(5) DENK, R.: Myxoedema circumscriptum praetibiale bei Hyperthyreose. Med. Welt *18* (N. F.): 1279–1280 (1967).

(6) EBERHARTINGER, CHR.: Das Problem des Erythema induratum Bazin. Arch. klin. exp. Derm. *217:* 196–254 (1963).

(7) FINE, R. M., and H. D. MELTZER: Chronic erythema nodosum. Arch. Derm. (Chic.) *100:* 33–38 (1969).

(8) GOTTRON, H. A., und G. W. KORTING: Zur Pathogenese des Myxoedema circumscriptum tuberosum. Arch. Derm. Syph. (Berl.) *195:* 625–649 (1953).

(9) GUMPESBERGER, G., und H. TIRSCHEK: Zur Klinik follikulärer und nodöser Epidermophytien an den Unterschenkeln. Z. Haut- u. Geschl.-Kr. *18:* 295–298 (1955).

(10) HÄLLSTRÖM, K., E. SAIRANEN and K. OHELA: A pilot clinical study on yersinioses in south-eastern Finland. Acta med. scand. *191:* 485–491 (1972).

(11) HAMMERSCHMIDT, E. E., und G. W. KORTING: Ulcerative tuberculides. Brit. J. Derm. *62:* 361–364 (1950).

(12) HEINDL, E.: Erythema nodosum staphylogenes bei Lymphogranulomatose. Hautarzt *16:* 453–455 (1965).

(13) KORTING, G. W.: Über cutane Periarteriitis nodosa unter besonderer Berücksichtigung begleitender Leberstörungen und der sogenannten Thrombophlebitis migrans. Arch. Derm. Syph. (Berl.) *199:* 332–349 (1955).

(14) KRANTZ, W.: Ulceröse Tuberkulide der Unterschenkel. Arch. Derm. Syph. (Berl.) *179:* 685–694 (1939).

(15) MALKINSON, F. D.: Hyperthyroidism, pretibial myxedema, and clubbing. Arch. Derm. (Chic.) *88:* 303–312 (1963).

(16) MONACELLI, M., and P. NAZZARO: Behçet's disease. Karger, Basel, New York 1966.

(17) MYGIND, N., and H. THULIN: Yersinia enterocolitica: a new cause of erythema nodosum. Brit. J. Derm. *82:* 351–354 (1970).

(18) RÖCKL, H.: Die Bedeutung der Histopathologie für die Diagnostik knotiger Unterschenkel-Dermatosen. Hautarzt *19:* 540–547 (1968).

(19) SCADDING, J. G.: Sarcoidosis. S. 57–64. Eyre & Spottiswoode, London 1967.

(20) SCHERMER, D. R., H. H. ROENIGK, O. P. SCHUMACHER and J. M. McKENZIE: Relationship of long-acting thyroid stimulator to pretibial myxedema. Arch. Derm. (Chic.) *102:* 33–67 (1970).

(21) SCHNEIDER, W., und W. UNDEUTSCH: Vasculitiden des subcutanen Fettgewebes. Arch. klin. exp. Derm. *221:* 600–601 (1965).

(22) SCHWEIER, P.: Zur Ätiologie des Erythema nodosum im Kindesalter. Münch. med. Wschr. *110:* 544–547 (1968).

(23) STRUPPE, A., und N. HOEDE: Über nodöse Erytheme an den Unterschenkeln bei Colitis ulcerosa. Med. Welt *20* (N. F.): 2745–2746 (1969).

(24) SZODORAY, L., und K. N. VEZEKÉNYI: Über die an Unterschenkeln junger Frauen auftretende Periarteriitis nodosa cutanea seu Vasculitis nodularis. Hautarzt *10:* 263–267 (1959).

(25) URTHALER, F., und E. TANNER: Löfgren-Syndrom. Vorkommen und Verlauf des akuten Morbus Boeck. Schweiz. med. Wschr. *100:* 111–113 (1970).

H. Migrating Erythemas

As migrating erythemas only erysipelas, erysipeloid, and erythema chronicum migrans will be discussed, although others, especially the annular erythemas (see later) may also be migratory.

1. Erysipelas essentially represents streptoderma cutanea lymphatica. It must be assumed that beta-hemolytic A-strepto-

Fig. 231. Erysipelas of the middle face.

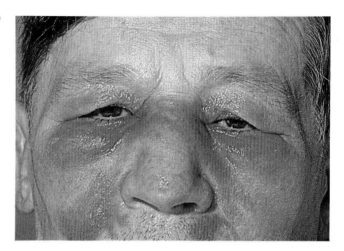

cocci are able to produce the disorder only when the skin has been sensitized to streptococci. To avoid recurrences, even minor portals of entry such as erosions on the nose or between the fingers or toes must be cured. Typically, after an incubation time of one to three days, but occasionally after only a few hours, a circumscribed erythema appears, which is sharply circumscribed only in the beginning. It is accompanied by mild itching or a sensation of tension or heat. Later on, the border becomes irregularly pointed or outreaching like the tongues of flames (Fig. 231, 232). In the erythema there is almost always a distinct edema, which may lead to multiple vesicles or formation of big blisters owing to increased cutaneous tension. In the next few days the erythema expands further but avoids firmly fixed bases such as the frontal hairline and chin area. After about five days, erysipelas in most cases comes to a halt (erysipelas fixum). The original fiery red color changes to blue and later to yellowish-brown, and is accompanied by simultaneous superficial desquamation. In first infections mostly, erysipelas is initiated by high temperatures (chill!) and painful swellings of the regional nearby lymph nodes.

An unusual course would show not only the vesiculobullous picture but also the even rarer hemorrhagic, phlegmonous, or gangrenous changes.

Fig. 232. Erysipelas.

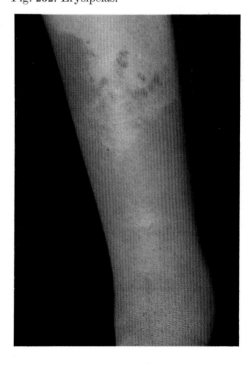

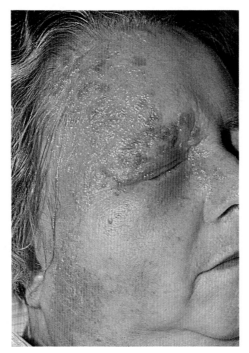

Fig. 233. Ophthalmic herpes zoster.

Primary erysipelas of the mucous membranes is rare. Tonsillitis, pharyngitis, or inflammation (for instance, from hypersensitivity to gold fillings), or an enanthema in scarlet fever or lupus erythematosus may have to be considered in the differential diagnosis.

Typical sequelae of habitual and already mitigated attacks of erysipelas are elephantiasic enlargements. After an attack loss of hair or activation of a seborrheic eczema may occur. But some conditions, among them malignant disorders, may be cured.

Only a few considerations are necessary for the differential diagnosis if one keeps in mind that in a recurrent attack, an originally sharp border has changed into a blurred border, and the drama of the first attack is gone. In uncoordinated and very old persons, however, even the first attack may be mitigated and the erythema appears pale or washed out. Furthermore, in

patients with anemia or hydrops, the redness of erysipelas is mild, comparable to that of the scalp in all cases. On the other hand, erysipelas of the scrotum and the periorbital region shows a special tendency to edema and consecutive elephantiasis. It should be mentioned in this connection that even common, acute eczemas and dermatitides may lead to massive swellings periorbitaly and on the scrotum.

Erysipelaslike redness and swelling occur, especially in the face, with beginning *herpes zoster* (Fig. 233). The characteristically grouped blisters of zoster together with mostly pronounced disturbances of sensibility (hypesthesia, hyperesthesia) appear later (after one to two days), facilitating the diagnosis. In addition, the limited segmentary and stationary site is typical for herpes, whereas erysipelas migrates especially rapidly, and often covers the entire face (except the chin area).

On the lower legs erysipelatous redness may occur, especially in acute, superficial thrombophlebitis. On careful palpation, however, the usually rather tender vein can be palpated. If this is impossible because of pronounced accompanying edema, one must wait until the edema subsides. In the course of thrombophlebitis there is no increase in the antistreptolysin titer as is typical for untreated erysipelas. It is easy to recognize *lymphangitides*, because they present long streaks. Perilymphangitic infiltrates create a plastic cordlike appearance.

The carcinomatous infarct of the lymph vessel of the skin in mammary cancer, *erysipelas carcinomatosum* or carcinoma erysipelatodes (Fig. 234), is discussed here, not alone because of its historic name. These metastatic disseminations may occasionally look like erysipelas because of their rapid development, migratory behavior, pointed borders, and flaming redness. At such a time in their course,

Fig. 234. Carcinomatous erysipelas in breast cancer.

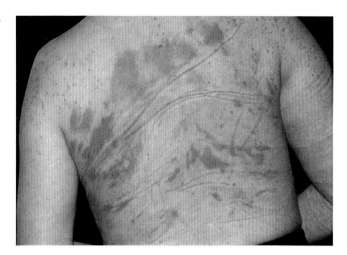

the nodose infiltration of the so-called "cancer en cuirasse" need not have been fully developed.

If one does not want to wait, a biopsy will decide doubtful cases. Some sequelae of smallpox vaccination show spreading ("area migrans") toward the elbow, extending flamelike toward the dorsum of the hand. In contrast to genuine streptococcic erysipelas, *postvaccinal erysipelas*, in which probably simultaneous or secondary contaminations of the vaccination site with streptococci play a role, may occasionally show residual pigmentations.[2]

2. Erysipeloid is characterized by its stereotyped predilection for the fingers as well as its occurrence in certain professions (for instance, butchers, fishermen, and housewives) and can, therefore, be distinguished from erysipelas. In general, erysipeloid is painless and often slightly pruritic, and, although exhibiting a certain migratory tendency, it does not extend beyond the palm (Fig. 235), even after weeks. It rarely reaches the wrist, as it is probably limited by the firm texture of the palm. Besides extension on the surface, spreading deep downward through con-

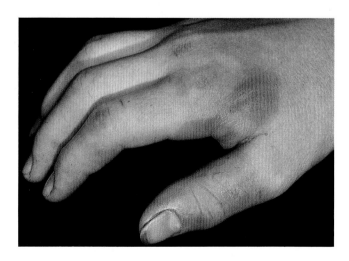

Fig. 235. Erysipeloid.

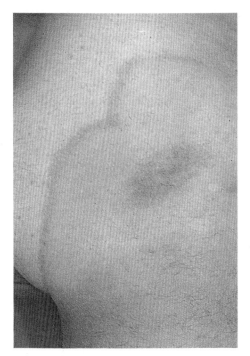

Fig. 236. Erythema chronicum migrans.

This eruption, however, has a different history (e.g., local recurrence following antipyrine or other drugs) and shows a rather dirty-grayish, brown color.

3. Erythema chronicum migrans is an erythema that shows little color saturation and is, therefore, pale and hardly infiltrated. It has an oval shape and later, by continuous centrifugal spreading, it assumes annular form. The erythematous ring is sharply demarcated but is washed out in the center (Fig. 236). In its center there is often a lymphocytoma, a residuum of a tick bite. Characteristic is the tendency to slow migration lasting months and the absence of fever and other general signs (such as headaches) as a rule, but it should be mentioned that ticks may transmit encephalitis. For the differential diagnosis it is important to remember that erysipeloid favors the hand and does not form rings. Erythema annulare centrifugum presents simultaneous, multiple, and smaller centrifugal migratory erythemas, whereas the so-called fixed drug eruption remains in the same place and, in cases of reexposure, recurs in loco and heals leaving hyperpigmentation.

tiguous structures is possible, leading to the characteristic involvement of the articular capsule. The only other differential diagnostic possibility, considering the typical bluish-red color of erysipeloid becoming centrally paler if it exists longer than two weeks, is a fixed drug eruption.

4. In a supplementary note, **larva migrans** (creeping eruption) must be men-

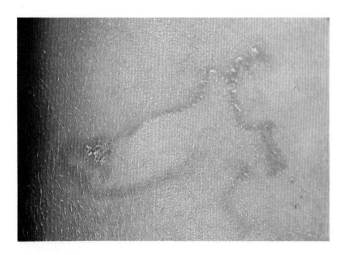

Fig. 237. "Creeping disease."

tioned. The larvae digging into the skin cause reddish ducts several millimeters in width. They can "creep" several centimeters in the course of a day (Fig. 237). This process is so characteristic that differential diagnostic considerations are unnecessary. It remains difficult, however, to decide which species of nematode has caused the "creeping eruption" in a given case, or whether the characteristic zigzag configuration has been caused by the larvae of a special order of flies.[1]

5. Erythrokeratodermia figurata variabilis will be extensively described in Chapter 22, A3).

(1) BRAUN, W., und G. SCHMIDT: Ein Beitrag zur Creeping disease (Larva migrans nematosa). Z. Haut- u. Geschl.-Kr. *42:* 913–918 (1967).
(2) WEBER, G., und W. RIESE: Hauterscheinungen nach Schutzimpfungen. Dtsch. med. Wschr. *88:* 1878–1886 (1963).

I. Annular Erythemas

1. Because **erythema annulare rheumaticum** favors children, it has been previously described in this chapter, page 218, under Erythemas in Childhood.

2. Erythema gyratum repens occurs chiefly in individuals between the fourth and sixth decades of life. The significance of this form of erythema lies in its high paraneoplastic properties. Up to now, all patients with erythema gyratum repens had simultaneous carcinomas (of breast, female genitals, pharynx, bronchi, and CNS). The eruption appears on the trunk and the proximal parts of the extremities as slightly infiltrated, pronounced urticarial, elevated, erythematous streaks, which are 1 to 2 cm wide, and are annular, gyrate, or show spiral constellations. This picture alone would be striking, but another unusual feature is the rapid (within hours and days) variability of the erythematous figures. At the border of the erythema, desquamation of the horny layer creates a scaling effect, which is again gyrate. On the face, neck, hands, and feet, however, often only plane, hyperkeratotically covered erythema exists. As a dermopathic reaction, lymph nodes near the affected skin may be indolently enlarged.

Histologically, the substrate of these changes is hyperkeratosis, some parakeratosis and acanthosis, and in the cutis, perivascular infiltrates of lymphocytes and histiocytes.[3, 9, 10, 12, 14]

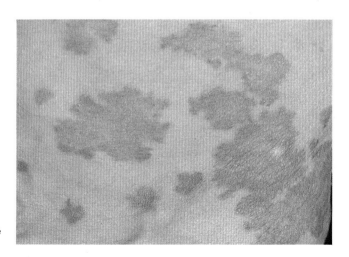

Fig. 238. Erythema annulare centrifugum.

3. In spite of the characteristic aspects of erythema gyratum repens, the differential diagnostic distinction from **erythema annulare centrifugum** may be difficult. These predominantly annular, multiple erythemas migrate only very slowly centrifugally. They consist of firmly infiltrated, sometimes almost keloidlike, large rings resembling those of granuloma annulare (Fig. 238). Besides the two main characteristic features (annular form and tendency to centrifugal migration) there are additional macroscopic-morphologic criteria. If they are in evidence, various special types such as indurated, squamous, vesiculobullous, and, finally, telangiectatic-purpuric have to be distinguished. The characteristic grainy woodlike aspect of erythema gyratum repens is completely absent. Also, in erythema annulare centrifugum, underlying malignant disorders (carcinomas, sarcomas, leukoses, and others) occur. In many instances, the course is "chronically protracted" except when drug-allergic influences (chloroquine derivatives) are the cause. Histologically, in erythema annulare centrifugum perivascular infiltrates, which surround the vessels like a cape, are preponderant. These infiltrates consist mostly of lymphocytes and are interspersed with only a few histiocytes. Rather frequently, these cell elements are associated with many eosinophilic granulocytes. The endothelium of the vessels is swollen and the entire vessel wall can be edematously enlarged. In addition, occasionally unusual lipoid storage is found. In the differential diagnosis, the possibility of dermatomycosis exists, especially if there is distinct scaling.[2, 5, 6, 8, 11, 13]

4. In some places of western Africa, a characteristic annular disorder, **granuloma annulare multiforme,** has been noted. It starts with itching on a circumscribed area. Soon a papule appears, the itching lessens, and the lesion widens to ringlike curved borders consisting of fine nodules.

In addition, arcs with atrophy and mild desquamation are present. The course is eminently chronic. Granuloma annulare multiforme favors the upper trunk, often symmetrically, of older women. In the differential diagnosis, tuberculoid leprosy must be ruled out. Histologically, similarity with granuloma annulare exists.[7]

5. Annular erythemas are observed chiefly in **sarcoidosis,** in which subepidermal infiltrates of epithelioid cells occasionally result in nodular elevations or, more often, lead to more confluent areas of diseased skin. Following central regression, unusual characteristic lesions of the face (frontal hairline) are formed (Fig. 239a). An annular form is also characteristic of lichen planus. Not too rarely, these annular formations develop from a single papule, but they also are formed by apposition of aggregated solitary papules. The favorite sites of *lichen ruber anularis* are the penis, scrotum, and sacral area (Fig. 241). Often the original papules disappear after some time, with the result that at first sight only annular erythemas or annular pigmentations seem to be present. Moreover, lichen planus often develops in an annular skin pattern as for instance, in cutis marmorata.

6. Only once has **familial annular erythema** been observed. It consists of intensely pruritic, circular, closed erythematous rings of various sizes. They develop from urticarial lesions which are small in the beginning. With increasing extension, they regress centrally, forming migrating rings. These erythematous configurations in various numbers are spread over the entire body but without any favorite sites. The mucous membranes may also be involved. In the patients observed up to now, these annular erythemas appeared a few days after birth and persisted until the death of the patient. It seems striking

Fig. 239. (a) Annular sarcoidosis. (b) Granuloma annulare.

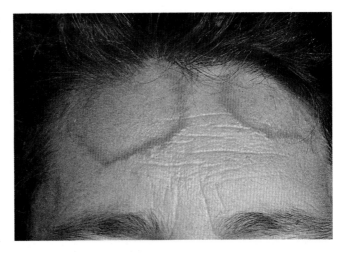

Fig. 239a.

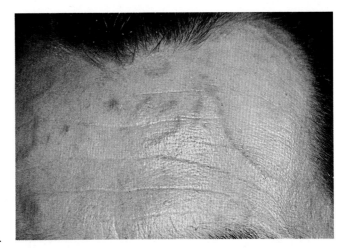

Fig. 239b.

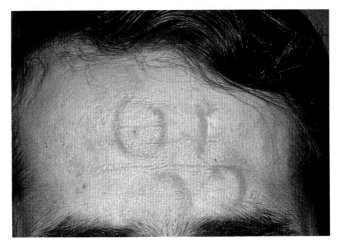

Fig. 240. Tuberculoid leprosy: annular erythema on the forehead.

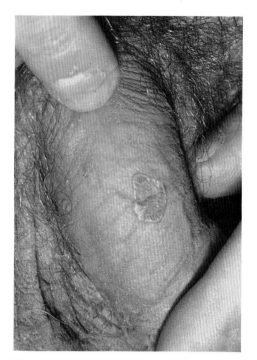

Fig. 241. Annular lichen planus.

that these patients succumb easily to infectious diseases. This may be explained by a defect of immune globulins, since in all probands in the serum an increase in alpha 1 and alpha 2 globulin fractions was found and as constantly a decrease in IgA globulins.

(1) BEARE, J. M., P. FROGGATT, J. H. JONES and D. W. NEILL: Familial annular erythema. An apparently new dominant mutation. Brit. J. Derm. *78:* 59–68 (1966).

(2) BREHM, G., und I. BREHM: Fixe Arzneimittelexantheme unter Anwendung des Zytostaticums »Trenimon«. Derm. Wschr. *147:* 134–141 (1963).

(3) GAMMEL, J. A.: Erythema gyratum repens. Arch. Derm. Syph. (Chic.) *66:* 494–505 (1952).

(4) GOTTRON, H. A.: Anulärer Lichen planus. Derm. Z. *59:* 164–165 (1930).

(5) KELLY, L. J., and E. KOCSARD: Congenital ichthyosis with erythema anulare centrifugum. Dermatologica (Basel) *140:* 75–83 (1970).

(6) KORTING, G. W., und H. EISSNER: Beitrag zur teleangiektatischen und purpurischen Erscheinungsform des Erythema centrifugum anulare (Typus Gougerot und Patte). Derm. Wschr. *138:* 854–863 (1958).

(7) KRAMPITZ, H. E.: Granuloma multiforme Leiker. Hautarzt *18:* 365–368 (1967).

(8) LAZAR, P.: Cancer, erythema annulare centrifugum, autoimmunity. Arch. Derm. (Chic.) *87:* 246–251 (1963).

(9) LEAVELL, U. W., W. W. WINTERNITZ and J. H. BLACK: Erythema gyratum repens and undifferentiated carcinoma. Arch. Derm. (Chic.) *95:* 68–72 (1967).

(10) MIGUÉRÈS, J., A. JOVER, M. LAYSSOL et J. RANFAING: Un syndrome para-néoplasique rare: l'érythème gyratum repens. Ses rapports avec le cancer bronchique. J. franç. Méd. Chir. thor. *21:* 313–324 (1967).

(11) NÖDL, F.: Zur Histopathogenese des Erythema anulare centrifugum. Arch. klin. exp. Derm. *202:* 407–423 (1956).

(12) PEVNY, I.: Erythema gyratum repens. Z. Haut.- u. Geschl.-Kr. *40:* 260–270 (1966).

(13) TAPPEINER, S.: Erythema annulare centrifugum Darier. Derm. Wschr. *130:* 1334–1339 (1954).

(14) THOMSON, J., and L. STANKLER: Erythema gyratum repens. Brit. J. Derm. *82:* 406–411 (1970).

K. Fixed Exanthems

1. The expression "**fixed drug eruption**" does not refer to an eruption present for a time but to recurrent lesions limited to about the same area as the original outbreak. As a rule these eruptions are sharply bordered, circular, or oval edematous

Fig. 242. Fixed bullous drug
eruption.

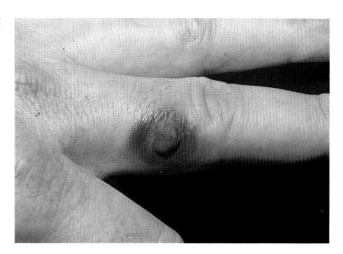

erythemas which assume quite early a
dusky bluish-red or dirty brown hue.
Seldom is there a change from an exudative
to an urticarial or centrally bullous reaction (Fig. 242). Almost always a residual
pigmentation remains for a long time;
with further recurrences in the same place
the color may assume a bluish-black hue
(for instance, the erythematous fixed
eruption due to antipyrine). This discoloration is seen especially after ingestion
of drugs containing phenolphthalein. Drug
eruptions of the mucous membranes of the
genitals or of the mouth show single or a
few multiple erythematous areas much
more rarely; symmetrically arranged eruptions hardly ever belong to a local exa-
cerbating cutaneous reaction caused by
drugs.

A fixed exanthem will seldom be accompanied by general signs such as fever,
hypotonia, or headaches. Fixed drug
eruptions appear only after a prolonged
period of ingestion of medications, especially of the antipyrine group. Other substances may give rise to instantaneous
paresthesias of the tongue or oral mucosa
upon first exposure (e.g., to phenolphthalein). Our own observations show that the
hands, the front and sides of the neck and
the genitals (especially of the male) are
sites of predilection of fixed drug eruptions
(Fig. 243). The list of triggering substances
includes, in addition to antipyrine and
phenolphthalein mentioned before, an

Fig. 243. Fixed drug eruption on the genitals.

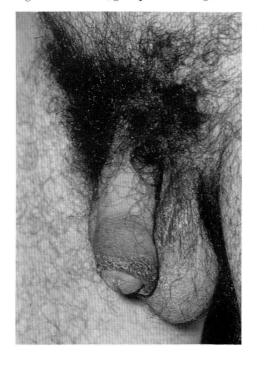

immense number of drugs, among others tetracycline, anticonvulsive drugs, and tranquilizers; also some foods, peaches, tomatoes, and especially legumes. From a differential diagnostic point of view there are few difficulties because usually the patient becomes aware of the connection between the medication and the eruption. Berloque dermatitis shows an intense brownish color and a droplike distribution. Today berloque dermatitis as such is hardly ever seen, but the local application of alcoholic solutions of furocoumarins* will have a similar effect. The sharply bordered, dark red, perianal dermatitis is caused by the transformation of the oral drug Istizin (danthron) in the intestine to Cignolin. Prolonged application of Cignolin in psoriasis causes cutaneous discoloring; the perianal skin shows the same dusky brown color after ingestion of Istizin.[1, 2, 4, 5]

2. Erythema dyschromicum perstans (ashy dermatosis) appears as ashy gray, disseminated, macular patches, which differ from fixed drug eruptions by their multiplicity. Especially in fresh "active" erythema dyschromicum perstans, aside from an inflammatory reaction with an abundance of melanophages, one finds distinct epidermal changes with vacuolization of the epidermal cells and hydropic degeneration of rete and basal cells. This differs from the findings in drug erythemas.[3]

(1) DERBES, V. J.: The fixed eruption. J. Amer. Med. Ass. *190:* 765–766 (1964).

(2) IPPEN, H.: Ätiologie und Pathogenese des sogenannten Istizin-Exanthems. Dtsch. med. Wschr. *84:* 1062–1063 (1959).

(3) KNOX, J. M., B. G. DODGE and R. G. FREEMAN: Erythema dyschromicum perstans. Arch. Derm. (Chic.) *97:* 262–272 (1968).

(4) NAEGELI, O.: Über fixe Arzneiexantheme. Klin. Wschr. *6:* 73–76 (1927).

(5) WISE, F., and M. B. SULZBERGER: Drug eruptions. Arch. Derm. Syph. (Chic.) *27:* 549–567 (1933).

L. Livid Erythemas

1. Cyanoses due to internal causes can be confused with discolorations caused by deposition of foreign substances (for instance, silver argyrosis). Among the internal causes, methemoglobinemia causes brown cyanosis; sulfhemoglobinemia gives rise to greenish-black cyanosis; and an increase in deoxyhemoglobin* results in blue cyanosis (a minimum of 5 grams of deoxyhemoglobin (reduced hemoglobin) in 100 cc of blood must be present). Cyanoses are differentiated into either centrally or peripherally caused forms. Clinically, one can distinguish the two conditions by rubbing the ear lobe to the point of appearance of capillary pulsation; in central cyanosis the ear lobe will remain blue, whereas in peripheral cyanosis it will not turn blue. Also, in central cyanosis but not in the peripheral type, the tongue will be cyanotic. In contrast to peripheral cyanoses the central type will frequently show clubbing of the fingers; this may, however, also occur as a familial or hereditary sign in connection with other syndromes (for instance, pachydermoperiostosis). Central cyanoses are either of pulmonary origin (pulmonary sclerosis) or of cardiac origin (arteriovenous shunt in congenital cardiac organic defects). Peripheral cyanoses, on the one hand, represent angiopathies caused by slowing down of the blood flow in the veins with simultaneous constriction of the arterial flow (dilatation of the subpapillary venous plexus together with arterial vasoconstriction); therefore, a spastic-atonic condition of inflow and outflow exists side by side.

---

* Psoralens. (Tr.)

* Formerly called reduced hemoglobin. (Tr.)

On the other hand, peripheral cyanoses are the result of throttled venous return flow, for instance in cardiac insufficiency.

2. Ordinary **acrocyanosis** shows symmetrical red to dusky blue cutaneous discoloration (Fig. 244) of the distal parts of the extremities, and sometimes also of the ears and buttocks. This cyanosis depends on the outside temperature and can be made anemic by finger pressure. Upon release of the pressure, the anemic area disappears immediately in the fashion of an iris diaphragm. Other characteristic signs of acrocyanosis are scattered cinnabar-red macules, the striking coldness of affected parts, and the tendency to hyperhidrosis. In both sexes acrocyanosis starts after puberty, with definite regression in women during the first pregnancy and recurrence during the climacteric.

The differential diagnosis must include especially deviations from the previously mentioned type of development or appearances because a separate etiology may be present. For instance, unilateral acrocyanosis could indicate lesions of nerves or vessels. Acrocyanosis occasionally may present minor paresthesias. However, in contrast to Raynaud's phenomena, real attacks of pain do not occur; in Raynaud's disease attacks of ischemia ("digitus mortuus") are followed by more or less pronounced acroasphyxia. However, acrocyanosis is not followed by further phenomena, for instance torpid paronychia or ulcerations. Acrodermatitis chronica atrophicans usually starts as unilateral erythromelalgia with sometimes bluish-red swellings which occur to a large extent independently of external thermal influences; after some time development of atrophy will permit the true diagnosis of this "acral cyanosis."

3. Erythrocyanosis crurum puellarum (acrocyanosis of the legs of girls) is a special type of acrocyanosis favoring the legs and represents a constitutional stigma

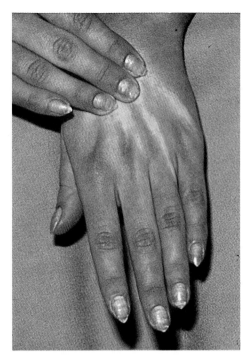

Fig. 244. Acrocyanosis.

Fig. 245. Eruption from cold hemagglutinins.

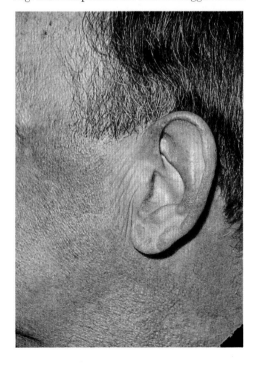

("thick red legs"). Marked follicular hypertrophy exists near the cyanotic zone ("perniosis follicularis"). In addition, doughy infiltrates appear, causing even more clinical resemblance to frostbite (perniosis). Application of heat results in the same type of improvement in erythrocyanosis crurum puellarum as in acrocyanosis. In the former, however, if perniosis is strongly developed (i.e., if succulent infiltrations are present as far down as the subcutaneous adipose tissue), a certain similarity to erythema nodosum or erythema induratum can be observed; only the latter will show ulcerations. In rare instances perniosis is less nodular but has more of a plaquelike infiltrative character, especially of the edges (perniosis marginata).[5]

4. Cold agglutinin disease may in rare instances be the cause of peripheral cyanosis. Acrocyanosis of skin exposed to cold may begin very quickly owing to marked clumping of erythrocytes in blood vessels, thereby establishing the diagnosis (Fig. 245). Sufficient proof is a cold agglutinin titer of more than 1 : 128. Agglutinated erythrocytes become hemolyzed frequently, causing anemia; also, hemoglobinuria should be looked for. The cause of cold agglutinin disease can be viral pneumonia, systemic lupus erythematosus, lymphogranulomatosis, or erythema multiforme. Idiopathic chronic cold agglutinin disease without an underlying cause is observed even more rarely. Such patients are endangered by the development of necroses of fingers, toes, ears, and nose.

The differentiation from **cryoglobulinemia** is important. In association with a less rapidly developing acrocyanosis on exposure to cold, the main signs are cold urticaria, purpura, Raynaud's phenomena, and necroses and ulcerations of the lower extremities. Serum proteins precipitated by cold belong to the class of alpha-2 or gamma globulins. Cryoglobulins occur with myeloma, lymphatic leukemia, macroglobulinemia, lymphogranulomatosis, systemic lupus erythematosus, and cirrhosis of the liver.[1, 7]

5. The **Klippel-Trenaunay-Weber** syndrome may present dark blue-red telangiectatic nevi simulating circumscribed cyanosis; these nevi are similar to those of the Sturge-Weber syndrome (see Chapter 18, F4) (Fig. 240). The complete Klippel-Trenaunay-Weber syndrome is characterized by hypertrophy of bones and related soft tissues and cutaneous varices of the affected extremity. In most cases thorough angiographic examination will show malformations of the arteries and the lymph vessels. The syndrome is not always fully complete, and at times only one or a few of the various manifestations may be present (Fig. 247). Beyond this, as rare variations, there may be hypoplastic instead of hypertrophic forms.[2, 4, 6, 8]

6. Adiponecrosis subcutanea neonatorum consists of subcutaneous fat induration with bluish-red, sometimes brownish, discoloration of the overlying skin. Further details of this disease are discussed in Chapter 16, B8.[3]

7. Phlegmasia caerulea dolens (blue phlebitis) shows severe dark blue cyanosis of one extremity (Fig. 248). (See Chapter 1, K8).

(1) BREHM, G.: Akrozyanose als Symptom einer Kälteagglutininkrankheit. Med. Welt *17* (N. F.): 1375–1376 (1966).
(2) FELLINGER, K., S. RAPTIS und G. ROTHENBUCHNER: Über eine Sonderform des Klippel-Trénaunay-Parkes-Weber-Syndroms. Klinische und chromosomale Studien. Wien. Z. inn. Med. *46:* 310–321 (1965).
(3) HERING, H., und W. UNDEUTSCH: Zur Klinik und Pathogenese der Adiponecrosis subcutanea neonatorum. Derm. Wschr. *134:* 917–921 (1956).

Fig. 246. Nevus flammeus in
the Klippel-Trenaunay-
Weber syndrome.

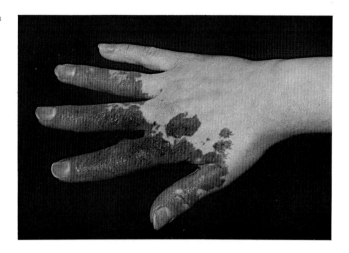

Fig. 247. Klippel-Trenaunay-
Weber syndrome: dysplasia
of the lymph vessels.

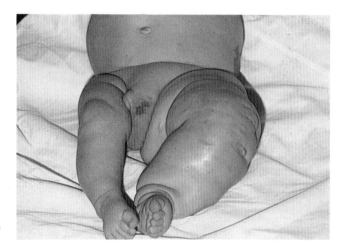

Fig. 248. Phlegmasia cerulea
dolens.

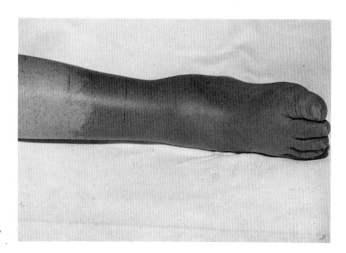

(4) Koch, G.: Zur Klinik, Symptomatologie, Pathogenese und Erbpathologie des Klippel-Trénaunay-Weberschen Syndroms. Acta Genet. med. (Roma) *5:* 326–369 (1956).

(5) Korting, G. W., und G. Weber: Perniosis marginata. Z. Haut.- u. Geschl.-Kr. *36:* LIII-LVI (1964).

(6) Lindemayr, W., O. Lofferer, A. Mostbeck und H. Partsch: Das Lymphgefäßsystem bei der Klippel-Trénaunay-Weberschen Phakomatose. Z. Haut- u. Geschl.-Kr. *43:* 183–191 (1968).

(7) Nödl, F.: Purpura bei essentieller Kryoglobulinämie. Arch. klin. exp. Derm. *210:* 76–85 (1960).

(8) Pevny, I., G. Becker und W. Zeisner: Lymphabflußstörungen beim Klippel-Trénaunay-Parkes-Weber-Syndrom. Isotopenlymphographische Untersuchungen. Hautarzt *24:* 58–62 (1973).

M. Skin Disorders of the Livedo Group

1. The etiologies of the several types of livedo are quite different; a reticular pattern of the cutaneous changes due to a deeper involvement of the blood vessels is common, in contrast to the patchy superficial areas of cyanosis. **Livedo reticularis** (cutis marmorata) represents an increased vascular response to cold stimuli in younger persons with a corresponding constitutional disposition (Fig. 249). In most cases, livedo reticularis is present symmetrically on the extremities; it may, however, involve the entire body with the exception of the face and neck. In any case, livedo reticularis will disappear when heat is applied and will reappear by corresponding cooling. The basis of this disorder is functional with no pathomorphological foundation.

Whenever livedo reticularis is present at birth or shortly afterward, it is called **cutis telangiectatica congenita** (Fig. 250). Up to the tenth year a definite regression can often be observed; it is probably due to a sinking of the vascular tree into deeper cutaneous layers combined with an increased development of fatty tissue. Persistent cutis marmorata can be seen in **Cornelia de Lange's syndrome** (see also Chapter 11, F2), and occasionally in patients with **Down's syndrome (mongoloids).** However, if the cutaneous vascular lesions are in a hypertonic phase the result will be **cutis marmorata alba,** which shows a white color of the reticulated pattern of these vascular areas. Circumscribed livedo reticularis may suggest regular application of warmth or heat (hot water bottle, heating pad, or poultices for lumbago). Such **livedo reticularis e calore** ("erythema ab igne") will soon produce brownish hues within the reticular pattern (Fig. 251), the result being a more or less brown network.

Histologically, these colors are caused by deposition of melanin within the epidermis and corium. The presence of livedo in acrodermatitis chronica atrophicans, mycosis fungoides, and several other cutaneous diseases is probably more or less accidental. Treatment with *amantadine*

Fig. 249. Livedo reticularis.

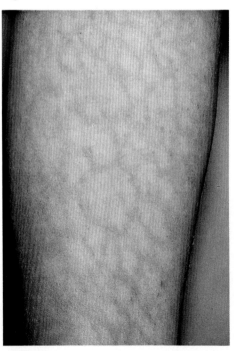

Fig. 250. Congenital telangiectatic skin.

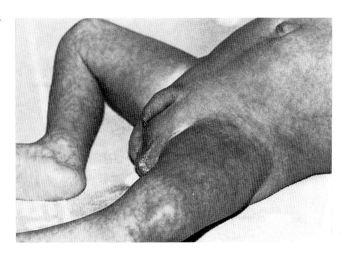

hydrochloride (NF) has caused reversible livedo reticularis in women. Within the group of collagen diseases, livedo phenomena are not infrequently observed as a partial sign in *systemic lupus erythematosus* and in *dermatomyositis*.[1-3, 5, 10, 11, 13, 14]

2. Livedo racemosa should be called **vasculitis racemosa** because of histomorphologic vascular changes as opposed to the sole functional changes observed in livedo reticularis. The pathologic-anatomic findings consist of granulomatous changes between endothelium and elastica together with perivascular infiltrations ("endophlebitis and endoarteriolitis racemosa"). Vasculitis racemosa has lightninglike or coarsely dendriticlike vascular cutaneous markings (Fig. 252), whereas livedo reticularis shows reticular erythematous figures of a more delicate outline.[1, 3, 12]

Even if cases of idiopathic vasculitis racemosa exist, the search for the etiology should be directed less toward discovering syphilis, tuberculosis, hypertension, or arteriosclerosis than on the recognition of **endangiitis obliterans** or **cutaneous periarteritis nodosa.** Vasculitis racemosa asso-

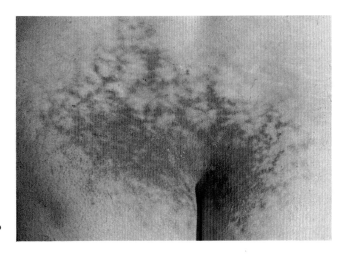

Fig. 251. Reticular livedo from heat.

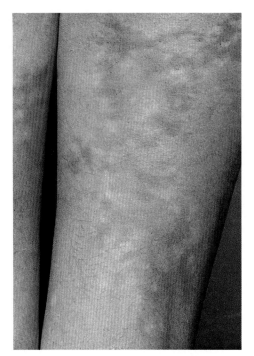

Fig. 252. Vasculitis racemosa.

Fig. 253. Summer ulcerations.

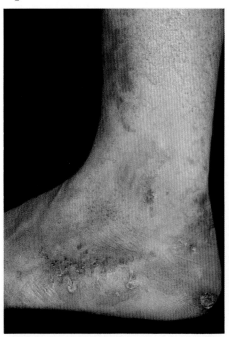

ciated with periarteritis nodosa should be considered when nodules are formed (either preceding other signs, simultaneously, or afterward) on the feet, legs, forearms, and other parts of the body. Sometimes these nodules are more easily palpated than seen. Occasionally the nodules are tender and are found along the course of blood vessels, revealing their vascular affinity; in rare instances they may even pulsate. "Livedo racemosa" may exist in association with cutaneous periarteritis nodosa without formation of nodes; general signs in such patients consist mostly of joint or muscle pains and additional cutaneous manifestations (such as urticarial erythemas, cutaneous apoplexia, or purpura). Regression of the nodes results in brownish pigmentation. Should other signs be absent it will be difficult to differentiate the condition from *nodular vasculitis* which is often the result of a drug allergy. Some patients (often young women) with vasculitis racemosa have poorly healing, shallow ulcerations with jagged borders around the ankles and edges of the feet in warm weather. The conspicuous seasonal limitation has led to the establishment of the term **summer ulcerations** (Fig. 253); this term, however, does not convey anything about the etiology.[4, 6-8, 16]

3. Localized or unilateral vasculitis racemosa lesions should always lead to an investigation for special conditions, as for instance a deep circulatory block (angiography); more rarely, central nervous factors such as a subdural hematoma or similar lesions may be involved. Since the start of intramuscular bismuth therapy, dermatologists have seen localized, dendritic, infarctlike necroses as localized livedo phenomena, the so-called **"embolia cutis medicamentosa"**(dermite livéoïde).[9, 15]

(1) CHAMPION, R. H.: Livedo reticularis. Brit. J. Derm. *77*: 167–179 (1965).

(2) COMEL, M.: Cutis marmorata alba. Dermatologica (Basel) *82:* 209–219 (1940).

(3) FARBER, E. M., and V. R. BARNES: Livedo reticularis. Stanford Med. Bull. *13:* 183–187 (1955).

(4) FELDAKER, M., E. A. HINES and R. R. KIERLAND: Livedo reticularis with summer ulcerations. Arch. Derm. Syph. (Chic.) *72:* 31–42 (1955).

(5) GOLDEN, R. L.: Livedo reticularis in systemic lupus erythematosus. Arch. Derm. (Chic). *87:* 299–301 (1963).

(6) GOLDSCHLAG, F., und A. v. CHWALIBO-GOWSKI: Über einen Fall von Periarteriitis nodosa mit ausgebreiteten Hauterscheinungen. Arch. Derm. Syph. (Berl.) *171:* 622–633 (1935).

(7) HERZBERG, J. J., und K. H. SCHULZ: Tuberkulöse Vasculitis unter dem Bilde einer Livedo racemosa. Hautarzt *7:* 442–448 (1956).

(8) KLÜKEN, N., und R. GERL: Ätiopathogenetische und klinische Beziehungen der Livedo racemosa und der Vaskulitiden zum Syndrom von O'Leary, Montgomery und Brunsting. Z. Haut- u. Geschl.-Kr. *47:* 807–825 (1972).

(9) KORTING, G. W., und H. LACHNER: Zur Kenntnis atypischer, einseitiger Livedo-Bilder. Z. Haut- u. Geschl.-Kr. *47:* 1–8 (1972).

(10) VAN LOHUIZEN, C. H. J.: Über eine seltene angeborene Hautanomalie (Cutis marmorata teleangiectatica congenita). Acta derm.-venereol. (Stockh.) *3:* 202–211 (1922).

(11) LYNCH, P. J., and A. S. ZELICKSON: Congenital phlebectasia, a histopathologic study. Arch. Derm. (Chic.) *95:* 98–101 (1967).

(12) NÖDL, F.: Livedo Vasculitis. Arch. klin. exp. Derm. *233:* 439–444 (1969).

(13) SALAZAR, F. N.: Dermatological manifestations of the Cornelia de Lange syndrome. Arch. Derm. (Chic.) *94:* 38–43 (1966).

(14) SHEALY C. N., J. B. WEETH and D. MERCIER: Livedo reticularis in patients with parkinsonism receiving amantadine. J. Amer. Med. Ass. *212:* 1522–1523 (1970).

(15) SNEDDON, I. B.: Cerebro-vascular lesions and livedo reticularis. Brit. J. Derm. *77:* 180–185 (1965).

(16) WINKELMANN, R. K., und H. MONTGOMERY: Über die cutane Periarteriitis nodosa. Hautarzt *11:* 82–86 (1960).

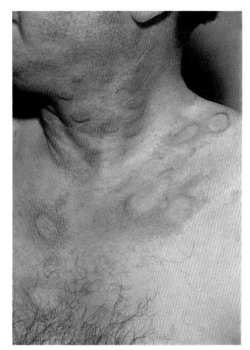

Fig. 254. Acute urticaria.

N. Urticarial Erythemas

Urticaria, strophulus (papular urticaria), and prurigo, pathologically and nosologically, are "related" cutaneous reactions. These diseases range from the fundamental lesion of the urticarial wheal, i.e., cutaneous diapedesis, to the acute papulovesicular lesion of strophulus, and finally to the cellular urticarial lesion of the prurigo papule. Here only urticaria will be discussed because strophulus and prurigo were dealt with in Chapter 2C. Recurrent swellings will be discussed in the subsequent chapter on swellings.

1. Acute urticaria, in which the cardinal sign is the urtica (wheal), is as a rule a highly fleeting and almost always pruritic disease process. According to the degree of filtration pressure the urticarial lesion may be "porcellanea alba," "anemica," "rubra," or sometimes also "vesicular" or "bullous;" rarely it may be hemorrhagic.

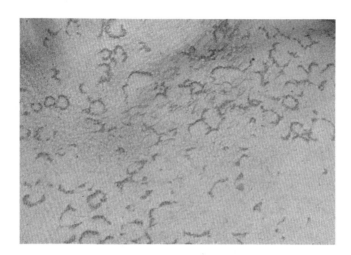

Fig. 255. Urticaria acuta figurata.

Receding urticaria shows central flattening of the individual lesion resulting in annular, garlanded, circinate, and gyrated erythematous lesions (Figs. 254, 255). These receding forms of urticaria are sometimes excoriated; however, the tops of fresh, highly hyperemic wheals hardly ever show scratches. A residual pigmentation of involuted urticarial areas (urticaria cum pigmentatione) seldom remains for long. An attack of urticaria may be accompanied by synchronous or alternating extracutaneous manifestations. Examples of such general signs are concomitant fever (most frequently after administration of penicillin, with a typical latent period of nine to ten days after medication), and gastrointestinal, tracheal, and cardiac complaints. To what extent such anginal signs are fleeting ischemic reactions or real myocardial signs can be ascertained only by repeated electrocardiograms. Quite frequently, again after penicillin urticaria, an increase in transaminase can be found, indicating involvement of the liver; signs pointing to irritation of the cerebrospinal fluid, including meningitis, are rare and are found mainly with the generalized type of so-called serum sickness.

Urticaria which, although the single lesion itself does not persist, shows recurrent lesions for weeks and months is called **chronic urticaria;** new lesions appear to an apparently inexhaustible degree. It is necessary to separate the so-called chronic urticaria from the **chronic intermittent type;** the latter usually is due to administration at certain times of antigens present in drugs or foods. Extremely rare is "**urticaria profunda dolorosa,**" which has boardlike swellings deep in the corium and subcutis together with neuralgias probably caused by these swellings.[13, 14, 16]

Histologically, acute urticaria shows extensive diapedesis; it corresponds to what is observed macroscopically. The middle of the corium also shows cellular involvement (histiocytes and, especially, granulocytes and lymphocytes), plus deposits of fibrinous material. In chronic urticaria, however, there will be an admixture of mast cells and plasmocytes, while eosinophils will appear more rarely (secondarily) when multilocular formation of vesicles takes place.

In acute urticaria a search for a trigger substance is necessary (analgesics, antibiotics, chemotherapeutic substances, hydantoins, and sedatives among others). Acute urticaria may occur also in the first stages of some viral infections – for instance, in viral hepatitis or infectious mononucleosis.[1, 7, 8]

Chronic types of urticaria should call special attention to gastrointestinal disturbances (subacidity and hypofermentation, ulcers, diverticulosis, fecal impaction, and intestinal parasites, among others). It is impossible to enumerate in this discussion the multitude of causes of chronic urticaria.

The urticarial lesion itself hardly ever points to the diagnosis of its cause. However, although nutritional or drug allergens causing urticarial attacks can not often be determined, the chance of finding the cause is much more favorable in *physical urticaria*.

2. Contact urticaria to cold can be easily diagnosed by its location on exposed parts of the body and its association with exposure to cold (Fig. 256). This diagnosis is supported by applying to the skin a metal cylinder filled with ice for one to five minutes. When positive, an urticarial wheal will appear at the site of contact. One can distinguish **idiopathic** from **familial** cold urticaria; the latter starts in early life and is seldom accompanied by pruritus. If urticarial wheals appear at locations different from those described earlier, a diagnosis of cold water urticaria as a special form of the idiopathic cold contact urticaria should be considered. The application of ice to a small area is not always sufficient to provoke a widespread attack of cold water urticaria, but immersion of both arms or both legs into a bath of about 15° C will cause such an outbreak. A cold tub bath or swimming out of doors in cold water may result in fatal shock. Cold urticaria may occur together with other signs of hypersensitivity such as Raynaud's phenomenon and purpura due to cold in cryoglobulinemia. The differential diagnosis must exclude panniculitis due to cold (discussed in Chapter 12, No. 8).

Another result of exposure to cold is the **cold reflex urticaria,** which shows very small (follicular) wheals favoring the trunk.

Local application of cold (ice water test) is not sufficient to provoke an outbreak, however; it is necessary to elicit a sensation of chilling. This can be accomplished by rapid cooling of several body regions, but it is not always possible to make a distinct separation from so-called cold water urticaria.[4]

Urticarial lesions observed within a few hours after bathing in lakes and ponds should raise the suspicion of an invasion of the skin by cercariae of schistosomes. Simultaneously an excessive itching occurs. (For further details see Chapter 2, C1.)

3. Similar to the various types of cold urticaria are forms of urticaria triggered by exposure to heat. This very rare **heat contact urticaria** is limited to the place of exposure to heat. A test can be performed by immersing an arm in warm water (38° to 40° C) for about 20 minutes. Wheals should appear only on the heated extrem-

Fig. 256. Cold contact urticaria after cold shower.

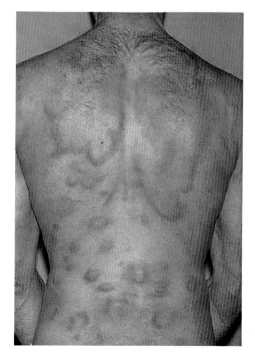

ity. **Heat reflex urticaria** (better known as cholinergic urticaria) consists of very small wheals on the trunk; the palms and soles remain free. The lesions may be induced in the susceptible patient by warm partial baths or by exercise (push-ups, climbing stairs, and so on).[4, 10]

4. In connection with cold and heat urticaria, it is important to mention the extremely rare **water contact urticaria.** Follicular urticarial lesions are confined to areas in contact with water; the wheals are independent of the temperature of the water. For testing one uses a wet compress of body temperature applied without pressure for about 10 to 40 minutes.[13]

5. Urticaria can also be produced by mechanical means. Well known is **factitious urticaria** caused by stroking of the skin; after a short latent period, an urticarial swelling will appear at the site of the stimulus. In contrast to dermatographia, factitious urticaria is accompanied by pruritus and thus may be self-perpetuating. Typically, patients complain about pruritic swellings caused by contact with undergarments (i.e., garters, tight belts, brassieres, and rough edges of clothing).

Although factitious urticaria represents urticaria with an immediate response, the so-called **pressure urticaria** shows a delayed reaction. The latter type is observed after prolonged compression of the deeper cutaneous layers. The appearance of a swelling on the palm after carrying a heavy suitcase is characteristic. These swellings, as a rule, are pruritic only in the beginning; later they become painful to pressure. The period of latency may amount to a few hours, so the patient may not be aware of the load-factor as the cause. The absence of both fever and migration and a careful history will prevent the physician from confusing the condition with erysipelas. Pressure urticaria can be provoked by applying a lead

cylinder weighing about 18 pounds to an area 4 cm in diameter for about 15 to 20 minutes.[3]

6. Idiopathic light urticaria (solar urticaria) is confined to unshielded or thinly covered skin. Corresponding to exposure to different wavelengths of the spectrum, there is an ultraviolet urticaria caused by shortwave rays (maximum effect at 3000 Å) and one caused by longwave rays (maximum effect between 3600 and 4500 Å). Window glass will protect against shortwave ultraviolet urticaria but will not prevent eruption of wheals in the presence of longwave ultraviolet rays. Urticarial wheals due to visible light (maximum effect at 5000 Å) occur by exposure to ordinary daylight, much less commonly to the rays emitted by filaments of electric bulbs. In some cases of idiopathic light urticaria, the spectrum triggering the eruption may extend over a very wide range (from about 2300 Å to 8000 Å).

In some cases, if the light exposure causes the formation of wheals beyond the area of contact and if, in addition, other cutaneous changes develop (i.e., edematous erythemas, bullae, varioliform scars, and hyperkeratoses), a diagnosis of **symptomatic light urticaria** or erythropoietic protoporphyria must be made. For further details of this disease, see also Chapter 2, C2, Chapter 17, C5, and Chapter 25, A10. Here it must be emphasized that not every erythropoietic protoporphyria presents light urticaria and that a patient may show definite seasonal fluctuations in the intensity of his urticarial attacks.

The diagnosis must be verified by determination of the protoporphyrins and coproporphyrins of the erythrocytes or by examination of the erythrocytes for fluorescence in a dry smear.[5, 17]

7. Exceptionally, **roentgen urticaria** may result from the effect of x-ray radiation at the site of treatment. This represents a definite late reaction with a latent period of about six hours.[18]

8. The simultaneous occurrence of diarrhea and an urticarial eruption is not always connected with food allergy or ingestion of contaminated or spoiled food. This association can also be observed in the **Verner-Morrison syndrome.** Clinically, this syndrome is characterized by diarrhea and coliclike abdominal complaints and hypokalemia. Hyperacidity of the gastric secretion and ulcers of the gastrointestinal tract are absent. The cause of this disease is a noninsulin-producing island cell adenoma of the pancreas.[9, 12]

9. Recurrent eruptions of wheals may be part of a special type of **hereditary idiopathic amyloidosis** associated simultaneously with deafness. (See Chapter 9, E.)[6, 11]

10. As an addendum **white dermatographia** should be mentioned. This is most likely a manifestation of an increased potential, congenital or acquired, for contraction of the cutaneous capillaries. This potential is one of the stigmas of the patient with atopic dermatitis. However, white dermatographia can be observed also in typhus and hypothyroidism and may be associated with ichthyosiform skin.

(1) COWDREY, S. C., and J. S. REYNOLDS: Acute urticaria in infectious mononucleosis. Ann. Allergy 27: 182–190 (1969).

(2) DENK, R.: Elektrokardiographische Untersuchungen bei Hautkranken. Arch. Kreisl.-Forsch. 60: 33–114 (1969).

(3) ILLIG, L., und J. KUNICK: Klinik und Diagnostik der physikalischen Urticaria. I. Teil. Hautarzt 20: 167–178 (1969).

(4) ILLIG, L., und J. KUNICK: Klinik und Diagnostik der physikalischen Urticaria. II. Teil. Hautarzt 20: 499–512 (1969).

(5) ILLIG, L., und J. KUNICK: Klinik und Diagnostik der physikalischen Urticaria. III. Teil. Hautarzt 21: 16–25 (1970).

(6) KENNEDY, D. D., F. D. ROSENTHAL and I. B. SNEDDON: Amyloidosis presenting as urticaria. Brit. Med. J. 1966: 31–32.

(7) LJUNGGREN, B., and H. MÖLLER: Hepatitis presenting as transient urticaria. Acta derm.-venereol. (Stockh.) 51: 295–297 (1971).

(8) LOCKSHIN, N. A., and H. HURLEY: Urticaria as a sign of viral hepatitis. Arch. Derm. (Chic). 105: 570–571 (1972).

(9) MARTINI, G. A., G. STROHMEYER, P. HAUG und W. GUSEK: Inselzelladenome des Pankreas mit urtikariellem Exanthem, Durchfällen sowie Kalium- und Eiweißverlust über den Darm. Dtsch. med. Wschr. 89: 313–322 (1964).

(10) MICHAËLSSON, G., and A.-M. ROS: Familial localized heat urticaria of delayed type. Acta derm.-venereol. (Stockh.) 51: 279–283 (1971).

(11) MUCKLE, TH. J., and M. WELLS: Urticaria, deafness, and amyloidosis: a new heredo-familial syndrome. Quart. J. Med. 31: 235–248 (1962).

(12) PABST, K., F. KÜMMERLE, H. H. HENNEKEUSER und G. MAPPES: Beitrag zum Krankheitsbild des Verner-Morrison-Syndroms. Dtsch. med. Wschr. 31: 235–248 (1962).

(13) PETZOLDT, D.: Ätiologische Faktoren bei chronischer Urtikaria. Med. Klin. 59: 1333–1336 (1964).

(14) SCHULZ, K. H.: Die chronische Urtikaria. Med. Welt (Stuttg.) 1965: 676–681.

(15) SHELLEY, W. B., and H. M. RAWNSLEY: Aquagenic urticaria. Contact sensitivity reaction to water. J. Amer. Med. Ass. 189: 895–898 (1964).

(16) STÜHMER, A.: Urticaria profunda dolorosa migrans. Derm. Wschr. 135: 272–279 (1957).

(17) SUURMOND, D., J. VAN STEVENINCK and L. N. WENT: Some clinical and fundamental aspects of erythropoietic protoporphyria. Brit. J. Derm. 82: 323–328 (1970).

(18) WEBER, G., und O. BRAUN-FALCO: Zum Entstehungsmechanismus urtikarieller Röntgenreaktionen. Derm. Wschr. 134: 892–895 (1956).

19. Erythematous Squamous Dermatoses

A. Psoriasis Vulgaris

Psoriasis vulgaris has few or multiple characteristic features involving the entire integument symmetrically. However, the knees, elbows, and sacral area are affected especially. In general, the face is spared; in those cases where it is not, exterior irritations or the light has a provocative, isomorphic effect. This "parakeratotic diathesis" has, by the way, created a dermatosis whose erythematous areas have an especially distinct and sharply circumscribed border (Figs. 257a and b). After removal of the lamellar stratified scales by methodical scratching and after the last of the scale is off, saturated red erythema with a dewlike drop of blood (Auspitz sign) (Fig. 258) becomes visible. In spite of this stereotypic single lesion the appearance of the disorder may vary due to changing dynamics and localizations. Thus the maximal erythrodermic (Chapter 22, C11), arthropathic (Chapter 7, B1), and pustulous (Chapter 1, C1) variants as well as the intertriginous forms deviate

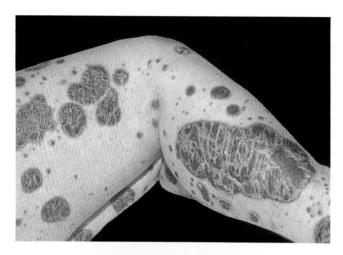

Fig. 257a. Psoriasis vulgaris: typical, sharply limited, multiple, erythemas with scales.

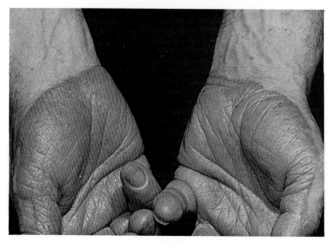

Fig. 257b. Palmar psoriasis vulgaris eruption, typically sharply circumscribed, after removal of the scales.

essentially in their appearance from typical psoriasis vulgaris (punctate, guttate, nummular, geographic, etc.).

Involvement of the nails, although not constant, occurs in various degrees in about 10 per cent of all psoriatics. It appears in the form of small pits (pitted nails) (Fig. 259a), or as a so-called oil spot (subungual, transparent parakeratosis) (Fig. 260), or as a completely broken down and crumbling nail (Fig. 261). The erythematous form of *psoriasis of the nails* extends from the subungual psoriatic nail (oil spot) and diffuse erythematous discolorations (subungual psoriatic erythema) to psoriatic onycholysis. The latter overwhelmingly represents the sequelae of a diseased nailbed itself and not the stippled nail of a diseased hyponychium. Additional nail changes, which are not characteristic

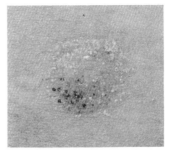

Fig. 258. Psoriasis vulgaris: bleeding points after removal of the last scale.

of psoriasis (for instance, longitudinal and transverse ridges), can be caused by accompanying psoriasis of the paronychium. It should be emphasized again that patients with psoriatic arthropathy show not only a considerably higher percentage

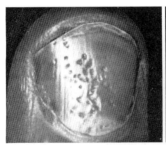
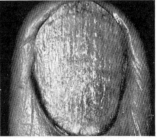

Fig. 259a. Pitted nails in psoriasis vulgaris.

Fig. 259b. Punctate onychosis in alopecia areata.

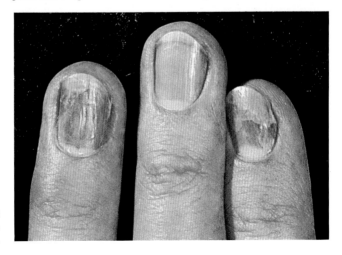

Fig. 260. Nail changes in psoriasis: subungual parakeratosis (so-called oil spot).

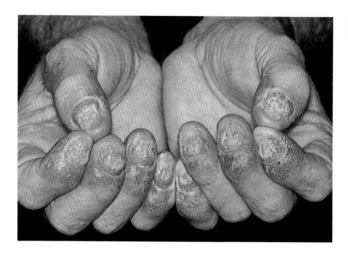

Fig. 261. Nail changes in psoriasis: crumbling nails.

(20 to 40 per cent) of nail involvement, but also more severe changes.[2, 6, 8, 9]

Frequently, inoculation with Candida occurs within the nail changes, whereas that with dermatophytes is rare.

Fig. 262. Intertriginous psoriasis vulgaris of the axillas and below the breasts.

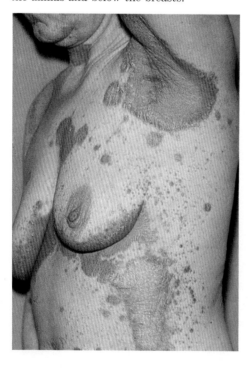

The most frequent sign among the nail disturbances in psoriasis is pitting. These typical pitted or thimble nails occur also in about 5 per cent of the normal population, so that, since many psoriatics do not show any nail changes, all that can be said is that typical pits occur more frequently in psoriatics than in nonpsoriatics. A similar, perhaps finer pitting (Fig. 259b) than in psoriasis occasionally accompanies alopecia areata (onychosis multi- et micropunctata). This sign is, of course, less important than the changes of the scalp but can still persist distinctly, years after the scalp changes have disappeared. Other characteristics of the "alopecia areata nail" are, besides the intensive, extremely fine, multiple pits, the loss of sheen and smoothness of the nail plate and the presence of a pale yellowish nail tone.

It was formerly believed that the psoriatic disturbance of keratinization occurred only on the scalp. Newer stereo-electron microscopic investigations, however, have found a psoriatic disturbance of keratinization represented on the surface of the skin in the form of chips of large cuticular scales.[5]

Etiologically, psoriasis has been recognized as an irregularly dominant, multifactorial, genetic disorder with a threshold

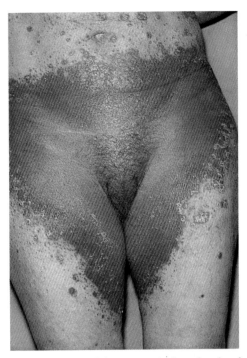

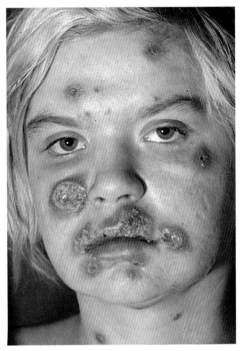

Fig. 263. Intertriginous psoriasis vulgaris of the inguinal and genital areas.

Fig. 264. Malignant syphilis, impetigolike facial lesions.

effect, as demonstrated by the distinct dependency of manifestations on internal changes and exterior influences on the patient.

Psoriasis vulgaris with its characteristic single lesions and typical localization

offers no differential diagnostic difficulties. The diagnosis is further proved by the following characteristics: stratified scaling; point-sized bleeding after removal of the last overlying skin; apparent isomorphic propagation; distinct sparing of the face,

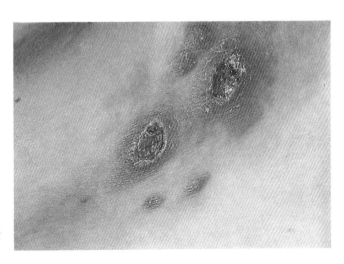

Fig. 265. Malignant syphilis: ecthymalike ulcerations of the trunk.

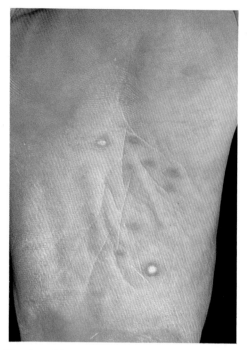

Fig. 266. Maculopapular secondary syphilis of the sole.

Fig. 267. Small macular plantar pigmentations in bare-footed blacks following trauma.

palms, and soles; the nail changes; and, sometimes, a familial occurrence. If, however, there are atypical localizations (typus inversus) (Figs. 262, 263) or mono-localizations, as for instance on the head or perianally or those which from the beginning are unusual (pustular, erythro-dermic, or limited to the nails), then even the experienced diagnostician can be in doubt.[7]

Psoriasiform, heavily scaling, **secondary syphilids,** which in "latent" psoriatics can easily assume the character of psoriasis vulgaris, are rare today. Psoriasis ostracea or rupioides can be mistaken for *malignant syphilis* (Figs. 264, 265), in which impetiginous-ecthymatous, ephemeral or destructive, superficial lesions are the expression of this special form of syphilis. For confirmation of the diagnosis of syphilis one has to look for changes of the oral mucous membranes ("plaques muqueuses"), loss of hair (alopecia areolaris), and enlarged lymph nodes and condylomas,

Fig. 268. Tylotic eczema.

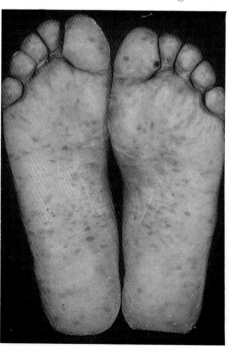

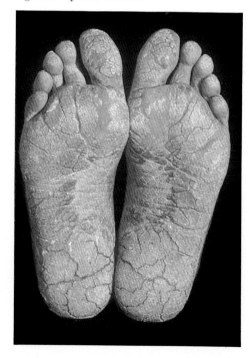

Fig. 269. Hyperkeratotic
fungus infection of the palms.

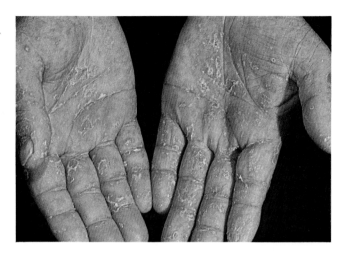

because, especially in malignant syphilis, the seroreactions and the Nelson test may remain negative or only mildly positive. Besides generalized syphilids, palmar and plantar syphilids occupy a favorite location; they are initially more papular than macular (Fig. 266). They are definitely dependent on mechanical influences. Lichenoid and lenticular lesions, the syphilitic clavi, are rare. Compared with the mostly light red or bluish-red, palmoplantar erythemas of psoriasis vulgaris, which are regular and profusely squamous, the palmoplantar syphilids are characterized by papular, nonscaling lesions and a saturated, coppery brownish-red coloring.[1, 4]

Tylotic or callous common *eczemas* of palms and soles (Fig. 268) are not sharply limited and extend over wide areas. They simulate rhagadiform, polygonal, *hyperkeratotic fungal* eruptions (Figs. 269, 270) from which differentiation is difficult. However, these eruptions will not easily be mistaken for psoriasis vulgaris (Fig. 257b) with its sharply limited, round, or polycyclic areas.

Psoriasiform *seborrheic dermatitides*, however, are hard to distinguish. One anticipates this difficulty from such concepts as "psoriasoid" or "dermatitis mediothoracica." In contrast to seborrheic

dermatitis, which is characterized by its location on the scalp, on the middle parts of the face, and in sweating areas, psoriasis vulgaris, with its completely different type of scales in isolated lesions, lacks peripheral maximal exudation. Histologically, psori-

Fig. 270. Hyperkeratotic fungus infection of the foot.

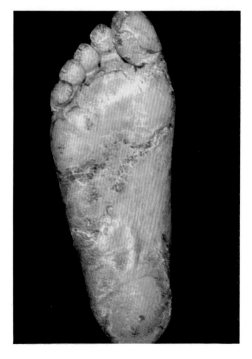

asis shows Munro abscesses, whereas seborrheic dermatitis is characterized by discrete spongiosis.

With regard to the face, involvement in both diseases is less than that in other places, but psoriasis is generally more distinctly limited and shows more scaling, especially in places which are not affected by much washing (upper eyelids). Seborrheic dermatitis in children is often connected with an enlarged pharyngeal tonsil. The dermatosis shows fine scaling and dry cutaneous inflammation (pityriasis alba and "dartre volante"). The decision will be in favor of psoriasis if, in spite of wide involvement of the scalp, the hair-lines are especially affected and if single, infiltrated, round areas show stratified scaling. In general, these psoriasiform areas will point to psoriasis if there is a distinct association with arthropathies.

The same can be said of distinctly pitted nails, although a few pits may be present in a patient severely affected with seborrheic dermatitis. On the other hand, a connection with pyogenic foci (furuncles, hidroadenitis, hordeolum, and otorrhea) and an association with intertriginous, bacterial infection point toward seborrheic dermatitis.

Areas of *pityriasis rosea* are finer and more delicate than petal-like seborrheic lesions. They are characterized by collar-ettes limited to the trunk and rarely present on the neck and extremities; they are distributed along the cutaneous tension lines with distinct accentuation of the inner armpits. Pityriasis rosea is much more irritable than psoriasis vulgaris or an eczematid. Moreover, the collarettes of pityriasis rosea have a less saturated red color and are less infiltrated than areas of

Fig. 271. Bowen's disease.

Fig. 272. Bowen's disease: massive acantho-sis, irregular arrangement of epidermal cells, multiple keratinizations of single cells and atypical mitoses. HE stain, 160×.

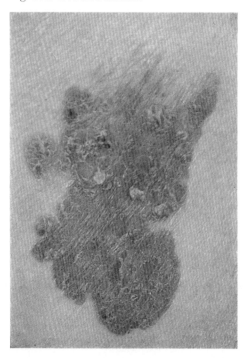

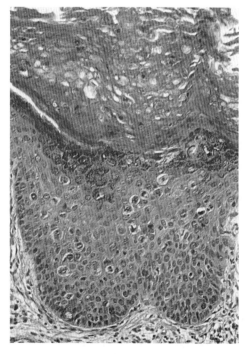

psoriasis. At the stage of the heraldic spot or in pityriasis rosea with few lesions, superficial trichophyton infections (evidence of fungi!) may have to be considered. On the scalp, round, ashy-gray, dusty areas with characteristically broken-off hairs point to a fungus infection, whereas psoriasis does not injure the shaft, at least not macroscopically.

If a solitary psoriasiform lesion remains for years localized at an atypical site, *Bowen's disease* (Figs. 271, 272) may be present. Its scales are white to yellowish, its surface smooth or granular but occasionally hyperkeratotic or crusted. Histologic evidence of "malignant dyskeratosis" will confirm the diagnosis. Large and glowing, saturated, psoriatic areas with only mild scaling on the glans or coronary sulcus must be distinguished from erosive secondary syphilis "en nappes" and from erythroplasia, which represents Bowen's disease of the mucous membrane and is, therefore, limited to one or a few lesions. It is characterized by velvety nodules.

On the genitals, in men (balanitis) as well as in women (vulvovaginitis), *thrush* has to be considered. Moreover, psoriatic skin is nowadays often treated with corticosteroids and occlusion, which in itself tends to favor a superinfection with Candida. Especially in intertriginous areas (submammary, inguinal, and genitoanal), candidiasis leads to shiny erythemas with a saturated red color. In contrast to intertriginous psoriasis, however, the diagnosis is indicated by the collarettes at the border and the satellitelike corymbiform propagation, as well as by the cultural evidence.

The lesions of **Reiter's syndrome** may also be psoriasiform. Besides the main signs of arthritis, conjunctivitis, and urethritis, parakeratotic circinate balanitis (Figs. 273, 274) is significant. The same can be said of so-called blennorrhagic keratoses, which are lentil-sized, spotted, and to some extent also confluent brownish-red erythemas, which are found especially

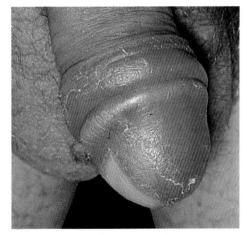

Fig. 273. Penile psoriasis vulgaris (psoriatic balanitis).

on the palms and soles (Fig. 275). In severe cases they may look like rupioid psoriasis or oyster shell-like crusts.[3]

In the course of *mycosis fungoides*, lesions simulating psoriasis may be encountered.

Fig. 274. Reiter's syndrome: parakeratotic circinate balanitis.

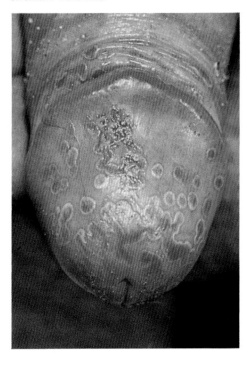

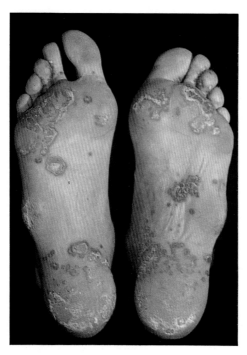

Fig. 275. Plantar keratodermas in Reiter's syndrome.

(3) HAUSER, W.: Zur Diagnostik der Reiter-schen Krankheit. Med. Welt (Stuttg.) *1964:* 2404–2409.

(4) HOLZMANN, H., und CH. DOBERKE: Lues maligna. Med. Welt (Stuttg.) *1965:* 2835–2836.

(5) ORFANOS, C., G. MAHRLE und R. CHRISTENHUSZ: Verhornungsstörungen am Haar bei Psoriasis. Arch. klin. exp. Derm. *236:* 107–114 (1970).

(6) SCHINAS, G., und R. BRUN: »Tüpfel« an den Fingernägeln. Dermatologica (Basel) *137:* 126–127 (1968).

(7) THEISEN, H.: Über einen Fall von Psoriasis follicularis spinulosa. Derm. Wschr. *134:* 1326–1329 (1956).

(8) WEBER, G.: Der »psoriatische Ölfleck« (Gottron), ein wenig bekanntes Symptom der Schuppenflechte. Derm. Wschr. *128:* 739–741 (1953).

(9) ZAIAS, N.: Psoriasis of the nail. Arch. Derm. (Chic.) *99:* 567–579 (1969).

Usually this reticulogranulomatosis, especially in its early stages, is fundamentally a polymorphic disease, so that disklike and circinate changes hardly ever appear as typically closed as in psoriasis vulgaris. Therefore, mycosis fungoides is associated with scales that are open, round or segmentary, distinctly marginated, and in no way regularly lamellar, as well as with attacks of subjective itching. In any case, these diagnostic difficulties will be encountered less frequently in relation to psoriasis vulgaris than in relation to the parapsoriasis group, especially Brocq's disease.

(1) ADAM, A., und G. W. KORTING: Lues maligna. Arch. klin. exp. Derm. *210:* 14–26 (1960).

(2) ALKIEWICZ, J.: Die erythematösen Formen der Nagelpsoriasis. Hautarzt *16:* 36–37 (1965).

B. Pityriasis Rubra Pilaris

The primary lesion of *pityriasis rubra pilaris* is a follicular, epidermal papule. Underneath a thin, often still transparent, plaster of paris-like scale a reddish-brown erythema develops, usually in the face (Figs. 276, 277) or over the elbows or knees (Figs. 278, 279). The simultaneous presence of closely aggregated, acuminated papules at the edges of the fingers and diffuse, although not excessive, palmo-plantar hyperkeratosis prevents the mistake of diagnosing psoriasis vulgaris. Typical cases of pityriasis rubra pilaris are more apt to regress than those with manifestations that are atypical from the beginning. Generally, the duration of the disorder can be expected to last months to years, and no sure results from modern treatment methods should be expected. Transition to erythroderma is always possible (see also Chapter 22, C14).

Formerly, the identity of pityriasis rubra pilaris with **lichen planus acuminatus** (lichen planopilaris) was assumed, but the latter is more acute. In general, lichen planopilaris is accompanied by an impairment of the general well-being and occasionally by erythema and edema in the neighborhood of disseminated and pointed nodules, which are often pierced by a hair (Fig. 280). But typical lichen planus occasionally shows, besides the usual polygonal flat or obtuse papules, singular acuminated or even pointed nodules. In contrast to pityriasis rubra pilaris, lichen planus spares the face, scalp, and armpits. All in all, predilection sites of lichen planus are more or less completely different. This is further illustrated by the initial involvement of the flexor sides of the forearms and wrists and frequent mucous membrane involvement. Histologically, lichen planus acuminatus, in spite of its planopilaris character, shows the typical picture of a mixed epidermocutaneous papule with bandlike round cell infiltrates in the corium and generalized orthohyperkeratosis. Cell infiltrates which characterize typical lichen planus are more or less distinctly related to follicles. Pityriasis rubra pilaris, however, shows a follicular epidermal papule with small infiltrates. In some cases, the differential diagnosis between the two der-

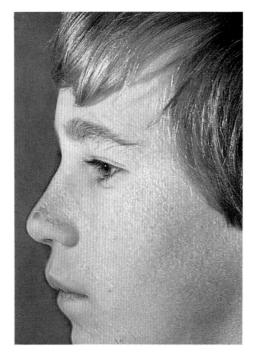

Fig. 276. Pityriasis rubra pilaris.

matoses may be difficult in the beginning.[1,2]

(1) SACHS, W., and G. DE OREO: Lichen planopilaris. Arch. Derm. Syph. (Chic.) *45:* 1081–1093 (1942).

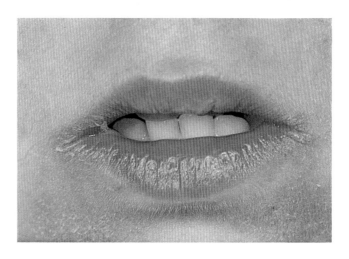

Fig. 277. Pityriasis rubra pilaris of the vermilion border.

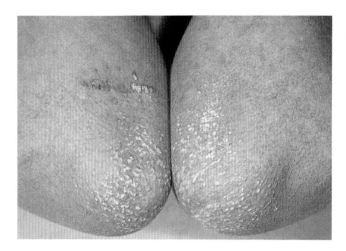

Fig. 278. Pityriasis rubra
pilaris.

(2) SILVER, H., L. CHARGIN and P. M. SACHS:
    Follicular lichen planus (lichen plano-
    pilaris). Arch. Derm. Syph. (Chic.) *67:*
    346–354 (1953).

C. Paraneoplastic Acrokeratosis

Large psoriasiform areas, especially on
the scalp and in symmetrical distribution
on the distal parts of the extremities, are
present in **paraneoplastic acrokeratosis.** On
the face, the lesions, which simulate those
of lupus erythematosus, are located on the
nose and the pinna of the ear, but the sharp
borderline characteristic of psoriasis is
missing. The nails are always affected,
showing longitudinal to transverse ridges
or even complete loosening of the nail
plates by underlying keratoses. Histologically, necroses of the capillaries, which are
surrounded by reticular or polynuclear
pyknotic cells, are paramount; the epidermis shows bowenoid features. In any case,
it is imperative in this acromelic keratosis
to rule out an internal neoplasm, especially

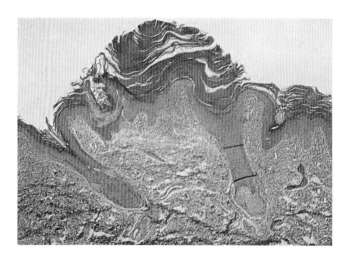

Fig. 279. Pityriasis rubra
pilaris: epidermocutaneous
papule with follicular hyperkeratosis. HE stain, 25 ×.

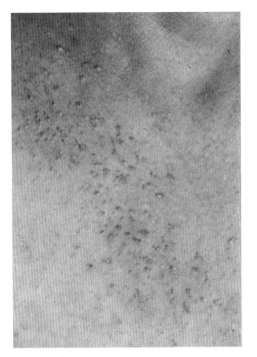

Fig. 280. Lichen planus acuminatus.

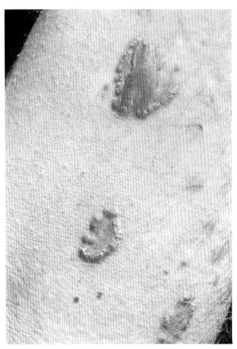

Fig. 281. Serpiginous elastosis perforans.

one of the gastrointestinal tract and the respiratory organs.[1,2]

(1) BAZEX, A., R. SALVADOR, A. DUPRÉ, M. PARANT, B. CHRISTOL, P. CANTALA et P. CARLES: Dermatose psoriasiforme acromélique d'étiologie cancéreuse (Entité paranéoplasique originale). Bull. Soc. franç. Derm. Syph. 74: 130–135 (1967).

(2) PUISSANT, A., und M. BENVENISTE: Das Bazex-Syndrom. Ein neues paraneoplastisches Syndrom. Münch. med. Wschr. 114: 19–22 (1972).

D. Hyperkeratosis Follicularis et Parafollicularis in Cutem Penetrans

Another dermatosis to be separated from psoriasis vulgaris is **hyperkeratosis follicularis et parafollicularis in cutem pene-** **trans** (Kyrle's disease). The primary lesion is a yellowish, later brownish-red, and sometimes verrucous nodule, which, by occasional confluence with similar lesions, may form larger polycyclic areas. The distribution of the lesions is as a rule arbitrary; however, hands, feet, and scalp are usually spared, although the disorder is usually eminently chronic. The legs are a favorite site. The main histologic characteristic is the penetration of orthokeratotic and parakeratotic substances into the connective tissue of the corium. Newer concepts consider this to be a dislocation of the keratinization level into deeper layers.

In the differential diagnosis of Kyrle's disease Darier's disease can be at once recognized histologically. However, lichen planus, pityriasis rubra pilaris, and follicular psoriasis (psoriasis follicularis spinulosa) will also have to be considered. More important still is the differentiation

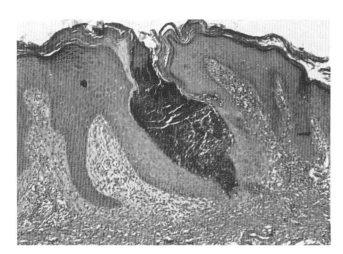

Fig. 282. Elastosis perforans serpiginosa. Perforation of amorphous keratotic masses through the epidermis. HE stain, 25 ×.

from **elastosis perforans serpiginosa*** which is occasionally wrongly identified as Kyrle's disease. Macroscopically, this perforating elastosis shows circinate or serpiginous lesions. The individual lesion is keratotically and conically acuminated and shows a rough surface with small elevations. The lesions are grouped polycyclically or in rings and are located predominantly on the neck or in the elbow region. Occasionally, the border gives the impression of a ledgelike prominence, especially since the center, surrounded by nodules, is moderately depressed owing to mild atrophy. Multiple occurrence is rare (Figs. 281, 282). Massive hypertrophic plugs as in Kyrle's disease are absent. One should look out for the tendency to syntropy with congenital anomalies (cutis hyperelastica, osteogenesis imperfecta, and congenital poikiloderma). Histopathologically, elastosis perforans serpiginosa shows a massive break through the epidermis of a substrate, staining like elastica and located in the corium. The histologic differentiation between Kyrle's disease and elastosis perforans serpiginosa is easy. In Kyrle's disease conelike hyperkeratosis ruptures into the epidermal layers below, whereas

in elastosis perforans serpiginosa the columnar "elastoma" tries to perforate the overlying epidermis.[1, 3-8]

If more collagenlike fibrillar substances break through, we are dealing with **reactive, perforating collagenosis.** It apparently develops frequently after the healing of scraped or torn wounds and shows multiple, small to lentil-sized, granulomatous nodules. This, therefore, is no primary perforating elastoma, but an elimination of thick collagenous fibers, accompanied by cellular detritus and leukocytes, with no proof that the cause for this process is scattered foreign bodies. (See also Chapter 29, B2).[2, 9]

---

* And also perforating folliculitis. (Tr.)

(1) BANDMANN, H.-J., und A. H. SCHMID: Zur Differentialdiagnose der Hyperkeratosis follicularis et parafollicularis in cutem penetrans (Morbus Kyrle) gegenüber der Elastosis perforans serpiginosa (Morbus Lutz-Miescher). Hautarzt *19:* 259–264 (1968).

(2) BOVENMYER, D. A.: Reactive perforating collagenosis. Experimental production of the lesion. Arch. Derm. (Chic.) *102:* 313–317 (1970).

(3) CARTER, V. H., and V. S. CONSTANTINE: Kyrle's disease. Arch. Derm. (Chic.) *97:* 624–632 (1968).

(4) Kocsard, E.: Un cas d'association de maladie de Kyrle et d'hyperkératose lenticulaire perstans de Flegel. Bull. Soc. franç. Derm. Syph. 77: 37–39 (1970).

(5) Korting, G. W.: Elastosis perforans serpiginosa als ektodermales Randsymptom bei Cutis laxa. Arch. klin. exp. Derm. 224: 437–446 (1966).

(6) Kyrle, J.: Über einen ungewöhnlichen Fall von universeller follikulärer und parafollikulärer Hyperkeratose. Arch. Derm. Syph. (Wien und Leipzig) 123: 466–493 (1916).

(7) Mehregan, A. H.: Elastosis perforans serpiginosa. A review of the literature and report of 11 cases. Arch. Derm. (Chic.) 97: 381–393 (1968).

(8) Tappeiner, J., K. Wolff und E. Schreiner: Morbus Kyrle. Hautarzt 20: 296–310 (1969).

(9) Woringer, F., und P. Laugier: Collagenoma perforans verruciforme. Derm. Wschr. 147: 64–68 (1963).

E. Hyperkeratosis Lenticularis

Hyperkeratosis lenticularis perstans presents nodular keratoses on the dorsum of the feet and on the legs and has no tendency to spontaneous cure; this genodermatosis is characterized by a chronic course extending over a period of years. It is transmitted as an autosomal dominant trait. A rare subtype shows disseminated distribution imitating psoriasis. Usually, however, there are micropapules of up to 0.5 cm in diameter with slightly depressed centers. After the lesion has been present for some time, it will form a firmly attached scale. This psoriasiform aspect is enhanced by the fact that removal of the scale will result in dewdrop-like bleeding and because larger lesions have a tendency to coalesce. This anomaly of keratinization with clinically distinctive hyperkeratosis has no resemblance to any other dermatosis and therefore, differential diagnostic difficulties should not arise; the disease may however, be mistaken for Kyrle's

disease, elastosis perforans serpiginosa, and Darier's disease (particularly the special type known as "acrokeratosis verruciformis"). Histologically, hyperkeratosis lenticularis perstans has an "inflammatory" character with bandlike or nodular infiltrates of round cells interspersed with many capillaries.[1-6]

(1) Bean, S. F.: Hyperkeratosis lenticularis perstans. Arch. Derm. (Chic.) 99: 705–709 (1969).

(2) Flegel, H.: Hyperkeratosis lenticularis perstans. Hautarzt 9: 362–364 (1958).

(3) Kocsard, E.: Un cas d'association de maladie de Kyrle et d'hyperkératose lenticulaire perstans de Flegel. Bull. Soc. franç. Derm. Syph. 77: 37–39 (1970).

(4) Kocsard, E., C. L. Bear and T. J. Constance: Hyperkeratosis lenticularis perstans (Flegel). Dermatologica (Basel) 136: 35–42 (1968).

(5) Müller, H., und H. Schleicher: Beitrag zur Hyperkeratosis lenticularis perstans. Derm. Wschr. 154: 577–583 (1968).

(6) Raffle, E. J., and J. Rogers: Hyperkeratosis lenticularis perstans. Arch. Derm. (Chic.) 100: 423–428 (1969).

F. Stuccokeratosis

Stuccokeratosis (keratoelastoidosis verrucosa) consists of scattered hyperkeratoses that are easily removed mechanically. Because these grayish-white or grayish-brown lesions, which favor the extremities and are found in older people, have no erythematous basis, there are no pathologic changes visible after removal of the thin scale.[2,4]

Macroscopically, there may be a certain similarity to *"papillomatose confluente et réticulée"* (Gougerot and Carteaud), which, however, affects primarily younger individuals and has other localizations (such as the inner aspects of the thighs and the epigastric region). The outer edges of some fingers may show marginal collagenous degeneration, presenting lesions similar to those of stuccokeratosis or hyperkeratosis lenticularis perstans. This **marginal keratoelastoidosis of the hands** has to be considered a special localization of senile elastosis; histologically, this is confirmed by degeneration of the collagen and elastica.[1, 3, 5]

(1) Kocsard, E.: Keratoelastoidosis marginalis of the hands. Dermatologica (Basel) *131:* 169–175 (1965).

(2) Kocsard, E., and F. Ofner: Keratoelastoidosis verrucosa of the extremities (Stuccokeratosis of the extremities). Dermatologica (Basel) *133:* 225–235 (1966).

(3) Korting, G. W., und J. Cabré: Papillomatosis Gougerot und Carteaud als ektodermale Randsymptomatik bei segmentärer Lipodystrophie. Arch. klin. exp. Derm. *215:* 422–437 (1963).

(4) Metz, J., und G. Metz: Die Stuccokeratosis, eine wenig beachtete Veränderung der alternden Haut. Z. Haut- u. Geschl.-Kr. *45:* 81–86 (1970).

(5) Ritchie, E. B., and H. M. Williams: Degenerative collagenous plaques of the hands. Arch. Derm. (Chic.) *93:* 202–203 (1966).

G. Pityriasis Rosea

The eruption of pityriasis rosea classically starts with a solitary primary lesion ("plaque primitive," "heraldic patch") with collarette scaling (Fig. 284); this area may remain solitary for up to two weeks. After the eruption has developed further, the heraldic patch usually remains as the largest lesion. The typical multiple lesions of pityriasis rosea are slightly elevated macules with a finely scalloped border. Much more rarely one sees lentil-sized small nodules (lichenoid pityriasis rosea). In ordinary pale red or reddish-yellow erythematous lesions the periphery enlarges rapidly while the central portion becomes depressed; at the same time there is fine wrinkling or rough splintering of the surface. Beyond this, the edge of the pityriasis rosea lesion is characterized by a fine scaly border ("coronella," "collarette"). Further toward the periphery there is a finely saturated reddish border, completing the picture of a medallion. These changes are best observed in the herald lesion. The single lesions show a distinct arrangement along the lines of cleavage of the skin (Fig. 283). A further characteristic of pityriasis rosea is a marked irritability of the lesions – for instance, after overly intense local therapy or maceration by sweat the faint reddish tone takes on a more yellowish hue as well as further signs of increasing exudation. Diagnostically important is the fact that the face and scalp are not involved regardless of the number of lesions elsewhere; there is also a tendency for projection of the lesions toward the middle of the axillae throughout the entire course (3 to 6 weeks) of the disease (Fig. 284). Enanthems are as rare as recurrence or complete healing with leukoderma. As a rule, there is only moderate pruritus. Occasionally, before the appearance of the lesions, the patient may complain of lassitude, headaches, painful throat, and mild fever. Most of the patients are in their second or third decade of life; very rarely will pityriasis rosea occur in infants before the age of 2 or in people over the age of 60 years. There may be a preponderance of outbreaks of pityriasis rosea in spring or fall, but in some regions, for instance, in Mainz, Germany, the authors see a certain epidemic frequency during the colder season (Fig. 285).

Laboratory tests in pityriasis rosea show only uncharacteristic "inflammatory signs" such as anemia or a shift of the white cells to the left, together with mild monocytosis or an increase in the ESR. These findings correspond with the classical conception of an infectious allergenic genesis of this exanthem. Formerly, wearing newly bought underwear impregnated with a

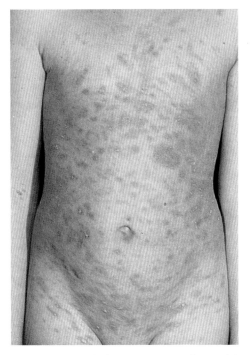

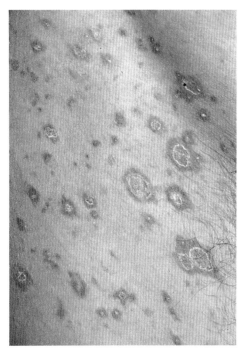

Fig. 283. Pityriasis rosea: eruption with herealdic spot.

Fig. 284. Pityriasis rosea: viewed toward the axilla, with typical collarette of the individual lesion.

finish or drinking raw milk were supposedly triggering factors. More recently, the possibility of an autoaggressive mechanism is being considered.

Histologically, pityriasis rosea presents an uncharacteristic dermatitis with epidermal changes (parakeratosis in places, moderate acanthosis, inter- and intra-

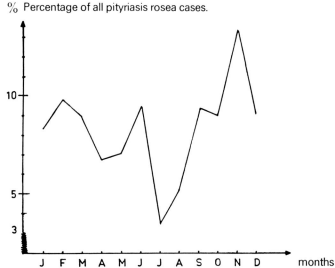

Fig. 285. Distribution of frequency of 266 instances of pityriasis rosea by month.

% Percentage of all pityriasis rosea cases.

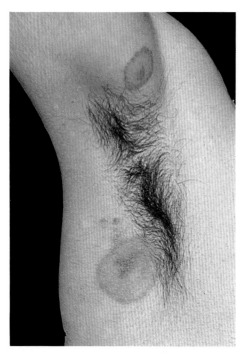

Fig. 286. Round lesions of tinea corporis with pronounced border.

of pityriasis rosea and parapsoriasis, there is a similar arrangement of the two diseases along the lines of cleavage. Secondary syphilis should be considered in pityriasis rosea-like elements of the nodular type before formation of scales has set in. The presence of a herald patch and a lack of palmar and plantar lesions point toward pityriasis rosea. When in doubt the serologic test for syphilis will decide the question. Pityriasiform lesions of some dermatomycoses (lesions of microsporon infections on the trunk will show fungi microscopically) show sharply marginated circular areas with a tendency to central healing (Fig. 286). The small macular, pityriasiform or seborrheic dermatitis lacks the herald patch and the marked arrangement along the lines of cleavage. Compared with pityriasis rosea, the course of seborrheic dermatitis is much more protracted and quiet. However, patches of seborrhea also have peripheral exudation but the typical marginal scales are lacking. Intertriginous areas of moniliasis have a dark red color with peripheral loose scales and corymbiform or satellite lesions in the vicinity; pityriasis rosea lacks similar satellite areas.[1, 2]

(1) Björnberg, A., and L. Hellgren: Pityriasis rosea. Acta derm.-venereol. (Stockh.) *42*, Suppl. 50 (1962).
(2) Burch, P. R. J., and N. R. Rowell: Pityriasis rosea. – an autoaggressive disease? Brit. J. Derm. *82:* 540–560 (1970).

cellular edema, and, to a lesser extent, subcorneal vesicles or abscesses). In addition, the upper cutis presents lymphocytic and histiocytic infiltrates, and sometimes also fibroblasts and eosinophils. All these cells are arranged perivascularly.

The differential diagnosis of pityriasis rosea versus psoriasis and parapsoriasis was discussed in relation to these two diseases. Apart from the different duration

20. Parapsoriasis Group and Mycosis Fungoides

Three disorders, morphologically quite distinct, are called parapsoriasis but do not resemble psoriasis at all. The three are: *pityriasis lichenoides seu acuta* (parapsoriasis guttata), *parapsoriasis en plaques* (Brocq's disease), and *parapsoriasis lichen-* *oides* (parakeratosis variegata). They involve mostly the trunk and only exceptionally the face. Parapsoriasis en plaques and parapsoriasis lichenoides demand a special differential diagnostic discussion with *mycosis fungoides*.

A. Pityriasis Lichenoides

1. Pityriasis lichenoides chronica presents rather monomorphic, exanthematous skin lesions. They are present for years, and therefore are "chronic." They consist of rice-corn-sized lesions, which may occasionally simulate syphilis; in the beginning they are reddish, brown-tinged, about lentil-sized infiltrations, later becoming more coppery red. In the later course of the disease they develop on top a cover, i.e., a whitish or silvery scale, which adheres only in the center and is loose toward the periphery. This creates the characteristic collodion or waferlike scale (Fig. 287). Additional characteristic signs are an absence of pruritus or only mild pruritus and an absence of mucous membrane lesions. Resistance to therapy is striking.

In the differential diagnosis of a typical exanthem psoriasis vulgaris will not be discussed since its chief signs (stratified, easily removable scales, Auspitz's and Koebner's phenomena, predilection for the extensor surfaces, and involvement of the scalp, nails, and sometimes joints) differ considerably from those of pityriasis lichenoides chronica. Signs in favor of maculopapular secondary syphilis are: rather coppery colored reddish brown papules (palms and soles), sensitivity to pressure with a probe,* and the absence of a covering scale. The presence of mucous membrane lesions, enlarged generalized lymph nodes, loss of hair (diffuse, areolar, or at the lateral eyebrows), and positive serology are unequivocally in favor of florid secondary syphilis. Papular or papulonecrotic tuberculids are not distributed indiscriminately but are grouped, favoring the lower half of the body to about the middle of the buttocks, and also the arms. The exanthems of sarcoidosis, if the individual lesions are small and irregu-

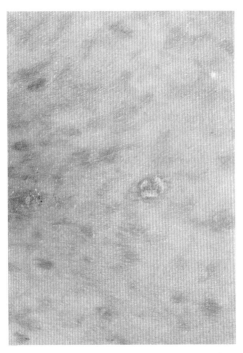

Fig. 287. Pityriasis lichenoides chronica: brownish-red papules with characteristic covering scale.

larly disseminated over the trunk (which they favor), are much smaller than the lesions of parapsoriasis guttata. They are in fact miliary-lichenoid. Besides, the characteristic covering scale is missing.

Lichen planus will have to be differentiated from pityriasis lichenoides chronica only if single lesions have assumed a polygonal aspect in areas that are more distinctly furrowed. Histologically, a distinction is easy.[7]

2. It is doubtful whether **pityriasis lichenoides (et varioliformis) acuta** is the acute form of pityriasis lichenoides chronica because the former is essentially a vasculitis, whereas the chronic form represents a primary disorder of the epidermis. On the other hand, in pityriasis lichenoides chronica vasculitis can occasionally be found histologically and clinically, and in spite of the chronic course

---

* Ollendorff sign. (Tr.)

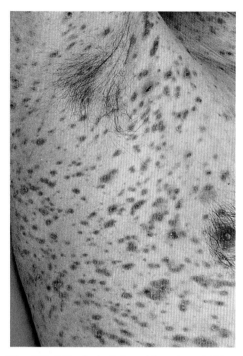 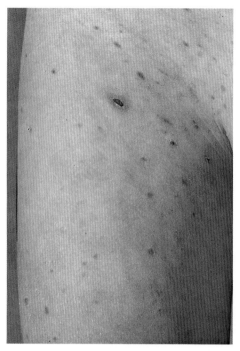

Fig. 288. Pityriasis lichenoides et varioliformis acuta.

Fig. 289. Pityriasis lichenoides et varioliformis acuta.

blistering stages may occur initially or intermittently without causing decisive diversion of such an instance of pityriasis lichenoides chronica from the usual picture.

In general, the course of pityriasis lichenoides acuta proceeds without fever (see also Chapter 1, K3). The apparently underlying "allergic vasculitides" begin in the course of catarrhal infections of the upper respiratory passages and disappear soon after they are healed, following antibiotic therapy. The many lesions appearing in attacks on the trunk and the flexor sides of the extremities show morphologic variations. Involvement of the face, palms and soles, and the mucous membranes is usually not severe, and if present, affects only a few areas. In general, there are in the beginning rice-corn-sized, rose-colored papules, which soon assume a vesicular character and heal with a small scar. In addition, pustular, hemorrhagic, and

necrotic elements of varying intensity can be found (Figs. 288, 289). However, a dramatically impressive course accompanied by large ulceronecrotic or ulcerocrusted lesions and above all, by fever, will only rarely occur.[2, 3, 6, 8, 9]

Histologically, pityriasis chronica lichenoides shows dilated capillaries in the corium, surrounded by masses of lymphocytes. The epidermis itself is edematous and loose and, occasionally, lymphocytes and erythrocytes are interspersed. This is often followed by increasing hemorrhagic infiltration of the epidermis, which finally becomes necrotic. Less acute cases show distinct eczematiform or mycosis fungoideslike substrates (microabscesses), so that the differential diagnostic decision has to be made from the clinical picture.

The predominant vesicular manifestations of pityriasis lichenoides acuta have to be differentiated from those of chickenpox.

The latter, like pityriasis lichenoides
chronica, spares the face and scalp in the
beginning. Chickenpox has no papular
lesions; on the other hand, the dimpled
blister formation is more pronounced.
Occasionally, small nodular, allergic drug
reactions, nodular reactions to insect bites,
multiple nodulo-ulcerating toxoplasmosis,
and necrotizing arteriolitides have to be
considered in the differential diagnosis.[1]

3. Morphologic (but not clinical) similarities can exist between pityriasis lichenoides acuta, *malignant atrophic papulosis*, and thromboangiitis cutaneointesti-
nalis disseminata. In this disorder there
are also eruptions of reddish to porcelain-
white papules of about lentil size. After a
few days, they sink in centrally and become
necrotic so that sharply outlined ulcerations result. The number of lesions varies,
and they are observed in various stages of
development over the entire integument.
Some weeks or months later extremely
painful intestinal signs begin, caused by
multiple microinfarcts of the intestinal
wall. Often also, similar cerebral, renal,
cardiac, or ocular complications occur. The
cause of the entire disorder is an obliterat-
ing and proliferating endovasculitis of the
arterial blood vessels. The medial and
exterior layers of the vessels and the
elastica interna remain unaffected. In the
beginning, necroses of the connective
tissue and deposits of mucin occur in the
neighborhood of the vascular changes;
later there is also fibrosis with only sparse
infiltrations, sometimes by lymphocytes.
In view of the changes of the basic substance a relationship to fibrosing mucinosis
is suggested. The combination with progressive scleroderma has also been observed. In some instances anomalies of the
immunoglobulins (IgA fraction) and increases in the levels of fibrinogen have
been noted.[4, 5, 10]

(1) ANDREEV, V. C., N. ANGELOV and N. B. ZLATKOV: Skin manifestations in toxoplasmosis. Arch. Derm. (Chic.) *100:* 196–199 (1969).
(2) BAZEX, A., A. DUPRÉ, B. CHRISTOL et H. RUMEAU: Érythème circiné pityria-sique bénin de l'enfant: Entité nouvelle? Ann. Derm. Syph. (Paris) *96:* 241–252 (1969).
(3) DEGOS, R., B. DUPERRAT et F. DANIEL: Le parapsoriasis ulcéro-nécrotique hy-perthermique. Ann. Derm. Syph. (Pa-ris) *93:* 481–496 (1966).
(4) DURIE, B. G. M., J. D. STROUD and J. A. KAHN: Progressive systemic sclerosis with malignant atrophic papu-losis. Arch. Derm. (Chic.) *100:* 575–581 (1969).
(5) EICHENBERGER, H., E. LANDOLT und W. WEGMANN: Papulose atrophiante maligne Degos. Schweiz. med. Wschr. *97:* 1639–1649 (1967).
(6) GARTMANN, H., und S. GOERGEN: Pityriasis lichenoides acuta vesiculosa. Arch. klin. exp. Derm. *222:* 115–126 (1965).
(7) MARKS, R., M. BLACK and E. WILSON JONES: Pityriasis lichenoides: a reap-praisal. Brit. J. Derm. *86:* 215–225 (1972).
(8) NASEMANN, TH., R. MARKOWSKI und K. JAKUBOWICZ: Zur histologischen Differentialdiagnose der Pityriasis lichenoides et varioliformis acuta Mucha-Habermann. Hautarzt *17:* 395–399 (1966).
(9) SZYMANSKI, FR. J.: Pityriasis licheno-ides et varioliformis acuta. Arch. Derm. Syph. (Chic.) *79:* 7–16 (1959).
(10) WINKELMANN, R. K., F. M. HOWARD, H. O. PERRY and R. H. MILLER: Malignant papulosis of skin and cere-brum. Arch. Derm. (Chic.) *87:* 54–62 (1963).

B. Parapsoriasis "en Plaques"

In **Brocq's disease** round, oval, and
sometimes polycyclic lesions are present;
they are yellowish-red with relatively
sharp borders. They are preponderantly
localized on the sides of the trunk in the

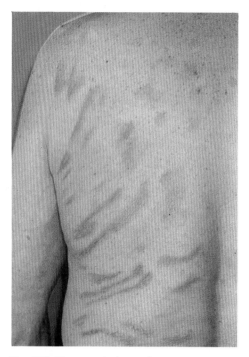

Fig. 290. Parapsoriasis en plaques.

lines of cleavage (Fig. 290). Usually, distinct infiltration is absent. The surface of the lesion is mostly "normal," i.e., smooth or occasionally somewhat rough (Fig. 291). In any case, pronounced scaling is missing. Of diagnostic importance if

present is pseudoatrophic wrinkling, which can be smoothed out if the skin is stretched. Pronounced genuine atrophies ("parapsoriasis atrophicans") are as unusual as pronounced infiltration or distinct pruritus; if these are present, the diagnosis should be in doubt. Rather frequently, however, one observes in the affected areas single, round, flat lichen simplex-like nodules with no roughening of the skin surface. Also significant are relatively frequent interspersions of tiny bleeding points or the apparent disposition to purpura factitia.[2,3]

Thus, a certain similarity to lesions of **progressive pigmentary purpura** (Fig. 292), especially those of the purpura annularis Majocchi type, is evident. It may occasionally appear on the upper half of the body with single lesions. Such purpuric lesions, however, lack the basic yellowish-brown erythematous areas and the atrophy of Brocq's disease. Because of the seborrheic erythematous character of Brocq's disease the differentiation from seborrheic dermatitis or psoriasiform seborrhea may be important. The yellowish-brownish erythematous areas of microbic-seborrheic dermatitis are, however, more sharply limited because there is a characteristic peripheral maximum exudation (discrete

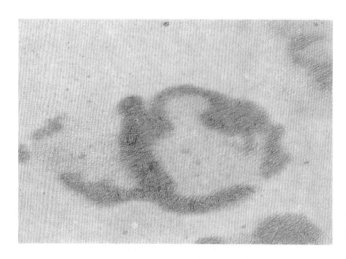

Fig. 291. Parapsoriasis en plaques with transition into mycosis fungoides.

spongiosis and parakeratosis). Moreover, it favors the anterior and posterior sweat lines and the medial facial parts or intertriginous regions and not the lines of cleavage. In addition, its development is quite often dependent on preceding pyogenic foci (furuncles, sweat gland abscesses, or others), whereas in parapsoriasis "en plaques" we are dealing with an eruption which from the beginning is adynamic and apparently independent of any other pathologic influences. Pityriasis rosea likewise is located along the lines of cleavage in the direction of the axillas and also spares the face but it is characterized by its heraldic spot, the special "collarette," and most of all by its short duration, whereas Brocq's disease persists torpidly for years.

Of practical importance is the differentiation from mycosis fungoides. This disorder is accompanied by an often unbearable, or at least severely interfering, itching and later shows a relatively rapid change of manifestations with regard to site and appearance. In this fashion an "eczematous mycosis stage" appears which may suggest Brocq's disease, especially if infiltrations or tumors are absent. If, in addition, instead of the usual clinical picture, streaks and only a few polycyclic

smooth erythemas are found in the first stages, the difficulty is increased. In such an instance severe eosinophilia of the blood strongly supports a decision in favor of mycosis fungoides. Even histologically, early Brocq's disease simulates mycosis fungoides, since both show the picture of a "dermatitis." (See the chapter on mycosis fungoides for additional microscopic differentiation.) In some ways, edema of the upper corium and areas of hydropic degeneration in the basal cell line are typical of Brocq's disease. Relatively monotonous lymphoreticular cell types may predominate in the dermal infiltrate with missing or only a few mast cells, which invade the epidermis only slightly.[1]

(1) ILLIG, L., und K. W. KALKOFF: Zum Formenkreis der Purpura pigmentosa progressiva (unter besonderer Berücksichtigung der Adalin-Purpura). Hautarzt *21*: 497–505 (1970).

(2) MUSGER, A.: Zur Frage nach der nosologischen Stellung der Parapsoriasis lichenoides Brocq. Hautarzt *17*: 280–284 (1966).

(3) SAMMAN, P. D.: The natural history of parapsoriasis en plaques (chronic superficial dermatitis) and prereticulotic poikiloderma. Brit. J. Derm. *87*: 405–411 (1972).

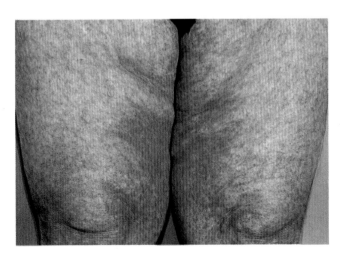

Fig. 292. Progressive pigmented purpura.

C. Parapsoriasis Lichenoides

In the disorder usually called **parakeratosis variegata,** but also reported as lichen variegatus, a mosaic of striated or reticular elements, not so much polygonal as roundish, is observed. Suggesting lichen planus papules, they are pinhead-sized, shiny or slightly scaling, and have a tendency toward regression with delicate atrophy (Fig. 293). During its course or in the end stage, the papular formations disappear and telangiectases together with pigmentations predominate in their place, so that more poikilodermalike changes develop. The course is extremely chronic, and itching or other disturbances of general well-being are usually absent. Rather striking, however, is the resistence to the usual treatment methods of this form of parapsoriasis also. It is possible that the changes described as parakeratosis variegata in some patients represent the

Fig. 293. Parakeratosis variegata.

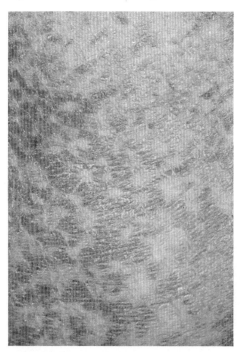

reticular change of pityriasis lichenoides. In other cases the origin seems to have been Brocq's disease. Quite often, however, development to mycosis fungoides occurs, so that in these cases parapsoriasis lichenoides is only a variant of mycosis fungoides. Corresponding with this macroscopic heterogeneity of the individual cases are the various histologic findings. The atrophic epidermis in places shows parakeratosis, the borderline between the epidermis and the corium is loose, and the basal cell line is hydropicly degenerated. The papillary layer shows infiltrates of lymphohistiocytes, which press against the epidermis and sometimes even invade it. Occasionally, neutrophils, plasma cells, or mast cells are also found in these cell masses. Rather regularly, a distinct dilatation of densely filled capillaries is present.

The fully developed picture of parapsoriasis lichenoides can, therefore, be easily diagnosed because of the manifestations listed, but occasionally changes of the single components are similar to those of lichen planus. However, the absence of mucous membrane lesions and the verrucous character of lesions on the legs and other locations always permit the correct diagnosis. It has already been mentioned that early mycosis fungoides may resemble parapsoriasis lichenoides. Not even the complete absence of pruritus or any infiltration can rule out the presence of a premycosis. Yellowish-brownish, streaky, and moderately infiltrated erythemas, interspersed with purpuric and telangiectatic lesions of the character of parapsoriasis lichenoides, were observed after repeated doses of nitrofurantoin (Fig. 294).[1]

(1) Korting, G. W., und R. Denk: Retikuläre Hyperplasie der Haut durch ein Hydantoin-Derivat. Derm. Wschr. 152: 257–262 (1966).

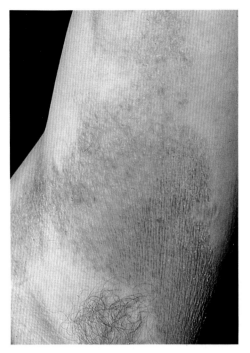 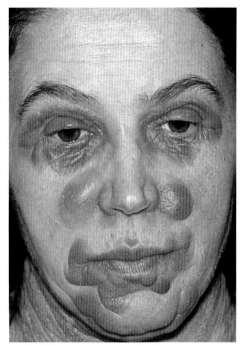

Fig. 294. Reticular hyperplasia from nitrofurantoin simulating parapsoriasis en plaques.

Fig. 295. Mycosis fungoides, tumor stage.

D. Mycosis Fungoides

Mycosis fungoides (granuloma fungoides) occurs in later life, starting between the fourth and sixth decades without preference to either sex. If the course is classic, the initial stage usually consists of violently itching eczematizations of varyingly pronounced prurigo character. Later, lichenifications and perhaps also spinulosism (with or without follicular mucinosis) may be present. The site and character of the manifestations can change astonishingly fast. After the stage of flat or nodose infiltrations of mycosis fungoides (Fig. 296), the third phase appears: tumors, which often are characteristically notched, develop and spill their contents overnight like spoiled tomatoes (Fig. 295). Only in rare cases does mycosis fungoides appear as flat erythroderma (see also Chapter 22,

C8). "Mycose d'emblée" seems to represent a reticuloendothelial sarcoma. In contrast to lymphogranulomatosis, of which mycosis fungoides has often been considered to be the cutaneous manifestation, enlarged lymph nodes are insignificant and eosinophilia, if it occurs at all, is transitory. Anemia and diarrhea, however, are present.[1,2]

Only in the beginning is a dermatitis present in the histologic picture. Only if the infiltration in the upper corium is pronounced does the epidermis react with irregular acanthosis, or, if the adjacent or invading infiltrate is more advanced, with atrophic flattening of the epithelial band. In addition, the epidermis of mycosis fungoides is characterized by formations of blisters and abscesses and an abundance of mitoses. Corresponding to this clinical polymorphism, the histologic picture shows

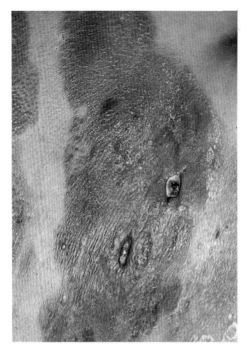

Fig. 296. Mycosis fungoides: plaquelike infiltrates with ulcerations and spinulosism.

cell masses consisting of lymphocytes, histiocytes, granulocytes, and plasma cells. Increased mitoses, which occasionally are present in inflammatory infiltrates with no specific character, are not as definitely pathognomonic as the presence of so-called mycosis cells. They are atypical reticulum cells characterized by large, irregularly contoured, and chromatin-dense nuclei. Pautrier's microabscesses of mycosis fungoides are composed of lymphocytes and histiocytes. They are predominantly present in the squamous cell layer, i.e., below Munro's neutrophilic microabscesses of the stratum corneum in psoriasis.

(1) BENNEK, J.: Mycosis fungoides innerer Organe. Zbl. Haut- u. Geschl.-Kr. *60:* 1–21 (1939).
(2) BETTINGEN, CH.: Über hochgradige Eosinophilie bei Mykosis fungoides. Med. Welt *18* (N.F.): 2507–2508 (1968).

21. Eczematous Cutaneous Changes

The diagnosis of "eczema" can be made with certainty only histologically. In the beginning the microscopic picture shows chiefly areas of suprabasal spongiosis, i.e., an intercellular edema of the epidermis. This spongiosis is followed by the development of vesicles. Other histologically less characteristic findings are areas of parakeratosis, acanthosis, development of edema of the upper layers of the corium, and migration of lymphocytes into the epidermis. From an etiologic and phenomenological point of view, the various forms of eczema, besides dermatitis, are divided into three main groups: (1) common eczema, (2) seborrheic dermatitis, and (3) atopic dermatitis (diffuse neurodermatitis). Eczematous erythrodermas will be discussed in Chapter 22, B.

A. Dermatitis

Macroscopically, **dermatitis** appears as superficial areas of continuous erythema

Fig. 297. Dermatitis following light sensibilization by
dimethylchlortetracycline.

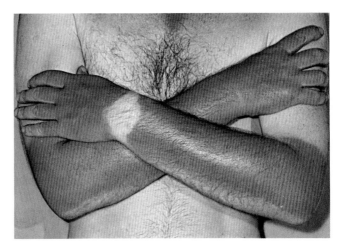

lacking interspersion with irregular nodular (papulovesicular) lesions (Figs. 297, 298).
Bullous and erosive lesions may be present
but we find in contrast to eczema, not a
juxtaposition of efflorescences of a different
character (synchronous polymorphism) but
a succession of reactive lesions (metachronous polymorphism). Because a dermatitis is always due to a contact agent,
the elimination of the noxious agent will
result in spontaneous remission. Therefore,
signs of acute exudative dermatitic inflammation will be confined to the site of
the damaging agent. If the history remains
unclear or doubtful as to the cause of the
dermatitis, epicutaneous patch tests will
be helpful. Corresponding to the localization of a dermatitis, different differential
diagnostic problems will arise; a compilation arranged in topographical order will
follow.

1. A dermatitis of the **face** may assume
monstrous edematous forms around the
eyes; i.e., a dermatitis due to cold-wave
applications which will also involve the
scalp. The face especially reacts to contact
substances applied accidentally by rubbing
with the hands which have been exposed
to noxious compounds (for instance, anti-
rheumatic creams). The thicker skin of the

hands, washed more frequently, may not
react to such a compound, and this fact
has to be considered when taking the
history. Perioral contact dermatitis may
be due to cosmetics such as lipsticks,

Fig. 298. Sunburn.

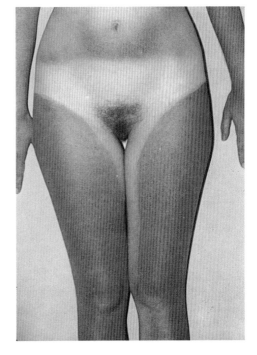

perfume, nail polish (especially in nail biters), drugs, or synthetic fabrics.

A differentiation from erysipelas can be made because this disorder will be accompanied by severe signs (chills and fever). A dermatitis will soon show "epidermal" participation (i.e., scale formation as an epidermal change), whereas erysipelas either lacks scaling or will show it very late. Necrotizing, gangrenous changes are characteristic in erysipelas of the aged.

Facial *herpes zoster* may start with a dermatitislike erythema. Concomitant or premonitory painful sensations, the early appearance of pinhead-sized vesicular lesions, and limitation of the erythematous reaction to one of the branches of the trigeminal nerve will easily permit a differentiation from a dermatitis.

Quincke's edema as a rule lacks an erythema and also fails to show participation of the epidermis; in addition, the edematous swelling is more homogeneous and not confined to the "softer" (periocular) regions (see Chapter 10, A1). For *perioral rosacealike dermatitis* see Chapter 18, E6 and Chapter 30, B2.

2. The region of the **ear** shows the so-called *otitis externa;* a voluminous collection of many nosologically heterogeneous conditions comprising a large number of possibilities for contact dermatitis; among others, earphone dermatitis, disinfectants, soaps, cosmetics containing perfumes, "ear drops" containing resorcin, mercury, phenol, antibiotics, benzocaine, and many more. An acute otitis externa might be caused by a beginning furuncle. Severe pain accompanying a furuncle and the early follicular formation of pus will quickly permit a correct diagnosis.

Recurrent inflammations of the cartilage of the pinna of both ears with inflammatory erythema are a leading sign of *polychondritis chronica atrophicans.* Within the framework of this systemic, autoaggressive disease of the cartilage, similar inflammatory signs are observed on the nose and joints (see also Chapter 1, J4). In addition, wine-red to steel-blue hues of the pinna with only moderate infiltration may suggest *frostbite. Vernal photosensitivity dermatitis* presents bullous elevated lesions containing serous fluid along the helix of the pinna.[2, 3, 4]

Circumscribed redness of the pinna is seen in the initial stage of herpes zoster oticus as part of the Ramsay Hunt syndrome. The subsequent vesicular eruption affects, in most cases, the inner region of the pinna or the preauricular region. Neurologic signs are facial paralysis, hemilateral disturbance of taste and of the vestibulocochlearis nerve.

3. Typical contact dermatitis of the **extremities,** especially of the axillae, is primarily caused by deodorants, soaps, dress shields, depilatories, perfumes, and many other agents. Thermometers put into the axillary fold may cause dermatitis due to traces of the disinfectant fluid used for sterilizing thermometers in a jar. The matchbook dermatitis that affects the upper thighs but not the scrotum is caused by phosphorsesquisulfide present on the striking surface of a matchbox carried in a trousers pocket.* Vesicular characteristics of a dermatitis point to the possibility of a *phytogenic cause* (acanthus leaves, parsnip, poison ivy, and similar plants). A linear bullous eruption is caused mostly by plants containing furocoumarins and subsequent sun exposure** (Fig. 299). However, contact with some parts of a plant may cause a dry, hyperkeratotic "eczematous dermatitis" from the beginning. Such "onion

---

* Or by loose matches carried in a shirt pocket near the chest. Both sites are more frequently affected in summer when no underwear is worn. (Tr.)

** Wild grasses and the plant families Umbelliferae, Rutaceae, and Moraceae. (Tr.)

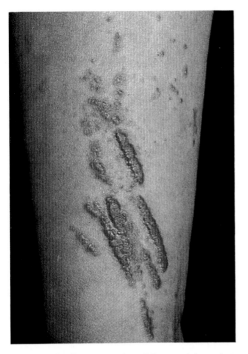

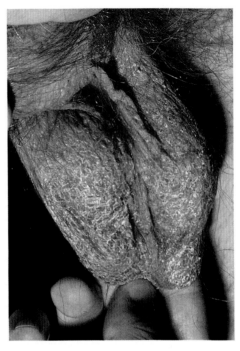

Fig. 299. Bullous streaks of dermatitis striata pratensis (from meadow grass [*Agrimonia eupatoria*]. Tr.)

Fig. 300. Pellagroid dermatitis of scrotum caused by deficiency of lactoflavin.

fingers" are caused by contact, not only with onions, but also with bulbs of tulips, hyacinths, or garlic or by peeling (not eating) citrus fruits.[1, 5, 6, 8, 9]

Grouped vesicular dermatitis may be caused by contact with caterpillars. Touching jellyfish causes aspiclike edematous reactions (dermatitis medusica).[7]

4. Contact dermatitis of the **genitoanal region** in the male was seen formerly quite frequently after the application of mercury ointments for the treatment of pubic lice. Similarly, scrotal dermatitis not infrequently is caused by contact with noxious substances present on the hands; the likelihood of such a substance being the cause is enhanced if there is a dermatitis venenata on some fingers at the same time. However, a contact dermatitis of the vulvar region will lead to a search for external causes

(cosmetics, intravaginally applied medicaments, contraceptive agents, pessaries, and others).

If the scrotum alone and not the genitocrural regions or the penis is affected by a dermatitis, it will be necessary to consider *pellagrous scrotal dermatitis* (Fig. 300). When prisoners of war in the Second World War presented such a dermatitis, it was diagnosed as "deficiency scrotal dermatitis"; in reality, however, it was an ariboflavinosis. In addition, other signs of vitamin-B deficiency are often present: angular stomatitis, folliculolichenoid hyperkeratoses of the nasolabial fold, and koilonychia. In contrast, pellagrous vulvitis has a dirty brown, thickly lamellar, scaling, rhagadiform-hyperkeratotic erythematous formation which is seldom observed even in endemic pellagrous regions. Such seborrheic dermatitis of the scrotum and vulva has been observed

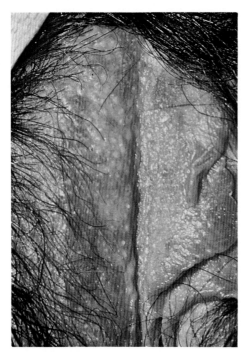

Fig. 301. Granular thrush vulvitis.

also after plentiful consumption of red beets.

Well known is the development of irritations of the genitals from dermatitic to eczematous processes (i.e., to a large extent they are autonomous continued disease processes) due to latent or manifest diabetes; the amount of sugar in the urine in addition to that present in perspiration and in the skin itself encourages the development of eczematous changes.

Vulvitis erysipelatosa acuta is a post-partum complication; otherwise, erysipelas of the genital region can be mistaken at first for an acute dermatitis. In erysipelas the soft vaginal tissue reacts with profound edema. Generalized signs, tenderness of the regional lymph nodes, and lack of epidermal changes from the beginning argue in favor of erysipelas.

Monilial vulvitis can also be confused with dermatitis venenata (Fig. 301); moniliasis of the vulva may occur without

diabetes and nowadays is especially frequent due to the application of vaginal sprays and medication with antibiotics. As a rule, monilial vaginitis develops after mycotic colpitis or an infection of a partner. The light- to dark-red edematous mucosa of the vulva shows plaquelike, grayish-white areas, usually combined with a considerable amount of whitish, crumbly, vaginal discharge. However, pustular lesions are seen less frequently. Small monilial areas arranged closely together like satellites show the characteristic fine scaly border. The genitocrural folds show more plaquelike, highly red, moist, shiny, erosive erythematous areas. A definite diagnosis is easily made by finding fungus elements microscopically stained by methylene blue.

Chronic *plasmacellular balanoposthitis* has blood-red or chocolate-brown patches on the mucosa of the genitals (see Chapter 38, I2). This condition must be differentiated carefully from Bowen's disease of the mucous membrane* (see also Chapter 38, I1).

(1) BRETT, R.: Neuere Beobachtungen über Streichholzschachteldermatitis. Z. Haut-u. Geschl.-Kr. *7:* 343–345 (1949).

(2) HARDERS, H.: Eine seltene Knorpel-erkrankung als Kollagenkrankheit. Acta med. scand. (Stockh.) *154,* Suppl. *313:* 442–445 (1956).

(3) LANG, H. D., D. MÜLLER und J. FINKE: Rezidivierende Polychondritis mit Aortenaneurysmen. Jaksch-Wartenhorst-v. Meyenburg-Altherr-Uehlinger-Syndrom. Dtsch. med. Wschr. *94:* 2033 bis 2040 (1969).

(4) NITZSCHNER, H., O. PETTER und K. SCHLENTHER: Polychondritis reci-divans et atrophicans. Derm. Mschr. *156:* 789–797 (1970).

(5) ROOK, A.: Plant dermatitis. The significance of variety-specific sensitization. Brit. J. Derm. *73:* 283–287 (1961).

_____

* And from erythroplasia Queyrat. (Tr.)

(6) ROOK, A.: Plant dermatitis in general practice. Practitioner *188:* 627–638 (1962).

(7) RORSMAN, H.: Caterpillar dermatitis. Acta derm.-venereol.(Stockh.)*50:*74–76 (1970).

(8) STOLTZE, R.: Dermatitis medicamentosa in eczema of the leg. Acta derm.-venereol. (Stockh.) *46:* 54–64 (1966).

(9) VERSPYCK MIJNSSEN, G. A. W.: Pathogenesis and causative agent of »tulip finger«. Brit. J. Derm. *81:* 737–745 (1969).

B. Common Eczema

Common eczema, primarily caused externally, macroscopically shows a distinctly nodular, discontinuous dermatitis. Although common eczema lacks a definite or singular primary lesion, the papular vesicle plays the main role as an intermediate characteristic lesion. The sliding scale of lesions seen with synchronous and metachronous polymorphic eczema is composed of erythematous, papular, vesicular, pustular, moist, crusted, squamous efflorescences. In contrast to these lesions, even larger, circumscribed eczematous areas will show, at least at the edge, the original discontinuity of isolated single lesions. Another characteristic of plain eczema is pruritus which is almost always present.

Like dermatitis venenata, common eczema is caused by an exogenous noxious agent brought into contact with the skin.* However, in contrast to dermatitis venenata in which only one contact is required to provoke the cutaneous response, common eczema calls for prior preparation of the skin. Therefore, the eczematous reaction is confined to the sensitized cutaneous area, and only after the hypersensitivity reaction has become more widespread will there be a response in other places. Diagnostic proof of a specific eczematous cause is furnished by patch tests. One must keep in mind that such a test requires 24 to 72 hours before the eczematous reaction takes place. On the other hand, the sensitization may still be confined to the eczematous area, with the result that the test site at a distance from the involved area will not have been sensitized. Therefore, it will be necessary to repeat the patch test later on the healed eczematous area.[2]

Histopathologically, the epidermis shows intercellular edema (spongiosis), minimal intracellular edema ("altération cavitaire"), and, above all, vesiculation and acanthosis with parakeratosis of many cells. In contrast to dermatitis herpetiformis with its lack of spongiosis, pronounced eosinophilia and subepidermal formation of vesicles are absent in common eczema.

Common eczema quite often shows considerable deviation from the usual appearance, with its acute polymorphous, principally nodular, manifestation and later in its monomorphous chronic phase. *Eczema vulgare rubrum* has a more or less chronic, moderately infiltrated and plaquelike eczematous appearance; in the main it resembles an erythema with a smooth, shiny surface.

Nummular eczema is characterized by a chronic, fixed, papulovesicular, plaquelike, sharply circumscribed, occasionally crusted or squamous eczematous area in contrast to the ill-defined border of common eczema. Nummular eczema shows centrally some regression, resembling a mycotic lesion in this respect. However, in contrast to real mycosis, it is especially remarkable that an external irritant will cause a papulovesicular flare-up of the previously healed center of an area of nummular eczema. If the clinical picture suggests beginning mycosis fungoides, histologic examination will show atypical histiocytes, mitoses, decayed

---

* Americans use the term dermatitis venenata when the causative agent has been in contact with the skin. In the following section "dermatitis venenata" has been used in place of "common eczema" when appropriate. (Tr.)

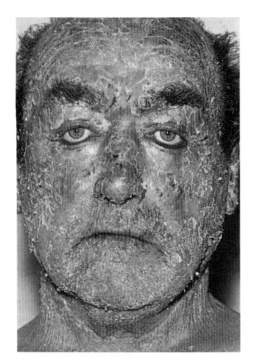

Fig. 302. Sun dermatitis.

hepatic porphyrias do not cause eczematous reactions.*

Solar eczemas are caused by a number of etiologically different disease processes; they all are limited to light-exposed skin and are aggravated by increased sunlight exposure. The face, front, side and nape of the neck and the radial aspect of the hands at first show macular, urticarial eruptions which then become papulovesicular. They quickly increase, becoming more widespread, highly edematous areas. After longer duration, the face especially will resemble a bulging infiltration with either a dry scaly surface or an erosive, moist, and secondarily pyodermic appearance (Fig. 302). Subjectively, solar eczema in accordance with its eczematous character is accompanied by severe pruritus. Histologically, an enormous lymphocytic infiltration, especially around the superficial vascular plexus, can be seen. An early phase shows only a pronounced erythematous and edematous change of the papillary body, occasionally with a slight vacuolization of the basal cell layer. Such cases, especially when follicular hyperkeratoses are lacking, may resemble chronic systemic lupus erythematosus. However, if the infiltrate shows marked cellular uniformity and less perivascular involvement toward the deeper corium one should consider in differential diagnosis actinic reticulocytosis (Fig. 303). Etiologically, in every case of solar eczema one must exclude pellagra (see also Chapter 24, D3), an erythrocytic disorder of porphyrin metabolism, photosensitivity due to drugs, and actinoreticulosis (see also Chapter 22, C6).

Actinic cheilitis with an acute beginning may have a certain eczematous character (Fig. 304). However, in most cases actinic cheilitis starts as a vesiculobullous eruption and will change into a chronic exfoliative condition only after longer duration. The

or clumped nuclei, and Pautrier's microabscesses. *Tylotic or callous eczema* is seen primarily on palms and soles. In addition to a small degree of inflammation, it presents an extended area of hyperkeratosis that causes considerable difficulty in differential diagnosis; see the section on lesions of the extremities, Chapter 21, B6.

The numerous differential diagnostic possibilites of common eczema will be discussed by grouping them from a topographical point of view. The number of potential noxious substances that might trigger an outbreak of eczema is so large that an attempt should be made to narrow the number down by defining the location of the lesions.

1. Eczematous lesions affecting the **face** are due above all to sensitivity reactions provoked by light. Such reactions may be the result of an endogenous increase of porphyrin, i.e., in *sideroachestric* (sideroblastic) *anemia*. In contrast, the different

---

* Protoporphyria may cause eczematous reactions. (Tr.)

seasonal character of actinic cheilitis points to its phototoxic cause. Chronic systemic lupus erythematosus is formed occasionally at the vermilion border of the lips. Here it appears as a cloudy epithelium with short radial lines interspersed with white hyperkeratotic punctate lesions, and the lips are also split by painful rhagades. In *systemic lupus erythematosus* the outer lips may have vesiculobullous or exudative crusted changes; however, in contrast to *erythema multiforme*, the erythematous color is not as darkly hemorrhagic and there is less formation of crusts. In addition, there is little excessive salivation or offensive mouth odor. Erythema multiforme may sometimes show a scalelike, pseudomembranous coating. Seriously ill patients with excessive salivation may have an eczematous dermatitis around the mouth caused by the macerating effect of the saliva.

Monilial cheilitis, seen in cachectic cancer patients or in patients with pemphigus, produces a generally granular appearance sometimes with membranous lesions resembling spilled milk; such a picture will exclude an ordinary eczema of the lips. In addition, such a monilia cheilitis either will be confined to the corners of the mouth or will start from these corners. In spite of this appearance,

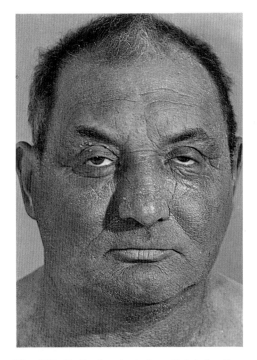

Fig. 303. Reticulocytosis from light, "actino-reticulosis."

one should not neglect to confirm the diagnosis by a search for monilia. Other causes of *perléche* in the adult are the aforementioned candidiasis caused by basic disorders such as subacidity or anacidity of gastric secretion, ariboflavinosis

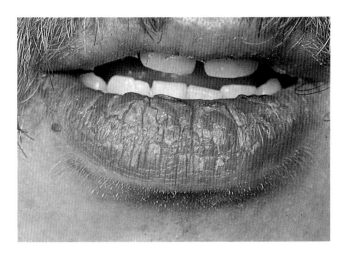

Fig. 304. Actinic cheilitis.

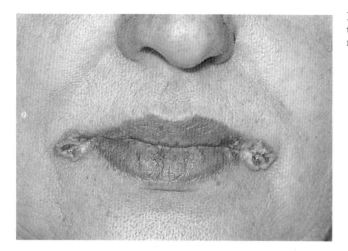

Fig. 305. Pemphigus vegetans at the angles of the mouth.

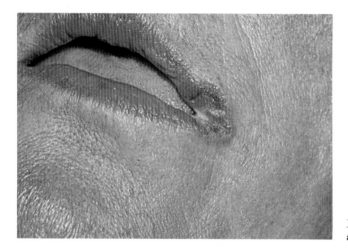

Fig. 306. "Perlèche" in agranulocytosis.

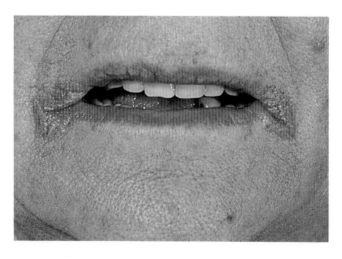

Fig. 307. Acanthosis nigricans at the angles of the mouth.

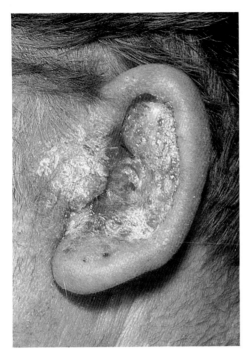

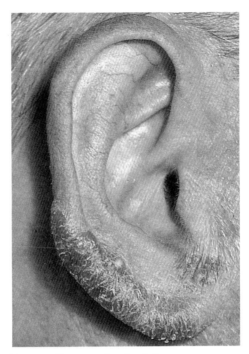

Fig. 308. Common eczema of the ear.

Fig. 309. Lupus vulgaris of the ear.

Fig. 310. Acanthosis nigricans of the inner part of the auricle.

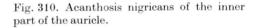

(for instance, with diabetes mellitus), badly fitting dentures, and other similar conditions. In especially stubborn cases, one must look for underlying congenital fistulas of the corners of the mouth. Children usually show a variation of pyoderma, streptococcic or otherwise (angulus infectiosus oris); strangely enough, rarely is there a simultaneous impetigo contagiosa of the face. A chronic exudative, crusted disease process of the lips with vegetating lesions extending into the oral mucosa, interspersed with many pustules, suggests *chronic pemphigus vegetans* (pyostomatitis vegetans) (Fig. 305).[13, 15, 17, 23]

2. Chronic eczematous changes of the **ear** may be due to *bacterial* or *mycotic* infections (Fig. 308). This eczematous reaction can be prolonged more or less indefinitely by the therapeutic application of potent medicaments. Occasionally, a markedly squamous *lupus vulgaris* may be

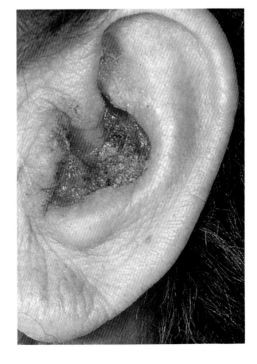

confused with eczema* (Fig. 309). *Chronic systemic lupus erythematosus* of the ear can also be confused with eczema. Lesions that healed with scar formation and especially with mutilation are not of eczematous origin. The pinna and the external auditory canal often show eczemalike cutaneous diseases easily diagnosed in other locations, but here they have lost their typical appearance; examples of such diseases are psoriasis vulgaris, dyskeratosis follicularis congenita, and acanthosis nigricans (Fig. 310). However, the solitary occurrence of these dermatoses confined to the pinna or the ear canal will hardly ever be observed; usually, the presence of the same cutaneous disease in other locations will help to establish the correct diagnosis.

3. The **trunk** itself shows areas of dermatitis venenata much more rarely than other parts of the body. Some possible causes are contact with metallic parts (nickel, chromium) of underwear, impregnation of clothing with dyes, synthetic fabrics, and substances used on the body

---

* The soft, specific infiltrate of lupus vulgaris is easily depressed with a blunt probe, which will painlessly sink into the tissue; diascopic examination shows apple jelly-colored infiltrates. (Tr.)

for personal hygiene. Marked symmetry of eczematous lesions may mask *dermatitis herpetiformis*. Lesions that occupy a place between eczema and dermatitis herpetiformis and lesions in the transitory monomorphous phase observed in prurigo and dermatitis herpetiformis are not subject to provocation by giving potassium iodide. In addition to the symmetrical appearance of lesions in dermatitis herpetiformis, the multiplicity of diseased areas, concomitant eosinophilia, appearance of vesicles, lack of proof of epicutaneous sensibilization, and the histologic picture will permit a definite differentiation from eczema.[6, 19]

Subcorneal pustular dermatosis is similar in its symmetrical distribution to dermatitis herpetiformis; during its course subcorneal dermatosis can be mistaken for common eczema. For further details see the chapter on pustular dermatoses (Chapter 26, H).

The differential diagnosis of the common eczema of the **mamillary region** requires special discussion. In its form as dermatitis venenata, it almost always affects both breasts and, like external dermatitis of the trunk, it may be caused by cosmetics, dyes, synthetic fibers, and externally applied medications (i.e., antibiotic oint-

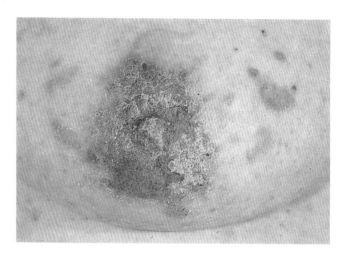

Fig. 311. Eczematized scabetic burrows of the mamillary region.

Fig. 312. Paget's disease.

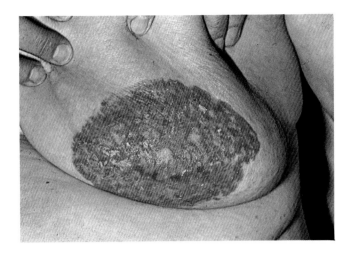

ments). Every mamillary eczema lasting more than six weeks without therapeutic response should have a biopsy in order to exclude malignancy. A unilateral eczematous lesion requires a biopsy at an earlier date. If the area is very pruritic, examination for scabies should be performed (Fig. 311). The elevated pruritic papular lesions of scabies are often difficult to see because of secondary pyodermic infection and may easily be mistaken for eczematous changes. However, a search for *Acarus scabiei* at the sites of predilection of scabies, chiefly the interdigital webs of the hands, the anterior axillary folds, and the penis, and in children also the soles and palms, will easily verify the diagnosis (see also Chapter 2, C1).

Fox-Fordyce disease, favoring the areolae of both breasts, presents small, pinhead-sized, level to conical, mostly flesh-colored, pruritic papules. Even after long duration, the follicular papules remain isolated and show neither lichenification nor pigmentation. In addition to the mamillary region, other regions with apocrine glands – i.e., the axillae, umbilicus, and anogenital region – can be sites of the disease; it affects women almost exclusively.

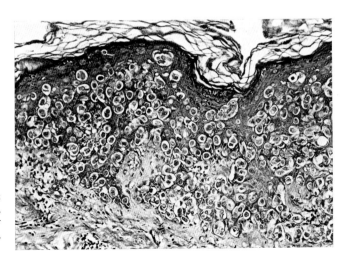

Fig. 313. Paget's disease: strictly intraepidermal, large, blisterous cells with visibly empty cytoplasm. HE stain, 150 ×.

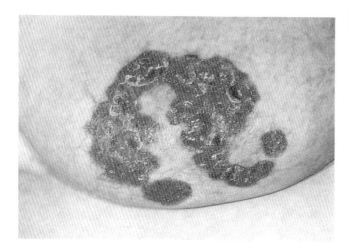

Fig. 314. Bowen's disease of
the mamillary region.

Paget's disease of the nipple starts usually unilaterally with redness, oozing, and desquamation, suggestive of a typical eczematoid dermatitis. There is an absence of pruritus and papulovesicular elements (Figs. 312, 313). The lack of obvious irritating substances as etiologic factors and the sharp outline of the affected area make it possible to differentiate this conditon from a common eczema. The Paget lesion keeps enlarging, and its dark red color sometimes suggests erysipelas; the eruption assumes curved, polycyclic, slightly elevated borders. The surface often is finely granular or oozing, and the nipple becomes increasingly retracted. In the rare extramammary location of Paget's disease that affects other apocrine regions there is sometimes a papillomatous, vegetating border. Histologically, one sees characteristic tumor cells growing intraepidermally. The typical Paget cell shows a large clear-staining, vesiclelike nucleus and a cytoplasm which is lighter than the surrounding (smaller) prickle cells. Intercellular bridges are absent. A peculiar feature of the Paget cell is the fact that it takes a PAS-positive diastase-resistant stain; this is due less to the presence of glycogen then to neutral mucopolysaccharides. In contrast to Bowen's disease, Paget's disease presents no dyskeratoses. It is important to distinguish Paget's disease from early melanoma. In Paget's disease, the cells are not arranged in nests; they occur in sweat and sebaceous glands, and also in the large lactiferous ducts. In addition, they show purely intraepidermal growth, are dopa-negative, and present the previously mentioned diastase-resistant PAS-reactivity.[10]

Clinically, at least at times, there is an undisputed similarity of Paget's disease and an eczema; in addition, the mammary as well as the extramammary location of Paget's disease must be distinguished from Bowen's disease; however, as a rule this distinction can only be done by histologic examination (Fig. 314).

Clinically, Paget's disease almost always favors the female sex, whereas Bowen's disease is not restricted to either sex. Beyond this, Paget's disease shows a marked predilection for the mammary region while Bowen's dermatosis is topographically a ubiquitous disease with no particular localization in the region of the breast.

Primary cancer of the nipple may start in the same fashion as Paget's disease with pre-eczematous changes; the location is always unilateral. During the course of the

Fig. 315. Neviform keratosis of the areola mammae.

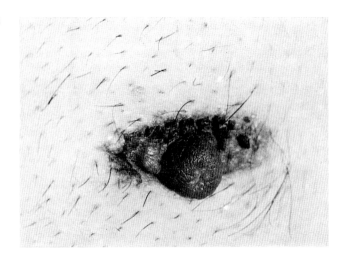

disease the nipple will enlarge and sometimes may ulcerate. Frequently, however, only hardening of the nipple can be palpated. Bloody or serous discharges are rather the exception than a regular finding. The clinical picture may suggest a diagnosis of cancer of the nipple but this must be proven histologically. This cancer may start either from keratinizing squamous epithelium ("deranged keratinocytes" of Pinkus) or from transitional cell epithelium. On the other hand, the epithelium of the mammary ducts or of sebaceous glands of the nipple may be the starting point for cancer.[3, 5]

The differential diagnosis of cancer of the nipple as opposed to erosive **adenomatosis** of the same organ can be extremely difficult clinically and histologically; however, a definite diagnosis is of great importance for the therapy. Like the previously mentioned pathological conditions, adenomatosis is located unilaterally; frequently it is misdiagnosed as one-sided eczema of the mamilla. Discharge of a secretion from the nipple, only slight in duration and of uncharacteristic redness and sometimes combined with erosions, presents an ambiguous clinical picture. The final diagnosis requires histologic examination.[7, 25, 27]

Circumscribed keratoses of the areola can be mistaken for eczema only when inspected superficially; these keratoses lack an erythematous base and papulovesicular elements. The nevoid **keratosis of the areola of the breast** is a nevoid birth defect almost always seen only in women. In this disease the areolar region proper shows light to dark-brown hyperkeratoses which usually appear for the first time during puberty (Fig. 315). The differential diagnosis must include development of keratoses of the mamilla due to application of ointments containing estrogenic hormone.[21, 22]

Otherwise, most skin diseases, especially erythrodermas, do not affect the areolar region. This is true not only for psoriasis vulgaris, pityriasis rubra pilaris, and circumscribed scleroderma but also for systemic leukoses (leukemias) and reticulogranulomatoses (i.e., mycosis fungoides); such lack of reaction of the areola of the breast (however, not without exception) is quite remarkable.[11]

4. The **axillae** may develop a dermatitis following contact with many substances. As examples of the innumerable possibilities one may mention deodorants, depilatories, hair dyes, and disinfectants (for

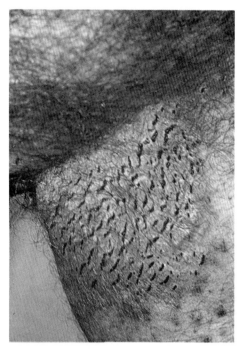

Fig. 316. Benign chronic familial pemphigus: macerated areas on the inner aspect of the thighs with rhagadiform erosions.

In addition, the axillae present an array of eczematiform cutaneous diseases of completely heterogeneous etiologic and pathologic origin. These conditions can be identified in most cases because they also occur in similar fashion in other locations, for instance, *Fox-Fordyce disease* discussed before with diseases of the mamilla.

In *chronic familial pemphigus*, characteristic manifestations are present especially in the axillae and the genitoinguinal region (Figs. 316, 317). Other favorite sites are the sides and back of the neck and intertriginous locations. Relatively sharply circumscribed erythemas, which are distinctly dependent on heat and humidity (thus, perspiration), are present; their epithelial cover is slightly darkened, and they are traversed by thin, parallel erosions. A collarette at the periphery and satellite lesions as in intertriginous candidiasis are missing. If there is a greater tendency toward sweating, groups of minimal blisters occur also on the trunk (mostly on the back). The blisters are usually observed later as small erosions

instance, mercury bichloride solutions used for sterilizing thermometers used in the axilla). Deodorant sticks contain zirconium, which causes inflammatory reactions with a granulomatous character.*[24]

* Zirconium deodorant granulomas. Zirconium salts should be avoided because they are sensitizers. (Tr.)

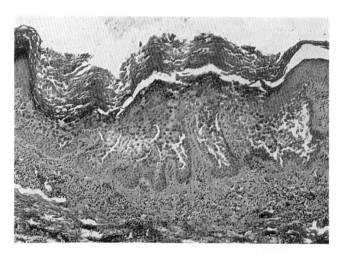

Fig. 317. Benign chronic familial pemphigus: preponderantly suprabasal intraepidermal acantholytic cleavage. HE stain, 25×.

covered with a crust. The explanation is that the appearance of the blister is always accompanied by itching and the patient rapidly excoriates it. Mucous membranes and mucocutaneous membranes remain unaffected. The Nikolsky sign is absent. If the growths are more pronounced and appear cockscomblike and shaggy, we are dealing with *pemphigus vegetans* (see also Chapter 25, A1) or if they are not so pronounced, with intertriginous *Darier's disease* (see also Chapter 29, A3). In these two latter entities, however, the sides and back of the neck are affected only if there is a wide extension of the lesions.[20]

If the clinical picture does not permit a definite diagnosis, histologic examination is helpful. It shows typical intraepidermal acantholytic clefts without acantholytic cells and eosinophilia. Darier's disease and benign familial pemphigus are both characterized by distinct dyskeratosis, which is, however, more pronounced in Darier's disease. On the other hand, acantholysis predominates in chronic familial pemphigus and does not remain restricted to the suprabasal region. Under the electron microscope, the functional architecture of the epidermis in chronic benign familial pemphigus seems disturbed by the interruption of the desmosomal continuity. The presence of distinct eosinophilia in the tissue favors a diagnosis of chronic pemphigus vegetans, which, in addition, shows pseudoepitheliomatous hyperplasia.

If, on the other hand, inflammatory signs are lacking and in their place papillary, darkly pigmented excrescences with hyperkeratoses prevail, *acanthosis nigricans* or *pseudoacanthosis nigricans* is present (see also Chapter 24, D20). Similar furrows and elevations of the axilla, although hardly eczematiform, occur in rare instances of hyalinosis cutis et mucosae. Psoriasis vulgaris of the axillas usually presents with few scales but with erosions. The single elements of pityriasis rosea tend to appear toward the middle of the axilla. In this area, their color remains unchanged

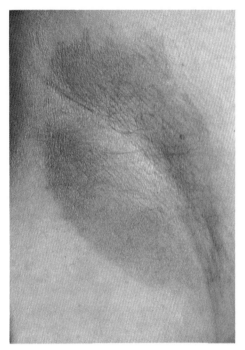

Fig. 318. Erythrasma of the axilla.

and they are dry, erythematous, and flat. In summary, the disorders mentioned here, because of their systemic character, will not offer any difficulties in the differential diagnosis against an isolated dermatitis venenata of the axilla.

More difficult can be the differentiation of dermatitis venenata from *erythrasma* (Fig. 318) or *tinea axillaris*. If the clinical signs, which will be extensively reported later (see page 321), do not permit the correct diagnosis, the result of the fungus examination must be decisive.

5. Diagnosis of the cause of common eczema in the **genitoanal region** must consider hypersensitivity reactions, often mentioned previously, to a large group of cosmetics or therapeutics that are applied externally (for example, balsam of Peru, benzocaine, and neomycin). In perianal contact dermatitis, an intolerance against drugs or vehicles in suppositories is possible. Distinct inflammatory signs with pronounced effects of excoriation may follow improper anal care, for example, the use of too abrasive or chemically irritating toilet paper. Dermatitis venenata of the sitting surface, in contrast to anal eczema, shows a more or less closed or circinate ring form on the periphery of this region, which points to the primary cause of this intolerance (contact with mahogany stains, synthetic material, polish or disinfecting material of the toilet seat). Purely moist or macerated phenomena are observed not only in the diaper rash of infants but also in adipose, profusely sweating adults or those with continuous incontinence of urine or stools (see also Chapter 28, A2). Eczematous changes in the anal region, regardless of their cause, are accompanied by rebellious itching, which can be provoked by cognac, coffee, cola, and food with strong condiments (pepper and cayenne pepper).

Fig. 319. Lichen planus of the vulva.

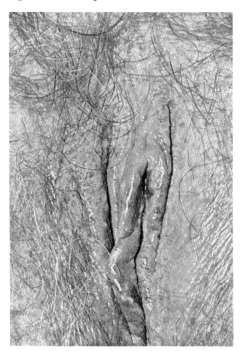

Since each attack of itching can lead to scratching, dermatitis may result from this defense mechanism alone, or if it existed already for other reasons, it may be prolonged. If no damaging contact agents can be found, the search for other disorders that lead primarily to itching, such as oxyuriasis, hemorrhoids, fibrosing folds of the peripheral anus, anal fissures, and inflammations and neoplasms of the rectum or prostate must be excluded. In a similar way, a common eczema can be caused or sustained by vaginal discharge, regardless of its origin.[14, 16]

In the female genital region it is most often *Fox-Fordyce disease*, which, because of its intense itching and the small papular lesions, can be mistaken for a common eczema. The differential diagnosis is discussed in this chapter (see page 314).

Sebaceous cysts (epidermoid cysts) also present clinically isolated and disseminated small nodular lesions of the female genitals. Their favorite site is the middle of the labia minora, but they may also be present on the labia majora and very rarely on the prepuce of the clitoris. Unilateral presence is rare, but in some instances this condition can be found simultaneously in the oral cavity as seboglandulia buccalis. Ectopic sebaceous glands of the female genitals are rare before puberty. In the menopause they usually regress, so that they are really observed only at the time of sexual maturity.

Lichen planus may also be mistaken for an eczema because of its itching, thus resembling Fox-Fordyce disease. In the genital region lichen planus is not characterized by polygonal, sharply circumscribed, solid, reddish-brown to slate-blue, faintly shiny, flat papules but instead shows mostly confluent areas or annular lesions (Fig. 319). Such rows of flat white papules are most distinct on the mucocutaneous surface.

Bullae or the remnants of bullous dermatoses may at times simulate eczema on the vaginal mucosa or the external genitals.

Fig. 320. Dermatophytosis
of the inguinal area.

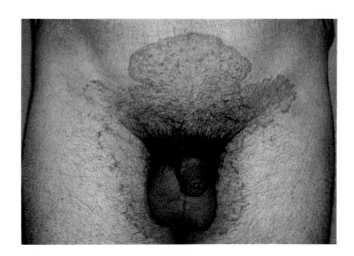

Pemphigus vegetans replaces blisters with vegetating proliferations, which at the periphery still show characteristic remnants of blisters. The favorite locations of these fetid, macerated, vegetating elevations are distributed in a bathing suit pattern on the genitocrural folds, the inner aspects of the thighs, and the anal region toward the sacrum. The skin of the genitals (vulva or scrotum) may develop edema simulating, if not thoroughly examined, a highly acute, oozing dermatitis or candidiasis.

Analogous to bullous dermatitides, papular eruptions located in the genital region often assume a special aspect, which may lead to the possibility of their being thought to be common eczema. In *dyskeratosis follicularis* on the vulva or scrotum, for instance, keratotic, crumbly, papular lesions become confluent and form papillomatous areas that are mushy, fetid, dirty, vegetating, and, moreover, often matted or cockscomb-like. In favor of dyskeratosis follicularis are, besides the extragenital changes, the characteristic serrated, splintering, keratotic thickening or longitudinal streaks of the nails. Furthermore, fingerprints of the thumb show a characteristic interruption of the pattern of the papillary lines on the tips of the fingers and the thenar eminences. *Acanthosis nigricans* in the intertriginous

areas of the genitals may be subject to considerable maceration, so that at first only a dark-brownish color is conspicuous. Observing other typical localizations of acanthosis nigricans permits a quick verification of the diagnosis (see also Chapter 24, D20).

The inguinal area and the inner aspects of the thighs are the favorite sites of *erythrasma*. In exceptional cases it may also be found in the axilla or the submammary region. The lesions do not cause any sensations. The affected areas are sharply limited and are a brownish-reddish color. Scratching reveals a thinly scaling surface. In contrast to tinea inguinalis, a central healing tendency and the accentuated periphery are missing. The red fluorescences of erythrasma under a Wood's light are typical. In this way, all atypically localized areas can be identified without difficulty. Compared with dermatitis venenata or lichen simplex chronicus, erythrasma is not pruritic; it lacks the papular elements and mildly suggestive lichenification. With regard to intertriginous anogenital candidiasis, see Section A4 (page 308) in this chapter.

Tinea inguinalis, as evident by its old name "eczema marginatum," is characterized by an inflammatory, sharply limited margin of the individual lesions. The lesions, often already healed in the center, are round or curved and often polycyclic at the periphery. They do not remain confined chiefly to the inner sides of the thighs like erythrasma (Fig. 320). Because of its greater pruritus, tinea inguinalis is much more often excoriated or covered with thin crusts than erythrasma. If pustules are present, candidiasis has to be ruled out.

Ulcerated eczemas in the anal region suggest above all ulcerated *tuberculosis of the mucous membrane* in primary intestinal tuberculosis. Reddish-yellow nodules and pustules usually precede the extremely painful, superficial ulcerations. Like exudative ulcerative perianal tuberculosis, *regional ileitis* may show dirty, indolent, anal ulcerations with undermined borders or fistulizations (see also Chapter 14, B9). It is important to differentiate Bowen's disease (see also Chapter 38, H1) and Paget's disease (see also this Chapter 21, B3) from the common eczema of the anogenital region because one seldom considers malignant tumors in this body area a diagnostic possibility.[18]

6. In an analysis of the common eczemas on **the extremities** one must consider hypersensitivity reactions of the hands. A classic example is the hand eczema of the mason. Chronic damage from alkaline soaps or detergents, cement, and many other agents, first causes destruction of the protective acid mantle of the skin. Gradually, a so-called abrasive dermatitis develops, opening the way to a sensitivity, e.g., to chromium, nickel, or dissolvers of fats. Also, chronic accumulation of irritations below the threshold may lead to the development of eczematous reactions, an event which is again particularly important in the hand region. Recurrent dermatitis can lead to eczematization, and therefore the causation of hand eczemas (Chapter 21, A3) is also important. Almost half of the eczemas of the hands start with dermatitis due to the use of irritating material. This type of

eczema is characteristic in women, 20 to 40 years old, who at this age come in frequent contact with many detergents. Morphologically important in such "degenerative" eczema is the scarcity of the nodular and papulovesicular character and the prevalence of confluent, hyperkeratotic, rhagadiform lesions (tylotic eczema). In contrast to common eczema, "degenerative" eczema does not "jump" or "scatter," as is characteristic of (covered) leg eczema; it does not persist (autonomy) after removal of the noxious irritation.[1]

Such pronounced scaling common eczema should be differentiated from *psoriasis vulgaris* (Fig. 321), although this dermatosis does not tend to eczematization and itching. The parakeratotic quality of psoriasis vulgaris is – especially on the hands – not very typical (frequent washing of hands); the basic erythema, however, still shows a sharp outline. In many cases the presence of other psoriatic lesions permits the correct diagnosis.

Hyperkeratotic ringworm of the palms may not be distinguishable morphologically from common eczema or psoriasis vulgaris (Fig. 322). Examination of the whole patient, the history, and tests may, however, not be helpful, so that the mycological examination must be decisive in these cases. It should be remembered that fungi may be difficult to detect because of the usual frequent washing, and, if the test is negative, it will have to be repeated several times. Diffuse *palmoplantar keratosis* should be recognized by its familial occurrence, a red margin, and hyperhidrosis. Moreover, it is usually not completely confluent and is limited in its extension (see also Chapter 28, B1). "Eczematiform" *chronic lupus erythematosus* (healing with atrophy) or eczematized *scabies* (burrows in the interdigital folds) will hardly ever be restricted to the hands.

However, the patient with *atopic dermatitis* rather often shows isolated lesions restricted to the hands, the lesions showing no characteristic features differentiating them from common eczema of the same location. Extensive confluent, strongly lichenified, and occasionally thickly lamellar scaling areas are mostly seen on the volar side of the carpal bones and occasionally even on the palms. These isolated eczematous areas are not recognizable as atopic dermatitis. Therefore, the course of the disorder or a history of asthma or hayfever will help in the diagnosis.

The question of eczema and *dyshidrotic eruptions* on hands and feet will be thoroughly discussed in Chapter 26, C.

Eczematous reactions on the legs occur with great morphologic variations, mostly in *stasis disorders*, which differ in the individual cases but are initially determined by the chief signs of hemosiderosis and dermatosclerosis. Gradually, eczematization will become the decisive factor. Eczema of the leg that develops on the basis of a chronic venous, or (less frequently), from a post-thrombotic syndrome is characterized by jumping and scattering as a sign of hypersensitivity against local therapeutics. On the other hand, eczemas with a tendency to generalization that arise from varicose and post-thrombotic states show intolerance to local therapeutic agents and are suspect of showing intolerance to bacteria as well (autosensitization eczema).[8, 9]

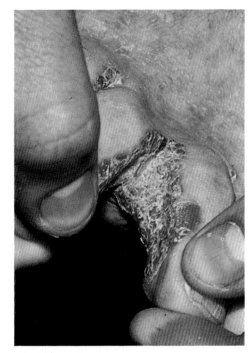

Fig. 321. Interdigital psoriasis vulgaris.

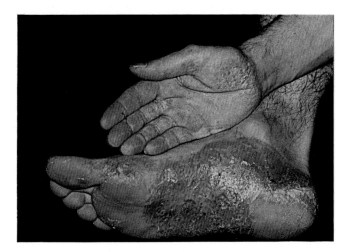

Fig. 322. Dermatophytosis of the feet and hands.

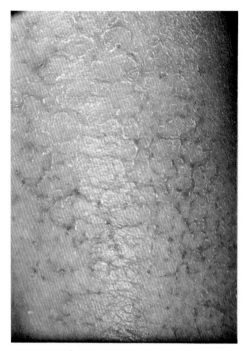

Fig. 323. "État craquelé."

In persons in whom the excretion of sebum is restricted, the pre-eczematous stage of "état craquelé" (Fig. 323) arises from frequent washing and the related additional loss of fat; it leads to the so-called exsiccation eczematides, which, with their increased hyperkeratotic tendencies, create diagnostic difficulties versus hyperkeratotic ringworm infections.[4, 12]

If, however, a discrete eczematous reaction with strong residual pigmentation is predominant, one should consider a special form of progressive purpura pigmentosa, so-called *"eczematidlike purpura."* Histologically, these hemorrhagically pigmented dermatoses are characterized by basal spongiosis and lymphohistiocytic infiltrates of the corium as well as by intrapapillary high-lying erythrodiapedesis and later subpapillary deposits of hemosiderin.[4, 12]

In the popliteal area and on the dorsa of the feet isolated areas of *atopic dermatitis* (see also Section D in this chapter, page 328)

as well as dermatitis venenata from synthetic stockings occur. Sensitivity to the dyes, not the raw material, is to be blamed.[26]

(1) AGRUP, G.: Hand eczema and other hand dermatoses in south Sweden. Acta derm.-venereol. (Stockh.) *49*, Suppl. 61 (1969).

(2) BANDMANN, H.-J., und W. DOHN: Die Epicutantestung. Bergmann, München 1967.

(3) CONGDON, G. H., and M. B. DOCKERTY: Malignant lesions of the nipple exclusive of Paget's disease. Surg. Gynec. Obstet. *103:* 185–192 (1956).

(4) DOUCAS, C., and J. KAPETANAKIS: Eczematid-like purpura. Dermatologica (Basel) *106:* 86–95 (1953).

(5) DREWES, J., und R. POCHE: Das primäre Karzinom der Brustwarze. Chir. Praxis *13:* 209–215 (1969).

(6) GORDON, S., and L. J. A. LOEWENTHAL: Chronic eczema as a variant of dermatitis herpetiformis. Brit. J. Derm. *61:* 359–378 (1949).

(7) HANDLEY, R. S., and A. C. THACKRAY: Adenoma of nipple. Brit. J. Cancer *16:* 187–194 (1962).

(8) HARTUNG, J., und P. O. RUDOLPH: Häufige Allergene bei Unterschenkel-Ekzematikern. Z. Haut- u. Geschl.-Kr. *47:* 375–378 (1972).

(9) HAXTHAUSEN, H.: Generalized »IDS« (»autosensitization«) in varicose eczemas. Acta derm.-venereol. (Stockh.) *35:* 271–280 (1955).

(10) HERZBERG, J. J.: Über den Morbus Paget. Hautarzt *6:* 67–71 (1955).

(11) HÖFS, W.: Zur Lokalisation der Psoriasis vulgaris an der Areola und Papilla mammae. Derm. Wschr. *153:* 25–33 (1967).

(12) ILLIG, L., und K. W. KALKOFF: Zum Formenkreis der Purpura pigmentosa progressiva (unter besonderer Berücksichtigung der Adalin-Purpura). Hautarzt *21:* 497–505 (1970).

(13) JANSEN, G. T., C. J. DILLAHA and W. M. HONEYCUTT: Candida cheilitis. Arch. Derm. (Chic.) *88:* 325–329 (1963).

(14) JENTSCH, M.: Das Gesäßekzem. Derm. Wschr. *116:* 282–285 (1943).

(15) KORTING, G. W.: Perlèche – als klinisches Leitsymptom bei Erwachsenen. J. med. Kosmetik *1953:* 322–328.

(16) KORTING, G. W.: Zur perianalen Erscheinungsweise der Crohnschen Krankheit. Hautarzt *19:* 553–556 (1968).

(17) McCARTHY, F. P.: Pyostomatitis vegetans. Arch. Derm. Syph. (Chic.) *60:* 750–764 (1949).

(18) MIESCHER, G.: Zwei Fälle von vegetierendem Morbus Paget der Genitalregion. Dermatologica (Basel) *108:* 309 bis 314 (1954).

(19) MUSUMECI, V.: Sui rapporti tra eczema e dermatite erpetiforme del Dühring. Minerva derm. *35:* 436–443 (1960).

(20) NÜRNBERGER, F., und G. MÜLLER: Elektronenmikroskopische Untersuchungen über die Akantholyse bei Pemphigus familiaris benignus. Arch. klin. exp. Derm. *228:* 208–219 (1967).

(21) OBERSTE-LEHN, H.: Hyperkeratosen im Bereich von Mamille und Areola. Z. Haut- u. Geschl.-Kr. *8:* 388–393 (1950).

(22) OBERSTE-LEHN, H., und M. KÜHL: Zur Kenntnis der Mamillar-Hyperkeratosen. Z. Haut- u. Geschl.-Kr. *15:* 345–347 (1953).

(23) RÖCKL, H.: Über die Pyodermite végétante von Hallopeau als benigne Form des Pemphigus vegetans von Neumann nebst einigen Bemerkungen zur Pyostomatitis vegetans von McCARTHY. Arch. klin. exp. Derm. *218:* 574–582 (1964).

(24) SHELLEY, W. B., and H. J. HURLEY: The allergic origin of zirconium deodorant granulomas. Brit. J. Derm. *70:* 75–101 (1958).

(25) SMITH, E. J., S. D. KRON and P. R. GROSS: Erosive adenomatosis of the nipple. Arch. Derm. (Chic.) *102:* 330–332 (1970).

(26) SUTER, H.: Untersuchungen über das Polyamidstrumpfekzem. Dermatologica (Basel) *130:* 411–424 (1965).

(27) TAYLOR, H. B., and A. G. ROBERTSON: Adenomas of the nipple. Cancer *18:* 995–1002 (1965).

C. Seborrheic Dermatitis

Seborrheic dermatitis has a constitutional background* similar to that of atopic dermatitis. In contrast to dermatitis venenata seborrheic dermatitis is characterized by sharply circumscribed, round or oval, erythematous plaques. Examination of a single lesion shows a faintly red to brownish-yellow, only slightly pruritic area (Fig. 324); its periphery shows a discrete amount of exudation and a

---

* Seborrheic diathesis. (Tr.)

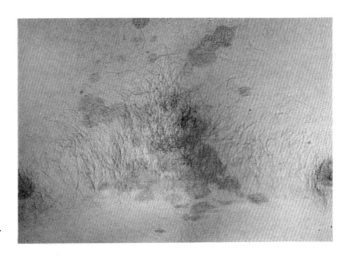

Fig. 324. Seborrheic dermatitis.

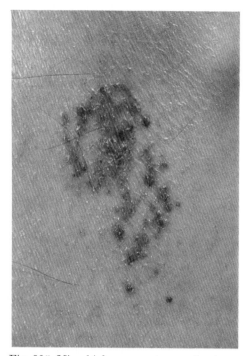

Fig. 325. Microbial eczema at an early stage.

of hypersensitivity against some kinds of bacteria. This points to a close relationship or even identity between seborrheic and *microbial eczema*. In the latter, intracutaneous testing is of fundamental importance in the demonstration of allergy to bacteria (foci!). Clinically, microbial eczema shows either ill-defined erythematous areas with a tendency to oozing, thick lamellar scaling, and crusting, or the formation of grouped papulovesicular lesions, sometimes with small hemorrhages (Fig. 325). Typical of microbial eczema is a tendency to dispersion or leaping from one place to another.[1-7]

1. The **facial regions** favored by microbial seborrheic dermatitis are the nasolabial folds, the vermilion border of the lips, and the retroauricular spaces. If the disease is in a more exudative phase, it shows oozing, crusted, scaling erythematous lesions. The more bland types present yellowish, brownish-red, washed-out erythemas.

A very slight degree of seborrheic dermatitis (a minimal variant) is represented by *pityriasis alba* of the cheeks; it usually occurs in children. The lesions consist of barely visible circular or maplike pseudoleukodermas with faint pityriasiform scaling. Simultaneous erythemas or papulovesicular lesions are lacking.

The differential diagnosis between microbial seborrheic dermatitis and **impetigo contagiosa** due either to streptococci or staphylococci is not difficult in most cases. However, occasionally it may be hard to distinguish between "eczematized" impetigo contagiosa and "impetiginous" seborrheic dermatitis. In such cases, the duration of the affection and the history will permit a definite diagnostic classification. The two types of impetigo start with a small erythematous macule which quickly turns from a vesicle into a pustule. The infection spreads peripherally, forming plaquelike or circinate areas with central healing. The high contagiousness leads to the development of numerous lesions of impetigo; poor

barely perceptible papule or vesicle. More marked infiltration and lichenification are not part of the clinical picture of seborrheic dermatitis. The lesion is covered with yellowish-white, crumbly, fatty scales. Preferred sites are the scalp, midface region, umbilicus, anterior and posterior axillary folds, and intertriginous regions. Seborrheic dermatitis more rarely may be confined to the follicular openings and their immediate vicinity, so one may speak of a follicular seborrheic dermatitis. Etiologically, seborrheic dermatitis is definitely exacerbated by excessive humidity of the air*; low vapor pressure results in more frequent outbreaks while the opposite is true when vapor pressure is high. In addition, there is a correlation between bacterial foci of infection and a high degree

---

* And the resulting increase in perspiration. (Tr.)

personal hygiene causes smear infections (i.e., scalp, genitals, umbilicus). Staphylococcic impetigo shows a slightly thicker wall of the vesicle or bulla than the streptococcic variety; the former, therefore, results in the appearance of vesicles and pustules of rather different size. After the wall of the pustule has ruptured, thin, varnished looking, covering crusts are formed (Fig. 326). The crusts of streptococcic impetigo are thick and irregularly arranged in layers. These morphologic differential possibilities can be applied only to a certain degree because quite often a simultaneous infection with staphylococci and streptococci takes place. The previously mentioned high contagiousness of the two types of impetigo is borne out by the frequency with which the same infection is observed among people in the immediate vicinity of the patient. An isolated case of impetigo in an adult requires exclusion of impetiginized rupioid secondary syphilis. Such manifestations of secondary syphilis favor the nasolabial folds, the corners of the mouth, the forehead, and also the scalp. However, such a crusted syphilid will always develop from a small nodular lesion, whereas impetigo contagiosa starts with a small erythematous macule or a very superficial erosion. If crusted angular cheilitis (perlèche) develops quickly in a patient of middle age, care should be exercised not to overlook a solitary, luxuriant, specific (syphilitic) papule.

For important differential signs in regard to perioral, rosacealike dermatitis, see Chapter 18, F6.

2. Microbial seborrheic dermatitis **of the scalp** becomes noticeable only by increased scaling and a faster rate of oiliness of the scalp hair or by an erythema covered thickly with crusts; a definite diagnostic classification often is not possible without careful attention to the history and the condition of the rest of the skin.

Differential diagnosis purely from a clinical point of view must consider exudative psoriasis vulgaris or pyoderma caused by

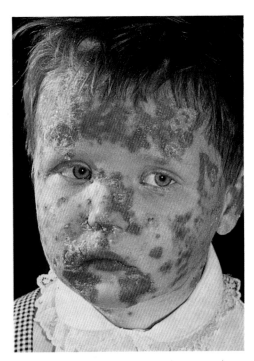

Fig. 326. Staphylococcic impetigo contagiosa.

infestation with head lice, especially of the nuchal region; heavy crusting here will result from the hair matting together into a pigtail-like condition. In addition, nits will be seen along the hairs. Psoriasis vulgaris of the scalp shows temporarily small macular lesions, unless the eruption is especially severe; however, seborrheic dermatitis starts with larger plaquelike lesions right from the beginning. Testing for psoriasis by removing a (multi-layered) scale to show the resulting pointlike capillary bleeding (Auspitz's sign) should take place only after the last thin scale has been removed; tearing off an entire, firmly attached, eczematous plaque will frequently be followed by a large drop of blood.

3. The **auricle** is the most frequent site of microbial seborrheic dermatitis. This type not infrequently depends on a pyogenic focus which causes spreading; it should be remembered that both forms of reaction (dermatitis and furuncle) may alternate with each other in such a fashion that the dermatitis appears when the furuncle disappears and vice versa.

If such a rhythm of manifestations is lacking and a rather persistent or torpid stationary condition prevails, one must consider *otomycosis;* this diagnosis requires proof of the presence of fungi either by microscopic examination or by culture. Because the normal auditory canal lacks dermatophytes or yeasts, a positive finding of such organisms is important. At present the candida group has to be considered first.

4. Cutaneous diseases affecting the **trunk** as a rule do not show variations of the sites of predilection. The preference of seborrheic dermatitis for the front of the chest and the midline of the back is well known. This preferential localization is shared among others by dyskeratosis follicularis and pemphigus erythematosus (Senear-Usher syndrome). Typically, seborrheic dermatitis develops rapidly after pyogenic cutaneous infections or after acute stress, for instance, with an acute attack of cerebral or cardiac disease accompanied by hyperhidrosis. The seborrheic patch presents, as mentioned previously, a certain peripheral zone of exudation, but it lacks the thin overhanging fringe of moniliasis or pityriasis rosea. The larger solitary area of *moniliasis* has typical small satellite lesions at the periphery. When in doubt, culture studies will permit the correct diagnosis.

Pityriasis rosea, besides the herald patch, differs from seborrheic dermatitis in the frequent symmetrical distribution along the lines of cleavage, the sparing of the face, and the involvement of the middle of the axilla (see also page 294). The clinician has a grave responsibility to make the correct differential diagnosis between seborrheic dermatitis of the trunk, parapsoriasis "en plaques" (*Brocq's disease,* see also Chapter 20, B), and *mycosis fungoides* in the premycotic stage (see also Chapter 20, D). The

presence of patches with fairly distinct borders on the sides of the trunk within the lines of cleavage, interspersed with discrete petechiae and round pinhead-sized papules, is in favor of parapsoriasis en plaques; pseudoatrophic wrinkling, long-term unchanging persistence, and an absence of pruritus are all further signs of this disease.

Multiple epitheliomas of the trunk, the so-called superficial "pagetoid" *basal cell epitheliomas,* may appear as thin-scaled, faintly red, barely brownish-yellow, erythematous patches. Although occasionally pruritus similar to an *"eczema"* is present, a pearly border with small, somewhat shiny nodules will permit a definite clinical diagnosis of epithelioma.

(1) Booken, G.: Die jahreszeitliche Häufigkeit des seborrhoischen Ekzems. Hautarzt *19:* 115–121 (1968).

(2) Nikolowski, W.: Über die differentielle Morphogenese des sogenannten seborrhoischen Ekzems. Arch. Derm. Syph. (Berl.) *196:* 501–600 (1953).

(3) Röckl, H.: Untersuchungen zur Klinik und Pathogenese des mikrobiellen Ekzems. II. Mitt. Hautarzt *7:* 14–23 (1956).

(4) Röckl, H.: Das mikrobielle Ekzem. Z. Haut- u. Geschl.-Kr. *42:* 475–484 (1967).

(5) Sönnichsen, N., P. Reich, E. Miemiec und A. Hochheim: Klinische und immunologische Untersuchungen zur Abgrenzung des sogenannten mikrobiellen Ekzems. Derm. Mschr. *157:* 553–563 (1971).

(6) Spier, H. W.: Zur Pathogenese des Ekzems. In: Fortschr. prakt. Dermatol. u. Venerol. Hrsg. A. Marchionini. Bd. V. S. 150–165. Springer, Berlin, Heidelberg, New York 1965.

(7) Tager, A., C. Berlin and R. J. Schen: Seborrhoeic dermatitis in acute cardiac disease. Brit. J. Derm. *76:* 367–369 (1964).

D. Atopic Dermatitis

Atopic dermatitis (neurodermatitis disseminata, endogenous eczema) shows polymorphous cutaneous lesions and is also accompanied by other allergic manifestations such as hay fever and asthma; however, not all cutaneous areas present the character of an atopic dermatitis. Typically, this dermatitis begins in infancy after the first three months; exceptionally, however, lateral facial erythema may be present at birth with subsequent further development into a full-fledged atopic dermatitis (Fig. 327). Exacerbation of this condition is seen with difficult dentition ("prurigo à feux de dents"*) or after smallpox vaccination. The elbow flexures (about 80 per cent) or popliteal spaces (about 40 per cent) are the typical sites of allergic eczema, especially during the preschool and school age years (Fig. 328). Such flexural eczema has a marked tendency to lichenification, both primary (with close aggregation of lichen simplex nodules) and secondary, the latter developing finally from the diminishing effect of repeated episodes of spongiosis. Such lichenification lacks the usual three-zoned configuration of chronic lichen simplex (outside, pigmentation; inside, round, plane, pinhead sized nodules; centrally, plaquelike thickening of the

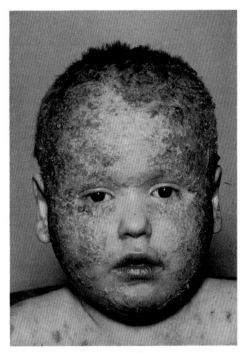

Fig. 327. Atopic dermatitis in infant.

* "Prurigo with fiery teething." (Tr.)

** With exaggeration of the normal markings showing quadrilateral facets. (Tr.)

epidermis).** A single lichenified area of the atopic patient shows typically a striated or rectangular plaque of reddish-gray color. The third phase of atopic dermatitis shows disseminated eczematous lichenoid manifestations with lichen simplex chronicus-like and common eczematous reactions occurring irregularly side by

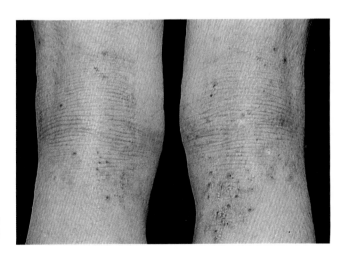

Fig. 328. Atopic dermatitis in typical localization in the flexures.

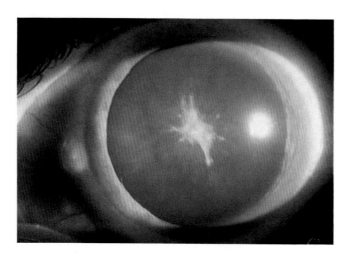

Fig. 329. Dermatogenous cataract in atopic dermatitis.

side. The final reactive stage of this disease is the monomorphic prurigo phase, which during the third decade of life appears more like chronic papular urticaria and later almost like prurigo nodularis.

Atopic dermatitis can be recognized even during an interval without lesions by perioral radial folds. However, differential diagnosis has to consider the similar formation of folds seen in progressive scleroderma and in congenital syphilis (Parrot's rhagades).

Because the reactive phases of atopic dermatitis can differ so widely, it is understandable that there is an absence of characteristic histologic features. Consequently, it is all the more important to consider the family history and extracutaneous equivalents of manifestations (synchronous or alternating occurrence of bronchial asthma in about 17 per cent, vasomotoric rhinitis in about 11 per cent of cases). Definite signs of atopy are a low hairline, giving the impression that the patient is wearing a fur hat, pale skin, white dermatographia, and thinning of the lateral part of the eyebrows (Hertoghe's sign). The so-called atopic cataract (neurodermatitic cataract) is an early axial cataract originating from the capsular epithelium and

characterized by an intensively white color and a disklike configuration; it occurs in about 1 to 20 per cent of patients suffering from extremely extensive and severe cutaneous changes (Fig. 329). Some questionable ophthalmic syntropies are keratoconus and retinal detachment. An abnormally small diameter of the aorta is a roentgenologically remarkable sign. Diagnostically important for atopic dermatitis – in contrast to other types of eczema – is pruritus when in contact with wool, improvement during the summer months, maximal activity in springtime, and frequently a distinct dependence on the climate. In spite of the sharply defined characteristics of atopic eczema, genotypical as well as phenotypical, and its hereditary fixation, it presents a few other confusing manifestations, apart from the differentiation from common and seborrheic dermatitis.[6, 7, 8, 10, 21]

2. Another sign of atopic dermatitis, especially in older patients, is xeroderma. The assumption that atopic dermatitis may occur in combination with **ichthyosis vulgaris** depends on the presence of typical disklike scales arranged in striae or rhombi. Besides, an ichthyosiform skin in an atopic individual will hardly ever be found in a small child, and in older patients as a rule it oc-

Fig. 330. Letterer-Siwe
disease.

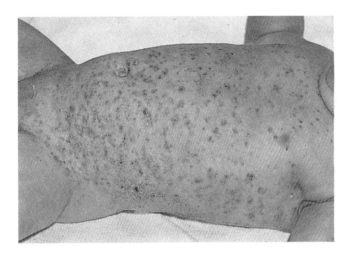

curs only on the lower half of the body. Another stigma of ichthyosis is a significantly low magnesium level in the erythrocytes in contrast to the normal level in an atopic patient. The special eczematous tendency of the flexures in ichthyosis and in the ichthyosiform atopic patient is accounted for by the simultaneous decreased resistance to alkali and a delayed neutralization of alkali; also in atopic dermatitis there is an increased tendency to cholinergic reaction in the flexures.[9, 12]

3. Ichthyosis linearis circumflexa (see also Chapter 27, A11) shows, soon after birth, annular or serpiginous erythematous ridges with double scaly borders. Within the erythematous areas, small papules or vesicles as well as eczematous lesions can be observed. Almost all patients show lichenification of the flexures of elbows and knees that has a certain similarity to an atopic dermatitis. Children with ichthyosis linearis circumflexa may show, at the same time, changes of the hairshaft suggestive of trichorrhexis invaginata; this combination is called *Netherton's syndrome*. The deformities of the hairshaft consist of nodular protuberances which are caused by pressure and invagination ("bamboo-hairs"). In addition, there are spindlelike thickenings of

the hair with torsion around the long axis. These two kinds of node formation are caused by a disturbance of the keratinization; both nodes may alternate on the same hair. In contrast to the almost equal involvement of both sexes in isolated ichthyosis linearis circumflexa, there is a large female predominance in Netherton's disease.[1, 3, 14, 18, 23]

4. Letterer-Siwe disease may in the early stages show cutaneous changes which may be mistaken for atopic or seborrheic reactions. Principally the scalp (external auditory canals) and the middle of the trunk show plaquelike seborrheic erythemas (Fig. 330), which then are successively interspersed with hemorrhagic, Darier's disease-like, scaly-crusted papules. Concomitant bouts of fever should always raise doubts about the proper classification of such an eczema and should elicit further investigation. Hepatosplenomegaly, enlargement of lymph nodes, areas of osteolysis, indefinite pyorrhea (for instance, otorrhea), and eosinophilic granulomas of the jaw are signs that establish the diagnosis of Letterer-Siwe disease. Histologically, one finds, according to the stage of the disease, histiocytic-proliferative, granulomatous, and xanthomatous tissue changes.[4, 17]

5. Another systemic disease of infancy with cutaneous changes similar to those of atopic dermatitis is the **Wiskott-Aldrich syndrome.** The face primarily, but also the upper trunk and the larger flexures of the joints show maculopapular, scaling, eczematous areas interspersed with petechiae. Concomitant respiratory, gastrointestinal, and cutaneous infections are indicative of the syndrome. Most of the children die of septic complications or of purulent meningitis. Another cardinal sign is constant thrombocytopenia (values of less than 50,000 cells). In spite of all these findings lethal complications from bleeding are very rare. The syndrome is inherited as a sexlinked recessive trait affecting boys exclusively; for homozygous girls it represents a lethal factor. Important for the pathogenesis is the absence of isoagglutinins and a low level of IgM immunoglobulins, while IgA immunoglubulins may be increased.[5, 11, 13, 22]

6. Atopic dermatitis-like eruptions have been observed occasionally with the **Pfaundler-Hurler syndrome** (see also Chapter 11, K9), with **phenyl pyruvic oligophrenia** (see also Chapter 24, A2), and in experimental **histidine deficiency.**[2, 15, 16, 17, 20]

7. There is a phenocopy of atopic dermatitis that is an occupational dermatitis caused by contact with substances containing potassium (so-called **pseudoatopic dermatitis**). In contrast to real atopic dermatitis, there is no familial history (bronchial asthma and others), and the first eruption occurs in adulthood. After the sensitizing substances (chromium, nickel, cobalt, formaldehyde, and animal hairs) have been discovered by patch testing and have been eliminated from further contact with the patient, proper therapy will have a much better chance of attaining cure than in an atopic individual. Women show such pseudoatopic dermatitis much more frequently than men.[19]

(1) ALTMAN, J., and J. STROUD: Netherton's syndrome and ichthyosis linearis circumflexa. Arch. Derm. (Chic.) *100:* 550–558 (1969).

(2) FLEISHER, T. L., and I. ZELIGMAN: Cutaneous findings in phenylketonuria. Arch. Derm. Syph. (Chic.) *81:* 898–903 (1960).

(3) GIANOTTI, F.: La maladie de Netherton. Étude de deux cas et des rapports avec les génodermatoses érythémato-desquamatives circinées variables. Ann. Derm. Syph. (Paris) *96:* 147–155 (1969).

(4) GLÄSS, A., und CH. KITLAK: Endogenes Ekzem als Fehldiagnose einer Abt-Letterer-Siweschen Krankheit. Kinderärztl. Prax. *37:* 287–293 (1969).

(5) DE GRACIANSKY, P., et G. SCHAISON: Le syndrome d'Aldrich. Ann. Derm. Syph. (Paris) *94:* 255–264 (1967).

(6) HARNACK, K., und U. LENZ: Familienprognose beim endogenen Ekzem. Derm. Mschr. *156:* 530–535 (1970).

(7) KORTING, G. W.: Zur Pathogenese des endogenen Ekzems. Thieme, Stuttgart 1954.

(8) KORTING, G. W.: Einige Wesenszüge des endogenen Ekzematikers. Dtsch. med. Wschr. *85:* 417–426 (1960).

(9) KORTING, G. W., H. HOLZMANN und B. MORSCHES: Über einen Unterschied des Magnesium-Gehalts der Erythrocyten von endogenen Ekzematikern und Kranken mit Ichthyosis vulgaris. Arch. klin. exp. Derm. *229:* 126–130 (1967).

(10) LEMKE, L., und A. JÜTTE: Augenbefall bei Neurodermatitis disseminata. Derm. Wschr. *152:* 921–927 (1966).

(11) MARCHAL, G., G. BILSKI-PASQUIER, M. BONNET-GAJDOS et M. SAMAMA: Le syndrome d'Aldrich (purpura thrombopénique familial, eczéma, infections récidivantes). Presse méd. *71:* 2621 bis 2624 (1963).

(12) MORSCHES, B., H. HOLZMANN und R. DENK: Zum Mg-Gehalt von Serum und Erythrocyten bei Kranken mit Ichthyosis vulgaris. Klin. Wschr. *45:* 316 (1967).

(13) NIORDSON, A.-M., and H. SCHMIDT: Aldrich's syndrome. Arch. Derm. (Chic.) *88:* 613–615 (1963).

(14) ORFANOS, C. E., G. MAHRLE und T. ŠALAMON: Netherton-Syndrom. Ichthyosiforme Hautveränderungen und Trichorrhexis invaginata. Nachweis eines krankhaft veränderten Cortexkeratins im Haar. Hautarzt 22: 397–409 (1971).

(15) PETERSON, R. D. A.: Immunologic responses in infantile eczema. J. Pediat. 66: 225–234 (1965).

(16) REILLY, W. A., and S. LINDSAY: Gargoylism (lipochondrodystrophy); review of clinical observations in eighteen cases. Amer. J. Dis. Child. 75: 595–607 (1948).

(17) ROSTENBERG, A., and L. M. SOLOMON: Infantile eczema and systemic disease. Arch. Derm. (Chic.) 98: 41–46 (1968).

(18) SCHNEIDER, W., R. COPPENRATH und H. D. BOCK: Ichthyosis linearis circumflexa (Comêl) bei familiärem Auftreten von Ichthyosis vulgaris. Arch. klin. exp. Derm. 215: 79–92 (1962).

(19) SHANON, J.: Pseudo-atopic dermatitis. Dermatologica (Basel) 131: 176–190 (1965).

(20) SNYDERMAN, S. E.: An eczematoid dermatitis in histidine deficiency. J. Pediat. 66: 212–215 (1965).

(21) STORCK, H., E. STREHLER und E. GYSLING: Abnorm geringe Aortenweite bei Patienten mit Neurodermitis disseminata. Arch. klin. exp. Derm. 222: 489–499 (1965).

(22) TYMPNER, K.-D., K. HAGER und P. SCHWEIER: Immunologische Untersuchungen beim Wiskott-Aldrich-Syndrom. Münch. med. Wschr. 110: 517–521 (1968).

(23) VINEYARD, W. R., L. R. LUMPKIN and J. C. LAWLER: Ichthyosis linearis circumflexa. Arch. Derm. (Chic.) 83: 630–635 (1961).

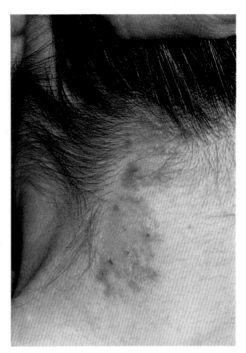

Fig. 331. Lichen simplex chronicus on the neck.

E. Lichen Simplex Chronicus

1. **Lichen simplex chronicus** (neurodermatitis circumscripta) is almost always restricted to a few patches – more than two or three are quite rare. Favorite locations are the back of the neck (Fig. 331), the inner aspects of the thighs extending to the genital region (vulva, scrotum), and also the extensor aspects of the forearms and legs. In contrast to atopic dermatitis, lichen simplex chronicus does not occur on a familial basis, it does not develop after infantile eczema, and it fails to appear with increasing frequency with hay fever or asthma. However, from an etiologic and pathological point of view lichen simplex chronicus may be connected with liver or gallbladder disease, constipation, anacidity of gastric secretion, and similar conditions. A typical single area of lichen simplex chronicus has three different zones: the central part shows plaquelike, primary lichenification; it is surrounded by a second zone of round, flat, obtuse, closely aggregated nodules, almost skin-colored or reddish-gray, and pinhead-sized or occasionally somewhat larger; the third peripheral zone has a washed-out, dirty-brown pigmentation. Although severe pruritus is al-

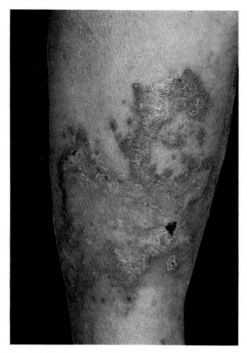

Fig. 332. Verrucous lichen planus.

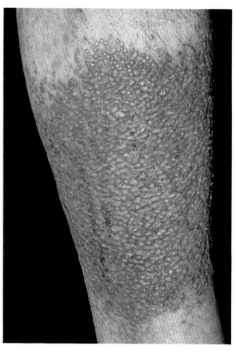

Fig. 333. Sarcoidosis resembling lichen simplex on the leg.

most always present, only few excoriations are seen. In the genital region the three-zoned structure, however, becomes indistinct, and only a plaquelike confluence of the single papules takes place ("lichenification géante"), accompanied by thinning or disappearance of the pubic hair. The legs, however, show increased hyperkeratosis of lichen simplex chronicus lesions; such a lesion may suggest a number of different diagnostic possibilities.[2, 3]

2. Verrucous lichen planus of the legs (Fig. 332) shows in its immediate vicinity a few typical, plane, polygonal papules. Isomorphically transformed scratch marks may be present as a result of the associated pruritus; this phenomenon is always absent in lichen simplex chronicus. Discovery of other lichen planus lesions (flexures of wrists, mucous membranes) will permit the correct diagnosis.

3. It is very difficult, if not macroscopically impossible, to differentiate **lichen amyloidosus** (see also Chapter 2, D5) from an isolated area of **cutaneous sarcoid** (Fig. 333). Lichen amyloidosus, which usually has sharply outlined areas that consist of frequently large obtuse papules, may extend like a stocking from the ankles to the knees. Important diagnostically is the Congo red reaction performed in histologic sections; intracutaneous or subcutaneous injection of a 1 per cent Congo red solution can be performed also, but the danger of persistent cutaneous discoloration should be kept in mind. Sarcoid simulating lichen simplex can be easily diagnosed histologically and also by the fact that sarcoid involves not only the skin but also many internal organs; the Kveim test is a further diagnostic help. Lichen planus and lichen simplex chronicus lesions of the legs in the early stages frequently are located on varicose protuberances or postphlebitic areas, whereas lichen amyloidosus and lichen simplex-like sarcoid will not show such a preference.[1, 4, 5, 7]

4. Prurigo nodularis appears primarily in women of middle age, showing extremely pruritic, firm, obtuse, bilateral but not very numerous, disseminated papules, especially on the extremities, more rarely only on the legs. There is no explicit connection with lichenification in the neighboring region. Histologically, the cutaneous nerves including Schwann's elements show proliferation and hypertrophic changes of the terminal elements of the vegetative nervous system; anomalous or gigantic lichenifications fail to show such changes of the nervous elements.[6]

(1) DENK, R., und N. HOEDE: Lichen simplex-artige Hautmanifestation eines Morbus Boeck. Med. Welt 18 (N.F.): 1881–1882 (1967).

(2) KORTING, G. W.: Zur Pathogenese des endogenen Ekzems. Thieme, Stuttgart 1954.

(3) LYNCH, F. W.: Suboccipital dermatitis. Arch. Derm. Syph. (Chic.) 60: 307–317 (1949).

(4) MARCHIONINI, A., und F. JOHN: Über lichenoide und poikilodermieartige Hautamyloidose. Arch. Derm. Syph. (Berl.) 173: 545–561 (1936).

(5) NOMLAND, R.: Localized (lichen) amyloidosis of the skin: report of two cases, with vital staining of the amyloid nodules by congored injected intracutaneously or subcutaneously. Arch. Derm. Syph. (Chic.) 33: 85–98 (1936).

(6) THIES, W.: Neurohistologische Studie zur Differentialdiagnose der Prurigo nodularis Hyde und anderer Formen umschriebener Lichenifikation. Arch. klin. exp. Derm. 201: 539–555 (1955).

(7) WEYHBRECHT, H.: Lichen amyloidosus unter dem klinischen Bild eines verrukösen Lichen chronicus Vidal. Derm. Wschr. 125: 460–464 (1952).

22. Erythrodermas

Erythroderma means extensive and therefore generalized redness of the outer integument, in most cases "from head to foot." The cutaneous change is usually associated with scaling, and, rarely, with vesicles or blisters. All in all, a more or less monotonous reaction is present; significantly, it remains "anonymous" with regard to etiology and is accompanied by the same monotonous reaction of the regional lymph nodes. Development toward an erythroderma takes place in the following manner: A cutaneous reaction, which apparently tends to chronicity, loses more and more of its original morphologic character during its course. But histologically such a chronic erythroderma is for the most part "anonymous" because through its long developmental phases, only the substrate of "chronic dermatitis" is present; if the dynamics of the disorder are subacutely increased, discrete spongiosis, parakeratosis, and "inflammatory" infiltrations may also appear. In the latter case, i.e., if a pronounced cutaneous infiltrate exists, the histologic analysis requires differentiation from reticulosis or reticulogranulomatosis.

On the other hand, there is now a tendency to restrict continuously the recognition of the formerly so-called primary generalized and exfoliating erythrodermas of the adult, so that at present only "desquamative recurrent scarlatiniform erythroderma" can be listed as a self-sustaining entity. Convincing arguments for a special niche for Hebra's pityriasis rubra (not to be confused with pityriasis rubra pilaris) as "primary" erythroderma are difficult to make, since the basic disturbance becomes apparent in the course of the disease process. Perhaps the so-called seborrheic old age erythroderma represents a special primary form. All erythrodermas, among them those, obviously, of secondary origin that follow such diseases as psoriasis vulgaris, lichen planus, "eczema," pityriasis rubra pilaris, mycosis fungoides, and so on, possess a pathologic mechanism that unites the group of erythrodermas. This special "vita erythroderma" is associated with loss of heat or hyperthermia and an extrathyroidal increase in the basal metabolism. There often exists a general tendency toward hypoproteinemia and dysproteinemia which cannot be explained by transcutaneous loss of protein (scaling). Clinically, loss of hair, loosening of the nails, and serious cachexia are evident. In any case, such continuous exertion, for which the patient cannot compensate after awhile, leads toward a gentle, slowly protracted death.[1, 2]

(1) Korting, G. W.: Über einige »anonyme« Krankheitszustände der Haut. Münch. med. Wschr. *108:* 973–978 (1966).
(2) Korting, G. W., H. Holzmann und E. Kallee: Zum Jodstoffwechsel der Erythrodermien. Arch. klin. exp. Derm. *216:* 155–160 (1963).

A. Congenital Erythrodermas

1. We shall discuss those erythrodermas that are associated with generalized or circumscribed hyperkeratoses and belong to the group of diffuse hereditary disturbances of keratinization.

Rather characteristic but with an intensity that varies greatly is the clinical picture of **collodion skin.** Erythroderma of varying intensity is already present at birth with large areas of parchmentlike, shiny, horny scales. The lack of flexibility of the skin can lead to deep tears (Fig. 234) at the body openings and flexures. In especially severe cases, an ectropion of the eyelids and lips and a fishmouth-like oral opening are present. The nails are malformed or absent. Hairs may also be underdeveloped or completely missing. Etiologically, this is no independent disorder but a variant of ichthyosis congenita, which is extensively described in Chapter 27 together with other forms of ichthyosis. Occasionally, a weakly developed collodion baby stage occurs in X-chromosomal recessive ichthyosis vulgaris and chondrodystrophia calcificans congenita (see Chapter 17, C7).[1, 9]

2. Congenital ichthyosiform erythroderma (bullous) is autosomally dominantly inherited, in contrast to ichthyosis congenita which is identical with congenital dry ichthyosiform erythroderma (Fig. 335). This disorder is either already present at birth or becomes manifest in the first weeks of life. The intensely red universal basic erythema with its large pieces of loose epidermis or bullous eruptions and its sore exudative character ("scalded children") is quite distinct from the drier or parchment paperlike appearance of collodion babies. Erythema and blisters are only facultative findings which, in addition, often exist for only a short time. In contrast to hereditary epidermolysis bullosa, the Nikolsky phenomenon, the limitation of blister formation to pressure points, and healing with scar formation are lacking. The mucous membranes always remain free from blisters. Even early in the course of the disease, the clinical picture will show partly hystrixlike hyperkeratoses (without basal erythema) on the palms and soles, on flexures, and in circumscribed arrangements on the trunk and extensor sides of the extremities (see also Chapter 27, A6). At this stage blister formation is often absent, so that from the appearance alone, a distinction from ichthyosis congenita may be impossible.

Fig. 334. Ichthyosis congenita (collodion baby).

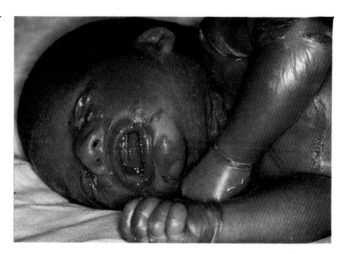

The histologic analysis is, therefore, decisive. In the area of the follicles the typical findings are granular degeneration of parts of the stratum spinosum and stratum granulosum, consisting of swelling of dyskeratotic cells and blurring of the cell borders, as well as deposits of basophilically tinged kernels of tonofilament and keratohyalin.[5, 7]

3. Erythrokeratoderma figurata variabilis (keratosis rubra figurata) is characterized by a typical association of erythrodermatic and keratotic features. Such erythrodermic, partly gyrated, partly "geographic," plaques are usually present from birth but may begin as late as the thirtieth year of life. They are symmetrical and are characterized by rapid changes in extension and intensity. Although the head and extremities are favorite sites, the palms and soles are spared in many patients. The keratotic plaques, however, react less intensely and less rapidly than the surrounding erythemas. After puberty and after the fiftieth year of life one may observe phases with a distinct tendency to spontaneous involution. This conspicuous change of extension and intensity alone distinguishes erythrokerato-

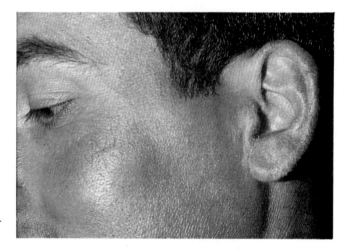

Fig. 335. Congenital ichthyosiform erythroderma.

derma figurata variabilis from the previously discussed ichthyosis vulgaris and
also from the erythroderma of pityriasis
rubra pilaris. Histologically, orthohyperkeratosis with acanthosis and papillomatosis is predominant. Granular degeneration,
in contrast to bullous congenital ichthyosiform erythroderma, is not present.[2, 6, 8]

4. In the few observations of **symmetrical erythroderma, congenital progressive,**
which seems to be transmitted as an autosomal dominant trait, erythrokeratodermic
areas are present. In these, erythemas form
merely a varyingly wide margin around the
hyperkeratoses. They develop in early
youth or as late as the beginning of adulthood and are located at the distal parts of
the extremities. This entity differs from
erythrokeratoderma figurata variabilis
mainly in the coexistence of erythema and
keratosis, the distinct persistence of the
erythemas, and the involvement of palms
and soles. Occasionally there are areas of
hyperpigmentation also which may show
point-shaped sparing of the follicular orifices and readiness to react isomorphically.
Histologically, islands of parakeratotic
horny formation are chiefly remarkable, as
well as orthohyperkeratosis, acanthosis,
and papillomatosis.[4]

5. Additional **(atypical) erythrokeratodermas** are characterized by either limited
localizations of distinct variability in the
same family or isolated occurrences. A sat-
isfying etiologic classification from a practical viewpoint is impossible at the present
time. A special report will therefore be
omitted here.

(1) BLOOM, D., and M. S. GOODFRIED:
Lamellar ichthyosis of the newborn.
The »collodion baby«: a clinical and
genetic entity; report of a case and review of the literature with special consideration of pathogenesis and classification. Arch. Derm. (Chic.) *86:* 336–342
(1962).

(2) GERTLER, W.: Lokalisierte Erythro-
keratodermien. Derm. Wschr. *136:* 1257
bis 1272 (1957).

(3) GREITHER, A.: Zur Klassifikation der
Ichthyosis-Gruppe. Dermatologica (Basel) *128:* 464–482 (1964).

(4) KOGOJ, FR.: Erythrokeratodermia extremitatum symmetrica et Hyperchromia dominans. Z. Haut- u. Geschl.-Kr.
20: 187–192 (1956).

(5) LAPIERE, S.: Les génodermatoses hyperkératosiques de type bulleux. Ann.
Derm. Syph. (Paris) *80:* 597–614 (1953).

(6) MENDES DA COSTA, S.: Erythro- et
Keratodermia variabilis in a mother
and a daughter. Acta derm.-venereol.
(Stockh.) *6:* 255–261 (1925).

(7) SCHNYDER, U. W.: Zur Histogenetik der
granulösen Degeneration. Pathol. et
Microbiol. (Basel) *27:* 486–493 (1964).

(8) SOMMACAL-SCHOPF, D., und U. W.
SCHNYDER: Über eine Familie mit 14
Fällen von Erythrokeratodermia figurata
variabilis. Hautarzt *8:* 174–176 (1957).

(9) WOLFRAM, G.: Ein Beitrag zur konnatalen Kollodiumhaut. Derm. Wschr. *137:*
650–657 (1958).

B. Forms of Erythrodermas Occurring Principally in Childhood

The differential diagnosis of the various
erythrodermas in infants and early childhood can be difficult and is sometimes possible only after a long period of observation.
Of the three types of eczema (common eczema, seborrheic dermatitis, and atopic
dermatitis), erythrodermic maximal development in small children can be expected
only in seborrheic and atopic dermatitides.

1. Erythroderma desquamativa represents
the maximal variant of seborrheic dermatitis in infants and small children and occurs more frequently in girls than in boys.
Its onset is between the first and second
months of life, apparently without pruritus
and without blister formation but with rapid extension of the cutaneous changes. They
are present first on the buttocks and the

head and constitute large, vividly red and yellowish-red erythemas with large areas of scaling. Enlarged lymph nodes are missing as a rule. In the later course of the disease, thin, mucous stools, tachycardia, enlarged liver, edema, and hypoproteinemia almost always become associated. Secondary infection with staphylococci or species of Candida has an important role in the diagnosis of the further course of the skin lesions as well as in the prognosis of these children. One can safely state that the differentiation between desquamative erythroderma with secondary Candida infection and erythrodermic candidiasis can be rather difficult. In the latter case, the first areas of involvement are principally the anal region and the intertriginous areas. The erythemas, which are at first round or polycyclic, subsequently present collarlike desquamation with satellite spreading of small elements around the older and larger involved areas. In contrast, Leiner's dermatosis shows large lamellar scales, no collars of scales, and corymbiform spreading. It takes less time to develop areas of redness, thus suggesting erythroderma from the beginning.

2. The other erythroderma in the eczematous child is **atopic erythroderma,** which arises from the constitution of the atopic dermatitis but is hardly ever observed in an adult. It starts in an infant around the fourth to twelfth week of life, corresponding to the time of a developing cradle cap, and characteristically spreads rapidly from an already existing atopic dermatitis. Only rarely is erythroderma the primary manifestation of the disorder. In addition, the skin is infiltrated with a distinct formation of scales. Pruritus is severe. Last but not least, atopic erythroderma is characterized by conspicuous involvement of the adjacent lymph nodes in the form of impressive, nonconfluent nodules, which are movable over their base and below the skin. In addition, leukocytosis with a high degree of eosinophilia is frequently present. Support-

ing a diagnosis of this form of erythroderma are a positive family history (atopic dermatitis, hay fever, and asthma) and subsequent development of reactive forms (flexural eczema, prurigo) characteristic of atopic dermatitis. As in exfoliative erythroderma, atopic erythroderma undergoes a development, according to its character as an eczema, which lasts for months and tends to recurrences (see also Chapter 1, C3). [1-4]

3. Exfoliative dermatitis of the newborn, which is nothing else but an extensive bullous staphylodermia, usually develops in the newborn. It starts around the mouth, with characteristic noninvolvement of the palms and soles. Extensive bullous separation of the skin then develops fulminantly, and eroded, red, and oozing areas or a general state of epidermolysis with a positive Nikolsky phenomenon remains. The epidermis is often tangentially separable as in an exfoliative scaly-crusted erythroderma or like

Fig. 336. Exfoliative staphylococcic dermatitis.

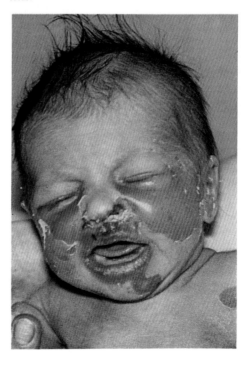

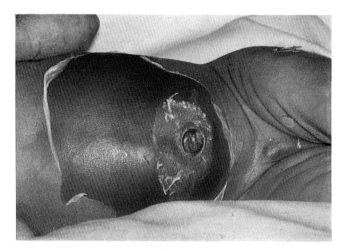

Fig. 337. Exfoliative staphylococcic dermatitis.

the skin of a ripe peach (Figs. 336, 337). The general condition of these children may sometimes appear undisturbed but, if septic complications develop, it may become life-threatening. This bullous superficial sta-

Fig. 338. Toxic epidermal necrolysis (Lyell's syndrome).

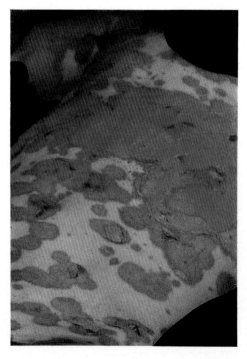

phyloderma, when it occurs in the adult, has been called *Lyell's syndrome* (see also Chapter 25, A8) or *toxic acute epidermolysis* (toxic epidermal necrolysis) (Figs. 338, 339, 340). In the adult, however, it seems that we are dealing in most cases with a "toxic-allergic," bullous epidermolytic exanthem, whereas in infants and children the sta-phylogenic origin is most important. There is some difference between the exfoliative dermatitis and Lyell's syndrome with regard to mucous membrane involvement: only in Lyell's syndrome does it reach excessive dimensions (oral cavity, esophagus, trachea, conjunctivae, and genitals).

So-called *measles pemphigoid* represents most probably a viral disease superimposed on acute toxic epidermolysis. If, however, irislike erythemas are present in addition to erythematobullous changes, differential diagnosis versus erythema multiforme is necessary, a decision that may be difficult in some cases since in Lyell's syndrome as well as in erythema multiforme, pluri-orifi-cial mucous membrane changes (conjunctiva, oral cavity, respiratory tract, and so on) are often present in the highest degree.*
[5, 6]

---

* The two diseases may be one and the same. (Tr.)

Fig. 339. Lyell's syndrome.

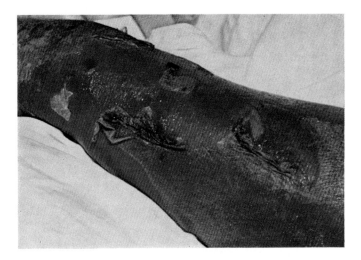

4. Only rarely does **urticaria pigmentosa** lead to diffuse infiltration of mast cells of almost the entire skin surface. The clinical picture is less that of an "inflammatory" reaction than of brownish color caused by increased brown melanin deposits. In other instances the color is more yellowish than brown in tone. Additional characteristics of such diffuse cutaneous mastocytosis are pachydermic thickenings of the skin with occasional superficial kernels or small nodose interspersion and increased skin markings, especially in the axillary and inguinal areas. Another characteristic of such mast cell reticulosis is the tendency to dermatographia, wheals, and bullae. Blisters not only are provoked by friction or thermic stimuli but form spontaneously without a recognizable outer cause. As in other dermatoses, the tendency to vesiculation is greatly diminished in the adult. Involvement of additional organs, especially the skeleton, is rare in mast cell erythrodermas, which do not always have an unfavorable outcome. Pruritus and fever, on the other hand, are relatively frequent.[2, 3, 8]

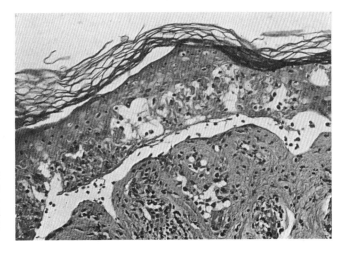

Fig. 340. Lyell's syndrome: beginning necrosis of the epidermis, hydropic degeneration, homogenization and suprabasal cleavage. HE stain, 160×.

(1) BANDMANN, H.-J.: Beobachtung zur Klinik und Therapie der Erythrodermia atopica Hill. Hautarzt *18:* 246–251 (1967).

(2) BURGOON, C. F., J. H. GRAHAM and D. L. McCAFFREE: Mast cell disease. A cutaneous variant with multisystem involvement. Arch. Derm. (Chic.) *98:* 590–605 (1968).

(3) HAENSCH, R., und H. IPPEN: Zur Klinik der Mastzell-Erythrodermie. Hautarzt *19:* 403–407 (1968).

(4) HILL, L. W.: Nomenclature, classification, and pathogenesis of »eczema« in infancy. Arch. Derm. Syph. (Chic.) *66:* 212–222 (1952).

(5) KÖTTGEN, U., und G. W. KORTING: Zur Frage des Masernpemphigoids. Dtsch. med. Wschr. *89:* 2318–2321 (1964).

(6) KORTING, G. W., und H. HOLZMANN: Universelle Epidermolysis acuta toxica. Arch. klin. exp. Derm. *210:* 1–13 (1960).

(7) MISGELD, V., U.-M. GROSS, J. KRATZER und K.-D. v. ROSENSTIEL: Zum Lyell-Syndrom (Toxic Epidermal Necrolysis). Med. Klin. *68:* 398–404 (1973).

(8) SAGHER, F., and Z. EVEN-PAZ: Mastocytosis and the mast cell. Karger, Basel, New York 1967

C. Erythrodermas, Chiefly of the Adult (Exfoliative Dermatitis)

1. With reference to age, infantile erythrodermas are at the opposite pole from the desquamative erythrodermas of old age, the so-called "**seborrheic**" **erythrodermas of the old** (Fig. 341). Such erythrodermas of old age start quite frequently as "seborrheic dermatitis," or sometimes as contact dermatitis (for instance, owing to turpentine sensitivity); this could be called autonomous eczematization. If the cause of development is not obvious, one has to accept a diagnosis of an autonomous exfoliative erythroderma. Should cachexia, pigmentation,

and swelling of lymph nodes become prominent, a diagnosis of benign hyperplastic cutaneous reticulohistiocytosis with melanoderma (Fig. 342) or subacute generalized exfoliative dermatitis can be made; however, such a diagnosis does not help to explain the etiology or pathogenesis, let alone the therapy. Because of the conspicuous swollen lymph nodes near the skin there was at one time a tendency to group such exfoliative erythrodermas with the "reticuloses."

Old age erythroderma itself appears as a dark red erythema with a tendency toward dark brown hues combined with bran-like and sometimes lamellar to coarse lamellar scaling. The scalp is almost always the site of thick scaling which can result in subtotal alopecia; however, if regression of the rest of the skin signs takes place, the alopecia is reversible. Sometimes there is thinning of the axillary hair and also most of the pubic hair. Likewise, there is loosening or loss of the fingernails, or the nails may show dystrophic transverse furrows. Depending on the activity of the eruption, the degree of infiltration and exudation of the skin varies; oozing may take place in intertriginous areas. Pruritus, fever, and severe chills with or without subsequent elevation of temperature are further, although variable, signs. After some months, a regular and prominent feature of erythroderma is development of cachexia, especially if there has been no treatment.

Histologically, there are no special findings. Besides orthokeratosis, hyperkeratosis, and parakeratosis, one sees acanthosis with somewhat irregular elongation of the rete pegs; however, the irregularity does not even come close to that in mycosis fungoides. A histologic diagnosis of old age erythroderma can be arrived at by observing perivascular lymphohistiocytic accumulations, sometimes mixed with eosinophils and giant cells, and an increase in the epidermal melanin, which is, more rarely combined with incontinence of pigment In most cases the axillary and inguina

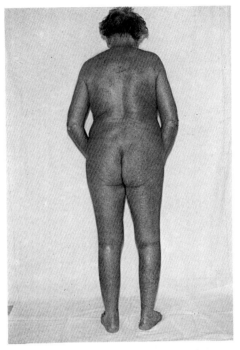

Fig. 341. Seborrheic old age erythroderma.

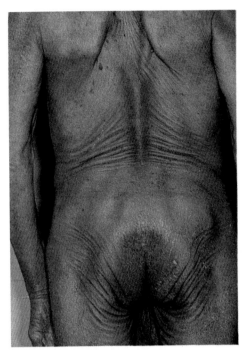

Fig. 342. Melanoerythroderma.

lymph nodes are definitely enlarged; they are indolent, hard, and freely movable against each other, against the epidermis, and against the underlying tissue. All this represents a basic lymphonodular reaction. The intensity of this enlargement of the lymph nodes depends on the varying degrees of involvement of the epidermis and is synchronous with the intensity of the erythroderma; in contrast, "*lipomelanotic reticulosis*" fails to show a specific reaction of the lymph nodes.

Histologically, this reticulosis shows follicular, lymphatic hyperplasia, large areas of reticulum cell hyperplasia near the cortical sinuses, deposition of isotropic lipids, melanin, and hemosiderin, and finally, a lacunalike dilatation of the cortical sinuses, together with plasma cells, eosinophils, and Russell bodies (Fig. 343). Finally, in addition to this reticulum cell proliferation, formation of new blood vessels occurs, giving a granulomalike appearance. In any case,

the normal basic structure of the lymph node remains intact; this dermopathic lipomelanotic lymphadenopathy obviously does not form a base for subsequent malignant lymph node development.[7, 8, 10, 19]

The previously mentioned *subacute generalized exfoliative dermatitis* does not differ clinically from seborrheic old age erythroderma. It is not justified to make a differential diagnosis of these two diseases only from the absence or presence of loss of hair and from disorders in the growth of nails. A differentiation based on the dynamics of the two diseases does not permit the establishment of two independent disease entities (on the one hand, generalized subacute exfoliative dermatitis may develop in a few days, and, on the other hand, seborrheic erythroderma of old age takes a protracted course). The diagnosis of subacute generalized exfoliative dermatitis establishes only a working basis until a definite etiologic clarification can be made.[20]

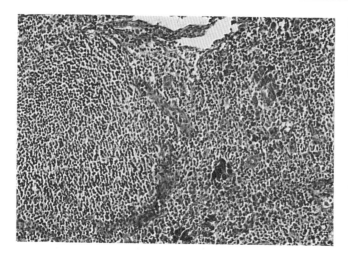

Fig. 343. So-called "lipomel-anotic reticulosis": lymph node with increased reticu-lum cells and focal melanin deposits. HE stain, 100×.

2. In cases of erythroderma of unknown etiology it is important to exclude the presence of a dermatosis simulating erythroderma caused by leukosis, reticulosis, or giant follicular lymphoblastoma. Among the chronic dermatoleukohemoblastoses, erythrodermatic forms such as **diffuse leukemia cutis** can be expected only with the chronic lymphadenoses. The question of whether cutaneous myelosis may present as universal erythroderma cannot yet be answered in the affirmative because there is not a sufficient number of case reports.

Apparently, the observations made so far show extremely close aggregations of cutaneous myelosis lesions without any definite connection with a specific erythrodermic base. The cutaneous areas show either an unspecific histologic picture (papular exanthem) (Fig. 344) or a specific structure (leukemid). The color of lymphatic erythroderma ranges from dark red to brownish-red; internally the disease presents hepatosplenomegaly and generalized enlargement of lymph nodes. The development may start primarily with a specific leukemic

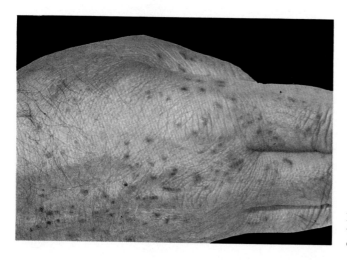

Fig. 344. Leukosis of imma-ture cells: unspecific papular eruption.

Fig. 345. Chronic lymphadenosis: Specific infiltrate of
the corium with free sub-
epidermal borderline. HE
stain, 25×.

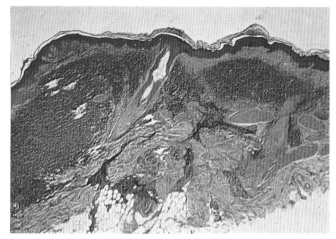

erythroderma or, on the other hand, an unspecific exfoliative erythroderma may develop finally into universal erythroderma composed of specific elements. Such a transition into specificity takes place so slowly that clinically only repeated biopsies will discover the true state of affairs. The magnitude of the specific leukotic cutaneous manifestations does not run parallel to the intensity of the leukemic changes of the blood. Very rarely one will observe the simultaneous presence of specific and non-specific infiltrates. Histologically, specific leukemic erythroderma frequently shows, below a free subepidermal borderline in the deeper regions, sharply bordered, dense nodules composed of relatively monotonous round cell infiltrates (Fig. 345) with occasional single lymphoblasts and plasmocytes. The main difficulty in differential diagnosis will be separation of the reticulogranulomatosis group from the erythrodermas.[5, 6]

3. Giant follicular lymphoblastoma (Brill-Symmers) infrequently shows cutaneous changes consisting of small nodules interspersed within an exfoliative dermatitis either as an unspecific reaction or as a specific disease effect. Histologically, reactive,

enlarged, giant-sized lymph follicles with relatively monomorphous cytology are seen together with considerable changes of the basic structure of the lymph node, an appearance that contrasts with that of follicular lymphatic hyperplasia. Otherwise, histologic examination of the skin shows no changes corresponding to the emphasis on the follicular aspect of the lymph nodes.[9, 18]

4. Reticuloses seldom take a predominantly erythrodermic course. The first sign may be pruritus, followed after some time by pruritic, eczematoid, psoriasiform, or parapsoriasiform areas; finally, a diffuse erythroderma will develop from head to foot. Depending on their location, there will be differences in the appearance of the lesions, with variations in the degree of erythema, pigmentation, and infiltration. Sometimes the lesions may start with edema and weeping or with dry desquamation. These two types later may show formation of nodules, and less frequently, interspersion with petechiae. In histologic examination such progressive irreversible proliferations of the reticulohistiocytic system show predominantly monomorphic periap-

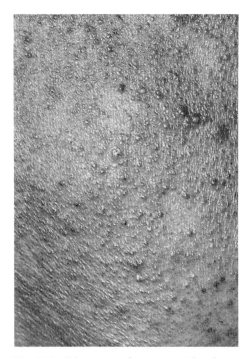

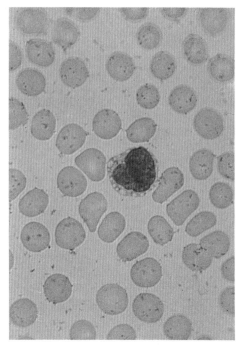

Fig. 346. Sézary syndrome: erythroderma consisting of small nodular infiltrates, limited to the follicles.

Fig. 347. Sézary-cell in peripheral blood smear. May-Grünwald stain, 1000×.

pendicular histiocytic masses of cells and only occasionally special cellular modulations (see also Table 15).[15, 16]

5. The Sézary syndrome is characterized by generalized erythema interspersed with mostly small nodular infiltrates, or, less frequently, with large nodular lesions (Fig. 346). The face in particular is covered by heavy infiltrates, giving the appearance of a leonine facies. Simultaneously there are severe pruritus, generalized superficial lymphadenopathy, and occasionally also dystrophic changes of nails and skin. Such erythroderma is accompanied by the presence of atypical mononuclear cells in the circulating blood and in the skin. Around the nucleus in these monocytoid cells, which resemble atypical reticulum cells, are vacuoles in a cerebriform arrangement

which contain a diastase-resistant, PAS-positive, polysaccharide material (Fig. 347). The Sézary syndrome can be classified as an intermediate form between erythrodermic mycosis fungoides and chronic lymphadenosis.[13, 24]

6. Some erythrodermas develop as abnormal reactions to sunlight. Cutaneous areas exposed to light are interspersed with micropapular lesions, which, surprisingly, on histologic examination show demonstrable reticular hematodermic infiltrates; these findings lead to the classification of such actinic erythroderma as **actinic reticulosis**. This dependency on light can also be demonstrated by a definitely diminished threshold to solar erythema. Sometimes the amount of urinary coproporphyrin is increased.[3, 12]

7. Reticuloendothelial proliferations of the skin depend on suitable stimuli and are therefore capable of regression; such proliferations can be called either orthopathic reticuloses or **reticulocytoses.** Occasionally, they have been observed as at least partially erythrodermic cutaneous reactions, sometimes also with small nodules and papules. Histologically, it is hardly possible to differentiate this eruption from a definite autonomous neoplastic reticulosis; a thorough history (especially as to drugs) and the benign course eventually will permit a diagnosis (see also Chapter 38, G8).[25]

8. Mycosis fungoides may have an erythrodermic or diffuse character which either follows a vague premycotic stage or may be an expression of a progressive intermediate phase (Fig. 348). In contrast to the classic Alibert-Bazin type of mycosis fungoides, mycotic erythroderma ("érythrodermie mycosique") appearing with universal redness (Indian skin, "homme rouge," "homme orange") or as a common "exfoliative dermatitis" cannot always be diagnosed with certainty by inspection only. Such mycosis fungoides erythroderma will occasionally develop in a short span of time; usually it is accompanied by pruritus, loss of hair, and loosening of nails — signs occurring also in other erythrodermas. In contrast to the lymphadenopathies observed in leukemic erythrodermas, mycosis

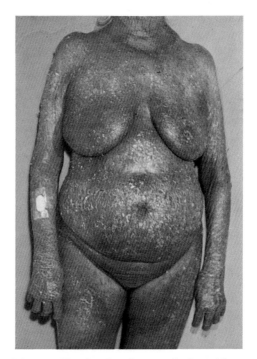

Fig. 348. Erythrodermic mycosis fungoides.

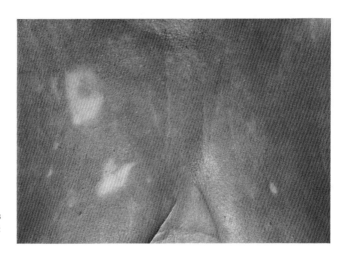

Fig. 349. Mycosis fungoides of the erythrodermic type: "nappes claires."

fungoides erythroderma as a rule lacks involvement of the lymph nodes. It is difficult to establish definite clinical signs for mycosis fungoides erythroderma. An increase in the consistency of the skin, accentuation of the normal cutaneous markings, varying degrees of desquamation, colors changing from dirty brown to red and deepening to bluish-violet on the lower extremities — all these changes can be observed in erythrodermas of different origin. Somewhat pathognomonic for the erythrodermic type of mycosis fungoides are small macular, triangular, or bizarre whitish patches of uninvolved skin ("nappes claires") within otherwise solid erythematous areas (Fig. 349).

9. An erythrodermic type of **sarcoidosis** is an uncommon occurrence; such a diagnosis requires confirmation by the observation of sarcoidal manifestations in other organs. To accept a case of sarcoidosis or Boeck-Besnier-Schaumann's disease as genuine, it is necessary to find epithelioid cell granulomas in many of the internal organs. A diagnosis of the erythrodermic form of sarcoidosis could be sustained by the simultaneous presence of other forms of cutaneous sarcoids (lupus pernio, uveoparotid fever, among others). The cases of sarcoidal erythroderma observed so far have demonstrated only minimal infiltration and lichenification, along with a distinct tendency to atrophy. In contrast to psoriatic erythroderma, there was an absence of capillary bleeding upon removal of the moderately thick scales. The erythema may show a perifollicular intensification that may persist for months and years without special symptoms except for occasional moderate pruritus.

Histologically, one sees discrete diffuse groups of epithelioid cells located periappendicularly; nodular lesions are less common. Like erythroderma of different genesis, the Boeck's type of erythroderma also shows vascular and perivascular infiltrations.[23,26]

Turning from the erythrodermas formerly known as "primary" and those either accompanying a systemic disease or specifically caused by such a disease, we will now proceed to what are still called "secondary" erythrodermas. It should be emphasized, however, that such a distinction is hardly tenable any longer.

10. In the manner of the erythrodermas previously discussed in connection with seborrheic dermatitis and atopic eczema (Chapter 22, B1, B2, and C1), **common eczema** may develop into a generalized dermatitis. When this takes place, the erythrodermic common eczema loses all of its former characteristic criteria and becomes transformed into the anonymity of a universal, more or less infiltrated, scaly or weeping dermatitis. Such erythrodermic common eczemas will eventually be complicated by other processes, such as lymphadenopathy or general cachexia, and finally will correspond to the so-called "lipomelanotic reticulosis."

11. Other common dermatoses may develop into really universal erythrodermas, which at first sight cannot be differentiated from erythrodermas of other origin. An example of such a difficult diagnosis is the **erythrodermic type of psoriasis,** if it is marked by an absence of scaling and nail changes and also by a lack of previous psoriatic manifestations (Fig. 350).

A special characteristic quality of psoriatic erythroderma is that when it finally begins to disappear, the skin will not return to normal immediately; instead, there will be an intermediate stage with development of lesions of psoriasis vulgaris. In addition, erythrodermic psoriasis often alternates with other manifestations of psoriasis such as arthropathic, exudative, or pustular phases. Less frequently, such phases may occur at the same time. Other manifestations are predominantly dry, pityriasiform lesions, and sometimes also thin, moist, exudative scaling areas appearing as weep-

ing, dusky red, cutaneous patches. Secondary pyodermas — for instance, subacute
abscesses or furuncles — are observed rather rarely and can be ascribed to injudicious
treatment with suppressive systemic drugs
without simultaneous antibiotic protec-
tion. A causative factor in the development
of psoriatic erythroderma might be a focal
infection (dental granulomas, amalgam fillings of dental cavities) or metabolic disturbances; another cause might be external
irritation from "too strong" local treatment. Also, medications known to provoke
psoriasis (chloroquine, gold) must not be
overlooked. However, occasionally psoriatic erythrodermas occur even when these
causes do not exist, in which case the development to erythroderma takes place without "provocation" by steady progressive
enlargement of the psoriatic areas.

Histologically, however, in spite of the
clinically uniform character of erythrodermic psoriasis, the typical structure of
psoriasis will remain intact (parakeratosis
with absence of the keratohyaline phase,
narrow pointed acanthosis, edema of the
apices of the papillae with abnormally long
capillaries, lymphocytic microabscesses).
The biopsy should not be taken from a
moist or "overtreated" region.

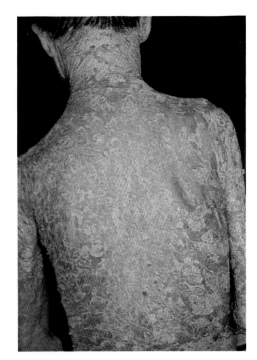

Fig. 350. Psoriatic erythroderma.

12. Within the group of parapsoriases,
Brocq's disease, although called an "erythroderma" with disseminated plaques, is
a chronic disorder which never develops
confluence of the lesions. These appear in
longitudinal streaks with a slightly saturated yellow-brownish color and often show
pseudoatrophic generalized areas in folds.
Only if the unvaried aspect of Brocq's disease reveals itself as mycosis fungoides will
confluence to partial or universal erythroderma develop, with simultaneous beginning polymorphism and polycyclism.

13. It is seldom that **lichen planus,** even
without external irritation (sulfur), devel-

ops into universal exfoliative erythroderma.
In such cases the lesions, which have been
isolated, coalesce to form still larger
plaques, so that the characteristic primary
lesion is perhaps still evident only at the
border of the erythroderma. In addition,
the erythroderma of lichen planus is often
interrupted by nonaffected streaks or netlike areas. In one of my own observations
lichen ruber pemphigoides of the skin occurred simultaneously. The reticulated lesions on the oral and genital mucous membranes may facilitate the diagnosis in unclear cases.

14. Another disorder that may develop
into universal erythroderma is **pityriasis
rubra pilaris,** which in a single instance may
be difficult to distinguish from lichen ruber
acuminatus. It may happen that at the
moment of examination no acuminated fol-

licular micropapules (on the extensor surfaces of the fingers or genitals), no psoriasiform areas on elbows and knees, no pityriasiform scaling of a facial erythema with the coloring of an American Indian and no palmoplantar hyperkeratoses are present, so that the classification of these erythematosquamous areas is difficult or even impossible. In general, however, the character of the scale in erythroderma of pityriasis rubra pilaris is like plaster of paris — fine and clinging — with no Auspitz's phenomenon being elicited when the scale, which is not stratified, is scratched off. Finally, the basic erythema of pityriasis rubra pilaris, apart from the slightly reddened face, is rather yellowish-red, so that on these criteria pemphigus erythematosus or psoriasis erythrodermica will be rejected. Sudden onset and rapid generalization of the cutaneous changes until the stage of fully developed erythroderma can occur in children as well as in adults.[2]

Fig. 351. Pemphigus foliaceus.

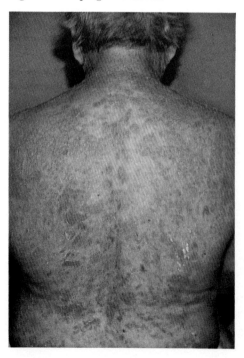

15. Within the group of pemphigus disorders **pemphigus foliaceus** is a subtype, which usually begins as pemphigus vulgaris and develops into exfoliating, squamous-crusted erythroderma (Figs. 351, 352). There are certainly cases without this change; their exfoliation starts with the onset of the disease. On the other hand, pemphigus foliaceus may revert to pemphigus vulgaris; this was known even before the introduction of cortisone for chronic pemphigus. Because the first locations of lesions of pemphigus foliaceus are the midface, scalp, chest, or the upper part of the back, a differential diagnosis against pemphigus erythematosus (Senear-Usher syndrome) must be considered in the beginning. The facial lesions above all are characterized by severe hyperkeratotic scaling. Moreover, the hyperkeratotic scales show tacklike projections corresponding to follicular funnels. This appearance may at times resemble lupus erythematosus. An easily elicited Nikolsky sign, however, favors pemphigus foliaceus. In addition, of all forms of pemphigus, pemphigus foliaceus especially seems to possess a peculiar penetrating fetor. In view of the extensive and severe epidermal maceration of this special form of pemphigus, this is understandable. The bad odor reminds one of that of severely macerated psoriasis erythroderma or of such psoriatic areas which have been treated for a long time with occlusive cortisone ointments.

16. Another disorder, which in certain cases may simulate chronic universal erythroderma by reason of its excessive, warty, and horny scaling, as well as its blood eosinophilia and absent itching, is **Norwegian scabies,** especially if lymph node involvement and cachexia are present. In general, however, after a period of time, when persons in contact with such "anesthetic" patients develop typical itching, the diagnosis of scabies will become evident.

Fig. 352. Pemphigus foliaceus.

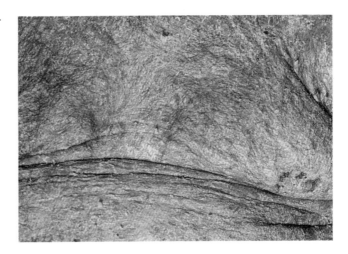

**17. Erythema scarlatiniforme desquama-
tivum recidivans** is another disorder which
is not limited to a special period in life. A
single bout is characterized by a scarlet
fever-like course. A generalized scarlatiniforme erythema is present at the beginning,
and is followed by typically large lamellar,
membranous or glovelike desquamation
(Fig. 353). In most cases the first signs of
redness of the skin are on the chest, face,
and the large body-folds. Characteristic of
this form of erythema, however, is its
strange mode of recurrence. Between the
periodic or irregularly spaced manifestations complete clearing may occur. Fever,
headache, and arthralgia may precede the
eruption. Involvement of the mucous membranes, reversible diffuse loss of hair, and
nail changes may or may not occur. The
typical raspberry tongue of the patient
with scarlet fever is missing. A kidney affection with proteinuria and microhematuria
may be present, increasing the character of
the disorder as scarlatiniform. Leukocytosis with eosinophilia and short-lasting increases of the ESR are noted. The differen-

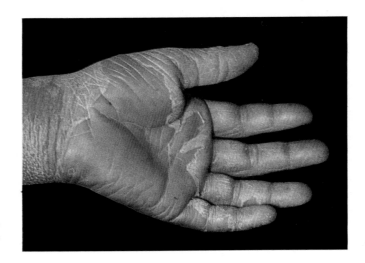

Fig. 353. Recurring des-
quamating scarlatiniform
erythema.

tial diagnosis against genuine scarlet fever or the extremely rare recurrences of scarlet fever may be difficult, especially if the patient is a child. Determination of the antistreptolysin titer may perhaps help to differentiate the disorder from genuine scarlet fever, in which the titer is positive in 80 to 90 per cent. In the adult, the Dick test may help to distinguish scarlet fever. A thorough history will facilitate the diagnosis of scarlatiniform erythrodermas following drugs (mercury, quinine, and hydantoin).Membranous scale does not occur as regularly, and apart from reexposures no recurrent attacks are observed.[4, 14, 21]

18. Exfoliating erythroderma in the course of **histoplasmosis** is rare. Usually several days to weeks after inhalation of the fungal spores, flu-like signs (pneumonia) appear and then take an unusually protracted course. When the organisms get

Fig. 354. Salvarsan erythroderma.

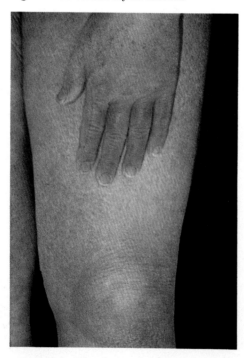

into the lymph and blood many organs can become affected. Most frequent are ulcerations of the mucous membranes. Histologic and cultural evidence of histoplasma capsulatum then confirm the diagnosis of such erythroderma.[22]

19. Different from the previously described dry and only occasionally oozing, almost always subchronically or chronically exfoliating erythrodermas are those vesiculoedematous erythrodermas which cover their vasculocutaneous origin by their acuity and severe epidermal alteration. They give the impression of dermatoses. The prototype of this group, the acute salvarsan damage of the skin, is usually called "dermatitis" and seldom **salvarsan erythroderma** (Fig. 354). It is dominated by waterlogged swellings, oozing, and vesicle formation. Usually such *toxic-allergic erythrodermas* (for instance, from gold and other heavy metals, quinine, mercury, barbiturates, or sulfonamides) start at a certain skin area and become rapidly generalized. This also occurs in salvarsan erythroderma after paravenous injection of the drug.

20. Apparently, acute vitamin-A **hypervitaminoses** (caused by either therapeutic error or ingestion of the livers of polar bears or certain fishes) with severe constitutional onset (nausea, drowsiness, tachycardia, increased need for sleep) can also cause vesiculoedematous redness, which later changes to the dry, lightly scaling reaction of erythema (Fig. 355). Only rarely do these erythemas increase to form areas of really universal erythrodermas.[1, 17]

(1) BODIAN, E. L.: Skin manifestation of Conradi's disease. Chondrodystrophia congenita punctata. Arch. Derm. (Chic.) *94:* 743–748 (1966).

(2) DAVIDSON, CH. L., R. K. WINKELMANN and R. R. KIERLAND: Pityriasis rubra pilaris. A followup study of 57 patients. Arch. Derm. (Chic.) *100:* 175–178 (1969).

(3) DEGOS, R., J. CIVATTE, H. AKHOUND-ZADEH, J.-Y. NOURY, F. DANIEL, M. LARRÉGUE et G. AUDEBERT: Actino-réticulose. Photo-allergie avec infiltrat hématodermique. Ann. Derm. Syph. (Paris) *97:* 121–134 (1970).

(4) FISCHBECK, R., und G. ZUCKER: Phenyl-hydantoin (5,5 Diphenylhydantoin)-Überempfindlichkeit unter dem klinischen Bild einer skarlatiniformen Erythrodermie. Dtsch. Gesundh.-Wes. *21:* 1273–1277 (1966).

(5) HARTMANN, E.: Über die Einteilung der myeloisch-leukämischen Erkrankungen der Haut vom dermatologisch-klinischen Gesichtspunkt. Derm. Z. *49:* 52–67 (1927).

(6) HERZBERG, J. J.: Die Pathogenese der Erythrodermien bei chronisch lymphatischer Leukose. Arch. klin. exp. Derm. *202:* 208–223 (1956).

(7) HOCHLEITNER, H.: Zur Klinik der Erythrodermien. Derm. Wschr. *148:* 653–666 (1963).

(8) KABOTH, W.: Die cutane Reticulo-histiocytose mit Melanodermie. Z. Haut- u. Geschl.-Kr. *33:* 69–76 (1962).

(9) KELLER, PH., und M. STAEMMLER: Erythrodermie und Brill-Symmerssche Krankheit. Hautarzt *3:* 101–107 (1952).

(10) KIESSLING, W., und H. TRITSCH: Die Melano-Erythrodermie mit Kachexie. Arch. klin. exp. Derm. *208:* 579–591 (1959).

(11) KNOTH, W., P. BREITWIESER und D. KLEINHANS: Zur Kenntnis unspezifischer Begleitdermatosen bei Lympho-granulomatose. Med. Welt *19* (N.F.): 170–177 (1968).

(12) KORTING, G. W.: Lichtbedingte retikuläre Hyperplasie der Haut. Med. Welt *22* (N.F.): 826–827 (1971).

(13) KORTING, G. W., und F. NÜRNBERGER: Sézary-Syndrom. Hautarzt *21:* 178–181 (1970).

(14) LAUSECKER, H.: Das Erythema scarlatiniforme desquamativum recidivans. Arch. Derm. Syph. (Berl.) *198:* 529–548 (1954).

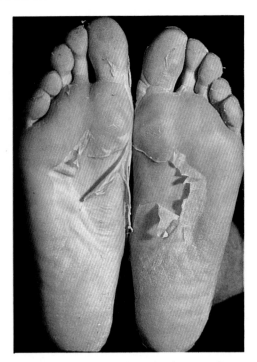

Fig. 355. Vitamin A intoxication: erythema with large lamellar scaling.

(15) MUSGER, A.: Erythrodermatische Haut-retikulosen. Hautarzt *17:* 148–152 (1966).

(16) MUSGER, A.: Hautretikulosen. Med. Klin. *62:* 1157–1160 (1967).

(17) NATER, J. P., and H. M. G. DOEGLAS: Halibut liver poisoning in 11 fishermen. Acta derm.-venereol. (Stockh.) *50:* 109–113 (1970).

(18) POLANO, M.K.: Über Hauterscheinungen beim Morbus Brill-Symmers. Hautarzt *8:* 136–138 (1957).

(19) REICH, H.: Die lipomelanotische Reti-culose. In: Dermatologie u. Venerologie. Hrsg. H. A. GOTTRON und W. SCHÖNFELD. Erg.- u. Reg.-Bd. S. 255–261. Thieme, Stuttgart 1970.

(20) RICHTER, R.: Zur Klinik der generalisierten exfoliierenden Erythrodermien. Arch. Derm. Syph. (Berl.) *179:* 611–638 (1939).

(21) RIEGEL, K., und G. W. KORTING: Zur
Kenntnis viscerocutaner Wechselwirkungen mit hoher Bluteosinophilie unter
dem Bilde des Löfflerschen Lungeninfiltrates und des Erythema scarlatiniforme   desquamativum   recidivans.
Arch. klin. exp. Derm. *205:* 235–244
(1957).

(22) SAMOVITZ, M., and TH. K. DILLON:
Disseminated histoplasmosis presenting
as exfoliative erythroderma. Arch.
Derm. (Chic.) *101:* 216–219 (1970).

(23) SCADDING, J. G.: Sarcoidosis. Eyre &
Spottiswoode, London 1967.

(24) TEDESCHI, L. G., and D. T. LANSINGER:
Sézary syndrome; a malignant leukemic
reticuloendotheliosis.   Arch.   Derm.
(Chic.) *92:* 257–262 (1965).

(25) UNDEUTSCH, W., und U. BALFANZ:
Kleinknotig-papulöse erythrodermische
lymphoretikuläre Hyperplasie der Haut.
Z. Haut- u. Geschl.-Kr. *37:* 231–243
(1964).

(26) WIGLEY, J. E. M., and L. A. MUSSO:
A case of sarcoidosis with erythroder-
mic lesions. Treatment with Calciferol.
Brit. J. Derm. *63:* 398–407 (1951).

23. Poikilodermas

Poikiloderma is characterized by checkered cutaneous changes consisting of atrophy, pigmentation (mostly in grouped or
reticulated arrangement), and telangiectases. Occasionally, mild scaling and purpuric
elements will be present; also, this condition almost always will be the final stage
of different, quite heterogeneous, pathological conditions. Acquired poikilodermas
are preceded by dyschromias, while telangiectases and atrophy occur later. The opposite is true for congenital poikilodermas
in which telangiectases in most cases are
the first sign of the later fully developed
poikilodermic picture; in addition, many
congenital defects may accompany this
condition.

A. Congenital Poikilodermas

1. The syndrome of Thomson and the
congenital dystrophy of Rothmund are
combined in present terminology as the
Rothmund-Thomson syndrome. The children, who are often the offspring of consan-
guineous marriages, are born with an apparently normal skin. Between the third
and twelfth month of life approximately,
pink patches will appear at first on the face
(Fig. 356), ears, and the dorsa of the hands.
These erythemas often resemble a sunburn;
later these areas develop into reticulated
and striated, small, yellowish-white atrophic lesions. Simultaneously, telangiectatic
cutaneous changes become more evident,
and the picture of poikiloderma is completed by the appearance of reticular brown
hyperpigmentations. During the later
course of the disease, the eruption spreads
from the face and hands to the arms, lower
extremities, and buttocks, with more localized areas on the trunk; the palms and soles
almost always remain free. Another conspicuous sign of this disease in many patients is a high sensitivity to light; a short
exposure to sunlight will result in the formation of bullae. The possibility of confusion with congenital porphyria exists but
this disorder can be excluded because increased secretion of urinary porphyrin is
absent. An adult with the Rothmund-

Thomson syndrome is marked by short stature combined with conspicuous acromicria. Additional marginal signs are anomalies of hairs, dystrophies of nails, disturbances of sweat secretion, hypogonadism, and skeletal defects. Involvement of the eye, which occurs in about 50 per cent of the cases, is particularly important. It consists of a rapidly progressive, simultaneous bilateral clouding of the lens, occurring usually between the third and sixth years of life.[6, 9, 12]

It is still undecided whether the joint occurrence of congenital poikiloderma with osteogenesis imperfecta is part of a syndrome or whether it represents a chance coincidence.[8, 10]

2. Dyskeratosis congenita, the Zinsser-Cole-Engman syndrome, requires differential diagnostic separation from the Rothmund-Thomson syndrome. In contrast to the Rothmund-Thomson syndrome, it affects the male sex almost exclusively. One of the first signs (occurring between the fifth and tenth years of life) is nail dystrophy accompanied by chronic paronychia and resulting almost always in complete loss of the nail. At about the same time the appearance of leukoplakias on the mucous membranes of the mouth and sometimes also of the anus, vagina, and urethra will serve as a guide to the diagnosis. Not until a few months later will dirty-brown reticulated deposits of pigment appear on the neck, upper arms, and thighs. Diffuse atrophies crisscrossed by telangiectases prefer the more distant parts of the extremities. In spite of marked palmoplantar hyperhidrosis, keratoses are absent in this location. A considerable percentage of patients will eventually suffer involvement of the hematopoietic system (hypersplenism, thrombocytopenias, anemias); the leukoplakias may show malignant degeneration even at a young age.

In the differential diagnosis pachyonychia congenita must be excluded. On the one hand, this disease will result in marked

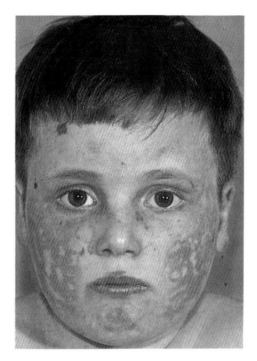

Fig. 356. Rothmund-Thomson syndrome.

onychodystrophies but not in the loss of nails, while, on the other hand, there is an absence of progression to poikiloderma. Frequently, enormous palmoplantar keratoses and follicular keratoses of the elbows and buttocks will be observed. At times pachyonychia congenita may be mistaken for incontinentia pigmenti, but both entities lack dystrophies of the nails, leukoplakias, and the syntropy with hemopathies.[7, 14]

3. The Hartnup syndrome may occasionally show poikilodermic changes of light-exposed areas during infancy. In accordance with an enzymatic defect in tryptophan metabolism, pellagroid cutaneous changes following exposure to sunlight take place. Clinically, cerebellar ataxia, intention tremor, and nystagmus are present. Neurologic signs precede the appearance of the first cutaneous changes. Laboratory tests show constant aminoaciduria without increase of the proline and oxyproline fractions; there is also secretion of large amounts of indican in the urine. After stress loading with tryptophan, secretion of indole bodies is retarded and prolonged.[1]

4. Bloom's syndrome. The originally named "congenital telangiectatic erythema resembling lupus erythematosus in Lorain-Levi dwarfs" is a more circumscribed type of poikiloderma. This syndrome is seen in male infants with low birth weight; later, proportionate dwarfism occurs, and during the first year of life telangiectases within the erythematous butterfly area of the face are evident. Sunlight leads to exacerbation. Further signs are a small face, high-pitched voice, and ichthyosis with follicular dyskeratosis. The prognosis is guarded because of the relatively high incidence of leukemia, a tendency which is also shown by an increased frequency of chromosomal breakage that is present in asymptomatic and heterozygotic genetic carriers as well.[3, 5]

5. Another rare type of poikiloderma is the **hereditary atrophic pigmentation of the legs**, which develops between the third and fourth decades of life. These lesions progress only slowly with a predominantly unilateral location on the distal third of the legs. Frequently the patients complain about the rapid fatigability of the lower extremities. The differential diagnosis must exclude melanodermatitis toxica lichenoides, lichen planus with atrophy (absent pruritus, no initial papular elements), dermatomyositis with final poikiloderma accompanied by adynamia, or an early manifestation of acrogeria, especially with familial incidence.[2, 11]

6. There exist two more types of congenital poikiloderma which, however, have been observed in only a few families; a proper classification of these diseases is therefore not yet possible. **Hereditary acro-**

keratotic poikiloderma begins soon after birth with formation of vesicles on the dorsal aspects of the hands and feet; their development is independent of external factors (such as trauma or light). A few months later eczematous changes affect the neck and the flexor aspects of the large joints. However, in contrast to atopic dermatitis, the face and scalp always remain free. During the first and second years of life, small macular areas of hyperpigmentation and depigmentation with telangiectases develop within the flexures of the joints without previous eczematization. The poikilodermatic transformation of the skin of the eyelids is conspicuous. The atrophic component is superficially reticular and quite insignificant. A fourth important sign is hyperkeratoses similar to arsenical keratoses on the dorsal and volar aspects of the hands, on the feet, and on the extensor sides of the elbows and knees.[16]

Hereditary sclerosing poikiloderma differs substantially in a few respects from the previously mentioned hereditary acrokeratotic poikiloderma. Up to the fifth year of life small macular hyperpigmentations, hypopigmentations, and depigmentations extend over the entire cutaneous surface including the eyelids but excluding the remainder of the face. Telangiectasis and slack atrophy are seen on the extensor sides of the elbows and knees, and on the backs of the fingers. However, the flexures of the large joints show cordlike sclerosis and partly reticular, partly linear, hyperkeratoses. The palms and soles show areas of sclerosis without involvement of the extensor aspects of the fingers, as seen for instance in progressive scleroderma.[15]

7. The clinical picture of **focal dermal hypoplasia**, the Goltz syndrome, also shows poikilodermic changes. According to our present knowledge this syndrome of malformations is found almost exclusively in girls. Already present at birth and only rarely lasting later in life, linear, reticular partly worm-eaten atrophies with telan-

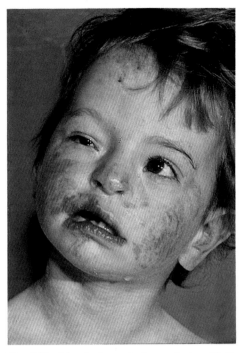

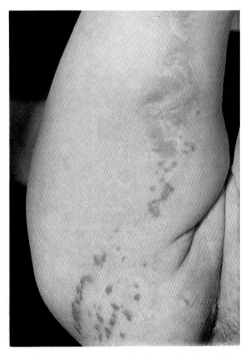

Fig. 357. Focal dermal hypoplasia (Goltz syndrome): poikilodermic features, microphthalmus, strabismus.

Fig. 358. Focal dermal hypoplasia (Goltz syndrome): hernialike protrusion of the subcutaneous fatty tissue; reticular atrophy covered with papules and an anal papilloma.

giectases and hyperpigmentations on the cheeks and extremities are characteristic of this disease (Fig. 357). In infancy the telangiectatic component is especially pronounced, with the result that the cutaneous changes preponderantly appear as erythema at first. Another typical sign is papillomas of the lips, the oral mucous

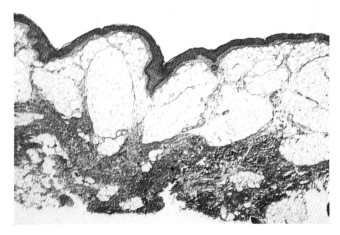

Fig. 359. Focal dermal hypoplasia (Goltz syndrome): high location of the fatty tissue caused by circumscribed aplasia of the fibrous tissue of the corium. HE stain, 60×.

membranes, or the anogenital region, and occasionally around the nails also; these papillomas appear, however, during the first few months of life. Within these atrophic areas (gluteal region) the subcutaneous fat may protrude like a hernia and lead to confusion with a superficial cutaneous lipomatous nevus (Figs. 358, 359). Another essential part of the Goltz syndrome is osseous malformations such as syndactylies, oligodactylies, and polydactylies, or anomalies of the clavicles and ribs. As in ectodermal dysplasia, there are malformations of the teeth, hypotrichoses, and dystrophies of the nails. More than half of the affected individuals have malformations of the eyes (colobomas, microphthalmus, or absence of the iris).[4, 13]

(1) CLODI, P. H., E. DEUTSCH und G. NIEBAUER: Krankheitsbild mit poikilodermieartigen Hautveränderungen, Aminoacidurie und Indolaceturie. Arch. klin. exp. Derm. *218:* 165–176 (1964).

(2) ENGMAN, M. F.: Hereditary pigmentation of the leg associated with atrophy. Arch. Derm. Syph. (Chic.) *8:* 483–486 (1923).

(3) GERMAN, J., R. ARCHIBALD and D. BLOOM: Chromosomal breakage in a rare and probably genetically determined syndrome of man. Science *148:* 506–507 (1965).

(4) GOLTZ, R. W., R. R. HENDERSON, J. M. HITCH and J. E. OTT: Focal dermal hypoplasia syndrome. Arch. Derm. (Chic.) *101:* 1–11 (1970).

(5) KORTING, G. W., und W. ADAM: Eine seltene Poikilodermie-Form: Lupus erythematodes-artige Hautveränderungen bei Minderwuchs. Arch. klin. exp. Derm. *207:* 508–520 (1958).

(6) MAEDER, G.: Le syndrome de Rothmund et le syndrome de Werner (étude clinique et diagnostique). Ann. Oculist. (Paris) *182:* 809–854 (1949).

(7) REICH, H.: Zinsser-Cole-Engman-Syndrom. Med. Klinik *68:* 283–292 (1973).

(8) REID, J.: Congenital poikiloderma with osteogenesis imperfecta. Brit. J. Derm. *79:* 243–244 (1967).

(9) ROOK, A., R. DAVIS and D. STEVANOVIC: Poikiloderma congenitale, Rothmund-Thomson-syndrome. Acta derm.-venereol. (Stockh.) *39:* 392–420 (1959).

(10) ROSCHLAU, G.: Rothmund-Syndrom kombiniert mit Osteogenesis imperfecta tarda und Sarkom des Oberschenkels. Z. Kinderheilk. *86:* 289–298 (1962).

(11) RUITER, M.: Eine ungewöhnliche, namentlich auf die Extremitäten beschränkte Form von Poikilodermie. Hautarzt *6:* 247–249 (1955).

(12) SILVER, H. K.: Rothmund-Thomson syndrome: an oculo-cutaneous disorder Amer. J. Dis. Child. *111:* 182–190 (1966)

(13) SUNDHAUSSEN, G.: Die Klinik der Fokalen Dermalen Hypoplasie. Inaug.-Diss. Mainz 1971.

(14) TEXIER, L., et J. MALEVILLE: La symptomatologic cutanée de l'anémie perniciosiforme de Fanconi. Ann. Derm. Syph. (Paris) *90:* 553–568 (1963).

(15) WEARY, P. E., Y. T. HSU, D. R. RICHARDSON, CH. M. CARAVATI and B. T. WOOD: Hereditary sclerosing poikiloderma. Arch. Derm. (Chic.) *100:* 413–422 (1969).

(16) WEARY, P. E., W. F. MANLEY and G. F. GRAHAM: Hereditary acrokeratotic poikiloderma. Arch. Derm. (Chic.) *103:* 409–422 (1971).

B. Acquired Poikilodermas

This chapter deals with those forms of poikiloderma that develop in the course of or following a nonhereditary or congenital basic disorder. So-called poikiloderma atrophicans vasculare, therefore, has no unique nosologic position. Instead, it represents end stages of burnt-out disorders (such as dermatomyositis or malignant lymphogranulomatosis, among others).

1. Circumscribed poikilodermic skin changes limited to the site of an exogenous injury usually occur after **radiologic**

treatments. Poikiloderma is limited to the exact size of the treated field. In addition, there are slack and taut atrophies with keratotic layers. All these signs permit a correct diagnosis (Fig. 360).

Poikilodermas of thermic or actinic origin are uncommon. They naturally favor the uncovered parts of the body such as the face, neck, hands, and forearms, and they do not show the sharp borderline of x-ray poikiloderma. Also of exogenous origin is "**poikilodermie reticulée pigmentaire** de la face et du cou" which, however, represents melanodermatitis toxica lichenoides interspersed with telangiectases (see Chapter 24, D1).

2. Of special significance is **dermatomyositis,** which sets the pace for universal poikilodermic changes of the outer integument. Frequently there is extensive hypertrichosis as well as calcifications of the skin, muscles, and connective tissue (Fig. 361). Since the muscle-specific enzymes in the serum usually do not show any increased activity at this late point in the course of the disease, tests for evidence of preceding dermatomyositis must be found electromyographically or by tolerance tests with peroral doses of creatine. Papular lesions on the neck may offer supportive evidence for the diagnosis in such patients. This sign has not been recognized often enough. Histologically, one sees PAS–alcian blue positive and perhaps also metachromatic structures without massive cellular masses as substrate of the papules.

Poikilodermas within the group of other systemic vascular connective tissue disease, as for instance in systemic **lupus erythematosus** or **progressive scleroderma,** are much rarer. The diagnosis results from additional clinical findings, which were discussed in Chapter 16.[1, 3]

Fig. 360. Poikiloderma caused by x-rays.

Fig. 361. Vascular atrophic poikiloderma as the final stage of dermatomyositis.

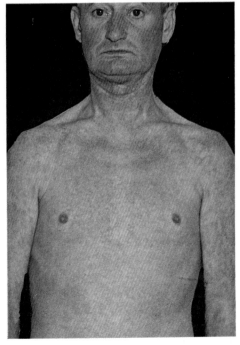

3. Among the storage diseases poikiloderma is known only in cutaneous **amyloidosis.** Besides a basic appearance similar to that of livedo racemosa and atrophies, it shows deposits of rust-brown points and fresh petechial cutaneous bleeding which convey a poikilodermatic aspect. Specific histologic investigations (congo red stain) result in the correct diagnosis.[2, 4]

4. A "poikilodermic state" can develop in parapsoriasis, especially in **parakeratosis variegata,** whose transformation to mycosis fungoides in some cases is not surprising.

Poikilodermas in the narrow sense in **malignant lymphogranulomatosis** or **reticulosis** usually do not occur until after the disappearance of the infiltrate. These at first "anonymous" poikilodermas can often be diagnosed only by histologic examination or by their accompanying signs such as pruritus (lymphogranulomatosis or mycosis fungoides) or lymph node enlargement (as in lymphogranulomatosis). Often, however, the development of typical changes will reveal the true character of the poikiloderma very early.[5-8]

5. Checkered reticular appearances were formerly observed after **salvarsan dermatitis** or after **lichen planus** (treated with arsenic?). In the latter, however, small pigmentations alone occur much more often than genuine poikiloderma.

(1) EVERETT, M. A., and A. C. CURTIS: Dermatomyositis; a review of nineteen cases in adolescents and children. Arch. intern. Med. *100:* 70–76 (1957).

(2) GROSSHANS, E., H. BERGOEND und A. KHOCHNEVIS: Die erblichen Haut-Amyloidosen. Die familiäre amyloide Poikilodermie. Münch. med. Wschr. *114:* 1183–1190 (1972).

(3) KREYSEL, H. W., und F. SCHANDELMAIER: Kreatin-Kreatinin-Studien sowie Fermentaktivitäts-Bestimmungen im Rahmen einer peroralen Kreatinbelastung bei der Dermatomyositis. Klin. Wschr. *42:* 1087–1093 (1964).

(4) MARCHIONINI, A., und F. JOHN: Über lichenoide und poikilodermieartige Hautamyloidose. Arch. Derm. Syph. (Berl.) *173:* 545–561 (1936).

(5) SAMMAN, P. D.: Survey of reticuloses and premycotic eruptions. Brit. J. Derm. *76:* 1–9 (1964).

(6) SIPOS, K., und I. DEME: Über einen Fall von Mykosis fungoides mit Parapsoriasis und Poikilodermie. Derm. Wschr. *141:* 669–675 (1960).

(7) THIERS, H., D. COLOMB, J. FAYOLLE et Mme PELLET: Atrophie cutanée à type de poikilodermie apparaissant au cours de l'évolution d'une réticulose à forme érythrodermique stabilisée par le cortancyl. Bull. Soc. franç. Derm. Syph. *66:* 732–733 (1959).

(8) TRITSCH, H., und W. KIESSLING: Poikilodermia atrophicans vascularis bei maligner Lymphogranulomatose Paltauf-Sternberg. Arch. klin. exp. Derm. *202:* 10–20 (1955/1956).

24. Pigmentary Disturbances

We shall discuss first those pathological, pigmentary, cutaneous changes which are also observed by the internist and the neuropsychiatrist. These are the disturbances which for the most part are not caused locally in an autochthonous manner but are primarily the result of endocrine-metabolic influences. However, benign or malignant nevus cell formations, which are essentially or facultatively caused by changes in the melanin synthesis, will be discussed in Chapter 38, B.

A. Leukopathias

The cause of genetically determined albinism is today no longer explained by a congenital deficiency of melanocytes in the skin and other pigment-containing organs but mainly by a deficiency or absence of melanocytic tyrosinase. This inability of tyrosine to change into melanin may be universally complete or incomplete as well as manifested in circumscribed areas.

1. A child with **universal complete albinism** shows immediately post partum a light pink-colored skin, white hairs, and a transparent vascular system (Fig. 362) showing faintly through the skin. Later, conspicuous light hypersensitivity develops, leading to reactive thickening of the skin, especially on the neck and the extensor surfaces of the arms. Since in albinos melanocytes show only a disturbance in the ability to form pigment, melanomas as well as small nevus cell nevi are occasionally found. Ophthalmologically, severe photophobia, horizontal nystagmus, and occasionally hypoplasia of the macula lutea are observed. Moreover, refractory anomalies, retinitis pigmentosa, and astigmatism are present, but disturbances of color perception and dark adaptation are lacking. Universal complete albinism is an hereditary autosomal recessive disorder. There are, however, exceptions to this mode of heredity (sex-linked recessive and dominant).[2]

Besides mental retardation, another anomaly in universal complete albinism is deafness. Another combination of universal and circumscribed albinism occurs in the simultaneous presence of pseudohemophilia (angiohemophilia) and ceroid-pigment storage in the bone marrow, a condition called **Hermansky-Pudlak syndrome.**[19, 38]

2. Albinoidism, i.e., universal incomplete albinism, is a quantitatively weaker form of complete albinism. In this type the skin is weakly pigmented and the hairs are not completely white. In addition, subsequent pigmentation occurs with advancing age. Ocular changes are much rarer than in com-

Fig. 362. Total albinism.

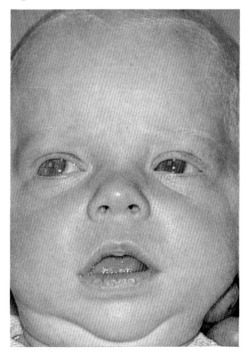

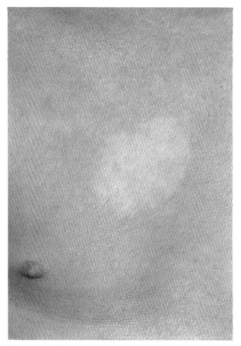

Fig. 363. Nevus depigmentosus.

plete albinism; however the transparency (diaphaneity) of the iris is always present. This makes possible a differentiation from secondary generalized hypopigmentation.

There is no difficulty in differentiating the alabasterlike skin color in **Sheehan's** **syndrome** from universal albinoidism. The pigment loss from the absent melanotropic hormone also affects the nipples and genital region. Tanning after sun exposure does not occur. Besides the loss of pigment another important sign is the loss of axillary and pubic hair and the lateral eyebrows. Similarly, in *eunuchism* the skin has little pigment and is devoid of all sexual hair.

In children with light complexions, the possibility of **phenylketonuria** should be considered. Besides the tendency to reduced pigmentation the skin is especially delicate and shows a tendency to eczematous reactions and follicular keratoses. Corresponding to the lack of pigment, there is an increased sensitivity to light. Pertinent laboratory examinations include the Guthrie test and the addition of a 10 per cent ferric chloride solution to the urine; if positive, a green color results.

3. Partial albinism is characterized by the presence of areas of absent pigment at birth. Such pigmentless areas of skin can be single or multiple and show a certain preference for the midline. In contrast to vitiligo, however, a pronounced hyperpigmented margin is missing. Other differentiating criteria are the duration of the manifestation, the distribution, and the "dynamics" of the individual lesions (see Table 3).

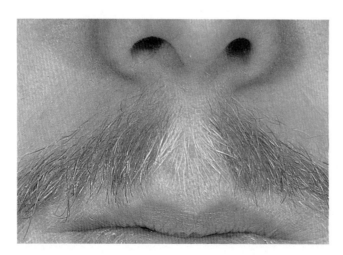

Fig. 364. Circumscribed poliosis.

Partial albinism is transmitted as an autosomal dominant trait. Only the lack of proof of heredity in the **nevus depigmentosus** differentiates these two entities (Fig. 363), so that the latter can easily be considered partial albinism. A rather conspicuous sign of partial albinism is white streaks of hair (circumscribed poliosis) (Fig. 364) on the forehead or the back of the neck. In association with such albinotic signs of the hair, areas of absent pigment on the chin, the back of the neck, the middle of the trunk, and the distal extremities are called the "**sixfield complex.**"

Waardenburg's syndrome consists of partial albinism, deafness, blepharophimosis, dystopia of the lower lacrimal points, and hypoplasia of the iris (with or without heterochromia). It is inherited dominantly with variable penetrance and expressivity (Fig. 365). For the differences between the dominant Waardenburg's syndrome and the recessively sex-linked partial *albinism with deafmutism* see Table 4.[22, 30, 37, 39]

Tietz's syndrome is the autosomal dominant combination of partial albinism and deafmutism. Other than absent eyebrows there are no ocular signs.[33]

The **Chediak-Higashi syndrome** is a combination of partial albinism of the skin and eye, hepatosplenomegaly, and generalized enlargement of the lymph nodes. The leukocytes show characteristic granulation, probably caused by abnormal lysosomes. Recurrent infections cause these patients to die before the tenth year of life. It is inherited as an autosomal recessive trait.[3, 35]

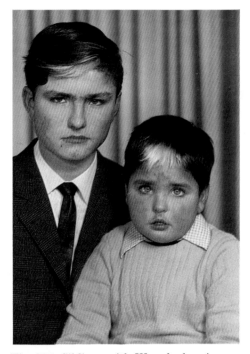

Fig. 365. Siblings with Waardenburg's syndrome.

The **Stargardt syndrome,** which includes, besides oligophrenia and nephropathy, progressive degeneration of the macula, bilateral central scotoma, and (in contrast to albinism) disturbances in the color perception, may in rare cases exhibit cutaneous changes like those of albinism.[32]

4. Hereditary, familial, **spotty dyschromia** (piebaldism) is characterized by mul-

Table 3

	Age at Onset	Size of Lesion	Favorite Localization	Border
Partial albinism	present at birth	constant	in midline and symmetrically on extremities	hyperpigmentation insignificant or absent
Vitiligo	predominantly around the 20th year of life	variable	symmetrically on extremities and anogenital region	distinctly hyperpigmented

Table 4

	Waardenburg's Syndrome	Partial Albinism with Deafmutism*
Skin	circumscribed absence of pigment	hyper- and hypopigmented areas
Hair	white forelock (17%)	white
Iris	partial or complete heterochromia (25%)	normally pigmented or partial heterochromia
Root of nose	hyperplastically wide (78%)	normal
Eyebrows	hypertrichosis of the medial parts (45%)	normal, but white
Canthi	lateral dislocation (99%)	normal
Faculty of hearing	congenital deafness or different degrees of partial deafness (20%)	congenital deafness
Bones	deformities may be present	normal
Intelligence	diminished**	normal
Mode of inheritance	autosomal dominant	male or female sex-linked recessive

* Deafness. (Tr.)
** Or normal. (Tr.)

Fig. 366. Depigmentations in Pringle-Bourneville's phakomatosis.

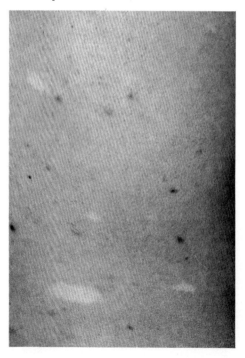

tiple, not sharply limited, and irregular hyper- and hypopigmented areas and is inherited dominantly. A white forelock is simultaneously present and facilitates confusion with Waardenburg's syndrome, but the latter has no areas of hyperpigmentation. Vitiligo can be ruled out by the absence of symmetry, vague borders, absent peripheral hyperpigmentation, and different localization. In addition, confetti-like depigmentations caused by hydroquinone monobenzyl ether or vitiligolike depigmentations must also be ruled out (see page 368).[34]

5. The ash-leaf-like hypomelanotic spots in patients with tuberous sclerosis (**Bourneville's phakomatosis**, Fig. 366) are different. Even in infants, they can, especially if they are weakly expressed, be made visible by a Wood's light. They precede the other dermatologic signs, such as adenoma sebaceum, periungual and perigingival fibromas, and

lumbosacral shagreen skin, sometimes by years. Cytologically, melanocytes in the hypomelanotic spots are altered and have diminished tyrosinase activity.[12]

6. Patients with **Darier's disease** show definite small leukodermas, which often are located at the opening of the follicles. Such depigmentations are not caused by the preceding manifestations and have no connection with the dyskeratotic papules. Histologically, there is only a diminished to absent pigment deposit in the basal cells. In contrast to idiopathic macular hypomelanosis a preference for light-exposed skin areas is not observed and the latter disease has no other cutaneous changes.[7]

7. The **idiopathic macular hypomelanosis** just mentioned occurs in patients with normal skin, appearing as angular, lentil- to fingernail-sized depigmentations. These porcelain-white areas, easily recognizable under Wood's light, occur on the extremities and the cheeks. Their number increases with increasing age, and they can be found relatively frequently from the fourth decade on. They do not favor either sex, however.[8]

8. An irregularly indented white area without peripheral hyperpigmentation is characteristic of **nevus anemicus,** which favors the anterior and posterior upper trunk. If rubbed, only the unchanged surrounding skin becomes red, so that the lesion becomes even more distinct by contrast. By this method it can easily be distinguished from a single nevus depigmentosus. Nevus anemicus does not represent hypopigmentation but is caused by a disturbed function of the motoric end plates of the smooth muscle cells of the blood vessels or by a neurally caused deficiency in their ability to dilate. The sweating function and the reaction of the pilomotors within the nevus are not altered. Since the function of the epidermal melanocytes is not impaired, tanning after sunlight exposure does not

differ from that of the surrounding skin. In the differential diagnosis a nevus anemicus, which, by the way, occasionally occurs in patients with von Recklinghausen's disease, differs with its indented or circinate borders from vitiligo with its smooth borders, and its normal consistency is conspicuously different from that of atrophic morphea plana.[13, 15]

9. In sun-exposed areas, e.g., on the extensor surfaces of the forearms and the lateral parts of the cheeks predominantly, older patients often show star-shaped, indented **depigmented pseudoscars** (Fig. 367). At first glance these depigmentations simulate the cutaneous changes seen following small wounds. Their location in skin that shows atrophy from old age and the presence of senile purpura is also typical. The depigmented pseudoscars, however, develop spontaneously without preceding injury. Histologically, they are characterized by a small band of absent elastica.[6, 27]

10. Vitiligo is acquired and primary and, therefore, not a leukoderma originating on the basis of a preceding change. It has sharply limited borders and is chiefly located on the hands and perianogenitally. A slowly developing disease, it is symmetrically distributed and its border is hyperpigmented (Fig. 368). Its location is not restricted to any neural or vascular distribution. In about 50 per cent of patients vitiligo starts before the twentieth year of life, and in about 20 to 30 per cent of cases there is a familial incidence.

This knowledge of by no means rare familial disposition to vitiligo therefore makes the accent on "hereditary" vitiligo completely superfluous and also eliminates a differentiation between hereditary and nonhereditary vitiligo.

In addition to a loss of function of the melanocytic tyrosinase, the pathogenetic mechanism seems to be the secretion of a melatoninlike substance at the peripheral nerve endings. This substance is supposed

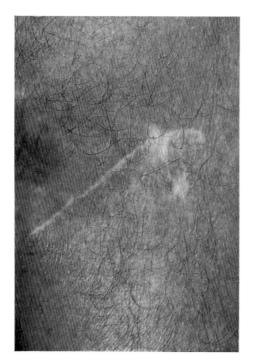

Fig. 367. Star-shaped pseudoscars of senile skin.

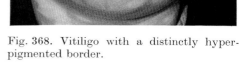

Fig. 368. Vitiligo with a distinctly hyper-pigmented border.

to lighten the pigment cell and hamper neomelanogenesis.

The relative frequency of vitiligo has led to a discussion of the relationship between vitiligo and pernicious anemia, diabetes mellitus, and an immunologically effective thyroid disturbance. Questions of a relationship between vitiligo and carcinoma and between vitiligo and melanoma have not yet been answered with certainty.[9, 10, 14, 17, 24, 26]

Perineval depigmentations as in *Sutton's nevus*, **leukoderma acquisitum centrifugum** (Fig. 369) represent either nevus pigmentosus et depigmentosus or perineval vitiligo.[11]*

The best-known complex vitiligo syndrome is the **Vogt-Koyanagi syndrome.** It consists of dysacusis, alopecia, circumscribed poliosis, and pronounced uveitis of nontraumatic origin. Rather similar is the

Harada syndrome with different ocular effects of an inflammatory process. Pathogenetically, allergic mechanisms (autoimmune reactions against the uveal pigment), or a viral infection are considered possible causes. The skin shows signs of canities or poliosis, especially on the eyebrows and lashes but also on the scalp, axillary, and pubic hair. In about 6 per cent of cases there is associated vitiligo. The loss of hair in a single area is hard to distinguish from alopecia areata, especially if round rather than bizarre spots of alopecia are present.

In **Mafucci's syndrome,** especially in the variant described by Kast and von Recklinghausen, vitiligo may also develop as well as pigmented nevi. However, it is possible that this is a coincidental occurrence.

In **porphyria cutanea tarda** extensive lesions of vitiligo may also occur; these, however, show a certain sclerosis in places (Fig. 370). Formerly, this occurrence was wrongly considered a syntropy of porphy-

* Rarely, a primary or secondary malignant melanoma is the center of the halo. (Tr.)

rinuria and progressive scleroderma. Today it is best called "sclerovitiligo" in porphyria cutanea tarda.[5, 25]

11. In contrast to vitiligo, **leukoderma** represents macules or areas of secondary whitening of the skin. It occurs most often after various dermatoses but also after contact with chemicals (e.g., hydroquinone benzyl ether).

Syphilitic leukoderma is found on skin that is otherwise unchanged, appearing as specific macular, lentil to penny-sized eruptions following and at the site of moderately sharply limited depigmentations. Favorite sites are the lateral and posterior areas of the neck, as the name "collier de Vénus" attests. The female sex is affected mainly. With increasing daylight, especially in summer, these depigmented areas become conspicuous owing to the tanning of the surrounding skin. In tertiary syphilis the melanodermic or vitiligolike depigmentations cover large areas.

In another treponematosis, namely **mal del pinto,** erythematous-squamous, whitish, and hyperkeratotic pintids occur two to six months after the first manifestation; these, especially in the late phase, lead to vitiligo-like achromias. In contrast to vitiligo, however, the margins of the lesions of pinto are not hyperpigmented and the predilection for periorificial locations is lacking. The presence of treponemas by darkfield examination in the lymph from affected areas may confirm the diagnosis, although the treponemas of pinta, syphilis, and frambesia are morphologically indistinguishable. The same thing can be said about the serology (including the Nelson test), so that one should be cautious in suggesting a diagnosis of pinto in patients with seronegative achromia.

Leprous leukoderma starts initially with point-sized perifollicular lesions and only later extends to wider areas. More characteristic, however, are its focal anhidrosis and, most important, its anesthesia which permit an easy differentiation of such areas from idiopathic vitiligo or another symptomatic leukoderma.

Like syphilitic leukoderma **psoriatic leukoderma** is limited to the site of a previous psoriatic lesion. As an achromic negative it is not too often observed in lesions which have regressed spontaneously. **Leukoderma psoriaticum verum** shows sharply indented, round or oval depigmentations, which are especially conspicuous in con-

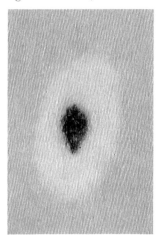

Fig. 369. Sutton's nevus.

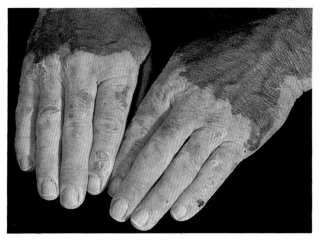

Fig. 370. Vitiligo and porphyria cutanea tarda.

trast to more strongly pigmented areas. They may last for months. Compared to vitiligo the intensity of the depigmentation of psoriatic leukoderma is not as strong.

The peripheral light halo (Fig. 371) of older psoriatic lesions is a clinically valuable sign of the (small) pressure of eruption of the psoriatic exanthem. These pseudo-atrophic zones of Woronoff are, by the way, not the result of a vasoconstricting effect but are a histochemically determined, structural change of the epidermis and corium in the lesion and its environment (Fig. 371).

More frequent is **pseudoleukoderma** (leukodermata psoriatica spuria) in the psoriatic patient treated with Cignolin. It sets the light, healed psoriatic lesions against the surrounding skin (Fig. 372).[20]

Additional leukodermas are observed most often after regression of pityriasis lichenoides chronica, pityriasis rosea, and dermatomycoses; less often after lichen scrofulosorum, chicken pox, dermatitis due to exposure to light, and many eczemas. Such contrasts are undoubtedly increased by sunlight or quartz light. This can be seen by the rapid repigmentation of skin areas formerly covered by scales.

Pityriasis versicolor alba most probably causes a leukoderma owing to the filtration effect of the preceding scales and a direct diminution of melanin formation by the causative organism (Fig. 373). The differentiation of this leukoderma from other depigmentations can be made by scraping off the scaling cover and performing the simple tests for evidence of the fungi.

Among the eczemas, the preseborrheic minimal variant **pityriasis alba** (Fig. 374) must be mentioned. The localized, vaguely limited, coin-sized areas, which are not too intensely depigmented, occur mostly on the face. In atopic dermatitis (disseminated neurodermatitis) small areas of depigmentation ("prurigo diathetica leukodystrophica") are present, mostly on the back of the neck. In addition, however, there are large areas with little or no pigment, and

these are easily distinguished from vitiligo because they are not sharply limited and are all located on lichenified skin.[23]

12. Chemical factors responsible for depigmentation are hydroquinone and its derivatives, chemicals retarding polymerization, derivatives of Furadantin, certain muscle relaxants (e.g., Myanesin), and above all, the chloroquine group. Especially after the application of monobenzyl hydroquinone ether a peculiar **confettilike depigmentation** may occur, composed of small areas of depigmented skin within the areas of application. Contact with materials containing rubber or synthetic fibers (such as brassieres, dress shields, Saran Wrap) can cause hyperpigmentation or depigmentation according to which factors are liberated. The same can be said for contact with phenol-containing disinfectants if they remain in contact with the skin for hours.[4, 21, 29, 31, 36]

Similar to confetti dyschromia but with no relationship to external or internal causes are the peculiar, noninfiltrated, nonscaling areas of depigmentation on the trunk and extremities that have been observed in Havana. The patients are always dark adults. The number of lesions (which are not hyperpigmented at the periphery) varies from a few to many hundreds. Fungi are not found and the seroreactions specific for treponemas are negative.[1]

13. In rare cases girls shortly after birth show reticular or macular, linear depigmentations on the extremities and lateral parts of the trunk. The loss of pigment has not been preceded by inflammation or blisters. Atrophies and telangiectatic vascular dilatations are also missing. Clinically, the skin corresponds to the negative picture of incontinentia pigmenti, so that we are dealing with **incontinentia pigmenti achromians.** The lesions are therefore accompanied by small areas of alopecia, ocular changes, and defects of intelligence. The cutaneous changes disappear completely

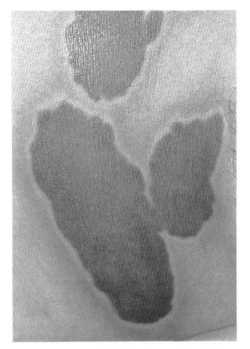

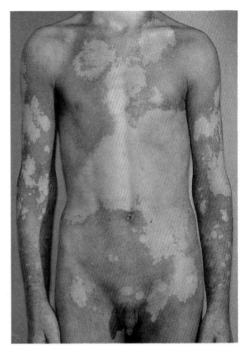

Fig. 371. Psoriasis vulgaris: perifocal clearing, so-called Woronoff's sign.

Fig. 372. Psoriasis vulgaris: pseudoleukoderma.

Fig. 373. Pityriasis versicolor.

Fig. 374. Pityriasis alba.

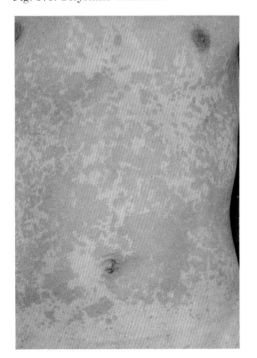

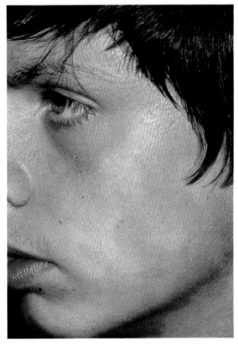

in later years and remain only rarely until adulthood. Histologically, inflammatory changes are also lacking, but there is a diminution of melanin deposits in the basal cell layer resulting from disturbed maturation of the melanocytes; occasionally a small increase in melanophages in the upper corium is found.[16, 18, 28]

(1) Argüelles-Casals, D., et Gonzáles: La leucodermie lenticulaire disséminée. Ann. Derm. Syph. (Paris) *96:* 283–286 (1969).

(2) Barnicot, N. A.: Albinismus in South-Western Nigeria. Ann. Eugen. (Lond.) *17:* 38–73 (1952).

(3) Bedoya, V.: Pigmentary changes in Chediak-Higashi syndrome. Microscopic study of 12 homozygous and heterozygous subjects. Brit. J. Derm. *85:* 336–347 (1971).

(4) Bleehen, S. S., and P. Hall-Smith: Brassiere depigmentation: light and electron microscope studies. Brit. J. Derm. *83:* 157–160 (1970).

(5) Bolgert, M., J. Canivet et J. Lépine: Lésions scléro-lichéniennes et scléro-vitiligineuses de la porphyrie cutanée de l'adulte. Ann. Derm. Syph. (Paris) *83:* 142–145 (1956).

(6) Colomb, D., J.-A. Pinçon et J. Lartaud: Individualisation anatomo-clinique d'une forme méconnue de la peau sénile: Les pseudo-cicatrices stellaires spontanées. Ann. Derm. Syph. (Paris) *94:* 273–286 (1967).

(7) Cornelison, R. L., E. B. Smith and J. M. Knox: Guttate leukoderma in Darier's disease. Arch. Derm. (Chic.) *102:* 447–450 (1970).

(8) Cummings, K. I., and W. I. Cottel: Idiopathic guttate hypomelanosis. Arch. Derm. (Chic.) *93:* 184–186 (1966).

(9) Cunliffe, W. J., R. Hall, D. J. Newell and C. J. Stevenson: Vitiligo, thyroid disease and autoimmunity. Brit. J. Derm. *80:* 135–139 (1968).

(10) Dawber, R. P. R.: Vitiligo in mature-onset diabetes mellitus. Brit. J. Derm. *80:* 275–278 (1968).

(11) Ebner, E., und G. Niebauer: Elektronenoptische Befunde zum Pigmentverlust beim Naevus Sutton. Dermatologica (Basel) *137:* 345–357 (1968).

(12) Fitzpatrick, T. B., G. Szabó, Y. Hori, A. A. Simone, W. B. Reed and M. H. Greenberg: White leaf-shaped macules. Arch. Derm. (Chic.) *98:* 1–6 (1968).

(13) Fleisher, T. L., and I. Zeligman: Nevus anemicus. Arch. Derm. (Chic.) *100:* 750–755 (1969).

(14) Friederich, H. C.: Vitiligo als unerwünschte Nebenerscheinung in der Melanombehandlung. Arch. klin. exp. Derm. *229:* 223–230 (1967).

(15) Greaves, M. W., D. Birkett and C. Johnson: Nevus anemicus: A unique catecholamine-dependent nevus. Arch. Derm. (Chic.) *102:* 172–176 (1970).

(16) Grosshans, E. M., P. Stoebner, H. Bergoend et C. Stoll: Incontinentia pigmenti achromians (Ito); étude clinique et histopathologique. Dermatologica (Basel) *142:* 65–78 (1971).

(17) Grunnet, I., J. Howitz, F. Reymann and M. Schwartz: Vitiligo and pernicious anemia. Arch. Derm. (Chic.) *101:* 82–85 (1970).

(18) Hamada, T., T. Saito, T. Sugai and Y. Morita: Incontinentia pigmenti achromians (Ito). Arch. Derm. (Chic.) *96:* 673–676 (1967).

(19) Hermansky, F., and P. Pudlak: Albinism associated with hemorrhagic diathesis and unusual pigmented reticular cells in the bone marrow: report of two cases with histochemical studies. Blood *14:* 162–169 (1959).

(20) Herrmann, F., G. K. Steigleder, Y. Kamei und J. H. Kim: Aminopeptidasen-Aktivität in der psoriatischen Papel. Derm. Wschr. *146:* 603–609 (1962).

(21) Kahn, G.: Depigmentation caused by phenolic detergent germicides. Arch. Derm. (Chic.) *102:* 177–187 (1970).

(22) KLEIN, D.: Les diverses formes héré-
ditaires de l'albinisme. Bull. Acad.
suisse sci. méd. *17:* 351–364 (1961).

(23) KORTING, G. W.: Zur Pathogenese des
endogenen Ekzems. S.18–21. Thieme,
Stuttgart 1954.

(24) KORTING, G. W.: Vitiligo und Karzinom.
Dtsch. med. Wschr. *81:* 911–912 (1956).

(25) KORTING, G. W., und H. HOLZMANN: Die
Sklerodermie und ihr nahestehende
Bindegewebsprobleme. Thieme, Stutt-
gart 1967.

(26) LASSUS, A., A. APAJALAHTI, K. BLOM-
QVIST, M. MUSTAKALLIO and U. KIISTALA:
Vitiligo and neoplasms. Acta derm.-
venereol. (Stockh.) *52:* 229–232 (1972).

(27) MIESCHER, G., L. HÄBERLIN und
L. GUGGENHEIM: Über fleckförmige
Alterspigmentierungen. Arch. Derm.
Syph. (Berl.) *174:* 105–125 (1936).

(28) OKUWA, H., and S. KITAMURA: Incontinentia pigmenti achromians. Jap. J.
Derm., Serie A *76:* 606 (1966).

(29) OLIVER, E. A., L. SCHWARTZ and
L. H. WARREN: Occupational leukoderma. Arch. Derm. Syph. (Chic.) *42:*
993–1014 (1940).

(30) REED, W. B., V. M. STONE, E. BODER
and L. ZIPRKOWSKI: Pigmentary disorders in association with congenital
deafness. Arch. Derm. Syph. (Chic.) *95:*
176–186 (1967).

(31) SIEMENS, H. W.: Beobachtung der
Dyschromia in confetti. Hautarzt *9:*
532–534 (1958).

(32) STARGARDT, K.: Über familiäre progressive Degeneration in der Macula-
gegend des Auges. Graefes Arch. Ophthal. *71:* 534–549 (1909).

(33) TIETZ, W.: A syndrome of deaf-mutism
associated with albinism showing dominant autosomal inheritance. Amer. J.
hum. Genet. *15:* 259–264 (1963).

(34) TOURAINE, A., et H. BOUR: Méche
blanche et dyschromies familiales. Bull.
Soc. franç. Derm. Syph. *45:* 835–839
(1938).

(35) UNDRITZ, E.: Die Chediak-Steinbrinck-
Anomalie oder erblich-konstitutionelle
Riesengranulation (Granulagiganten)
der Leukozyten. Schweiz. med. Wschr.
88: 996–999 (1958).

(36) VOLLUM, D. I.: Hypomelanosis from an
antioxidant in polyethylene film. Arch.
Derm. (Chic.) *104:* 70–72 (1971).

(37) WAARDENBURG, P. J.: A new syndrome
combining developmental anomalies of
the eyelids, eyebrows and nose root with
pigmentary defects of the iris and head
hair and with congenital deafness. Amer.
J. hum. Genet. *3:* 195–253 (1951).

(38) ZIPRKOWSKI, L.: Total albinism and
deaf-mutism due to a recessive autosomal gene. XIII. Congress Internat.
Dermat. München 1967. Bd. II, S.1418.

(39) ZIPRKOWSKI, L.: Partial albinism and
congenital deafness due to a recessive
sex linked gene. XIII. Congress Internat. Dermat. München 1967. Bd. II,
S.1418.

B. Diffuse Yellow Pigmentations

1. Jaundice (icterus) is characterized by
universal impregnation of tissue with dissolved bile pigments; the blood serum in
jaundice shows a level of bilirubin of at
least 1 mg per cent. Even before icterus
develops, yellow dermatographia can occasionally be elicited, or a histamine wheal
will show a preicteric yellow color; these
observations prove an increase of the capillary permeability to bilirubin of the icteric
skin. The icteric discoloration is first seen
on the conjunctivae and the soft palate,
and even after regression remains there
longer. Frequently the upper half of
the body shows more intense discoloration.
As far as the shades of color are concerned
a *ruby tint* is supposed to be a sign of a diffuse hepatitis, whereas the greenish *verdin*

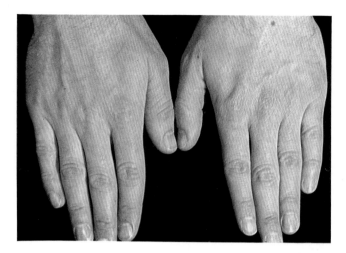

Fig. 375. Aurantiasis of the skin of the right hand; the left hand is that of a normal person.

icterus may indicate mechanical obstruction of the flow of bile, i.e., cholestasis. A *"melas icterus"* (black jaundice) is observed in cachectic patients suffering from cirrhosis of the liver or hepatic tumors. Hemolytic anemias or massive blood decomposition of different forms show a straw yellow *"flavin tint."*

An increase of the icteric color in the palmoplantar region and also in the axillae and chest area is typical of the saffron yellow *icterus juvenilis Meulengracht*, with the exception of some cases of pseudoicterus; the same discoloration is seen in posthepatic intermittent hyperbilirubinemias.

A rupture of the choledochus duct may result in a slight icteric discoloration, especially of the periumbilical region. However, a cutaneous discoloration of the umbilical area that is more bluish-green than yellow-reddish is a sign of intraperitoneal hemorrhage. This so-called *Cullen-Hellendahl sign* is seen also in acute hemorrhagic pancreatic necrosis; the skin has a lattice or livedo reticularis-like pattern. Infectious hepatitis shows jaundice first, pruritus later; however, in obstructive jaundice and cholestatic jaundice pruritus precedes the appearance of icterus.[1]

2. Discolorations simulating icterus with its genuine diffusion of tissue with bilirubin can be caused by certain **drugs.** Jaundice-like colors may be produced intentionally as artefacts by derivatives of acridine, picric acid, or dinitrophenol; however, in most cases the conjunctivae will not be affected.

3. Aurantiasis cutis or **xanthosis** (from the Latin *aurantium*, orange) (Fig. 375), also known as carotenemia, is a canary, ochre, or sulfurlike cutaneous discoloration; in children it may be due to excessive eating of carrots. In normal times it can be observed in adults after consumption of too many carrots, oranges, or tomatoes; in times of hunger or food shortage it may be caused by wild spinach (orach) or the European nettle. In addition, carotenemia occurs in diabetes as the result of prolonged hyperlipemia with increased values of serum lipoids, and also in nephrosis, hypothyroidism and primary hypercholesterol-emic xanthomatosis. Such excess deposition of carotenoids is especially noticeable for streaklike saturated yellow pigmentations of the nasolabial or other facial and skin folds as well as for flat spreading on palms and soles. Axillae and flexures can also show more intensive yellow discoloration. Impregnation of the nailplate, especially of the lunula, takes place less often. Diffuse cutaneous aurantiasis spares the conjunctivae and most of the other mucous membranes, permitting a differentiation from jaundice. Histologically, a distinct yellow permeation of the entire epidermis, especially of the horny layer with its abundant lipoids, can be seen. The ducts of the sweat glands show marked yellow impregnation.

(1) KORTING, G. W.: Die Beziehungen zwischen Haut und Leber mit ihren diagnostischen und therapeutischen Möglichkeiten. Therapiewoche *12:* 19–26 (1962).

C. Diffuse Melanodermas

1. Hemochromatosis with its bronze pigmentation of the skin is caused by synchronous deposits of hemosiderin and melanin; however, the overproduction of melanin and simultaneous thickening of the epidermis furnishes the larger amount of the deposit. Some patients with this iron storage disease may not show the brown skin color. Sometimes the brownish color of hemochromatosis may take on a bluish hue, especially on the face, neck, flexor aspects of forearms, and genitals (Fig. 376). Mucous membranes show pigmentation that is more spotted than diffuse. Diagnostically, histochemical proof of the presence of iron in the skin is of no help because the percentage of iron is normally subject to considerable variation. More important for the diagnosis is the histologic analysis of the liver, the plasma iron concentration, and the serum's high capacity for binding iron.[4]

2. The patient with **porphyria cutanea tarda** often shows a conspicuous dark color of the exposed parts of the skin and considerable darkening of the otherwise abundantly well developed hairs of the scalp and eyebrows and of the ears. Inspection of the skin of the patient with hepatic porphyria as contrasted to that of a patient with hemochromatosis will show vivid conjunctival redness, except for the characteristic formation of bullae of the light-exposed areas. An exception occurs in *melanodermic porphyria*, which shows marked universal Addison-like melanoderma without the formation of bullae. The diagnosis is supported by an increased urinary secretion of porphyrin and red fluorescence of freshly prepared liver biopsy material.[3]

3. Addison's disease shows melanodermic darkening of exposed skin areas, especially during the summer months (knuckles of fingers and palms) or in such areas that tend physiologically to possess more pigmentation already (Fig. 377).

In contrast to melanodermic "neviform" keratosis of the areola — for instance, after application of estrogenic ointments to the mamillae — the hyperpigmentation of the areolae in Addison's disease lacks additional cornification.

Frequently, scars are especially hyperpigmented, and in general, the intensity of the bronze color of the patient with Addison's disease is not at all diffusely homogeneous. Pigmentations of the mucous membranes, frequently in hues of blue or smoke-gray, are seen inside the mouth or in the anogenital region. However, corresponding pigmentations of the conjunctivae are extremely rare. Some patients may present marked pigmentation of the nailbed or the terminal phalanges of the fingers. In addition, pre-existing ephelides become more pigmented during the course of Addison's disease. The recognition of the patient with Addison's disease is facilitated by the light color of his fingernails; however, they are not always porcelain-white. Occasionally, sparseness of the hairs of the axillae and pubis may be present, as well as a tendency to increased perspiration.

Histologically, the Addison color corresponds to a suntan; its basis is a deposition of melanin in the basal cells of the

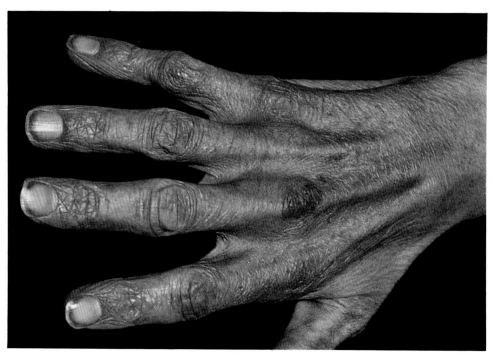

Fig. 376. Hemochromatosis.

Fig. 377. Diffuse melanin pigmentation in Addison's disease.

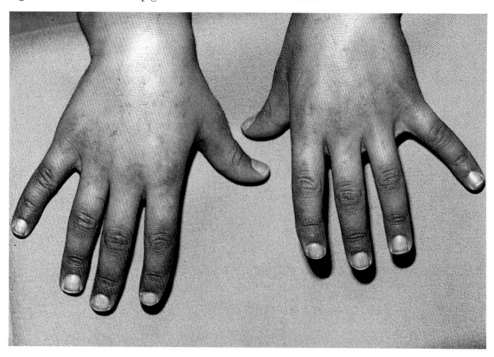

epidermis and the cranially adjacent lower cellular layers of the stratum spinosum. The corium takes part in the melanotic pigmentation only in the papillary body, if at all. The Addisonian pigmentation shares this cutaneous reaction with arsenical melanosis; however, there is a more dustlike interspersion of the melanin within the epidermis and a widening of the stratum corneum in the latter. In contrast, in chronic pellagrous dermatitis the melanin appears as coarse grains all through the epidermal layers, while in Addison's disease, finer grains are observed. In Riehl's melanosis, however, the melanin deposits are characteristically found in the upper third of the corium separated from the epidermis by a free papillary zone.

4. Arsenical melanosis differs clinically from Addison's disease in that it does not present a diffuse homogeneous increase of pigment but shows multiple confluent, partly angular, pigmented macules. The axillary regions and the abdomen show greatly increased arsenical pigmentation. Mucous membranes remain almost always unaffected. The absence of asthenia excludes Addison's disease; other signs characteristic of chronic arsenical intoxication are hyperkeratoses, multiple epitheliomas of the trunk, and cutaneous changes resembling those of acrodermatitis chronica atrophicans.

5. Extreme diffuse hypopigmentations have been observed in association with tumors of the **thymus** or with **mediastinal cancers.** These tumors produce ACTH or MSH (melanocyte-stimulating hormone).[16]

6. Gaucher's disease does not cause very characteristic cutaneous changes. When present they are seen mostly in older patients as ochre- to yellow-brown melanin pigmentations. The lesions prefer the exposed parts of the skin; e.g., on the face they resemble chloasma and on the legs

they have an asymmetrical reticular pattern, while the soles, heels, and toes remain free. In addition to these reticulated melanodermas small macular or linear pigmentations can be observed. Diagnostically important is the sharp outline of such pigmentations immediately below the malleoli. The skin of the legs may be glossy with a smooth shiny surface, and sometimes it shows scales and ulcerations. The mucous membranes in rare cases may take part in the melanin pigmentation. The conjunctiva characteristically shows wedge-shaped, pinguecualike, brownish-yellow macules with a broad base at the limbus of the cornea.[8]

7. Niemann-Pick's disease also shows a special yellow-brownish or faintly brownish skin color, distinctly more marked in cutaneous areas exposed to light. The patient with this disease has a color that is, on the whole, more saturated than that of the patient with Gaucher's disease. Pigmentations of the oral mucosa, seen more rarely, have a brownish-black color.

Histochemically, melanin and hemosiderin occur together as pigment deposits in both Gaucher's and Niemann-Pick's diseases.

8. Argyria or argyrosis are names given to an irreversible cutaneous impregnation with silver or a silver salt. This condition is found locally in employees working with silver; it can be caused by absorption of silver solutions applied locally (eyedrops), and, finally, it may result from long-term absorption of drugs containing silver* and throat disinfectants containing silver compounds. The bluish or dirty-gray discoloration of the skin caused by storage of silver remains throughout life, generally causing no ill effects; it may appear suddenly, for

---

* Inunction treatments with silver solutions are used in Germany for stomach ulcers; in the United States silver nitrate solutions per os are used. (Tr.)

instance, after intensive exposure to sun. Impregnation of the conjunctiva with silver by instillation of solutions containing silver salts causes a bluish-gray discoloration. Also, the nailbed appears typically blue and the lunules of the nails are azure blue. The generalized discoloration at first may suggest cyanosis, especially in adults, while in children the intensity of such a pseudo-cyanosis may lead one to suspect a congenital cardiac defect.

Histologically, the precipitated silver particles are easily visible by dark-field examination; the disappearance of this phenomenon upon application of a 1 per cent potassium cyanide solution (KCN) is quite characteristic. Another quality of deposited metallic silver is its affinity for the elastic fibers of the basal membrane of the sweat glands and for the connective tissue border areas of hair follicles and sebaceous glands. Silver granules in tissue are relatively inert, so that inflammatory or reactive responses to resorption of silver do not take place in this storage disease; as a rule subjective complaints are absent.[15,17]

9. Ochronosis has been mentioned before in connection with arthropathias as ochronotic arthropathy; ochronosis also shows cutaneous pigmentations. Even in early infancy the voided urine is dark and turns black on standing; it causes diapers to turn dark. However, clinical manifestations as a rule do not become noticeable before the third decade in life. Endogenous alkaptonuria due to an enzymatic defect in the metabolism of phenylalanine and tyrosine can be recognized by examining the urine with ferric chloride, which produces an evanescent blue or green discoloration, or by the reduction tests of *Trommer* or *Fehling*, or by paper chromatography. Light-exposed photographic paper will be blackened by a drop of such urine (Fischberg test). Essential alkaptonuria will not be checked by giving ascorbic acid.

The above tests are necessary because not every case with *darkened urine* indicates the presence of alkaptonuria. Dark urine may also be melanuria caused by melanoma or resorption of potent therapeutic drugs such as pyrogallol, creosote, or guaiac or some tars, as well as by ingestion of salicylates and derivatives of resorcin.

Alkaptonuria is known to follow chronic intoxication with phenol (carbolochronosis).

Clinically, endogenous ochronosis causes changes in the cartilage, darkening of the urine, and externally visible pigmentations. Such pigment anomalies are seen on the sclerae (Osler's sign) and the cartilage of the ear and nose. High diagnostic value is ascribed to transillumination of the pinna of the ear; if this sign is positive, there will be a lack of transparency in places. Otherwise, the color hues observed on the visible cartilage (e.g., nasal cartilages) can differ widely; there may be greenish-yellow to dark gray or brownish-black macules. In addition, the affected cartilaginous parts may sometimes lack elasticity and are thickened. The sclerae within the palpebral fissure present grayish-blue spots characterized less frequently by diffuse hues than by sharply outlined triangular or sickle-shaped macules. Involvement of the cornea or the fundus of the eyes takes place much more rarely. In contrast to the pigmentations of the ear and sclerae, cutaneous ochronosis of other areas is not as infrequent as was believed formerly. Predominantly macular ochronotic pigmentations occur mostly on the face and neck. Much more rarely, bluish-green, diffuse pigmentations are seen within the axillary and genitocrural folds. Premonitory changes of the skin, for example, nevus cell nevi, may be the sites of increased deposits of ochronotic pigment. Other rare locations of pigmentation are the oral mucous membranes, such as the exits of Stensen's duct, or the nails.

Histopathologically, it is demonstrable, as the clinical references previously given have shown, that the bradytrophic tissues are storage organs for pigment. As a rule one finds coarse lumps of pigment or deposits within the skin; they probably represent degenerated collagen, which has an affinity for homogentisic acid. The light brown pigment reacts with polychromic methylene blue by turning blackish, but it cannot be stained with silver nitrate as melanin can.[5, 7, 10, 11, 12]

10. Exogenous ochronosis (chronic carbolic intoxication) as a rule does not reach the same degree of cutaneous and articular involvement as seen in endogenous ochronosis.

A dirty gray cutaneous color is sometimes seen in cases of chronic **phenacetin addiction;** the deposits consist of pathological derivatives of hemoglobin and lipofuscinlike mixtures.[2]

11. Asthma melanodermicum is a disease entity involving diffuse melanin hyperpigmentations; there is a definite connection with preceding asthmatic attacks. When combined with such a diffuse increase of melanin, existing nevus cell nevi and lentigines become darker and definitely more numerous.[14]

12. Catatonic **schizophrenia** shows occasionally an Addison-like pigmentation with no indication of adrenal insufficiency. Certain cutaneous areas, e.g., the neck, shoulders, and lips, show various degrees of dark pigmentary disturbances. In addition, pigmentary stimulation is definitely increased when the skin is exposed to light (bronze catatonia). Pigmentary masks in brain tumors (ependymomas) are even rarer; the postencephalitic brown ring of the forehead is not so infrequent.[6]

13. Hepatolenticular degeneration (Wilson's disease) occasionally shows various kinds of pigmentation — for example, that around the malleoli and the extensor aspects of the legs — caused by increased solar tanning. As a rule, cutaneous light-exposed areas are considerably more pig-

mented. Pigmentations due to hemosiderin as well as to melanin can also be found on some internal organs (spleen and kidneys). Almost always the pigmentations are accompanied by the greenish-brown or greenish-gray *Kayser-Fleischer corneal ring;* this ring is an early, highly characteristic sign of Wilson's pseudosclerosis.[13]

14. Metastatic melanoma (Fig. 378) in rare cases may cause generalized blue-gray cutaneous hyperpigmentation together with involvement of the mucous membranes. At the same time there is often a definite increase in melanogen in the urine (Fig. 379). Histologically, deposits of melanin are found in the histiocytes and also extracellularly throughout the entire corium. In the differential diagnosis argyrosis can be excluded by proving the lack of response of light-exposed cutanous areas and the absence of silver particles in histologic preparations.[1, 9]

15. Melanoerythroderma with cachexia is the same condition as *lipomelanotic reticulosis;* see the discussion of erythrodermas, Chapter 22, C1 (page 342).

(1) ALBEAUX-FERNET, M., R. LAUMONIER et P. COLLART: Un cas de tumeur mélanique du foie avec mélanodermie généralisée. Presse méd. *1949* II: 941–942.

(2) BERNEIS, K., und A. STUDER: Ablagerung farbiger Lipide in der Haut als Folge von Phenacetinabusus. Virchow's Arch. Abt. B. (Zellpath.) *2:* 311–317 (1969).

(3) BRUGSCH, J.: Melanodermie – Porphyrie (Porphyrie mit Melanodermie). Z. ges. inn. Med. *11:* 5–8 (1956).

(4) CAWLEY, E. P., T. HSU, B. T. WOOD and P. E. WEARY: Hemochromatosis and the skin. Arch. Derm. Syph. (Chic.) *100:* 1–6 (1969).

(5) COOPER, J. A., and TH. J. MORAN: Studies on ochronosis. I.Report of a case with death from ochronotic nephrosis. Arch. Path. (Chic.) *64:* 46–53 (1957).

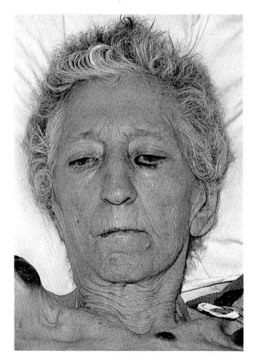

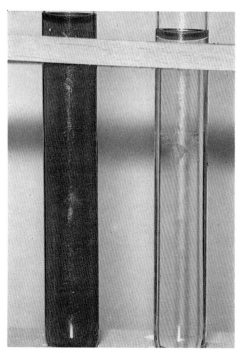

Fig. 378. Diffuse melanosis in metastasizing malignant melanoma.

Fig. 379. Melanuria in metastasizing melanoma.

(6) DERBES, V. J., G. FLEMING and S. W. BECKER, Jr.: Generalized cutaneous pigmentation of diencephalic origin. Arch. Derm. Syph. (Chic.) 72: 13–22 (1955).

(7) DIHLMANN, W., H. GREILING, R. KISTERS und W. H. STUHLSATZ: Biochemische und radiologische Untersuchungen zur Pathogenese der Alkaptonurie. Dtsch. med. Wschr. 95: 839–844 (1970).

(8) EAST, T., and L. H. SAVIN: Case of Gaucher's disease with biopsy of typical pingueculae. Brit. J. Ophthal. 24: 611–613 (1940).

(9) FITZPATRICK, T. B., H. MONTGOMERY and A. B. LERNER: Pathogenesis of generalized dermal pigmentation secondary to malignant melanoma and melanuria. J. invest. Derm. 22: 163–172 (1954).

(10) FLECK, F.: Zur Symptomatik und Entstehung der endogenen Ochronose. Derm. Wschr. 134: 1317–1326 (1956).

(11) FRIDERICH, H., und W. NIKOLOWSKI: Endogene Ochronose. Arch. Derm. Syph. (Berl.) 192: 273–289 (1951).

(12) LAYMON, C. W.: Ochronosis. Arch. Derm. Syph. (Chic.) 67: 553–560 (1953).

(13) LEU, M.L., TH. STRICKLAND, C.C.WANG, T. S. N. CHEN: Skin pigmentation in Wilson's disease. J. Amer. med. Ass. 211: 1542–1543 (1970).

(14) LOEWENTHAL, L. J. A., and S. SHAPIRO: Asthma melanodermica. Arch. Derm. (Chic.) 78: 210–213 (1958).

(15) SIEMUND, J., und A. STOLP: Argyrose. Z. Haut- u. Geschl.-Kr. 43: [71–74] (1968).

(16) STEENO, O., und P. DE MOOR: Extreme Hyperpigmentierung bei Cushing-Syndrom mit ACTH-produzierendem Tumor der Lunge. In: Wachstumshormon und Wachstumsstörungen; 11.Symp. dtsch. Ges. Endokrinologie. Hrsg. E. KLEIN. S.165–167. Springer, Berlin, Heidelberg 1965.

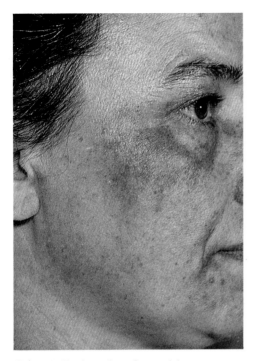

Fig. 380. Toxic melanodermatitis.

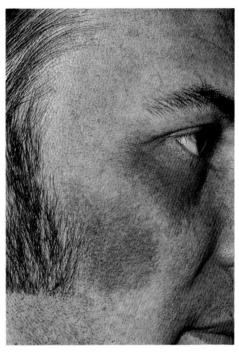

Fig. 381. Pigmentation after contact with bromethylalanin.

(17) WHELTON, M. J., and F. M. POPE: Azure lunules in argyria. Arch. intern. Med. *121:* 267–269 (1968).

D. Circumscribed Hyperpigmentations

1. Riehl's melanosis and its equivalent, melanodermatitis toxica lichenoides (et bullosa), which has been observed mainly in times of hunger and malnutrition, show grayish-brown or faintly saturated, violet-brown cutaneous discolorations (Fig. 380). Most of the localized pigmented areas have no sharp borders and blend with the surrounding skin; the forehead, sides of the face and neck, and less frequently, the arms and sides of the trunk are involved. The mucous membranes always remain free.

Within such conspicuous areas of discoloration there are many perifollicularly and follicularly arranged, millet-sized hyperkeratoses. Occasionally, a pellagroid character may be simulated by this lamellar or flourlike desquamation or rough hyperkeratotic surface.[44]

In the pathogenesis of Riehl's melanosis endogenous factors such as a deficiency syndrome or enteric disorder are considered primarily. Melanodermatitis toxica has more inflammatory lesions that depend on the effect of light. In addition, exogenous contacts with tar and derivatives of lubricating oils should be considered (Fig. 381).

Histologically, Riehl's melanosis shows a special pattern of distribution of pigmentary deposits. The papillary body and the basal cellular line do not show an increase of pigment in a typical case; however, below the papillary body there is a free zone

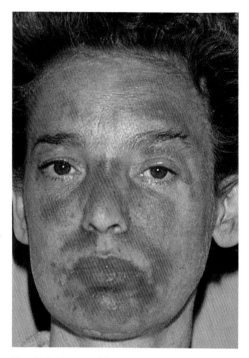

Fig. 382. Acute pellagra.

will soon change from the "phrynoderma" (toadskin) caused by vitamin-A deficiency to the chessboard pattern of bleeding points of folliculitis scorbutica hemorrhagica. With further exacerbation, cutaneous petechiae and hemorrhages follow especially on the legs or other places of special muscular stress; in addition, spongy, dusky red swellings of the interdental papillae develop.

3. Patients suffering from chronic **pellagra,** especially those who have suffered seasonal manifestations of pellagra for several years, show different, partly Addison-like, macular, chloasmalike, spotty or pointed brown pigmentations. These pigmentations manifest themselves within the areas of former cutaneous lesions and spread further away from them. Clinically typical of pellagra are the four D's (diarrhea, dermatitis, dementia, and death). The first cutaneous changes consist of occasionally edematous but only rarely exudative, symmetrical, sharply outlined, erythematous areas (Fig. 382), which after some time assume a mahogany brown color. This change is followed by thin and small lamellar desquamation which in the beginning is still flourlike and fine; this appears chiefly in the middle of the erythematous areas. Later, the originally peripheral parts show hyperkeratotic dirty borders, especially on the medial aspect of the arms. The sites of predilection of this pellagrosis are chiefly the hands and forearms, then the dorsa of the feet, the neck, and the sternal region (Casal's necklace). The palmar aspects of the hands have a marked yellow discoloration simultaneously with thick keratinization. The presence of filiform lesions or folliculopapular keratoses on the nasolabial folds, like the seborrheic erythematous changes of the genital region, is more likely a manifestation of ariboflavinosis. The vermilion border of the lips of the pellagrin is sore and looks as if it is covered with lacquer, and the tongue is highly red or bluish-purple, somewhat re-

which is contiguous to deposits of melanin concentrated less extracellularly but mostly in the melanophages; melanin appears in unusually coarse clumps. Further attributes of Riehl's melanosis are inflammatory infiltrates in the corium, especially where vacuolization of the basal cells has taken place at the same time; this could be a sign of epidermal damage. Apparently the epithelial cells have lost their physiological pigment, which then has been taken up in the deeper sections of the papillary body by the macrophages.

2. Compared with the marked melanodermic brown line of Riehl's melanosis the color of vitamin-A avitaminosis is a peculiar ashy gray tone that comes close to the coloration of argyrosis; at the same time, avitaminosis shows follicular keratoses. **Scurvy,** or rather pre-scurvy, can show a certain cutaneous melanodermic dark hue. Pre-scurvy follicular keratosis, however,

sembling Möller's glossitis or the so-called beefsteak tongue. Especially characteristic of pellagrins is profuse salivation.

During the last few years symptomatic pellagra caused by alcohol abuse has been observed by the authors in adults. Secondary pellagra has been observed in association with stomach cancers or after stomach resection, and with carcinoid of the intestine. It has also been seen as a iatrogenic disease after prolonged medication with broad-spectrum antibiotics, and especially after protracted intake of isoniazid, and to a lesser extent after therapy restricted to one component of the vitamin B complex.

4. In **chloasma uterinum** there are sharply bordered or angular, dark brownish and mostly macular facial pigmentations that prefer the forehead, cheeks, and chin. Characteristically, exposure to light will enhance the difference from the rest of the facial skin (Fig. 383). In contrast to Riehl's melanosis chloasma lacks any history of exogenous irritants (with the exception of estrogenic ointments), the neck always remains free, and there is no reaction of the surface of the epidermis. Synchronously with the increase of facial pigmentation, the linea alba of the abdomen becomes the linea nigra of pregnancy; the nipples, the axillae, and the genitoanal region turn dark. Chloasma uterinum is caused chiefly by hormonal factors (estrogens). Such factors are pregnancy, the ingestion of contraceptive pills (they cause a small speckled and less saturated pigmentation), and ovarian tumors. Menopause may give rise to *climacteric chloasma*, and at the time of the first menstrual period normal young girls show the *perioral chloasma of virgins;* this pigmentation in most cases is located exclusively around the mouth and is typically separated from the vermilion border by a small light area. *Erythrosis pigmentata faciei* (Brocq's name, "érythrose peribuccale pigmentaire") is marked by the addition of a faint telangiectatic erythema to the perioral chloasma with extension to the chin and

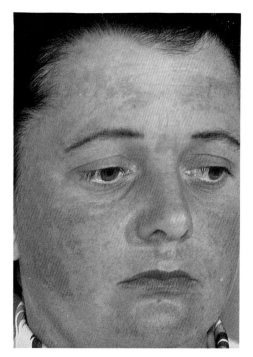

Fig. 383. Chloasma uterinum.

nasolabial folds. The erythema can become so intense that a preponderantly dark red to brown skin color will result, sometimes with mild desquamation. The development of additional papular seborrheic lesions will

Fig. 384. Periocular pigmentation with medial accentuation in hyperthyroidism.

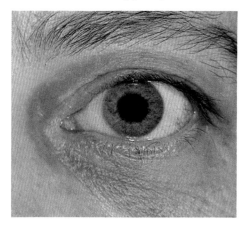

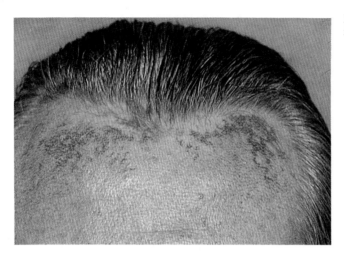

Fig. 385. So-called brown forehead ring.

form a transition to the *perioral rosacealike dermatosis*, which almost always is seen in the female sex.[42, 46]

Some forms of chloasma are not confined to the female sex but may occur after protracted medication with *hydantoin* and *chlorpromazine*.[16, 25]

Some special forms of chloasma are confined to circumscribed facial areas and lack any connection with specific gynecological disorders. The periorbital region may show *hepatic chloasma*, or biliary mask ("masque biliaire"). This fairly sharply bordered, periocular hyperpigmentation is seen mostly in brunette, pyknic women. The skin around the eyes is a light coffee-brown or a dirty walnut-brown; it may extend up to the eyebrows, medial to the bridge of the nose, lateral to the outer border of the orbit, and below to about the zygoma. Such a biliary mask is not present in every woman suffering from biliary disease; inversely, not every patient with a biliary mask has a corresponding disease of the bile ducts.[38]

Jellinek's sign (Fig. 384) describes increased hyperpigmentation, especially around the internal canthi; this sign supposedly indicates hyperfunction of the thyroid as seen in Grave's disease. Another kind of discoloration is the blue-blackish color of the orbit seen in younger patients with a history of long-standing allergic rhinitis; this condition is probably due to stasis of the marginal venous arcades.[18]

Periorbital hyperpigmentations may be observed without any other concomitant disease as a genetic disorder of pigmentation.[13]

The so-called *brown ring of the forehead* (Fig. 385) should be considered an abortive chloasma. This markedly brown hyperpigmentation of the frontal region occurs mostly during or after encephalitis. The differential diagnosis must take into consideration dermatitis caused by a hatband or by wearing protective glasses made of rubber at work.[15, 47]

Other diffuse facial hyperpigmentations can be observed in patients with chronic enterocolitis, tuberculosis of the lung, or the various rheumatic diseases.[24]

5. Erythromelanosis interfollicularis colli presents a more or less bilateral, ill-defined, faint or blue-reddish erythema interspersed with many pinhead-sized macules arranged in a finely reticulated network. Sometimes the lighter colored macules, which in reality are sebaceous glands, are arranged in streaks which form horizontal or wavy lines. Under diascopic pressure this erythrosis is blanched out, revealing telangiectatic dilatations of the subpapillary vascular net as its causative factor.

Erythrosis follicularis prefers the sides of the neck and almost always spares the submental region. This disease is composed of small papules and erythemas; however, when there is additional epidermal hyperpigmentation one uses the expression *"erythromelanosis follicularis faciei et colli."* Not only the skin of the neck but also the preauricular region may be involved.[28, 31]

Reticulated or isletlike **dyschromias of the sides of the neck** may be caused by external stimuli but also by internal disorders of the hematopoietic or neurohormonal system. In addition, toxic-infectious factors combined with the disposition of the individual play a role. In any case, dyschromias of the sides of the neck have diverse origins caused by many factors and require individual analysis in each case.[10]

6. Larger macular **hyperpigmentations**, especially on the exposed areas of the skin, may be due to photosensitization, and may sometimes develop into exudative and bullous reactions. As a rule, not only straight hyperpigmentation but also alternating areas of hypopigmentation will be present. The most common example of such photosensitivity is **berloque dermatitis,** caused by perfumes such as eau de Cologne applied before and during sun exposure, especially while perspiring. The perfume drops running down from the neck or the nuchal region cause a dermatitis at first; later, the characteristic streaky hyperpigmentation (Fig. 386) results. One of the photosensitizers is bergamot oil, an ingredient of eau de Cologne; this oil contains furocoumarin, a potent photosensitizer.

7. Not uncommon, although not as frequent as berloque dermatitis, are the residual **hyperpigmentations** that occur after **phytophotodermatoses,** for instance, **dermatitis bullosa striata pratensis** (grass or meadow dermatitis) due to contact with the

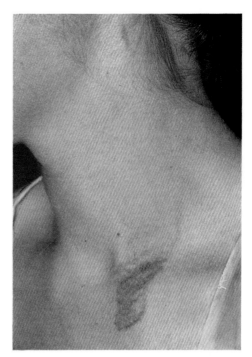

Fig. 386. Berloque dermatitis.

sap of heraculeum* and after contact with *tar products, acridin dyes,* and so on. Other possibilities of allergic photosensitization are oral antidiabetic preparations, antimycotic drugs, and blancophores; however, only *phenothiazines* show subsequent hyperpigmentation. **Chlorpromazine** taken for a very long time, even years, may cause in light-skinned patients brownish-yellow or slate-gray pigmentations of the face, dorsa of the hands, and, if exposed to light, also of the legs.

Histologically, the upper corium shows an increase in melanophages but is separated below by a free papillary strip; this histologic picture corresponds to that seen in Riehl's melanosis.

High doses of the anti-anginal drug **Amiodarone** given for some months may cause gray to bluish-black pigmentations

_____
* *Agrimonia eupatoria.* (Tr.)

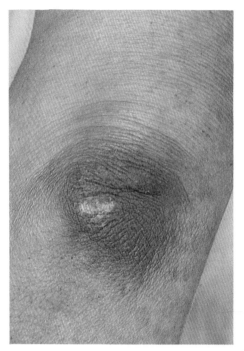

Fig. 387. Pigmentations due to bleomycin therapy.

in a small number of patients. These discolorations affect only light-exposed cutaneous areas such as the face, the back of neck, and dorsa of the hands; discontinuance of the drug results in complete re-

gression. Because the hyperpigmentation is caused by photosensitization, the intensity of sun exposure is an important factor in the degree of pigmentation. Histologically, there is not so much an increase of melanin as an intensive intracellular accumulation of lipofuscin-like substances. The differential diagnosis must consider argyrosis (histologic proof of the presence of silver) and hyperpigmentation due to intake of phenothiazine.[32, 48]

8. Atabrine treatment may cause blue-black hyperpigmentations that are not dependent on light exposure on the hard palate, legs, and subungual area, sometimes near the lips and also on the nasal and auricular cartilages. **Chloroquine** derivatives (such as Resochin) cause similar deposits of dirty gray-white pigment on the back of the neck, legs, and genitals, for example; in addition, hairs of the scalp and pubic region become depigmented. Histochemically, not only are deposits of melanin increased but also part of the storage consists of hemosiderin. Perhaps such hemosiderin pigmentation due to Resochin takes place via a hemorrhagic capillaritis.[27]

Treatment with **bleomycin,** an antibiotic with antineoplastic properties, may cause circumscribed, macular, dark brown hyper-

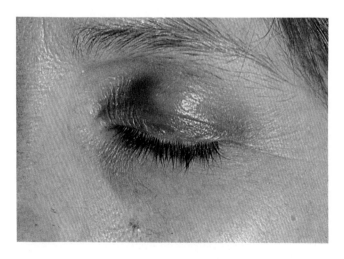

Fig. 388. Hydrargyrosis of the skin.

pigmentations (Fig. 387), which regress after conclusion of the treatment.

9. Hyperpigmentations may occur after **overdosage** as well as after chronic doses of **vitamin A.** Manifestations of hypervitaminosis-A are, by the way, rather similar to those of the vitamin-A deficiency syndrome. Membranous desquamation, however, is observed only after acute vitamin-A overdosage.

10. Finally, simple external irritations such as rubbing, pressure, or heat can stimulate the skin to increased pigmentations. Well known are the **postlesional hyperpigmentations** after secondary syphilitic eruptions (secondary syphilis nigricans), lichen planus, psoriasis, and even after impetigo contagiosa and some eczemas, especially circumscribed neurodermatitis.

11. Circumscribed slate-gray to blackish-blue pigmentations may occur after long application of **mercury-containing substances** (e.g., bleaches). They are limited to the site of the application. A distinct accentuation of the body folds is observed (Fig. 388).

Histologically, a finely granular deposit of pigment is present in the upper corium. It cannot be stained with the yellow-brownish silver and iron staining methods.

In the differential diagnosis argyrosis must be ruled out. This is achieved by evidence of noninvolvement of the conjunctivae and absence of dependency on light.[26]

After the application of **estrogen-containing salves,** as in the treatment of pruritus vulvae, dark brown hyperpigmentations that are limited to the site of application may occur (Fig. 389). Additional development of flat hyperkeratoses (see Chapter 31, B3) is possible.

12. In **erythema dyschromicum perstans** ("ashy dermatosis"), observed until now only in South and North America, we are dealing with oblong pigmentations. They

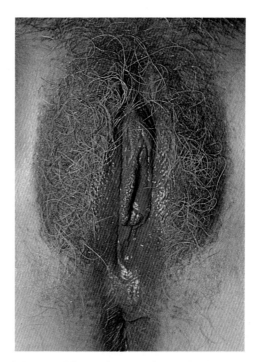

Fig. 389. Hyperpigmentation following application of salve containing estrogen.

start as small spots with little infiltration and peripheral elevation of the lesion. In the course of the dermatosis mild follicular keratosis may occur. Fungi are always absent. These changes are located mainly on the trunk and the upper extremities, leaving the scalp, palms, soles, and the mucous membranes unaffected. The histologic appearance is similar to that of the substrate of Riehl's melanosis due to hydropic degeneration of the basal cell line and to a certain pigmentary insufficiency. Certain features such as thin perivascular infiltrates by round cells, histiocytes, and especially melanophages should be emphasized.

In the differential diagnosis other persisting erythemas with subsequent pigmentation such as occur with malignant visceral tumors, intestinal parasites, or some rheumatic affections like the Felty syndrome, must be considered. Dirty-brownish fixed drug eruptions do not have so many lesions; they occasionally have a tendency

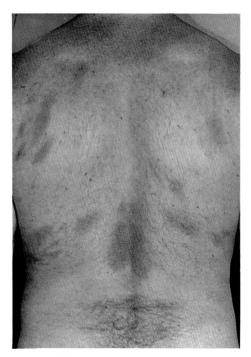

Fig. 390. Idiopathic atrophoderma.

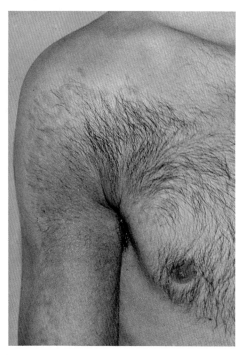

Fig. 391. Neviform melanosis.

to bullous changes and heal after discontinuance of the drug. Pityriasis alba of the face usually shows more distinct scaling and, above all, a raised margin is lacking. [5, 21, 43]

13. If, however, we are dealing with faintly saturated hyperpigmentations, which are occasionally sunken-in and rather homogeneous and may be as large as the palm, **idiopathic atrophoderma** must be considered (Fig. 390). It can be said that any circumscribed scleroderma can be followed by more or less extensive areas of hyperpigmentation.[17, 19]

14. Melanosis neviformis is the name of an always unilateral, palm-sized or larger, brown pigmentation with "archipelagolike loosening" of the marginal zone and often distinct hypertrichosis. A favorite location of this melanosis is the upper part of the thorax (Fig. 391). Histologically, this con-

genital, nevuslike melanosis shows acanthosis, increase of pigment in the basal cells, and an increase of clear cells. Therefore, a differentiation of melanosis neviformis from a pigmented nevus is not possible on histologic grounds. Pityriasis versicolor can be easily identified by the presence of fungi.[12, 41]

15. The pale blue or grayish-blue and usually single **Mongolian spot** is variable in form and is only exceptionally raised above the level of the skin; occasionally it may be covered with hair. It is usually located in the sacral, lumbar, or coccygeal areas. A ventral location is extremely rare. The intensity of the color of the lesion varies, as do its borders, which are sometimes sharp, sometimes vague. The dermal melanocytosis is usually palm-sized. This nevus favors the male sex and, within a family, the first child or children with dark hair and dark eyes.

Hyperpigmentations of the corium on any part of the trunk are usually larger and more irregularly limited than a typical Mongolian spot, and are light blue to blue-gray in color (so-called *light blue nevus of Yamamoto*) (Fig. 392). **Nevus fuscocaeruleus acromiodeltoideus** in the shoulder-back region occurs in this special location in Japanese and black women. Clinically, the **nevus of Ota (nevus fuscocaeruleus ophthalmomaxillaris)** is a predominantly unilateral, only rarely bilateral, dark bluish, sharply limited, discoloration of the sclerae, lids, forehead, and cheeks; the lips and the middle of the forehead usually remain free (Fig. 393). Occasionally, greater deposits of pigment are observed in various parts of the eye. The nevus of Ota is usually present at birth and may regress somewhat in later life without fading altogether. Familial incidence is rare. All these nevi favor the Mongolian race and occasionally blacks.

Histologically, the nevus of Ota and the Mongolian spot, aside from the obvious relationship to the nervous system, show an increase of melanocytes and freely lying interstitial melanin in the upper to middle layers of the corium. An aggregation of large melanocytes in the depth of the corium occurs similarly in nevus caeruleus. There are, however, no strict differences according to layers. It is only a relative observation that the dermal melanocytes in a blue nevus appear larger and more elongated than those in the nevus of Ota.[8, 23, 50]

The **diffuse mesodermal melanodermas,** which also occur in some cattle and horses, constitute the greatest rarity among mesodermal pigmentations. They manifest themselves as multiple, light to black-blue spots of different sizes. They are raised insignificantly or not at all above the level of the skin. Histologically, they present ag-

Fig. 392. So-called light blue nevus Yamamoto.

Fig. 393. Nevus Ota.

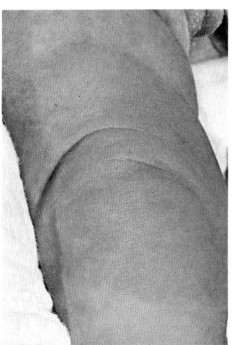

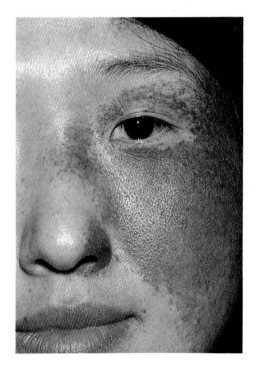

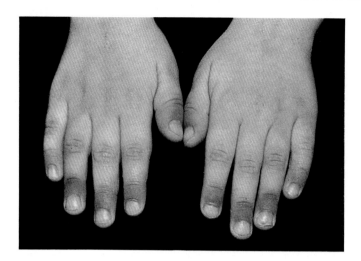

Fig. 394. Physiologic
acropigmentation.

gregations of melanocyte in the corium as in a blue nevus.[4, 37, 51]

16. Among the circumscribed hyperpigmentations the most important topographically is **acropigmentation.** It is physiologic in children up to the sixth year of life. This is a slowly regressing, dark brown coloring of the terminal phalanges of the fingers and, to a lesser degree, of the toes (Fig. 394). Children manifesting the hyperpigmentation have dark coloring, judged by their hair color and that of the iris. A similar hyperpigmentation is imitated by a deficiency of vitamin B_{12} and by rheumatoid arthritis of the joints of the fingers.

In **progressive pigmentary dermatosis** an increase of brownish-black pigmentation on the dorsa of fingers and toes begins a few months after birth. Later, it extends over the thighs, perineum, popliteal spaces and the testicular region.[11]

Symmetrical acropigmentation or **hereditary symmetrical dyschromatosis** also starts in early childhood. Especially on the face and on the dorsa of the hands and feet, symmetrical, widespread, small, hyperpigmented spots occur, similar to freckles or xeroderma pigmentosum. They are occasionally mixed with leukodermic areas. The intensity of the pigmentation is subject to

seasonal variations. This pigmentary anomaly, which has so far been observed only in Japanese and Koreans, shows a distinct familial incidence, but the genetic mechanism may vary.[22]

17. Reticular pigmentations on the neck, chest, and body folds are always present in **congenital dyskeratosis** (the Zinsser-Cole-Engman syndrome). If vascular dilatations and atrophies occur, the hands, feet, elbows, and knees assume a poikilodermic aspect. In addition, there are always leukoplakic changes of the mucous membranes and severe dystrophy of the nails leading to the loss of the nails. In general, the disorder starts with the changes of the nails and the mucous membranes, while the hyperpigmentations occur for the first time in the succeeding years; all manifestations are fully developed as late as the twentieth year of life. Palmoplantar hyperhidrosis, disturbances in the hair growth, and dental anomalies are facultative manifestations. In contrast to pachyonychia congenita palmoplantar keratoses are always absent. In pachyonychia congenita the distinct tendency toward involvement of the male sex is missing. Quite often, the leukoplakias of the esophagus, rectum and urinary bladder give rise to malignant tumors. Disturbances of the hematopoietic system, such as anemia or leukemia, may occur in later years.

The familial combination of congenital dyskeratosis and Fanconi's anemia (constitutional infantile panmyelopathy), the **Fanconi syndrome,** shows, in addition to the previously mentioned cutaneous changes, abnormal erythrocytes with a high color index, a shortened life span, and variable contents of the fetal hemoglobin. The bone marrow shows lymphoid plasmacellular mastocytic hyperplasia. Strikingly often, malformations of the skeleton coexist with endocrine disturbances. Congenital dyskeratosis of the dermatologist doubtless simulates Fanconi's syndrome of the pediatrician, but the hematologic findings differ somewhat.[7, 36, 45]

18. Vaguely limited, pretibial pigmentations of the legs, even if papular elements are absent, suggest isolated **cutaneous amyloidosis.** Pruritus, if present, is not intense. The diagnosis can be ascertained only with evidence of amyloid in the histologic picture. Since this form of amyloidosis always remains limited to the skin, a rectal biopsy offers no diagnostic clue. In the differential diagnosis similar pigmentation of the legs in diabetics play a role.[3, 14, 49]

19. These **pretibial pigment spots** occur predominantly in diabetics and indicate a general microangiopathy. They are flat oval deposits of brown pigment, measuring about 0.5 to 3.5 cm in size (with the long axis either lengthwise or crosswise) and located in the area near the edges of the tibia (Fig. 395). In exceptional cases they may also be located on the trunk or the upper arms. Besides the pigmented spots, which arise from flat, slightly scaling, erythematous lesions, faintly atrophic and depressed scars are present. They are about the same size as the pigment spots but show no increase of pigment.

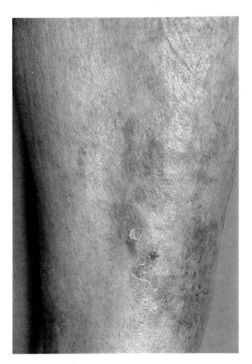

Fig. 395. Pretibial pigment spots in diabetes mellitus.

Histologically, pretibial pigment spots show enlarged vessels in the upper and middle corium. Vessels in this area are surrounded by a dense infiltrate of lymphocytes with only a few histiocytes and neutrophil granulocytes. Necrobiotic areas or striking changes of the vascular walls are not present. The pigment gives a positive iron reaction.

In the differential diagnosis progressive purpura pigmentosa should be considered first. A distinction is possible. First, progressive purpura pigmentosa originates from punctate bleeding areas; second, it affects the entire leg; and third, it is progressive. Deposits of hemosiderin in the course of a "stasis dermatosis," located in the ankle region, prefer a different part of the leg; moreover, the skin shows chronic stasis (varicose veins and edema).[1, 20, 29]

20. Circumscribed hyperpigmentation is a characteristic sign of the diseases of the

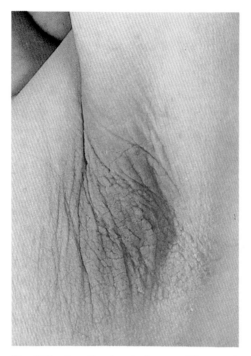

Fig. 396. Acanthosis nigricans with gastric carcinoma.

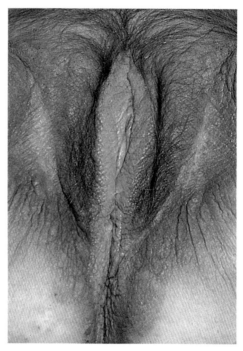

Fig. 397. Acanthosis nigricans with gastric carcinoma. Brownish black acanthosis in the genital region.

acanthosis nigricans group. In this well-defined dermatosis, papillomatous warty growths of various intensities are located primarily in the body folds, the axillae, genitoanal region, and on the umbilicus. The degree of pigmentation extends from light caramel to dark brown. Inflammatory signs are absent and the transition to normal skin is fluent and without peripheral sharp limitation. The palms and soles show extensive hyperkeratoses in some patients. In the differential diagnosis different forms of acanthosis nigricans must be recognized. **Benign acanthosis nigricans** in some patients is present at birth or appears at the latest at puberty. After puberty the dermatosis is at least arrested or complete regression takes place. In contrast to malignant acanthosis nigricans the mucous membranes are affected only rarely. In some families benign acanthosis nigricans ap-

pears in several successive generations. At present the genetic mechanism is considered to be irregularly dominant. In numerous patients there are accompanying developmental disturbances.* The *Seip-Lawrence syndrome* shows acanthosis nigricans and connatal lipoatrophy and often also insulin-resistant diabetes. The *Miescher syndrome* is the name given to the combination of acanthosis nigricans, mental retardation, hypertrichosis, and diabetes mellitus. In conjunction with acanthosis nigricans, endocrine disturbances in the sense of primary hypogonadism may occur. Furthermore,

---

* In another type, "acanthosis nigricans as part of a syndrome," the Seip-Lawrence syndrome is mentioned, among others, whereas benign acanthosis nigricans itself is not accompanied by endocrine or developmental disturbances. (Tr.)

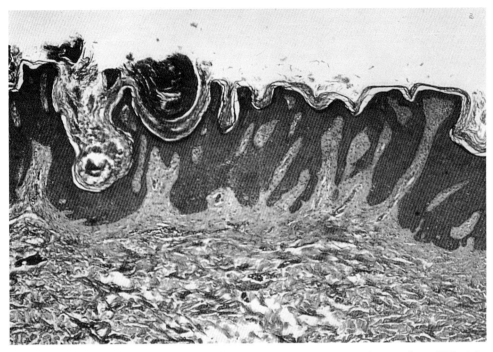

Fig. 398. Acanthosis nigricans: distinctly acanthotic epidermis with horny plugs. HE stain, 30×.

the simultaneous occurrence of acanthosis nigricans and cutis verticis gyrata has been mentioned.[2, 6, 9, 33–35, 39, 40]

Malignant acanthosis nigricans indicates the occurrence of acanthosis nigricans with a malignant tumor (Figs. 310, 396, 397, 398).

In the overwhelming number of patients the tumor is an adenocarcinoma (stomach, prostate, breast, and pancreas)*

_____

* Also ovaries, gallbladder, uterus, and lung, among others. (Tr.)

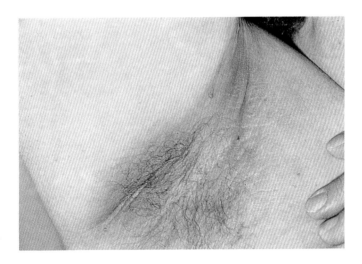

Fig. 399. Pseudoacanthosis nigricans in obesity.

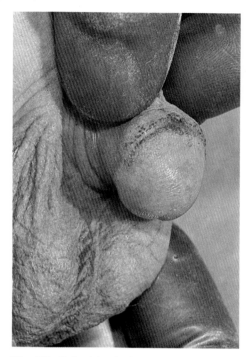

Fig. 400. Balanitis nigricans.

which usually becomes manifest simultaneously. In some patients the cutaneous changes precede the proven tumor by many months. After removal of the malignant tumor acanthosis nigricans regresses. If the tumor recurs, so does the dermatosis. Both sexes are equally affected, and the age of manifestation is in general about the fortieth year of life, corresponding to the age at which the number of tumors increases. But any acanthosis nigricans occurring in an individual of normal weight after puberty must be considered a paraneoplastic syndrome, unless the contrary can be proved.* [9, 35]

Likewise, **pseudoacanthosis nigricans** has been described without limitation to age. It develops in the typical locations in obese individuals (Fig. 399). With the regression of the overweight, of any etiology, the cutaneous changes disappear. Since a clinical distinction between pseudoacanthosis nigricans and malignant acanthosis nigricans is impossible, a search for a tumor should not be omitted in these patients.[34]

21. In the region of the genital semi-mucous membranes, pigment-forming bacteria or fungi (e.g., **balanitis nigricans**) can cause black-brown attached hyperkeratoses (Fig. 400).

(1) Bauer, M., and N. E. Levan: Diabetic dermangiopathy; a spectrum including pigmented pretibial patches and necrobiosis lipoidica diabeticorum. Brit. J. Derm. *83:* 528–535 (1970).

(2) Beare, J. M., J. A. Dodge and N. C. Nevin: Cutis gyratum, acanthosis nigricans and other congenital anomalies. A new syndrome. Brit. J. Derm. *81:* 241–247 (1969).

(3) Brownstein, M. H., and K. Hashimoto: Macular amyloidoses. Arch. Derm. *106:* 50–57 (1972).

(4) Carleton, A., and R. Biggs: Diffuse mesodermal pigmentation with congenital cranial abnormality. Brit. J. Derm. *60:* 10–13 (1948).

(5) Convit, J., F. Kerdel-Vegas and G. Rodriguez: Erythema dyschromicum perstans. J. invest. Derm. *36:* 457–462 (1961).

(6) Davis, J., and M. Feiwel: Lipoatrophy, gigantism and hyperlipemia with xanthomatosis and acanthosis nigricans. Brit. J. Derm. *69:* 229–230 (1957).

---

* Several amplifying comments may be added to this discussion of malignant acanthosis nigricans. In the first place, in some patients, the dermatosis manifests itself after the tumor has been present for some time. After removal of the tumor the disease does not always regress, and if it does. the regression is not always complete. Recently, the possibility that prolonged use of the "pill" can cause acanthosis nigricans in adults has been recognized. Obese patients with malignant acanthosis nigricans would not long remain overweight, a fact to be noted in differential diagnosis of pseudoacanthosis nigricans (following paragraph). (Tr.)

(7) FANCONI, F.: Die familiäre Panmyelo-pathie. Schweiz. med. Wschr. *94:* 1309–1318 (1964).

(8) FITZPATRICK, T. B., R. ZELLER, A. KU-KITA and H. KITAMURA: Ocular and dermal melanocytosis. Arch. Ophthal. *56:* 830–832 (1956).

(9) FLADUNG, G., und H.-J. HEITE: Häufig-keitsanalytische Untersuchungen zur Frage der symptomatologischen Ab-grenzung verschiedener Formen der Acanthosis nigricans. Arch. klin. exp. Derm. *205:* 282–311 (1957).

(10) FLECK, F.: Zur Entstehung und Be-handlung von Dyschromien im seit-lichen Halsbereich. Derm. Wschr. *138:* 1133–1145 (1958).

(11) FURUYA, T., and Y. MISHIMA: Progres-sive pigmentary disorder in Japanese child. Arch. Derm. (Chic.) *86:* 412–418 (1962).

(12) GARTMANN, H., D. NEUHAUS und H. TRITSCH: Melanosis naeviformis. Z. Haut- u. Geschl.-Kr. *43:* 973–984 (1968).

(13) GOODMAN, R. M., and R. W. BELCHER: Periorbital hyperpigmentation. An overlooked genetic disorder of pigmenta-tion. Arch. Derm. (Chic.) *100:* 169–174 (1969).

(14) GRUPPER, CH., et J. CIVATTE: Amyloi-dose cutanée localisée primitive, à forme exceptionnelle, maculeuse. Bull. Soc. franç. Derm. Syph. *65:* 270–272 (1958).

(15) HAXTHAUSEN, H.: Skin changes in chronic encephalitis. Acta derm.-vene-reol. (Stockh.) *13:* 408–416 (1932).

(16) HAYS, G. B., C. B. LYLE, Jr. and C. E. WHEELER, Jr.: Slate-gray color in patients receiving chlorpromazine. Arch. Derm. (Chic.) *90:* 471–476 (1964).

(17) JABLONSKA, S., and A. SZCZEPANSKI: Atrophoderma Pasini-Pierini: is it an entity? Dermatologica (Basel) *125:* 226–242 (1962).

(18) JELLINEK, S.: Ein bisher nicht beach-tetes Symptom der Basedowschen Krankheit. Wien. klin. Wschr. *17:* 1145 (1904).

(19) KEE, CH. E., W. S. BROTHERS and W. NEW: Idiopathic atrophoderma of Pasini and Pierini with coexistent mor-phea. Arch. Derm. (Chic.) *82:* 100–103 (1960).

(20) KERL, H., und H. KRESBACH: Prätibiale atrophische Pigmentflecke. Ein mikro-vasculär bedingtes Hautsymptom des Diabetes mellitus. Hautarzt *23:* 59–66 (1972).

(21) KNOX, J. M., B. G. DODGE and R. G. FREEMAN: Erythema dyschromicum perstans. Arch. Derm. (Chic.) *97:* 262–272 (1968).

(22) KOMAYA, G.: Symmetrische Pigment-anomalie der Extremitäten. Arch. Derm. Syph. (Berl.) *147:* 389–393 (1924).

(23) KORTING, G. W.: Haut und Auge. Thieme, Stuttgart 1969; translated by CURTH, W., CURTH, H. O., URBACH, F., and ALBERT, D.: The Skin and Eye. W. B. Saunders Co., Philadelphia, 1973.

(24) KORTING, G. W., und H. HOLZMANN: Dermatologische Veränderungen beim Felty-Syndrom. Arch. klin. exp. Derm. *210:* 472–484 (1960).

(25) KUSKE, H., und A. KREBS: Hyper-pigmentierungen vom Typus des Chlo-asmas nach Behandlung mit Hydan-toin-Präparaten. Dermatologica (Basel) *129:* 121–139 (1964).

(26) LAMAR, L. M., and B. O. BLISS: Localized pigmentation of the skin due to topical mercury. Arch. Derm. (Chic.) *93:* 450–453 (1966).

(27) LANGHOF, H., G. GEYER und H. BAR-THELMES: Hyperpigmentationen und Retinopathie durch Chlorochindiphos-phat. Derm. Wschr. *151:* 185–193 (1965).

(28) LEDER, M.: Erythrosis interfollicularis colli. Dermatologica (Basel) *89:* 132–138 (1944).

(29) MELIN, H.: An atrophic circumscribed skin lesion in the lower extremities of diabetics. Acta med. scand. *176,* Suppl. *423:* 1–75 (1964).

(30) MIESCHER, G.: Zwei Fälle von kongeni-taler familiärer Akanthosis nigricans kombiniert mit Diabetes mellitus. Derm. Z. *32:* 276–305 (1921).

(31) MISHIMA, Y., and E. RUDNER: Erythro-melanosis follicularis faciei et colli. Dermatologica (Basel) *132:* 269–287 (1966).

(32) MORAND, P., J. BENATRE, G. VIAU, C. CARLI-BASSET, J. L. LAINE, J.-L. NEEL, M. BROCHIER et R. RAYNAUD: Étude clinique et histologique (ultra-structure) de la pigmentation par le chlorhydrate d'amiodarone. Sem. Hôp. Paris *48:* 553–563 (1972).

(33) OGAWA, A., and F. BABA: Miescher's syndrome in siblings. Acta paediat. Jap. *73:* 730–739 (1969).

(34) OLLENDORFF-CURTH, H.: Die Probleme der Acanthosis nigricans. Hautarzt *15:* 433–439 (1964).

(35) OLLENDORFF-CURTH, H., A.W. HILBERG and G. F. MACHACEK: The site and histology of the cancer associated with acanthosis nigricans. Cancer (Philad.) *15:* 364–382 (1962).

(36) ORFANOS, C., und H. GARTMANN: Leukoplakien, Pigmentverschiebungen und Nageldystrophie, Zinsser-Cole-Engman-Syndrom – sog. Dyskeratosis congenita. Med. Welt *17* (N.F.): 2589–2594 (1966).

(37) PARISER, H., and H. BEERMAN: Extensive blue patchlike pigmentation. Arch. Derm. Syph. (Chic.) *59:* 396–404 (1949).

(38) PHLEPS, R.: Die klinische Bedeutung der periokulären Hyperpigmentierung (»Pigmentlarve«). Münch. med. Wschr. *96:* 1186–1188 (1954).

(39) REED, W. B., R. DEXTER, C. CORLEY and C. FISH: Congenital lipodystrophic diabetes with acanthosis nigricans; the Seip-Lawrence syndrome. Arch. Derm. (Chic.) *91:* 326–334 (1965).

(40) SCHIRREN, C.: Acanthosis nigricans benigna und Zusammenhang mit primärem Hypogonadismus. In: Wachstumshormon und Wachstumsstörungen. 11. Symp. dtsch. Ges. Endokrinologie. Hrsg. E. KLEIN. S. 251–253. Springer, Berlin, Heidelberg 1965.

(41) SIEMENS, H. W.: Die naevusähnliche Melanose. Hautarzt *18:* 299–303 (1967).

(42) STEIGLEDER, G. K., und A. STREMPEL: Rosaceaartige Dermatitis des Gesichts. Hautarzt *19:* 492–494 (1968).

(43) STEVENSON, M. J. R., and M. MIURA: Erythema dyschromicum perstans (Ashy dermatosis). Arch. Derm. (Chic.) *94:* 196–199 (1966).

(44) STORCK, H.: Über Riehlsche Melanose. Dermatologica (Basel) *92:* 246–258 (1946).

(45) TEXIER, L., et J. MALEVILLE: La symptomatologie cutanée de l'anémie perniciosiforme de Fanconi. Ann. Derm. Syph. (Paris) *90:* 553–568 (1963).

(46) TRITSCH, H., und A. GREITHER: Erythrosis pigmentata faciei. Arch. Derm. Syph. (Berl.) *199:* 221–227 (1955).

(47) VOLHARD, F.: Über chronische Dystrophien und Trophoneurosen der Haut im Anschluß an kasuistische Mitteilungen. Münch. med. Wschr. *50:* 1108–1111 (1903).

(48) WANET, J., G. ACHTEN, G. BARCHEWITZ, C. MESTDAGH et M. VASTESAEGER: Amiodarone et dépots cutanés. Étude clinique et histologique. Ann. Derm. Syph. (Paris) *98:* 131–140 (1971).

(49) WOLF, M., and J. A. TOLMACH: Macular amyloidosis. Arch. Derm. (Chic.) *99:* 373–374 (1969).

(50) YOSHIDA, K.: Nevus fusco-caeruleus-ophthalmo-maxillaris Ota. Tohoku J. exp. Med. *55*, Suppl. I: 34 (1952).

(51) ZARFL, M.: Neue Beiträge zum Studium der blauen Geburtsflecke (Mongolenflecke). Z. Kinderheilk. *41:* 356–369 (1926).

E. Small Macular Pigmentations

Spotted pigmentations are often generalized and are called "pigmented nevi." The substrate of such circumscribed increases in pigment, however, is not uniform, so that more exact determinations are necessary.

1. Ephelides are multiple, irregularly circumscribed, smooth spots of pigmentation. They are especially numerous in individuals with a light skin and are characteristically diffusely distributed on the face and extensor aspects of the arms. The midface region, however, remains relatively free, and involvement of the mucous membranes and palms and soles is always absent (Figs. 401, 402). Ephelides are not present at birth but appear in childhood and regress at advanced age. The German name Sommersprossen (summer freckles) indicates the enlargement and darkening of the individual maculae that occurs from the effect of sunlight.

Histologically, the epidermis has a normal structure with no increase in melanocytes. Increased activity of the mel-

Fig. 401. Ephelides.

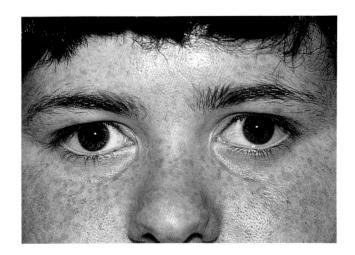

Fig. 402. Ephelides.

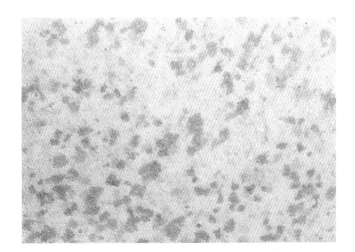

Fig. 403. Lentigo: pigmentary deposits, acanthosis, and increased number of melanocytes. HE stain, 100×.

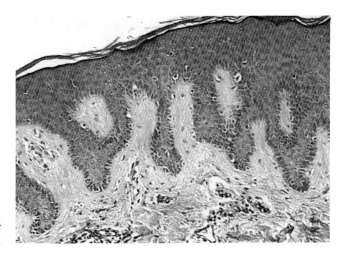

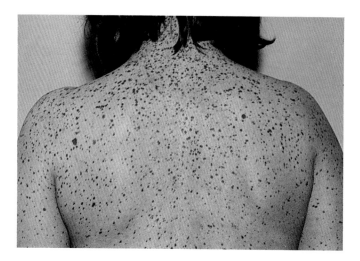

Fig. 404. Lentiginosis profusa.

anocytes, however, leads in places to an aggregation of pigment in the basal cells.

Inverse ephelides are ephelides with a special tendency of grouping in the middle of the face. Here also the mucous mem-

Fig. 405. Lentiginosis perigenito-axillaris.

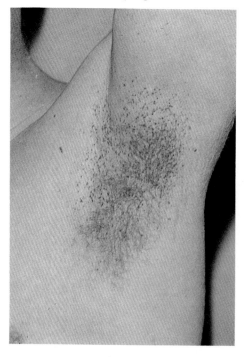

branes are unaffected. Occasionally the vermilion border shows pigmentation.

2. Lentigines can be differentiated clinically from ephelides only with difficulty. They are, however, somewhat darker and have a smoother margin than ephelides. Lentigines are often present at birth or manifest themselves shortly afterwards. An essential influence from sunlight irradiation is lacking, so that lentigines do not show a favorite location on the sun-exposed areas.

Histologically, there are increased deposits of pigment in the basal cells and, in contrast to ephelides, elongation of the rete pegs and an increase in melanocytes (Fig. 403).

The existence of generalized or circumscribed increases of lentigines has led to the definition of special dermatoses. In *lentiginosis centrofacialis* the individual lentigines are densely grouped around the facial openings. As with ephelides, however, the mucous membranes always remain free. Also there are the following differences from inverse ephelides of the first perinatal manifestation: a darker color, an almost nonexistent dependency on light, and the previously mentioned different histologic features.

In combination with lentiginosis centro-facialis the existence of a progressive hereditary keratosis of the extremities with dominant heredity has been observed.[13]

Lentiginosis profusa (Fig. 404) shows an abnormal increase of lentigines. The entire skin (but not the mucous membranes) is covered with lentil-sized pigment spots, which, however, have no tendency toward grouping. In addition, there are solitary larger pigmentations such as "café-au-lait" spots and typical nevus cell nevi. As in lentiginosis centrofacialis, involvement of the mucous membranes and dependency on light are missing.

In rare cases lentiginosis profusa may be arranged in a mosaiclike pattern on the skin.[6] If lentiginosis profusa occurs in individuals of small stature, and if at the same time hypertelorism, inner ear deafness, malformations of the genitals, and pathological findings of the heart are present, we are dealing with the **leopard* syndrome**. With regard to the cardiac findings, there is narrowing of the exit of the pulmonary artery rather than endomyocardial fibroelastoses. In the electrocardiogram disturbances of conduction, a branch block pattern and nonspecific intraventricular conduction abnormalities can be seen in almost all patients. In several instances familial occurrence of the fully developed syndrome or only individual features were present.[12, 29, 36]

Lentiginosis perigenito-axillaris (Fig. 405) is limited to the area of apocrine sweat glands and can be considered an abortive form of lentiginosis profusa. It needs, however, careful differentiation from the axillary freckling that occurs in neurofibromatosis.[22]

---

* **L**entigines, multiple; **e**lectrocardiographic conduction defects; **o**cular hypertelorism; **p**ulmonary stenosis; **a**bnormalities of the genitals; **r**etardation of growth; and **d**eafness, sensorineural. (Tr.)

3. A nevus spilus is in most cases a congenital spot of hyperpigmentation with a completely smooth surface. Such nevi spili are mostly single; they have sharply limited margins and may be located on any part of the body. Macroscopically, they cannot be differentiated from the so-called café-au-lait spots of generalized neurofibromatosis.

Histologically, however, there are distinct differences. In the nevus spilus, the number of melanocytes in the hyperpigmented area is lower than in the unchanged epidermis, whereas conditions in generalized neurofibromatosis are exactly the reverse. In contrast to lentigo, a nevus spilus can be diagnosed microscopically by the absence of extension of the rete pegs and the absence of an increase in melanocytes.[18]

4. On the face and on the extensor surfaces of the arms and hands, that is, in the areas exposed to sunlight, **old age pigmentations** occur.

In the ephelid stage of *circumscribed melanotic precancerosis* there is a pigment spot with a completely smooth surface. It is polycyclic and slow-growing, and in the beginning is milk-coffee-colored but later has various brownish speckles. Infiltrations and inflammatory manifestations are lacking. Such hyperpigmentations are about the size of a 50-cent piece and are almost always observed as single lesions.

Histologically, the epidermis has few characteristic features but is atrophic. Increased pigment is found only in the basal cells. At this stage, nests of melanocytes characteristic of circumscribed melanotic precancerosis do not yet occur. Also absent is the typical increase of melanocytes in the long extended rete pegs of lentigines.

The diagnosis can be made only by considering the clinical findings of a slowly enlarging pigment spot on a light-exposed area in aged patients and the histologic findings as well. If the surface of such an old age pigmentation has small papular elements or especially dark pigmentary de-

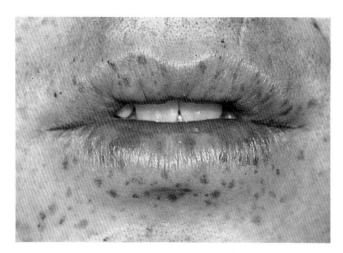

posits, the full picture of circumscribed melanotic precancerosis has appeared. If the surface, however, is crumbly and faintly glistening, we are probably dealing with a senile wart, which lacks a distinctly verrucous surface, especially on the scalp. Only the histologic features are different in the three dermatoses just described.[1, 26]

Besides the isolated spotted pigmentations of old age there are also *multiple small-spotted pigmentations of old age,* which like ephelides are present on the extensor surface of the forearms and dorsa of the hands and on the face, but in contrast to ephelides do not affect the shoulders and upper arms. Pigmentations of old age also lack the darkening and expansion that follow sunlight exposure of ephelides. Small spotted pigmentations of old age are observed predominantly on skin areas atrophic by age. They often occur simultaneously with streaks or star-shaped depigmentations or senile purpura.

Histologically, increased pigment is present only in the basal layer. The entire epidermis is thin without many changes. Pigment may occasionally occur in single squamous cells but without a simultaneous increase of melanocytes. In the upper parts of the corium there is an explicit basophilic degeneration with loss or rarefaction of the

net of elastic fibers in areas with pseudo-scars.[16, 26]

5. Among the small spotted pigmentations in the facial region, spotted pigmentary polyposis, or the so-called **Peutz-Jeghers syndrome,** is important. In this autosomal, dominantly inherited phakomatosis there are round or oval pigment spots grouped around the facial openings (Figs. 406, 416). The most important diagnostic criterion is the extension of these pigment spots to the mucous membranes of the lips and cheeks. Also located on the extensor surfaces of the extremities, this pigmentary anomaly shows a tendency toward grouping that permits a differentiation from the more disseminated ephelides. The occurrence of pigment spots on the palms and soles* is characteristic. In contrast to ephelides, however, the Peutz-Jeghers syndrome favors individuals with dark complexions, so that a conspicuous influence of light is missing. Pigmentations, especially of the mucous membranes of the cheeks, either are already present at birth or appear in the first years of childhood.

Histologically, there are no uniform tissue changes which would permit a diagno-

---

* And on the digits. (Tr.)

sis. The structure of the pigment spots is similar in part to that of ephelides, in part to that of lentigines, with the addition of speckled nests of nevus cells.

The second important sign of this disorder is polyposis of the small intestine. Although the jejunum is favored, polyposis can establish itself in any part of the intestines from the stomach to the colon. Complaints relating to the polyposis appear in the second to third decades of life under the guise of acute invaginations, intestinal bleedings, and secondary iron-deficiency anemia. Malignant degeneration of the polypous intestinal hamartomas is rare but should be kept in mind, especially if gastric polyposis is present. Changes of other inner organs are ovarian cystomas and papillomas of the milk duct; both of these may possibly undergo malignant degeneration.

Ophthalmologically, extension of the pigmentation to the conjunctiva and sclera may occur.[21, 23, 33]

The most important and leading sign of **Gardner's syndrome,** another autosomal dominant hereditary disorder, is intestinal polyposis. In this disorder there is a simultaneous occurrence of subcutaneous fibromas, sebocystadenomas, and, infrequently, lipomas and leiomyomas. Occasionally, extensive atheromatous formations are present on the scalp. Multiple osteomas occur predominantly on the skull, especially on the mandible. In contrast to the Peutz-Jeghers syndrome the polyps are mostly located in the colon. Their malignancy rate is about 40 per cent.[11, 20]

The **Canada-Cronkhite syndrome** is another familial syndrome showing polyposis. Its cutaneous changes include universal alopecia, onychodystrophy, and skin pigmentations. They occur especially on the palms and soles in the form of single, pinhead-sized, round, and brownish lentigines. The disorder first manifests itself after the fortieth year of life. Besides the gastrointestinal polyposis, which extends from the esophagus to the rectum and exhibits

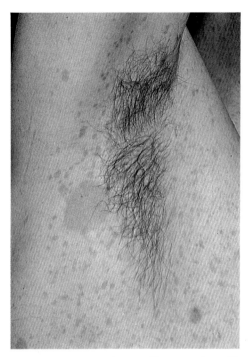

Fig. 407. Generalized neurofibromatosis: café-au-lait spot and axillary freckling.

histologically benign adenomas, intense hypoproteinemia exists. This syndrome does not seem to constitute a specific disorder, but the consecutive skin changes are caused by intensely changed enteral resorption conditions caused by the intestinal polyposis and leading to watery and voluminous stools.[28]

6. Another ectodermal dysplasia is the **Berlin* syndrome.** It exhibits small macular to reticular gray-brown pigmentations, preponderantly on the extremities. The hyperpigmentations are already present at birth and increase in intensity during puberty. Several patients show hyperkeratoses of palms and soles. Lanugo hairs are sparse or are absent completely, while sexual hair does not appear and the hair of the scalp is thin and tends to premature gray-

---

* Named for Chaim Berlin, an Israeli dermatologist. (Tr.)

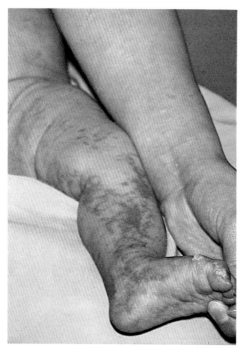

Fig. 408. Incontinentia pigmenti: spattered pigmentary deposits in the healing stage.

ing. Nails can be hypoplastic, there may be hypodontia and delayed eruption of teeth, and the function of sweating may be diminished. Stunted growth and absent sexual maturation are additional features of this not yet well defined syndrome.[2]

7. As mentioned before, axillary freckling is a frequent pigmentary manifestation of **generalized neurofibromatosis**. However, this diagnosis should not be made unless typical molluscoid tumors or at least six café-au-lait spots larger than 1.5 cm in diameter are present on the entire integument (Fig. 407). Since café-au-lait spots are only the first manifestation of this phakomatosis starting in childhood, it is unnecessary to establish a special form (Leschke's syndrome, pigment spots without tumors). These spots are located almost exclusively on the trunk and show a smooth border. Histologically, an accumulation of pigment and an increase of the melanocytes are seen in the basal cell layer.

The predominantly multiple cutaneous tumors of neurofibromatosis are lipomas and fibromas and, to a great extent, neurinomas; they are often found along the nerve trunks. Characteristically, the tumors can be invaginated through a ring in the skin by pressing with the finger as if pressing a bell button. Because of their tendency to become generalized, neurofibromas are found on many internal organs, and complications arising from them have been found in the eye, the gastrointestinal tract, the vessels of the kidneys, the heart, and especially, the acoustic nerve. The skeletal system shows asymmetry of the body frame, deformities of the spine, and hyperostoses, especially below the large paunchlike pendulous tumors of the extremities. Malignant degeneration takes place in about 15 per cent of neurinomas. This disease is of autosomal dominant inheritance, and although fertility is reduced, genetic counseling of these patients seems necessary.[18, 23]

To be distinguished from neurofibromatosis is another dominantly inherited syndrome with *multiple*, smooth bordered *café-au-lait spots* but no tumors. Such patients regularly show temporal dysrhythmias in the electroencephalogram. Other signs are forgetfulness, learning disability, headaches, depressions, and *cerebral epileptic seizures*.[35]

8. Polyostotic fibrous dysplasia is accompanied in about 50 per cent of cases by café-au-lait-like pigmentations. However, in contrast to neurofibromatosis, these pigmented spots show an irregularly outlined, zigzag border; the lesions occupy larger areas and show a certain segmental arrangement. Frequently these café-au-lait spots are seen in close proximity to multiple, focal, mostly unilateral osseous dysplasias. Gross pathological differences in the calcium and phosphorus metabolism are not found. In females the combination of pubertas praecox with polyostotic fibrous dysplasia is called *Albright's syndrome*.[3, 10, 17]

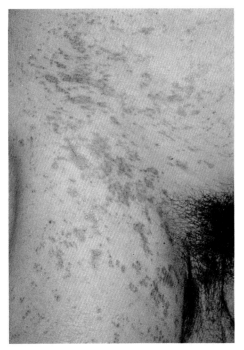

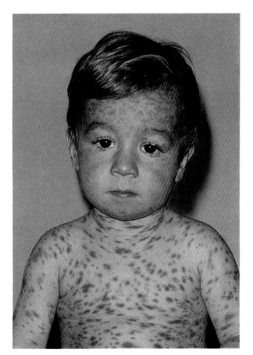

Fig. 409. Heavily pigmented, exanthematic lichen planus.

Fig. 410. Urticaria pigmentosa.

9. A special characteristic pigment dermatosis of childhood is **incontinentia pigmenti,** which is known to occur in two well-delineated subtypes. The *Bloch-Sulzberger* type occurs predominantly in girls. At birth or during the first weeks of life successive crops of pinhead- to lentil-sized papuloverrucous lesions or lineally arranged bullous lesions appear. Simultaneously, high eosinophilia of the blood and tissues occurs without impairment of the general well-being. After the inflammatory cutaneous lesions have disappeared, persistent, spattered, rarely reticulated, light-to-dirty brown pigmentations remain for years (Fig. 408). About a quarter of the cases show cicatricial loss of hair that resembles pseudopelade. Occasionally these changes are present at birth, apparently as the result of intrauterine presence of the disease; the hairs themselves are normal, however. The development of teeth shows many anomalies, ranging from absence to formation of peg-shaped teeth. Special importance must be attached to ophthalmic disorders (25 to 35 per cent), among them uveitis of the posterior portion of the eye, postneuritic atrophies of the optic nerve, and pseudogliomas. Just as frequent are cerebral defects involving mental retardation, microcephaly, epileptic seizures, spastic paralyses, and similar conditions. In the differential diagnosis one must consider dermatitis herpetiformis during the early bullous stage of incontinentia pigmenti.

Histologic examination shows primarily intraepidermal and subcorneal vesicles with many eosinophils. Around the vesicles there is spongiosis of the epidermis with acanthotic widening and keratinization of some single cells. The corium sometimes shows eosinophilia also, but in general there is a predominantly lymphocytic infiltration. During the regressive phase, loss of stored melanin of the basal cell layer results in deposit of considerable amounts of mel-

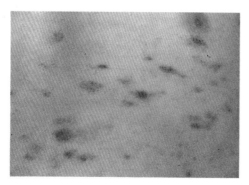

Fig. 411. Telangiectasia macularis eruptiva perstans.

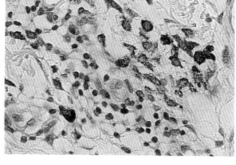

Fig. 412. Urticaria pigmentosa: mast cells situated perivascularly.

anin within the melanophages of the corium.

The other kind of incontinentia pigmenti, the *Franceschetti-Jadassohn* type (synonyms are familiar chromatophore nevus of Naegeli and dermatose pigmentaire réticulée), affects both sexes equally. Beginning about the second year of life, with no preceding inflammatory changes, reticular increases of pigment of diverse brown intensity appear on the trunk and extremities. In addition, palmar and plantar keratoses are found almost regularly. The hair and nails fail to show any changes, but the teeth may present developmental abnormalities including conspicuous yellow discoloration. The presence of anhydrosis is important, because at times of bodily stress the absence of perspiration will result in febrile episodes. So far, pathological manifestations of the eyes and central nervous system have not been observed.[9, 34] Between the two types of incontinentia pigmenti, however, transitional forms are occasionally encountered. The resulting mixed types cannot be differentiated with any more certainty.[14]

10. Small macular pigmentations must be examined with regard to their deuteropathic genesis (i.e., secondary to some other disease). As a rule, **pigmented lichen planus** develops only in long-standing lesions; however, in rare instances it may appear without any preceding papule as a reticulated or punctiform, pruritic, graybrown pigmentation (Fig. 409). The final diagnosis in such cases will depend on the concomitant or later finding of at least a few typical lichen planus lesions on the skin or mucous membranes.

11. Whereas the tendency to pigmentation of lichen planus definitely belongs to the clinical picture, other dermatoses may show residual pigmentation only occasionally. As a rule, urticaria regresses without residual signs, but in rare cases late pigmentation may indicate the sites of original wheals. Another causative factor of **urticaria with pigmentation** is the hemorrhagic suffusion of the lesions during the acute stage. In contrast to urticaria pigmentosa, intensive rubbing of the pigmented spots of urticaria with pigmentation will not result in any more wheals. Finally, histologic examination will establish the absence of an increase in mast cells, thereby excluding urticaria pigmentosa.

12. The presence of lentil- to coin-sized, multiple, flat or slightly elevated lesions raises the possibility of a diagnosis of **urticaria pigmentosa** (Fig. 410). The degree of saturation of each lesion with brown pigment differs markedly. Fresh lesions in general tend to be lighter in tone. Sometimes only the middle of each lesion shows an increase of pigment. Markedly nodular lesions that are distinctly yellow-brownish in tint occur in urticaria pigmentosa xanthelasmoidea. However, compared with their normal surroundings the individual brown spots as a rule are hardly more succulent or otherwise different in consistency. Additional phenomena such as pruritus, dermatographia, and spontaneous fleeting formation of wheals appear only irregularly; these signs can be provoked by additional stimuli such as differences in temperature (hot baths or, less often, exposure to cold) or mechanical insults. In this connection a warning is necessary against the intravenous medication of urticaria pigmentosa patients with short-acting narcotics of the histamine liberator type (propanidid); such medication may result in severe shock. Single lesions or several lesions seldom show a bullous element. In any event a demonstrable urticarial swelling of such a small brown macular lesion by rubbing will offer clinical help. This phenomenon is not present in every case, and after rubbing there is a certain refractory interval before renewed provocation will be successful. In adults one can expect as a rule an exanthema characterized by a few small lesions and conspicuous primarily by pigmentation. The typical appearance of urticaria pigmentosa may be changed greatly by intrafocal bleeding and telangiectases; the latter, the so-called *teleangiectasia macularis eruptiva perstans*, persists for many years and affects adults primarily (Fig. 411). The differential diagnosis of this form must consider above all the group of progressive pigmented purpuras. The appearance of punctate bleeding within a macular and usually reddish patch that is typical of the initial lesions of Schoenlein's purpura cannot be used against the clinical diagnosis of urticaria pigmentosa because in this disease extravasation of blood within a single lesion may take place either spontaneously or conditionally on other causes — for instance, the occurrence of fever or

bruising. Finally, urticaria pigmentosa may appear as a diffuse cutaneous *mastocytosis* with cobblestonelike thickenings or infiltrations of large areas, especially of the large body folds, and a yellow color or café-au-lait appearance. Such a picture of pseudolichenification, especially if it is interspersed with prurigolike infiltrations, keloidlike bars and arches, as well as excoriations and ulcerations, will at first hardly suggest a diagnosis of urticaria pigmentosa or a diffuse mast cell infiltration. The same applies also for more erythrodermic manifestations.

These manifestations on histologic examination may also show during the course of the disease an absence of mast cell conglomerates either as tumors or in a perivascular arrangement. As a rule, especially in children, tumorlike accumulations of mast cells can be found below a free subepidermal zone, corresponding to a macroscopically typical single lesion (Fig. 412). Adult cases that begin after puberty, however, usually show only scattered, sparse, perivascular conglomerates of mast cells. In such cases the diagnostic decision, therefore, cannot be made only by histologic examination, especially when one considers that mast cells can be found also in other reactions of the stroma, for instance, around inflamed areas or a tumor.

An infiltrate may occasionally be composed in part of mast cells in lichen planus, chronic lichen simplex, some vascular inflammations, pretibial myxedema, scleromyxedema, and also during the course of early scleroderma. In addition, mast cells are formed in the vicinity of carcinomas, fibromas, neurofibromas, and lipomas. The occurrence of eosinophils during the course of urticaria pigmentosa is shared with the entire group of so-called histiocytosis-X diseases. However, in contrast to histiocytosis X and also mycosis fungoides, urticaria pigmentosa histologically lacks obtrusion or immigration of cells into the epidermis.

In such clinically and histologically equivocal cases decisive diagnostic importance

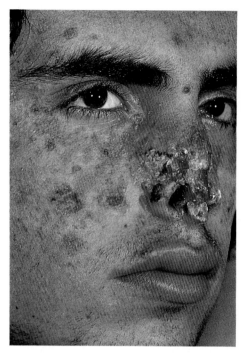

Fig. 413. Xeroderma pigmentosum: spots of hyperkeratotic pigmentations, scleroderma-like basaliomas, and mutilating basalioma of the nose.

should be accorded to gastrointestinal findings, flush syndrome, and above all to skeletal changes. The most frequent sign of pathological generalization of mast cells is hepatosplenomegaly, which is clinically impressive because of the hard consistency of the involved organs. Development of cirrhosis of the liver is possible. The skeletal changes of urticaria pigmentosa are easily diagnosed; they consist of either local or generalized as well as endosteal scleroses, and also osteoporoses. The gastrointestinal changes give rise to complaints of a "nervous" character, such as sensations of indistinct fullness, or of colic and diarrhea. These subjective complaints are supplemented by cardiovascular sensations such as precordial compression, rapid pulse, a peculiar sensation of cold or heat, or other vasomotoric phenomena. Such flush phenomena of urticaria pigmentosa can be clinically differ-

entiated only with difficulty from the carcinoid syndrome. Hematologically, basophilic leukocytes of the peripheral blood are occasionally increased in number. Transitions to basophilic leukemia of tissue apparently start primarily from mast cell reticuloses. A diagnosis of such malignant mast cell reticulosis with its rapidly fatal course should be made only if there are completely unequivocal malignant mast cell proliferations involving the bones, lymphatic system, and other organs; as mentioned before, there is a leukemic aspect to this disease. Not to be overlooked is the fact that generalized benign urticaria pigmentosa as well as malignant mast cell reticulosis shows quite similar organotropism; in addition, phenomenologic isomorphism makes a quick differentiation difficult.

To a certain degree cytologic criteria can be used for differential diagnosis: signs of malignancy of the proliferating cells (mitoses, cell- and nuclear polymorphism, displacement of the nuclear and plasma reaction); the solubility of mast cell granules (typical urticaria pigmentosa granules are not water soluble); and above all, the histochemical finding of sulfated acid mucopolysaccharides and 5-hydroxytryptophan in the mast cell granules. Staining with buffered toluidine-blue at acid pH will reveal the metachromatic granules more clearly; progressive ripening of the granules will result in increased color intensity.[4, 24, 31, 32]

13. Xeroderma pigmentosum also shows small spotted, ephelidelike increases of pigment (Fig. 413). The time of manifestation of such pigmentations depends to a large extent on the type of course and the stage of illness. As far as localization is concerned, the cutaneous changes of xeroderma pigmentosum typically involve the sun-exposed areas of the body; however, generalized and also strictly circumscribed variants exist. In the usual course of the disease the first exposure to the sun (wavelengths 280 to 310 nm) will result in the development of erythema and edema with possible formation of bullae. The erythema will soon heal with mild desquamation; however, with each successive reexposure to light the erythema will last longer and finally will heal with formation of pigmented spots. The pigmented lesions may be as large as lentils and are distributed in varying degrees of density. Each spot has zig-zag borders and a smooth surface and varies in color from light to dark brown. Morphologically, the individual lesion can hardly be distinguished from freckles; however, xeroderma pigmentosum lacks the tendency to spread and the pigmentation activity that are dependent on exposure to sunlight.

Histologically, increased deposition of melanin pigment is found in the basal cell layer and partly also in the spinous layer of the epidermis. As in incontinentia pigmenti, the upper corium shows extracellular and also intracellular increases of pigment (melanophages). The number and structure of the melanocytes are normal.

Some patients with xeroderma pigmentosum also show pigmented spots on the lips and oral mucosa. During the later stages a poikilodermic appearance becomes increasingly evident because multiple telangiectases and small hypopigmented or depigmented, easily folded areas of atrophy will have developed. The complete picture of the disease will then appear: badly healing, sometimes deep ulcerations, multiple "senile" keratoses, and many benign and also malignant epithelial and mesodermal tumors (Fig. 414). The various types of xeroderma pigmentosum each take different courses that are responsible for the time of life at which the first manifestation appears or a certain stage of the disease will prevail. The acute form has an accelerated course in which the first cutaneous changes appear within a few weeks after birth and death occurs at a very young age due to cachexia and generalized metastases of tumors. The classical (subacute) and also most common form also begins during the first year of life; however, the separate stages last considerably longer,

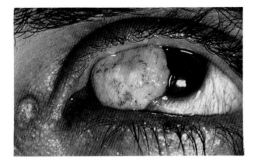

Fig. 414. Xeroderma pigmentosum: Bowen's disease of the conjunctiva bulbi.

so that the transformation of cutaneous changes into malignant tumors can be expected only in adults. Finally, in the tardive, abortive type — at present called *pigmented xerodermoid* — the first cutaneous changes may begin to appear after puberty and quite often very much later. Only incidentally it should be mentioned that xeroderma pigmentosum may occasionally exist without pigment. Constant or more than coincidental involvement of internal organs is lacking, with the exception of neurologic-psychiatric disturbances. Consequently, the combination of xeroderma pigmentosum, oligophrenia, hereditary spinal ataxia, hypogonadism, and proportionate dwarfism is called the *DeSanctis-Cacchione syndrome*.

The mode of inheritance of xeroderma pigmentosum and the De Sanctis-Cacchione syndrome is at present thought to be autosomal recessive, although a few observations indicate an autosomal dominant mode. Recent investigations have shown that xeroderma pigmentosum is due to a defect in the "dark repair enzyme system" that causes diminished activity of one of the two DNA-polymerases. [5, 7, 8, 15, 19, 27, 30]

(1) ANTON-LAMPRECHT, I., U. W. SCHNYDER und W. TILGEN: Das »Stade éphélide« der melanotischen Präcancerose. Arch. Derm. Forsch. *240:* 61–78 (1971).

(2) BERLIN, CH.: Congenital generalized melanoleucoderma associated with hypodontia, hypotrichosis, stunted

growth and mental retardation occurring in two brothers and two sisters. Dermatologica (Basel) *123:* 227–243 (1961).

(3) BOENHEIM, F., und TH. H. McGAVACK: Polyostotische fibröse Dysplasie. Ergebn. inn. Med. Kinderheilk. N. F. *3:* 157–184 (1952).

(4) BRINKMANN, E.: Mastzellenreticulose (Gewebsbasophilom) mit histaminbedingtem Flush und Übergang in Gewebsbasophilen-Leukämie. Schweiz. med. Wschr. *89:* 1046–1048 (1959).

(5) CLEAVER, J. E.: Defective repair replication of DNA in xeroderma pigmentosum. Nature *218:* 652–656 (1968).

(6) DAVIS, D. G., and M. W. SHAW: An unusual human mosaic for skin pigmentation. New Engl. J. Med. *270:* 1384–1389 (1964).

(7) EL-HEFNAWI, H., M. EL-NABAWI and A. RASHEED: Xeroderma pigmentosum. I. A clinical study of 12 egyptian cases. Brit. J. Derm. *74:* 201–213 (1962).

(8) ELSÄSSER, G., O. FREUSBERG und F. THEME: Das Xeroderma pigmentosum und die »xerodermische Idiotie«. Arch. Derm. Syph. (Berl.) *188:* 651–655 (1950).

(9) FRANCESCHETTI, A., et W. JADASSOHN: A propos de l' « incontinentia pigmenti »; délimitation de deux syndromes différents figurant sous le même terme. Dermatologica (Basel) *108:* 1–28 (1954).

(10) FRENK, E.: Etude ultrastructurale des taches pigmentaires du syndrome d' Albright. Dermatologica (Basel) *143:* 12–20 (1971).

(11) FUHRMANN, W., U. W. SCHNYDER, K. H. KÄRCHER und H. PFEIFER: Gardner's syndrome without polyposis? Humangenetik *5:* 59–64 (1967).

(12) GORLIN, R. J., R. C. ANDERSON and M. BLAW: Multiple lentigines syndrome. Amer. J. Dis. Child. *117:* 652–662 (1969).

(13) GREITHER, A.: Über drei Generationen vererbte, auf Frauen beschränkte Keratosis follicularis mit Alopecie, Hypidrose und abortiven Palmar-Plantar-Keratosen in ihren Beziehungen zur Hypotrichosis congenita hereditaria. Arch. klin. exp. Derm. *210:* 123–140 (1960).

(14) GREITHER, A., und R. HAENSCH: Anhidrotische retikuläre Pigmentdermatose mit blasig-erythematösem Anfangsstadium. Schweiz. med. Wschr. *100:* 228–233 (1970).

(15) HADIDA, E., F.-G. MARILL et J. SAYAG: Xeroderma pigmentosum (à propos de 48 observations personnelles). Ann. Derm. Syph. (Paris) *90:* 467–496 (1963).

(16) HODGSON, C.: Senile lentigo. Arch. Derm. (Chic.) *87:* 197–207 (1963).

(17) JESSERER, H.: Erkrankungen und Probleme aus den Grenzgebieten der Inneren Medizin. XII. Fibröse Knochendysplasie. Med. Klin. *55:* 225–230 (1960).

(18) JOHNSON, B. L., and D. R. CHARNECO: Café au lait spot in neurofibromatosis and in normal individuals. Arch. Derm. (Chic.) *102:* 442–446 (1970).

(19) JUNG, E. G., und U. W. SCHNYDER: Xeroderma pigmentosum und pigmentiertes Xerodermoid. Schweiz. med. Wschr. *100:* 1718–1726 (1970).

(20) KÄRCHER, K. H.: Die Röntgen-Symptomatologie des Gardner-Syndroms. Fortschr. Röntgenstr. *107:* 90–95 (1967).

(21) KLOSTERMANN, G. F.: Pigmentfleckenpolypose. Thieme, Stuttgart 1960.

(22) KORTING, G. W.: Lentiginosis profusa perigenitoaxillaris. Z. Haut- u. Geschl.-Kr. *42:* XIX–XXII (1967).

(23) KORTING, G. W., und G. BREHM: Über partielle Hyperostosen und Periostosen bei Neurofibromatose und Cutis laxa. Arch. Derm. Syph. (Berl.) *199:* 183–196 (1955).

(24) LENNERT, K.: Zur pathologischen Anatomie von Urticaria pigmentosa und Mastzellenreticulose. Klin. Wschr. *40:* 61–67 (1962).

(25) MANEGOLD, B. C., J. F. BUSSMANN und H. S. FÜRSTENBERG: Klinischer Beitrag zum Peutz-Jeghers-Syndrom mit Befall des Magendarmtraktes, der oberen Luftwege sowie beider Mammae. Med. Welt *20* (N. F.): 1435–1439 (1969).

(26) MIESCHER, G., L. HÄBERLIN und L. GUGGENHEIM: Über fleckförmige Alterspigmentierungen. Arch. Derm. Syph. (Berl.) *174:* 105–125 (1936).

(27) MÜLLER, W. E. G., R. K. ZAHN, G. BREHM and G. W. KORTING: Activity and kinetics of DNA dependent DNA and RNA polymerases in xeroderma pigmentosum and in normal human skin. Arch. Derm. Forsch. *240:* 334–341 (1971).

(28) NISHIYAMA, S., S. MORI und S. HARADA: Gastrointestinale Polyposis mit universeller Alopecie, Onychodystrophie und Pigmentation der Haut. Arch. klin. exp. Derm. *221:* 144–161 (1965).

Fig. 415. Physiologic pigmentation of the gingiva.

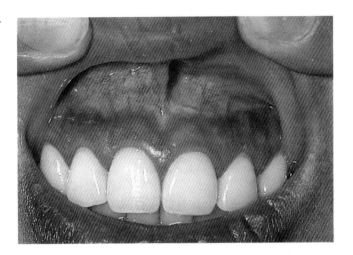

(29) PICKERING, D., B. LASKI, D. C. MC-MILLAN and V. ROSE: "Little Leopard" syndrome. Description of 3 cases and review of 24. Arch. Dis. Childh. *46:* 85–90 (1971).

(30) REED, W. B., B. LANDING, G. SUGARMAN, J. E. CLEAVER and J. MELNYK: Xeroderma pigmentosum; clinical and laboratory investigation of its basic defect. J. Amer. med. Ass. *207:* 2073–2079 (1969).

(31) REMY, D.: Gewebsmastzellen und Mastzellen-Reticulose. Ergebn. inn. Med. Kinderheilk. N.F. *17:* 132–189 (1962).

(32) SAGHER, F., and Z. EVEN-PAZ: Mastocytosis and the mast cell. Karger, Basel 1967.

(33) SCULLY, R. E.: Sex cord tumor with annular tubules; a distinctive ovarian tumor of the Peutz-Jeghers-syndrome. Cancer *25:* 1107–1121 (1970).

(34) UEBEL, H., A. LUDWIG und G. W. KORTING: Zur Kenntnis der Incontinentia pigmenti Bloch-Sulzberger. Arch. Derm. Syph. (Berl.) *190:* 114–124 (1950).

(35) VERNER jr., J. V., J. H. JOHNSON and F. L. MERRITT: Café au lait spots, temporal dysrhythmia, and emotional instability. Int. J. Neuropsychiat. *2:* 179–187 (1966).

(36) WALTHER, R. J., B. J. POLANSKY and I. A. GROTIS: Electrocardiographic abnormalities in a family with generalized lentigo. New Engl. J. Med. *275:* 1220–1225 (1966).

F. Pigmentations of the Oral Mucosa

1. In order to assess hyperpigmentations of the mucous membrane within the oral cavity, one must rule out **physiologic pigmentations of the mucous membrane,** which

Fig. 416. Peutz-Jeghers syndrome: pigment spots on the buccal mucosa.

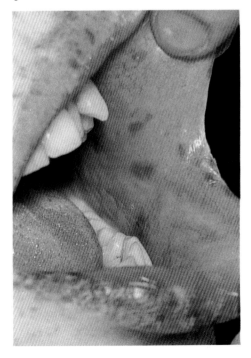

occur predominantly in individuals with dark skin color. Their manifestations vary greatly, appearing as streaklike or macular melanin deposits. On the gingiva, however, the marginal border is always uninvolved (Fig. 415). This alone is an important differential diagnostic point against the findings in heavy metal poisonings.[9]

2. Macular hyperpigmentations, mostly of the buccal mucosa and the mouth opening, may be caused by a physiologic variant but require the exclusion of a phakomatosis. As on the skin, café-au-lait-like pigmentary increases may occur on the mucous membrane in **generalized neurofibromatosis** and **Albright's syndrome.** In the **Peutz-Jeghers syndrome** small macular pigmented spots (Fig. 416) occur on the lips and the oral mucosa. For the diagnosis additional findings are naturally important (see page 398). If pigmentations are limited to the vermilion border without simultaneous pigmentations of the oral mucosa, one should be cautious in diagnosing the Peutz-Jeghers syndrome.[5]

3. Nevus cell nevi may occur on the oral mucosa but are rare in this location compared to their frequency on the outer integument. In addition, because of their small size and the few symptoms they elicit, they are frequently missed, unless one especially looks for them in a large group of patients. In most cases intraoral nevus cell nevi present intradermal growths which are often pigment-free. Like melanomas they favor the hard palate, so that nevus cell nevi of the buccal mucosa should be diagnosed with caution. Although it is possible that "juvenile melanomas" can occur in the oral cavity, such nevi have been accepted with this diagnosis only with reservations. Rather, we are dealing with **circumscribed precancerous melanosis** of the oral mucosa. These "melanoplakias" increase by confluent extension or by partially exophytic nodular growth; their development toward

melanoma is evident at the latest when satellites appear. Precancerous melanosis occurs mostly on the gingiva and palate. Circumscribed, and especially slightly protuberant lesions of a bluish color suggest a **blue nevus** of the oral mucosa.[1–4, 6]

4. Among the endocrinopathies the pigmentations of **Addison's disease** of the oral mucosa are most important, since such macular or streaky, sometimes diffuse pigmentations may precede other signs of the disorder. Since in Addison's disease pigmentations can be provoked by common traumatic or actinic irritations, pigmentations of the lips of the patient suffering from the disorder occur more often than those on the buccal mucosa or the gingiva, where they may give the impression of a lead pencil line. Pigmentations similar to those of Addison's disease occur also in **Whipple's disease** and **sprue.** Occasionally, however, a very old person, especially a cachectic one, shows addisonoid pigmentations of the oral mucosa even without Addison's disease, sometimes without a history of heavy use of tobacco (especially chewing tobacco).

Compared to the findings in Addison's disease, pigmentations of the oral mucosa in other endocrine disorders, especially pituitary changes or other internal diseases, remain unconfirmed, if one discounts the dark colors caused by deposits of metals in **hemochromatosis** and **Wilson's pseudosclerosis.** Hyperpigmentations in these disorders, which also include **Gaucher's disease** and **Niemann-Pick disease,** are most probably of a more complex nature (melanin-, hemosiderin-, and lipopigment).

Urochromogens and derivatives of indole are responsible for the occasional light brownish mucosal pigmentations seen in terminal and azotemic kidney insufficiency. In the various forms of icterus the imbibition with bilirubin of the oral mucosa is expressed in various tones of yellow, most pronounced on the soft palate and the gingiva.

5. Pigmentations of the oral mucosa also demand a thorough analysis to determine whether they are exogenous. Rather well known are the pigmentations of the gums caused by **heavy metals** such as drugs (localized argyrosis, brown stone formation following potassium permanganate, slate-gray borders from lead and bismuth; if the borders are red, they suggest copper). Gingival impregnation of mercury, however, appears "inflammatory," i.e., red and edematous or bluish-edematous and dirty-looking, so that we are actually faced with mercurial gingivitis, which characteristically affects root stumps or defective teeth. Only if mercury is given in protracted doses and in very small amounts may one sometimes be able to see narrow blue-violet or gray-black borders. Brown-black discolorations of the gingiva and oral mucosa have been observed in workers handling tin or bronze; brownish pigmentations appear in those working with iron, whereas chronic arsenic poisoning leads to inflammatory processes, or even ulcerations and loosening of the teeth. Since most of the penetrating metal compounds cause relatively similar reactions on the oral mucosa and on the gingiva, the processes, which are polarized between stomatitis on the one hand and reaction-poor metal impregnation on the other hand, demand thorough professional or iatrogenic histories and the study of additional manifestations on the skin or other organs. The substance responsible is usually inorganic. It should not be forgotten that subgingival deposits (exogenously colored tartar) may suggest a metallic border. Recently, hyperpigmentations of the oral mucosa have been found to be caused by the various **antimalarial** drugs, especially resochin* and estrogen-containing **birth-control pills.** The two drugs usually show only part of the hyperpigmentations on the oral mucosa. Compared with the effects from these drugs, oral pigmentations from

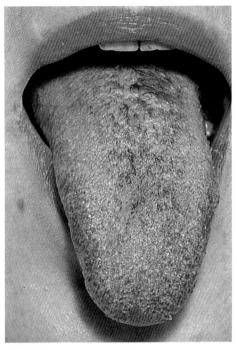

Fig. 417. Black hairy tongue.

phenolphthalein, chlorpromazine, or quinine are probably much less frequent.[7, 10]

6. Spots of dark color in the area of filled teeth can be caused by **amalgam** particles which were set free by corrosion. After a tooth extraction amalgam particles may remain in the alveola and may lead to blue-black areas of pigmentation. Roentgenologic evidence of metal particles is helpful in arriving at a diagnosis. However, if a tooth extraction was done a long time previously, the x-ray picture is not always helpful.[8, 9]

7. The changes accompanying a **black hairy tongue** (Fig. 417) may be mistaken for pigmentary deposits. In the former we are dealing with villous hyperplasia of the horny elongations of the filiform papillae. The first lingual changes occur on the back portion of the dorsum of the tongue and extend toward the tip. The discoloration of a so-called black hairy tongue is most

---

* Chloroquine. (Tr.)

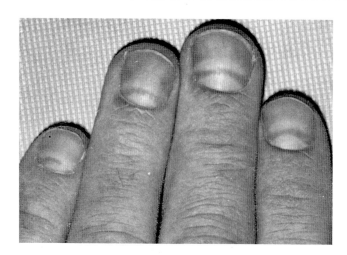

Fig. 418. Mees's nail bands
in thallium poisoning.

probably caused by pigment-provoking
bacteria or fungi. It vacíllates between
yellowish-brown   and   brownish-black.
Treatment with antibiotics may have
caused the eruption, but diabetes mellitus
and infections with Candida are also
possible causes.

(1) ACEVEDO, A., and C. D. LANE: Nonpig-
    mented intradermal nevus of the gingiva.
    Arch. Path. (Chic.) *85:* 448–449 (1968).

(2) BREUCKMANN, H.: Über Melanome der
    Mundschleimhaut. Derm. Wschr. *110:*
    36–40 (1940).

(3) GRIMMER, H.: Naevuszell-Naevus des
    harten Gaumens. Z. Haut- u. Geschl.-
    Kr. *35:* XLIX–LII (1963)

(4) JERNSTROM, P., and G. E. APONTE:
    Juvenile melanoma of the tongue. Amer.
    J. clin. Path. *26:* 1341–1347 (1956).

(5) KLOSTERMANN, G. F.: Pigmentflecken-
    polypose. Thieme, Stuttgart *1960.*

(6) KOCH, H.: Blaue Naevi der Mund-
    schleimhaut. Dtsch. zahnärztl. Z. *25:*
    1022–1026 (1970).

(7) LANGHOF, H., G. GEYER und H. BAR-
    THELMES: Hyperpigmentationen und
    Retinopathie durch Chlorochindiphos-
    phat. Derm. Wschr. *151:* 185–193
    (1965).

(8) OVERDIECK, H. F.: Amalgam-Täto-
    wierungen der Gingiva. Zahnärztl.
    Rdsch. *73:* 351–355 (1964).

(9) STRASSBURG, M., und G. KNOLLE: Pig-
    mentierungen und Tätowierungen der
    Mundschleimhaut. Dtsch. zahnärztl. Z.
    25: 1014–1021 (1970).

(10) TUFFANELLI, D., R. K. ABRAHAM and
    E. I. DUBOIS: Pigmentation from anti-
    malarial therapy. Arch. Derm. (Chic.)
    88: 419–426 (1963).

G. Color Changes of the Nails

1. Completely white nails occur in the
dominantly inherited *total leukonychia.*
The keratin of the nail is also disturbed.
The nails of patients suffering from
cirrhosis of the liver may be porcelain-
white; the color change, however, does not
affect the nailplate, only the nailbed. Also
limited to the nailbed are the paired white
streaks which run parallel to the lunula in
chronic hypoalbuminemia. In patients with
Addison's disease the mother-of-pearl-like
nail contrasts greatly with the generalized
yellow-brownish skin color. Patients suffering from *anemia* have white or pale nails
caused by the diminished blood supply of
the nailbed.[6, 10, 12]

2. Circumscribed whitening of the nailplate is called *punctate* or *striated leuko-*

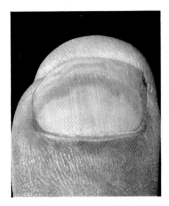
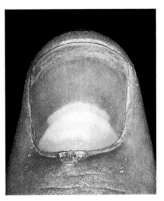
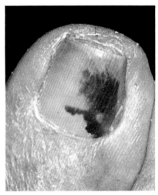

Fig. 419. Transverse band of   Fig. 420. Double lunula.   Fig. 421. Onychomycosis
the nail in pellagra.   nigricans.

nychia. The transverse bands on the nail-plate are several millimeters wide. Their color corresponds to that of the lunula. These *Mees's transverse bands* (Fig. 418) are considered characteristic of arsenic poisoning. Similar light streaks, accompanied occasionally by softening of the nailplate in the area of the band, occur after other local or generalized injuries or damage such as that following manicures, cauterization with acids, thallium intoxication, or severe brain trauma. *Onychomycosis (mycotic leukonychia)*, however, may cause longitudinal white marks with thickening of the nailplate. On the free border they have an elderberrylike aspect.

Often, patients with severe or recurrent *pellagra* present strange wide, milky-white, and sharply limited transverse bands (Fig. 419) parallel to the free border of the nail.[4]

Partial whitening of the fingernails occurs in about 20 per cent of patients with chronic kidney insufficiency. This is a rather characteristic whitening of the proximal half of the nailplate, with red or brown coloring of the distal half. The borderline between the two is relatively sharp, so that these nails are also called *"half-and-half nails."* The nailplate shows no other changes besides the differences in color.[9]

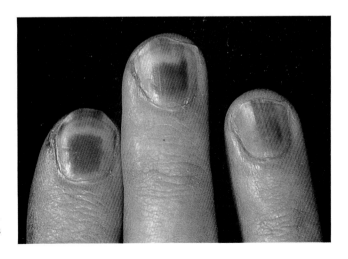

Fig. 422. Brownish discoloration of the fingernails caused by film developer.

3. Strikingly **yellow nails,** i. e., a yellow color of the entire nail *("yellow nail syndrome")* have been observed in conjunction with permanent slowing-up of nail growth in lymphedema. In these cases the nails seem thickened; they are more distinctly arched than they would be normally. They also may become loose at the sides. The nail changes often precede the formation of edema; in such nails fungi are usually not found.[5, 11]

4. Brownish-black, mostly spotty **color changes of the nail** may have arisen from infections of the nailbed, such as with *Proteus mirabilis* or *Pseudomonas aeruginosa,* and may lead to a black nail *(onychomycosis nigricans)* (Fig. 421). It is simple to confirm thé diagnosis by evidence of fungi or bacteria.[3, 14]

Dark brown to blackish longitudinal streaks are most likely *striated nevus cell nevi.* The differentiation from a beginning subungual *melanoma* may be extremely difficult since, if a melanoma is suspected, a biopsy is out of the question.* Rapid growth, inflammatory signs, or pain as well as a special dark brown color or definite differences in the intensity of the brown color tone are in favor of a melanoma. A subungual *hematoma* may present equal differential diagnostic difficulties if a direct connection with trauma is not elicited. In doubtful cases careful trepanation of the nail above the suspected hematoma may produce blood and thus the correct diagnosis. The presence of *subungual* streaks of blood of the *splinter hemorrhage* type is not limited to a special dermatosis or internal disease.[3, 7, 8] Occasionally, brown longitudinal streaks of the nailplate occur in patients with *Addison's disease.* These pigmentary deposits regress gradually with corticosteroid substitution therapy.[2]

---

* In the United States a biopsy is not always excluded. (Tr.)

Diffuse brown coloring of the nailplate is also found in chronic malaria, long-lasting exposure to heavy metals (arsenic, gold), and occasionally in pregnancy or thyrotoxicosis.

5. A blue-reddish color of the nailbed is a sign of *cyanosis* of the patient with a cardiac disease. *Argyrosis* and *Wilson's pseudosclerosis* may likewise be accompanied by bluish discolorations of the lunula. Light blue to blue-black discolorations of the nails may also be caused by *drugs* (atabrine, chloroquine, and phenolphthalein). The color changes of the nail or lunula in *ochronosis* are rather bluish-green.[1, 13]

6. Normally, the nailplate shows weak bluish-violet **fluorescence** under the ultraviolet light. After long-lasting atabrine doses it appears yellow-green, and after dimethylchlortetracycline, red.

(1) BEARN, A. G., and V. A. McKUSICK: Azure lunulae. J. Amer. med. Ass. *166:* 904–906 (1958).

(2) BISSELL, G. W., K. SURAKOMOL and F. GREENSLIT: Longitudinal banded pigmentation of nails in primary adrenal insufficiency. J. Amer. med. Ass. *215:* 1666–1667 (1971).

(3) BREHM, G.: Zum Thema »Pseudomelanom«: Onychomycosis nigricans. Med. Welt *18* (N.F.): 2923–2924 (1967).

(4) DONALD, G. F., G. A. HUNTER and B. D. GILLAM: Transverse leukonychia due to pellagra. Arch. Derm. (Chic.) *85:* 530–531 (1962).

(5) FÖLDI, M., M. SZEGVÁRI, I. SZÁDECZKY, A. LAKOS, L. VARGA und D. BARA: Zum »Syndrom der gelben Fingernägel«. Z. klin. Med. *158:* 501–507 (1965).

(6) JUHLIN, L.: Hereditary leukonychia. Acta derm.-venereol. (Stockh.) *43:* 136–141 (1963).

(7) KORTING, G. W.: Drei Demonstrationen zum Thema Melanom und Pseudo-Melanom. Med. Welt *18* (N. F.): 917–918 (1967).

(8) KUSKE, H.: Splitterblutungen der Nagelplatte. Dermatologica (Basel) *123:* 219–226 (1961).

(9) LINDSAY, P. G.: The half-and-half nail. Arch. intern. Med. *119:* 583–587 (1967).

(10) MUEHRCKE, R. C.: The finger-nails in chronic hypoalbuminaemia, a new physical sign. Brit. med. J. *1956/I:* 1327–1328.

(11) SAMMAN, P. D., and W. F. WHITE: The "yellow nail" syndrome. Brit. J. Derm. *76:* 153–157 (1964).

(12) TERRY, R.: White nails in hepatic cirrhosis. Lancet 1954/I: 757–759.

(13) WHELTON, M. J., and F. M. POPE: Azure lunules in argyria. Arch. intern. Med. *121:* 267–269 (1968).

(14) ZUEHLKE, R. L., and W. B. TAYLOR: Black nails with proteus mirabilis. Arch. Derm. (Chic.) *102:* 154 (1970).

25. Bullous Dermatoses

A. Dermatoses Characterized Primarily by Blisters

1. Within the group of skin diseases showing primarily blisters **chronic pemphigus** with its three variants, vulgaris, vegetans, and foliaceus, has always occupied a special phenomenological place. This position is based upon the development of at first firm, easily destroyed, unilocular blisters arising from unchanged skin or mucous membrane; these lesions show tangential displacement (Nikolsky sign). The individual blisters are distributed in an irregular manner and do not show, like dermatitis herpetiformis, a special tendency to form groups. Involvement of the mucous membranes is found in almost all patients. The intraepidermal position of the blister results in healing without scarring, occasionally with residual slight pigmentation. Not infrequently, chronic pemphigus starts with a circumscribed bullous area (for instance, on the mucous membranes of the mouth or genitals, or on the flexor aspects of joints); this area will soon develop crusts, with the result that the diagnosis of pemphigus is overlooked. Only with increasing generalization will the true character of the disease become evident. As far as age is concerned, the group between 30 and 60 is most frequently involved, but as a general principle individuals of any age may be affected. Before the era of corticosteroids and immunosuppressive drugs most patients died of septic complications or chronic marasmus.

Pemphigus vegetans frequently begins with ulcerous eroded lesions of the oral mucosa or as pemphigus vulgaris; only later during the course of the disease will areas of vegetating lesions favor the larger flexor aspects of the joints and the intertriginous areas (Fig. 423). Foul-smelling,

Fig. 423. Pemphigus vegetans.

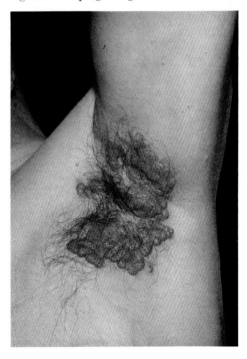

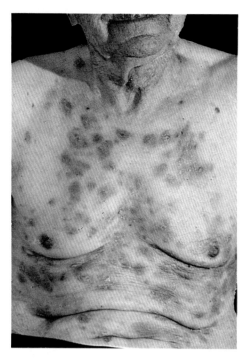

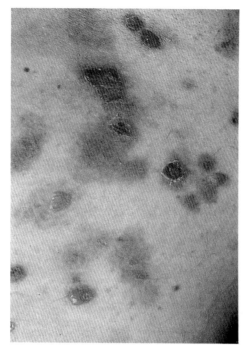

Fig. 424. Senear-Usher syndrome.   Fig. 425. Senear-Usher syndrome.

crusted, relatively well circumscribed granulations show blisters and pustules only in peripheral areas. Healing takes place without scar formation as it does in pemphigus vulgaris. The differential diagnosis has to exclude hypertrophic tertiary syphilis or vegetating bromoderma; these two diseases not only prefer the same localizations as pemphigus vegetans but also lack remnants of blisters at the edge of their vegetating proliferations.

Pemphigus foliaceus resembles pemphigus vulgaris at first with large, flaccid blisters that quickly form crusts. Finally, blister formation is so extremely rapid that only weeping, gluey, macerated, crusted, scaling lesions predominate. In contrast to the other two variants of pemphigus, large macular erythematous areas become preponderant and soon change into a universal erythroderma (see also Chapter 22, C15). The clinical picture itself permits a definite diagnosis only with qualifications. There are no laboratory

tests which are helpful. However, finding circulating immunofluorescent antibodies that attach to the intercellular substance of the stratum spinosum is an important step. It has to be kept in mind that in a certain percentage of tests falsely positive pemphigus-immunofluorescence may occur.

The intraepidermal formation of blisters in chronic pemphigus results from the lack of adherence (acantholysis) of the tonofibrils. The blister formation of the various forms of pemphigus starts with an intercellular edema of the lower strata of the epidermis; in pemphigus vulgaris this progresses to typical suprabasal acantholysis. The appearance of the blister brings about the presence of acantholytic cells* lying free in the bullous cavity. These cells are conspicuous by their rounded, hyperchromatic nuclei. The PAS-positive basal membrane zone remains unaffected. In

_____

* Tzanck cells. (Tr.)

pemphigus foliaceous the subcorneal formation of acantholytic blisters appears
much higher in the epidermis. Sometimes
only the upper layers of the epidermis
become separated, with no proper formation of bullae. Histopathologically, pemphigus vegetans is characterized by intraepidermal acantholytic formations of clefts
and development of massive acanthosis
and papillomatosis, together with eosinophilic abscesses.[5, 7, 20, 39, 44]

**2. Pemphigus erythematosus or sebor-
rhoicus** (Senear-Usher syndrome) resembles lupus erythematosus in that it affects
the face with formation of a butterfly-like
crusted erythema.

In addition, the scalp and the middle of
the chest and back show erythemas with
greasy-crumbly scaling and a few crusts
(Figs. 424, 425). There are also recurrent
separate bullae, on either erythematous or
unchanged skin. The mucous membranes
are seldom affected. Histologically, pemphigus foliaceus produces intra-epidermal
blisters in the upper strata. This differentiates it from lupus erythematosus, which
seldom shows blisters and then in a subepidermal location. Circulating immunofluorescent antibodies can be found directed at
the intercellular substance of the stratum
spinosum and also the basal membrane.[47]

3. Cases of **familial benign chronic pemphigus** (Hailey-Hailey disease) must be
differentiated from pemphigus vegetans.
In contrast to pemphigus vulgaris Hailey-
Hailey disease lacks involvement of the
mucous membranes and produces bullae
on the rest of the skin, only occasionally
preferring intertriginous regions (axillae,
groins, peri-genital areas) and especially
the sides of the neck. Only rarely does one
see clear, grouped vesicles on unchanged
or slightly erythematous skin (Figs. 316,
426). Because of the accompanying pruritus these small vesicles are quickly destroyed, with the result that only circinate,
pointlike or pinhead-sized excoriations
remain. However, the intertriginous areas
show a relatively sharply circumscribed,
dark red erythema with a macerated
surface. Stretching such an area permits
visualization of mostly parallel, coxcomb-
like, small vegetations. The presence of one
or only a few isolated areas suggests eczema or circinate impetigo. However, Hailey-
Hailey disease is definitely influenced by
heat and humidity and appears in places
atypical of eczema. Histologic examination shows acantholysis characteristic of
the substrate of pemphigus, but, in contrast to pemphigus vulgaris, the acantholytic cells are still loosely connected with
their intercellular bridges, so that usually

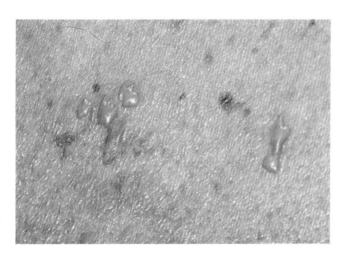

Fig. 426. Blisters on the trunk
in familial benign chronic
pemphigus.

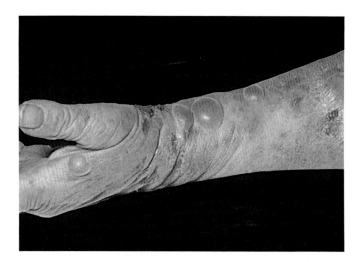

Fig. 427. Bullous pemphi-
goid.

even in a bullous cavity only a few separated acantholytic elements with pyknotic
nuclei can be found. In addition, examinations so far have not shown a definite type
of immunofluorescence for familial benign
chronic pemphigus. Familial occurrence of
this type of pemphigus, which is transmitted as an irregular autosomal trait, is
an important sign of the disease; however,
patients will seldom give statements
spontaneously about the hereditary aspect.
Histologically, there can be close similarities between familial benign chronic
pemphigus and **bullous dyskeratosis follicularis** (Darier's disease). The presence of
so-called "corps ronds" and "grains," however, favors a diagnosis of Darier's disease.
Clinically, there are also distinct differences
between familial benign chronic pemphigus and bullous Darier's disease; the latter
favors the face and the midlines of the
chest and back. In addition to small,
flaccid, vesiculous pustules, typical follicular horny papules can be found. Interruptions of the normal palmar creases can be
found in both diseases, although in Hailey-
Hailey disease these interruptions are not
as marked as they are in Darier's disease.
For further details about Darier's disease
see Chapter 29, A3.[31]

4. Bullous pemphigoid (parapemphigus
of old age) is characterized by large, taut,
frequently hemorrhagic bullae, which do
not rupture as easily as do those of pemphigus vulgaris; also, the Nikolsky phenomenon is not present. These facts are
explained by the subepidermal location
of the bullae and the absence of acantholysis. Bullous pemphigoid appears in
eruptions, with bullae developing mostly
on an erythematous or urticarial base and
only rarely on normal skin (Fig. 427).
Quite often the bullae show a tendency toward grouping, and at the time of eruption
they are accompanied by pruritus. Sites of
predilection are the axillae, the flexor
aspects of the upper arms, the umbilical
region, and the inner aspects of the thighs;
however, there is no typical pattern of
distribution as in erythema multiforme.
The mucous membranes are rarely affected. In the differential diagnosis there are
two difficulties: first, the differentiation
from chronic pemphigus vulgaris, which
can be done by histologic examination. In
bullous pemphigoid there is the subepidermal location of the bulla and the absence
of acantholysis. The indirect immunofluorescent test demonstrates antibodies
against the basal membrane zone of the
epidermis but, in contrast to pemphigus

vulgaris, fails to show them against the intercellular substance of the stratum spinosum. Whereas the difficulty of separating chronic pemphigus from bullous pemphigoid exists only macroscopically, in the second diagnostic problem, the differentiation from dermatitis herpetiformis, the difficulty extends to the histology as well. In both entities there is a subepidermal bulla, but in bullous pemphigoid the contents of the bulla shows fewer cells (eosinophils) than in dermatitis herpetiformis. Further, the latter has a leukocytic infiltrate with a tendency to leukocytoclasis in the upper corium; such a condition is found in bullous pemphigoid only to a very limited degree. The most important differential point, histologically, is the presence of papillary microabscesses within the peribullous region. Dermatitis herpetiformis almost always shows such microabscesses regularly, whereas they are absent in pemphigoid. It should be men-

tioned that a definite separation between bullous pemphigoid and dermatitis herpetiformis is not always possible even with the aid of histologic or immunofluorescent methods, and therefore the existence of intermediate forms must be considered.[4a, 5, 20, 23, 32, 37, 39, 44, 48, 50]

5. Dermatitis herpetiformis typically shows a tendency to polymorphism. Subjectively, most patients complain of severe pruritus and, if they are able to analyze their sensations, a feeling of burning. Such perceptions as a rule accompany the appearance of fresh cutaneous lesions. Although formations of vesicles or bullae are the most frequent manifestations, erythemas, wheals, and prurigo lesions are not at all exceptional (Figs. 428, 429). In contrast to the lesions of chronic pemphigus, the bullae do not arise on normal skin and cannot be moved tangentially because of their subepidermal location. Important

Fig. 428. Circinate dermatitis herpetiformis with large blisters.

Fig. 429. Dermatitis herpetiformis with large blisters.

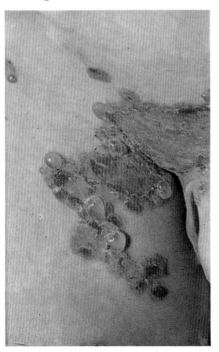

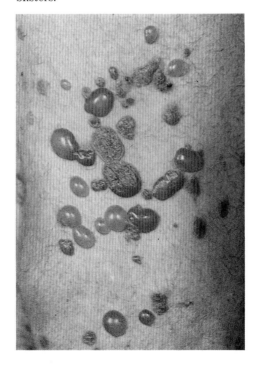

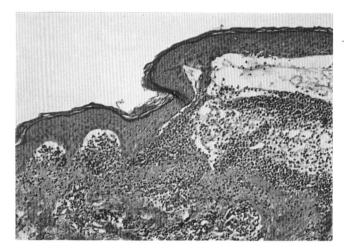

Fig. 430. Dermatitis herpetiformis: subepidermal blister
and peribullous papillary abscesses. HE stain, 25×.

signs of the presence of dermatitis herpetiformis are symmetrical arrangement of
lesions, a preference for the anterior
axillary fold, and the tendency to grouping
of the individual lesions. Involvement of
the mucous membranes is as rare as it is in
bullous pemphigoid; the diagnostic differentiation of the latter from dermatitis
herpetiformis in a single case, especially in
childhood, may cause considerable difficulty. The histologic criteria are the same
as those described in the previous paragraphs on bullous pemphigoid. Marked
eosinophilia of the circulating blood and
increased retention of bromsulphthalein
during the eruptive phase are signs in
favor of dermatitis herpetiformis. Characteristic among the primary dermatoses with
formation of bullae is, if present, an idiosyncrasy toward iodine in dermatitis herpetiformis. Indications of such an idiosyncrasy
are a history of an increase of cutaneous
lesions following ingestion of salt water
fish or iodized salt, roentgenologic contrast substances containing iodine, and iodine applications in the treatment of thyroid conditions. Idiosyncrasy to iodine can
be shown by patch-testing with 30 per cent
potassium iodide vaseline or by a peroral
dose of 10 to 20 drops of Lugol's solution.

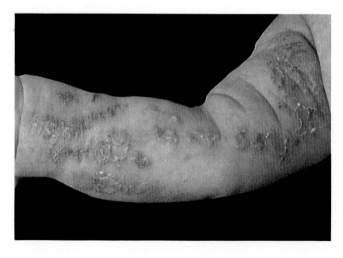

Fig. 431. Incontinentia pigmenti: bullous and striated
initial stage.

Histologically, the subepidermal bullae of dermatitis herpetiformis develop from a marked subepidermal edema; the edematous tips of the dermal papillae show an eosinophilic and neutrophilic exudate (Fig.430) even before the bullous stage or degeneration of the collagen. In addition, dermatitis herpetiformis shows a granular pattern of immunofluorescence of the basal membrane within the peribullous papillary abscesses, in contrast to the homogeneous continuous fluorescent line seen in bullous pemphigoid.

Some patients with dermatitis herpetiformis suffer from disturbances of the small intestine. At present it is uncertain whether these disturbances are part of the dermatitis herpetiformis complex; however, when present, an attempt should be made to clarify their etiology. For involvement of the joints, see Chapter 7, H2.

In rare cases dermatitis herpetiformis may involve only a circumscribed cutaneous area (Cottini type). This type favors the extensor aspects of the knees and elbows. Clinically one sees only individual, grouped bullae, as large as rice grains, some with an erythematous halo. A histologic examination will prevent confusion with herpes simplex because it will show the previously mentioned typical histologic findings of dermatitis herpetiformis.[8, 13, 17, 23, 24, 32, 37, 39, 40, 48, 54, 60]

In infancy the initial vesicular stage of **incontinentia pigmenti** (Bloch-Sulzberger type) may resemble dermatitis herpetiformis. Small vesicular changes may exist for weeks before the typical characteristic picture of incontinentia pigmenti develops (Figs.408, 431, 460). In any case, in the vesicular stage the striated, reticular pattern of distribution with later pigmentation can be recognized. There is no impairment of general health, however, and a high degree of eosinophilia of blood and tissue is present as in dermatitis herpetiformis (Fig.432). Further details are discussed in Chapter 24, E9).[3, 6]

6. Benign mucosal pemphigoid, which was formerly called, somewhat erroneously, ocular or conjunctival pemphigus, occupies an autonomous position strictly separating it from other bullous dermatoses. The disease has a certain tendency to affect persons of either sex between the ages of 40 and 70. The oral mucosa is always affected, and it is here that the majority of patients show the first signs of the disease as a desquamative gingivitis. The next most frequent sites of disease are the conjunctivae and the genital

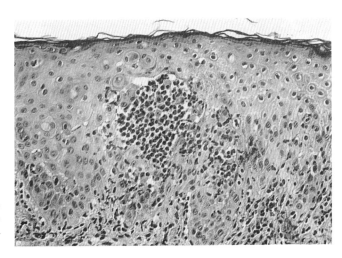

Fig.432. Incontinentia pigmenti: intraepidermal pustule, rich in eosinophils. HE stain, 100×.

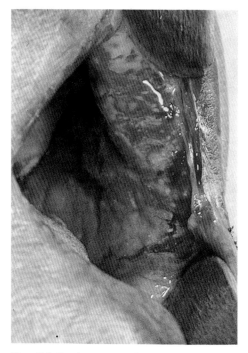

Fig. 433. Benign mucosal pemphigoid.

mucosa; however, the mucosa of the nose, urethra, and rectum may be affected also. Further, it is important to note that individual bullae may be found on the skin. The oral mucosa may show, in addition to the previously mentioned desquamative gingivitis, bullae with a distinct erythematous

halo; these persist for a few days before they undergo changes into aphthae (Fig. 433). Essentially the same changes take place on the conjunctivae. Cicatrization may result in progressive shrinkage of the lids, corneal opacities, and subsequent blindness (Fig. 434). Histologically, in contrast to chronic pemphigus vulgaris, subepidermal bullae with inflammatory infiltration (lymphocytes, plasma cells, some granulocytes) are seen in the upper corium. Direct immunofluorescence reveals antibodies in the basal membrane zone.*

The differential diagnosis between benign mucosal pemphigoid on the one hand and chronic pemphigus vulgaris (and also erythema ·multiforme) on the other hand is not difficult. If the diagnosis cannot be made by clinical examination alone, microscopic studies will produce a definite answer. Erythema multiforme seldom affects the gingiva but in the vast majority of cases prefers the lips and the entrance of the mouth. Very problematical, if not impossible, is the differentiation from bullous pemphigoid. In favor of bullous pemphigoid is the presence of many cutaneous bullae. According to our present

---

* Rarely; one case published in the American literature. (Tr.)

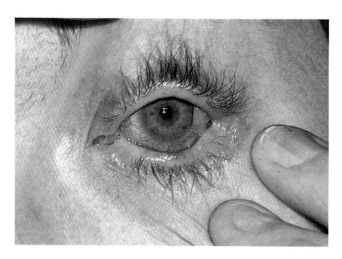

Fig. 434. Benign mucosal pemphigoid: conjunctival synechiae.

knowledge only immunofluorescent examination will permit a definite distinction because bullous pemphigoid shows typical antibodies in the basal membrane zone. The differential diagnosis against a pemphigoid lichen planus is also difficult. If there are typical cutaneous lesions, reticulated mucous membrane changes, or gray-blue papules of the tongue, desquamations of the gingiva and vesiculoulcerous changes of the mucous membrane can be attributed to lichen planus without hesitation. However, if these signs are absent, the diagnosis will depend on the positive histologic findings of liquefaction of the basal cell layers, invasion of round cells into the epidermis, and a relatively sharp line of demarcation of the infiltrate of the corium toward the deeper layers. For further details about pemphigoid lichen planus see Section B3 of this chapter.[4b, 49]

7. Erythema multiforme with its entirely polymorphous clinical picture shows as its initial lesion a small, flat, and above all exudative papule. The originally edematous lesion will show peripheral enlargement with formation of a central bulla, creating the diagnostically characteristic iris or target lesion (Fig. 435). The lips soon show hemorrhagic, blackish crusts, and although the oral mucosa itself does not

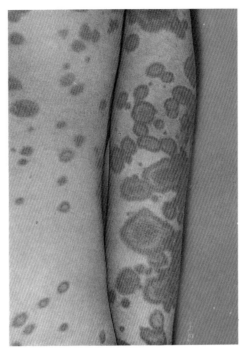

Fig. 435. Erythema multiforme: herpes-iris forms.

develop such dried up lesions owing to the increase in salivation, erosive lesions covered with whitish-yellow material are formed instead. The individual cutaneous lesions appear in crops, so that the different

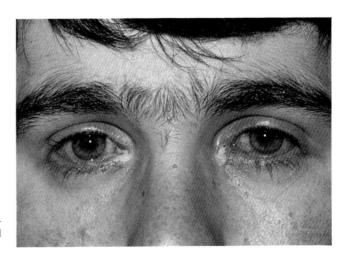

Fig. 436. Erythema multiforme: pronounced bilateral conjunctivitis.

stages of development can be seen simultaneously. Frequent recurrences are another conspicuous sign of erythema multiforme; typically, the extensor surfaces of the arms, and also the face and genitals are affected. However, the inverse type favors the flexor aspects of the extremities, including the palms and soles. If the disorder takes a severe course, pseudomembranous lesions on the conjunctivae and nasal mucosa will appear, as well as lesions of the oral and genital mucosa (Fig. 436). Such extensive forms of erythema multiforme are accompanied by an increase in body temperature and are called the **Stevens-Johnson syndrome** or "acute mucocutaneous ocular syndrome"; however, these names do not emphasize any special etiology. Myocarditis or myositis are rare complications of erythema multiforme, while atypical pneumonias occur somewhat more frequently. These internal manifestations may present so few signs that they are easily overlooked unless one searches for them especially. Laboratory tests do not yield any special findings, with the exception of an increase of the sedimentation rate and the occasional presence of cold agglutinins; the latter may indicate an atypical pneumonia.

The etiology of erythema multiforme is still unknown. Suspected are infections with the virus of herpes simplex or mycoplasma pneumoniae; however, toxic-allergic reactions (i. e., drugs) play a role which should not be underestimated. The differential diagnosis must include dermatitis herpetiformis, chronic pemphigus vulgaris, and bullous pemphigoid. If characteristic herpes iris lesions are present, the decision is facilitated. However, the differentiation from Lyell's syndrome (toxic-epidermal necrolysis) may be difficult. Only an exact analysis of the various cutaneous manifestations will help, because the pattern of distribution, involvement of the mucosa, fever, and histologic findings are the same in both diseases to a great extent. However, Lyell's syndrome produces flat and more diffuse separations of the epidermis similar to a second degree burn.

Erythema multiforme shows subepidermal bullae with adjacent lymphohistiocytic infiltrates and a few neutrophils or eosinophils. The fluid of the bullae contains cellular elements of a predominantly polymorphous character. However, in every case at any given time there are sufficient differential diagnostic criteria to make possible a certain histopathological separation between erythema multiforme, bullous pemphigoid, and dermatitis herpetiformis.[11, 19, 23, 25, 48, 65]

8. Lyell's syndrome requires further differential diagnostic consideration (see also Chapter 22, B3). This syndrome in the adult represents in most cases a maximal type of "toxic-allergic" bullous epidermolytic exanthem. However, in infants and small children Lyell's syndrome apparently represents a bullous staphyloderma.

"Pemphigus acutus febrilis gravis," or so-called febrile butcher's pemphigus, probably has a bacterial origin*. At first there are only circumscribed formations of bullae (formerly called "pemphigus neonatorum" in infants), followed by fulminant development of extensive bullous separation of the epidermis with flat, red, weeping erosions. The Nikolsky sign is positive in the vicinity of the bullae and erosions. The mucous membranes are also involved in this generalized epidermal necrolysis; when healing takes place the result can be formation of extensive adhesions. Patients with a beginning, still prebullous Lyell's syndrome frequently complain of a strange sensation or burning within the areas of later epidermolytic lesions. With regard to accompanying fever see Chapter 1, L2.

Histologically, Lyell's syndrome shows the characteristic sign of epidermal necrol-

---

* This type is not recognized any longer. (Tr)

ysis. However, this necrolysis is found also with such other skin diseases as bullous fixed drug eruptions, allergic vasculitis, and erythema multiforme; the latter dermatosis requires consideration of the whole clinical picture (herpes iris lesions with emphasis on the extensor aspects and the upper half of the trunk, as well as circumorificial extension in the inversed type). Histologically conspicuous in Lyell's syndrome is the small amount of cellular reaction that occurs in the beginning.[2, 30, 42, 46]

Purely from a clinical point of view **burns** and **scaldings** look similar to the skin changes in Lyell's syndrome. However, in burns and scaldings the Nikolsky sign cannot be produced in perilesional areas. Besides, the history would give the necessary information.

9. If in infants and small children blisters appear on sites of pressure, **hered-**

itary epidermolysis has to be considered. This disorder is based on a gene-conditioned structural weakness in the area of the basal cells and neighboring layers. Essentially, this is a "mechanical bullosis," although in certain special forms an association with hot weather or warm baths has been noted in addition. Clinical and genetic biotypes recognized today are: epidermolysis bullosa hereditaria simplex, the dominantly inherited epidermolysis bullosa dystrophica, the recessively inherited epidermolysis bullosa dystrophica, and hereditary dystrophia bullosa.

The main characteristic of **epidermolysis bullosa hereditaria simplex** is blisters (Fig. 437), which appear a short time after a firm mechanical irritation. Healing is generally achieved in a few days without residual scar formation. Disturbances of nail growth, hair anomalies, and changes

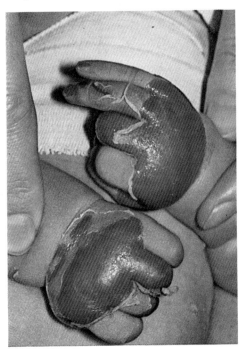

Fig. 437. Epidermolysis bullosa hereditaria simplex.

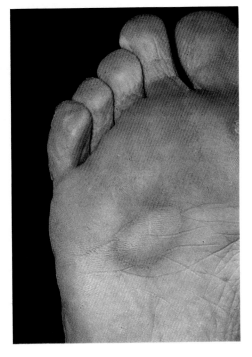

Fig. 438. So-called recurrent blisterous eruption of the feet.

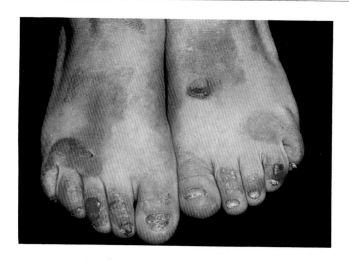

Fig. 439. Epidermolysis bullosa hereditaria dystrophica: blisters and nail dystrophies.

in the bones or the teeth are absent. The mucous membranes remain free, with the exception of the oral mucosa, which regularly becomes traumatized during food intake. A clinical variant is the so-called recurrent **blisterous eruption of**

Fig. 440. Epidermolysis bullosa albopapuloidea.

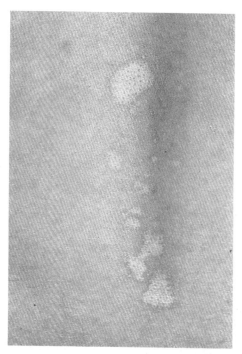

the feet. The blisterous attacks remain confined to the feet, and their manifestations are increased by heat in particular (Fig. 438). Small blisters on the hands and the body appear only rarely. Both variants of epidermolysis are autosomal dominant traits.[28, 63]

In the dominantly inherited **epidermolysis bullosa hereditaria dystrophica** the blister formation is located subepidermally so that healing progresses with scar formation and milia. The scars are of either atrophic or hypertrophic character. In contrast to epidermolysis hereditaria simplex, however, a high proportion of nail dystrophies occurs (Fig. 439). Follicular and palmoplantar keratoses are rare. The oral mucosa is often affected. The presence of residual leukoplakias after healing of the blisters indicates previous involvement. Striking mutilations on the extremities and stenoses of the esophagus are absent.
[16, 26, 55]

Epidermolysis bullosa albopapuloidea is clinically and genetically identical with the dominant form of epidermolysis bullosa hereditaria. The sole difference is the manifestation of perifollicular, ivory-colored, flat papules, which are independent of the blisters. The papules, which may be as large as lentils and are partly confluent, are often located in the lumbosacral region (Fig. 440). Although they do not develop before the tenth year of life, they remain permanently unchanged thereafter. Confusion with *lichen sclerosus et atrophicus* or lumbosacral cobblestone nevi can be avoided by the history and the characteristic clinical findings.

The forms of epidermolysis bullosa hereditaria that have been mentioned so far show autosomal dominant heredity. **Recessive** (or polydysplastic) **epidermolysis bullosa dystrophica,** however, shows an autosomal recessive mode. Biochemically, increased cutaneous collagenase activity in blisterous as well unchanged areas may be present. Corresponding with these findings is a structural defect of the anchoring fibers of the entire skin that can be seen with the electron microscope. In this disorder the tendency to spontaneous blister formation manifests itself very soon after birth.

The adherence of the epidermis to the corium is so loose that in many patients a positive Nikolsky phenomeon can be elicited. Cicatrizations and the growing together of adjoining areas result early in limited mobility and severe mutilations. In contrast to these features, any tendency to reepithelialization of large blister defects is missing at other sites (Fig. 441). Nail dystrophies and milia are always present. If the patients reach a certain age, one must watch for the possible development of cancer within the firm scars. Quite often, however, the patients succumb – like patients with severe burns – to sepsis or the sequelae of an esophageal stenosis (Fig. 442). Involvement of the conjunctivae, mucous membranes of the oral cavity, pharynx, esophagus, and genitals is rather severe in this polydysplastic form. A cicatricial shortening of the frenulum linguae can be observed in almost all patients. The tongue and the gingivolabial

Fig. 441. Epidermolysis bullosa dystrophica (recessive type).

Fig. 442. Esophageal stricture in epidermolysis bullosa hereditaria dystrophica.

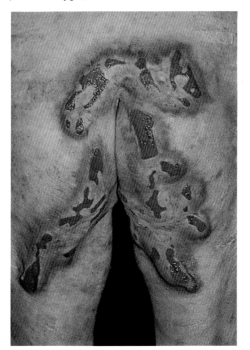

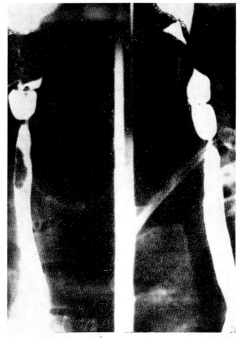

mucous membranes often grow together. The esophageal stenoses are vital, however, and therefore need special attention. A differentiation between the recessive and dominant dystrophic epidermolyses cannot always be made with certainty on clinical grounds because of the latitude of variation in both forms.[29, 61, 64]

So-called **epidermolysis bullosa letalis** is also inherited as an autosomal recessive trait. The histologic analyses, however, suggest that this is not a uniform disease. Most of the observations suggest that we may be dealing with early fatal cases of recessive epidermolysis hereditaria dystrophica. Even in the uterus or a few hours or several days after birth the skin is raised in large areas. Nail dystrophies may already be present at birth but usually develop in the first weeks of life. The absence of milia and scarred healed areas cannot be considered as evidence against the diagnosis of recessive epidermolysis bullosa hereditaria, since it takes weeks or months before they appear. A differentiation of these two disease forms cannot be made solely from the clinical picture in the first days of life. The subsequent course must be awaited and the hereditary conditions must be analysed.

In the newborn the differential diagnosis must include the possibility of bullous impetigo of the exfoliative dermatitis type. In this disorder mechanical irritation does not elicit blisters, and accompanying inflammatory signs point to the bacterial origin. Large blisters rarely ever develop, and the perioral onset with noninvolvement of the mucous membranes differs basically from hereditary epidermolysis. Bullous impetigo also lacks nail dystrophies and scarred healed areas. The nowadays extremely rare bullous syphilid of the newborn generally develops in the first days of life; the lesions are surrounded by other flat syphilids. Especially in the palmoplantar region it may become rupioid. Hypertrophic oozing processes are

often observed simultaneously around the body openings or on areas that touch each other. Here, *Treponema pallidum* can be demonstrated. The Wassermann and Nelson reactions are positive.[27, 38]

Acquired bullous epidermolysis is rare. Occasionally there have been reports of a clinical picture of epidermolysis bullosa hereditaria dystrophica which became manifest as late as adulthood and showed no hereditary aspects, even under the most careful investigation. However, before this diagnosis is made, other blister-forming dermatoses such as bullous drug eruptions, dermatitis herpetiformis, pemphigus, pemphigoid, and porphyria cutanea tarda must be ruled out. It is striking that in many cases of acquired epidermolysis bullosa internal accompanying disorders such as diabetes mellitus, multiple myelomas, tuberculous lymph nodes, amyloidosis, and intestinal disorders are present.[41, 53]

Dystrophia bullosa hereditaria of the macular type also manifests blisters in early childhood. Absence of hair is already apparent at birth; the blisters, however, do not appear before the second month of life. This tendency to spontaneous blister formation continues until about the fourth year of life and then disappears completely. In contrast to epidermolysis bullosa hereditaria the mucous membranes always remain free. The blisters heal leaving tender, atrophic, white spots, which form a distinct contrast to the reticular, brown pigmentations on the extremities and the face. For further details see Chapter 11, A21.[43, 66]

10. The **porphyrias** and the hereditary epidermolyses show mechanically triggered development of blisters, which heal with atrophy and milia. According to the different biochemical disturbances of the synthesis of porphyrin the following clinical pictures are differentiated. Among them only porphyria acuta intermittens is unaccompanied by cutaneous changes.

A. Erythropoietic porphyrias
   1. Congenital erythropoietic porphyria
   2. Erythropoietic protoporphyria
   3. Erythropoietic coproporphyria
   4. Erythropoietic porphyria lenta

B. Hepatic porphyrias
   1. Porphyria acuta intermittens
   2. Porphyria cutanea tarda
   3. Porphyria variegata
   4. Hereditary coproporphyria

C. Symptomatic porphyrias
   1. Hexachlorobenzol-porphyria
   2. Paraneoplastic porphyria
   3. Drug-induced porphyrias
   4. Porphyrin-producing hepatic tumors

Congenital erythropoietic porphyria is extremely rare. Its mode of heredity is autosomal recessive. The first cutaneous changes of the affected children are considered by the parents to be itching erythemas caused by light. In these erythemas blisters soon appear, healing with scar formation and leading to mutilations and contractures. Relatively early a conspicuous red color of the urine appears, caused by the large amount of excreted porphyrin. If exposure to light continues, blister formations are accompanied by cicatricial loss of hair and loss of nails. The teeth assume a dirty brown hue and show in ultraviolet light (like the urine) a distinct red fluorescence (erythrodontia). A number of peripheral erythrocytes and, most important, erythroblasts show the same phenomenon of fluorescence. In addition, many patients have hemolytic anemia. The clinical findings of pronounced sensitivity to light (observed in similar fashion only in some forms of xeroderma pigmentosum), in combination with erythrodontia and the red color of urine permit the correct diagnosis without difficulty. Among the laboratory tests strongly increased excretion of uroporphyrin and coproporphyrin of the isomere chain I is typical. In the erythrocytes uroporphyrin I, coproporphyrin I, and, to a lesser extent, protoporphyrin I are increased.[18, 51, 62]

Erythropoietic protoporphyria is characterized by a substantially smaller light hypersensitivity. The mode of heredity is autosomal dominant. The skin shows mostly formation of blisters and wheals after exposure to sunlight (Fig.443). A single blister does not become especially large, and after healing it leaves a small retracted scar. In some patients the sun-exposed skin shows only reddened edema with sporadic petechiae. The hyaline deposits, which suggest hyalinosis cutis et

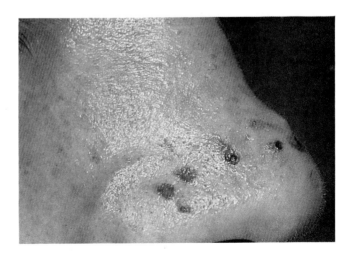

Fig. 443. Erythropoietic protoporphyria.

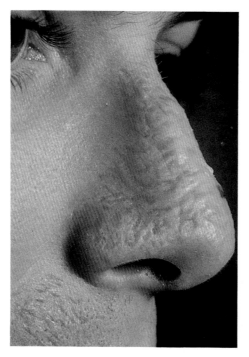

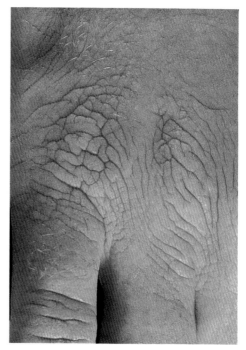

Fig. 444. Erythropoietic protoporphyria with deposits of hyaline masses on the dorsum of the nose.

Fig. 445. Erythropoietic protoporphyria with deposits of hyaline masses on the dorsum of the hand.

mucosae, are conspicuous on the face and hands (Figs. 444, 445). However, the characteristic involvement of the mucous membranes in hyalinosis is always absent. Likewise, the pachydermias assume a brownish-red color in the course of time.

Electron-microscopically, the so-called hard clods in the finely fibrillar, concentric sheaths of the vessels of the papillary bodies are absent in erythropoietic protoporphyria, in contrast to the findings in hyalinosis cutis et mucosae.

As in congenital erythropoietic porphyria, but much less intensely, red fluorescence of the erythrocytes (10 to 25 per cent) can be shown in peripheral blood smears (Fig.446). The red color of the urine, however, is absent, since no porphyrinuria is present. Erythrodontia and hemolytic anemia are lacking, but lethal liver cirrhosis can be observed. In the erythrocytes themselves protoporphy-

rin and coproporphyrin of the isomere type III are distinctly increased. Both substances are also increasingly excreted in the feces. (See also Chapter 2, C2 and Chapter 17, C5.)[1, 14, 34, 58]

Erythropoietic coproporphyria also becomes manifest in earliest childhood. It seems to be transmitted as an autosomal dominant trait. After exposure to sunlight, erythemas with small blisters as well as itching edemas develop, but real urticarial reactions are not present. Red fluorescent erythrocytes are again evident in blood smears. Red urine, erythrodontia, and hemolytic anemia do not occur. In the erythrocytes an increase in coproporphyrin III and protoporphyrin III prevails, the reverse condition of that found in erythropoietic protoporphyria. In the urine only the coproporphyrins are slightly increased.

It has not been decided whether or not **porphyria erythropoietica lenta** is a definite

Fig. 446. Fluorescence of erythrocytes in erythropoietic
protoporphyria.

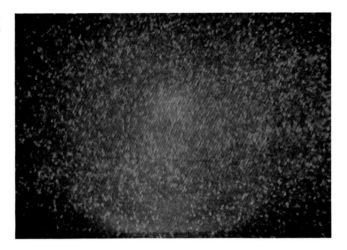

disorder sui generis. The disease first
begins in adulthood and is accompanied
by mild hypersensitivity to sunlight. Only
a few blisters and a marked brown pigmentation and hypertrichosis of the light-
exposed parts of the skin appear. Erythrodontia is missing, but the red color of the
urine and hemolytic anemia as in congenital erythropoietic porphyria are present.
In the erythrocytes coproporphyrins and
protoporphyrins of the isomere chain I are
distinctly above normal. Conditions of
concentration within the erythrocytes are,
therefore, the reverse of those found in
congenital erythropoietic porphyria. Increased excretion of porphyrin in the urine
affects coproporphyrin I and uroporphyrin
I.[57]

Of all porphyrias **porphyria cutanea
tarda** is probably the most frequent form.
In contrast to the other erythropoietic
forms already mentioned, the first signs
of the disorder appear as late as the fourth
and fifth decades of life. Only exceptionally do children develop the disorder. Male
patients are so much more affected than
female patients that instances of the
disorder in females suggest paraneoplastic
or drug-induced porphyrias. On cutaneous
sites that are chronically exposed to

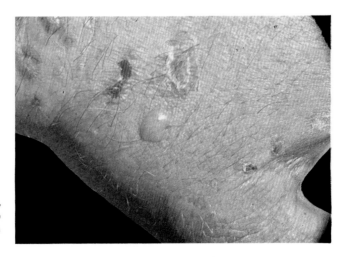

Fig. 447. Porphyria cutanea
tarda: typical conglomerate
of blisters, erosions, and fresh
scars.

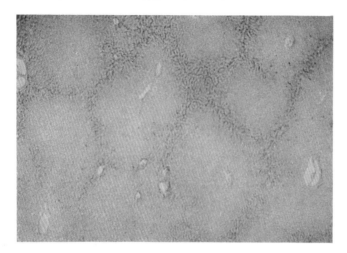

Fig. 448. Siderosis of the liver in porphyria cutanea tarda. Berlin-blue reaction, 155×.

sunlight such as the face, neck, and backs of the hands, small, itching blisters appear after common mechanical insults, and soon develop into large blisters. Since the small blisters on the face are scratched,

Fig. 449. Porphyria cutanea tarda: red fluorescence of a cylindrical specimen obtained by liver puncture.

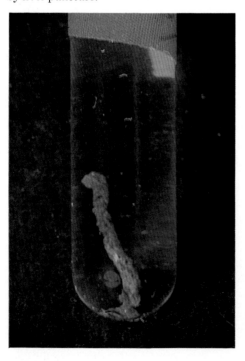

only relatively large ulcerations covered by hemorrhagic crusts develop there. Since the site of the blister is subepidermal, healing always results in scar formation. On the backs of the hands there is a conglomeration of fresh blisters, flat ulcerations, depigmented scars, and milia (Fig. 447). Numerous scars on the hands, especially on the fingers, can lead to firm attachment of the skin. This has given rise to the concept of scleroporphyria, but since this name may lead to the assumption that porphyria is associated with scleroderma, its use is not recommended. Besides the generalized dark skin color, hypertrichosis of the face on the eyes, ears, and cheeks is conspicuous. Increased light hypersensitivity leads to chronic conjunctivitis in many patients, making them look like habitual drinkers. The urine, in accordance with the increased excretion of porphyrin, assumes a dark brown-red color (like Coca-Cola). Every patient with porphyria cutanea tarda has some liver damage, which occurs in various degrees such as fatty liver, chronic persistent hepatitis, and others (Fig. 448). The cylinder of tissue obtained by liver puncture is fluorescent under an ultraviolet light in glowing orange-red (Fig. 449). The same can be said for specimens prepared by suction of the stomach and for urine specimens, but there is no erythrodontia. The erythrocytes are likewise not fluorescent. The frequent association with diabetes mellitus is striking. Laboratory tests will show hepatic damage (LDH [lactic dehydrogenase], gamma-GTP [glutamine transpeptidase], Bromsulphalein retention, and protein electrophoresis) and the simultaneously occurring hypersiderinemia with lack of transferrin. In the urine coproporphyrins and uroporphyrins of both isomere chains (I and III) are liberally excreted, but not porphobilinogen. Improvement of the skin progresses* parallel with decreased excretion of porphyrin. Although we have been dealing mainly with single observations in porphyria cutanea tarda, a genetic disposition must at least be postulated, as not every patient with liver disease has porphyria, and instances of the disorder occur in several generations of a family although the cause of their liver damage varies (i. e., arsenic, alcohol, and hepatitis); the increased presence of a disturbed red-green color sense is also seen occasionally.

In the differential diagnosis the symptomatic porphyrias, which may imitate perfectly the clinical picture of porphyria cutanea tarda, must be considered. First, a careful drug history (i. e., barbiturates, estrogens, stilbesterol, and griseofulvin) must be taken, and tumors of the liver and biliary tract must be excluded. A definitely lowered level of the serum iron and an unusual age for the disorder point to the possibility of the presence of such a **paraneoplastic porphyria.** Another disorder that does not differ clinically from porphyria cutanea tarda is hexachlorobenzol porphyria, which has occurred in Turkey after consumption of poisoned grain.[9, 10, 12, 22, 52, 62]

Another disorder to be differentiated from porphyria cutanea tarda is **porphyria variegata** (mixed porphyria, protocopro-

porphyria). It shows a mixture of signs of acute intermittent porphyria (chronic obstipation, colicky "acute abdomen," hypertonia and tachycardia, neurogenous pareses, ataxia, paralysis of breathing, epileptic fits, and psychoses) and those of porphyria cutanea tarda. Both sexes are about equally affected and the mode of inheritance is autosomal dominant. In contrast to porphyria cutanea tarda, however, the first typical cutaneous manifestations appear in the second decade of life. Acute crises are somewhat dependent on the menstrual cycle (premenstrual phase) and pregnancy. Most important, however, is the fact that severe general signs may be provoked by drugs containing barbiturates. Evidence of delta-aminolevulinic acid and porphobilinogen in the urine confirms the diagnosis. Particularly high values are present during the "attack" and a small increase of delta-aminolevulinic acid only is found in the so-called free interval. This does not influence the simultaneously present porphyria cutanea tarda-like constellation of porphyrins. Evidence of porphobilinogen is quickly obtained with the Watson-Schwartz test: to 5 ml of urine are added 5 drops of Ehrlich's reagent; if a red color appears, 5 ml of chloroform are added and the whole mixture is vigorously shaken. If after waiting a short while the red color is present in the watery (upper) part, this is positive proof of the presence of porphobilinogen. If the chloroform (lower) part is colored red, the presence of urobilinogen is proved.[51, 62]

In **hereditary coproporphyria** large quantities of coproporphyrin III are excreted in stools and urine, usually without special clinicals signs. After ingestion of barbiturates, estrogens, or sulfonamides, or with the onset of pregnancy, however, severe manifestations, simulating those of acute, intermittent porphyria may occur. During such crises the concentrations of the intraerythrocytic coproporphyrins and protoporphyrins may increase slightly and

---

* Sometimes. (Tr.)

Table 5

	Normal	Porphyria Cutanea Tarda	Porphyria Variegata	Porphyria Erythropoietica Congenita	Erythropoietic Protoporphyria	Erythropoietic Coproporphyria
Erythrocytes	UP III Trace CP III 0–1.9 µg/100 ml erys PP 19.4–53.5 µg/100 ml erys	normal	normal	UP I ++++ CP I ++++ PP IIIn → (+)	UP III (+) CP III + PP III +++	UP III + CP III ++++ PP III +
Fluorescence of erythrocytes	0	0	0	++	+++	+++
Bone marrow		normal	normal	UP I +++++ CP I +++++		
Fluoroblasts	0	0	0	++++	++	++
Liver	UP 0,05–0.18 CP 0.1 –0.29 } µ/g dry residual PP 0.3 –1.4 } mass	UP III ++ CP III + PP III (+)	PBG ++ UP III ++ CP III + PP III (+)	UP I +++	CP III + PP III ++	normal
Urine	ALA 2217 ± 534 PBG 1513 ± 444 UP 6.24 ± 10.44 } µg/24 h CP 72.6 ± 62.6 PP 10.9 ± 10.36	ALA normal PBG normal UP I ++ UP III +++ CP I ++ CP III ++	ALA n → ++ PBG n → ++ UP III n → +++ CP III n → +++	ALA normal PBG normal UP I ++++ CP I ++++	ALA PBG UP } normal CP PP	ALA (+) PBG (+) UP normal CP normal → + PP normal
Stools		UP I + UP III (+) CP I + CP III +++	UP III +++ CP III ++++ PP III ++++	UP I ++ CP I +++	CP III +++ PP III ++++	UP normal CP normal PP normal → (+)

ALA = delta-aminolevulinic acid, PBG = porphobilinogen, UP = uroporphyrin, CP = coproporphyrin, PP = protoporphyrin, n = normal

increases of aminolevulinic acid and porphobilinogen in the urine may occur. Increased sensitivity to light of the skin with formation of erythemas and blisters does not occur regularly. With the onset of acute signs hepatic damage (icterus and an increase in the transaminases) may become evident. In contrast, erythropoietic copro-porphyria, whose manifestations are limit-ed to the skin, does not show the high rate of excretion of coproporphyrin in the stools. These same findings also permit a differentiation from acute intermittent porphyria and porphyria variegata.[21]

11. Concerning **congenital** (bullous) **ichthyosiform erythroderma,** see the chap-ter on erythrodermas (Chapter 22, A2).[36]

12. Ichthyosis linearis circumflexa with blister formation is discussed in the chapter on ichthyoses (Chapter 27, A11) and the chapter on eczematiform skin changes (Chapter 21, D3).[15]

13. Herpes simplex is an eruption of grouped blisters characterized mainly by its tendency to recur. According to its main localizations, the face (see also Chapter 33, B1) and the genital region (see also Chapter 33, C2), two viral types separated by their different antigenic structures can be established. Herpes simplex is rarely accompanied by distinct fever (see also Chapter 1, E1). A recurrent attack is usually initiated by sensations of tingling or a feeling of tension or burning. The blistering eruption itself is usually located on a base which is distinctly ede-matous and erythematous in the beginning. The transition of blisters to pustules is the rule but does not always occur. Other changes, such as hemorrhagic, disseminat-ed, or zosteriform extensions are the excep-tion. Frequent local recurrences may be followed by long-lasting swellings (see also Chapter 10, A4). Recently, cortisone or other cytostatic immunosuppressive drugs

favoring herpetic eruptions have gained practical significance. If the genital blis-ters are distinctly eroded, a primary syph-ilitic lesion must be ruled out (see also Chapter 33, C1 and C2).

In contrast to herpes simplex the **Pospi-schill-Feyrter aphthoid** occurs mainly in infants and small children, mostly as a primary manifestation and usually in a negative-anergic phase after whooping cough, measles, scarlet fever, or other diseases. At the height of development of this secondary disease "vagante," annu-lar or serpiginous blisters develop; they are confluent and sometimes also hemor-rhagic and flabby. They extend to the vestibule of the mouth or toward the pharynx. This serious condition also includes fever, enlargement of the regional lymph nodes, and profuse salivation.[45]

14. Herpes zoster (shingles), which has the same causative organism as the virus of varicella, shows at the height of its development a disseminated eruption of blisters conspicuously limited to the segments of the areas of projection of the affected nerves. This eruption is preceded by red papules, small in the beginning, that are located on an equally segmentary erythematous and occasionally edematous base (see also Chapter 18, H1). Before they appear, prodromal subfebrility and little malaise are noted, but high temperatures would be exceptional (see also Chapter 1, E2). Not too infrequently, however, hemorrhagic, necrotizing, or gangrenescent changes can be observed (see also Chapter 33, A13). In former times shingles affected mainly adults, but today juvenile patients with herpes zoster are observed. They should be carefully scrutinized for the presence of an underlying malignant dis-order. Other important diagnostic criteria are, besides unilateral involvement and segmental extension, remarkable neuralgic complaints (see also Chapter 5, B1), which should suggest herpes zoster alone among all other blistering eruptions. The enlargement of the regional lymph nodes is, on the contrary, an uncertain sign, especially if it has to be distinguished from herpes simplex. An important prognostic sign is the aberration of single blisters *(herpes zoster generalisatus seu varicellosus)*, which sometimes first occurs several days later. It is usually associated with a disturbance of the immune resistance (leukoses, reticulogranulomatoses, and dysproteinemias, among others). Generalized herpes zoster may simulate varicella, unless there is still an original conspicuous segmentary limitation. Moreover, the "map of stars" of varicella has stages yet is more polymorphous than the generalized herpes zoster. The preeruptive or posteruptive diagnosis of herpes zoster is especially difficult if it is seen for the first time when pain alone is present. Because of its segmentary limitation this pain can simulate pleurisy, otitis, cholecystitis, cystitis, or other conditions.[59]

15. The sweat retention syndrome of **miliaria** is caused by the keratotic plug of the sweat gland duct in a single lesion. According to the site or level of such sweat gland retention one can differentiate miliarias crystallina (sudamina), rubra, and pustulosa or profunda. The manifestations differ; if sweat secretion is increased (sunlight without wind) or in feverish patients without sufficient sweating, explosive and irregularly distributed groups of many water-clear or slightly turbid blisters appear; they are of pinhead size and soon dry up. Such phenomena can be observed under adhesive tape dressings. The usual site of miliaria is the trunk, whereas the face is almost always spared. A further characteristic is the appearance of small blisters with no general or perifocal base reaction. Subjectively, moderate itching or "prickly" skin may be present. Secondary infections (Staphylococci and Candida species) (Fig. 450) can cause redness and pustules.

(1) ANTON-LAMPRECHT, I., und A. BERSCH: Histopathologie und Ultrastruktur der Haut bei Protoporphyrinämie. Virchows Arch. path. Anat. Abt. A *352:* 75–89 (1971).

(2) ARBUTHNOTT, J. P., J. KENT, A. LYELL and C. G. GEMMEL: Studies of staphylococcal toxins in relation to toxic epidermal necrolysis (the scalded skin syndrome). Brit. J. Derm. *86:* Suppl. *8:* 35–39 (1972).

(3) ASBOE-HANSEN, G.: Bullous keratogenous and pigmentary dermatitis with blood eosinophilia in newborn girls. Arch. Derm. Syph. (Chic.) *67:* 152–157 (1953).

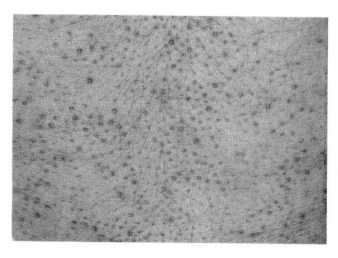

Fig. 450. Miliaria rubra.

(4a) BARTHELMES, H.: Zur Immunologie der blasenbildenden Dermatosen. 1. Mitt.: Der Parapemphigus (bullöses Pemphigoid von Lever) und die kombinierte Immunofluoreszenzmethode. Derm. Mschr. *155:* 507–517 (1969).

(4b) BEAN, S. F., M. WAISMAN, B. MICHEL, CH. I. THOMAS, J. M. KNOX and M. LEVINE: Cicatricial pemphigoid. Immunofluorescent studies. Arch. Derm. (Chic.) *106:* 195–199 (1972).

(5) BEUTNER, E. H., R. E. JORDON and T. P. CHORZELSKI: The immunopathology of pemphigus and bullous pemphigoid. J. invest. Derm. *51:* 63–80 (1968).

(6) CARNEY, R. G., and R. G. CARNEY jr.: Incontinentia pigmenti. Arch. Derm. (Chic.) *102:* 157–162 (1970).

(7) CORMANE, R. H., and D. PETZOLDT: Immunofluorescence studies on the affinity of pemphigus antibodies to epithelial intercellular substances. Dermatologica (Basel) *140:* 1–8 (1970).

(8) COTTINI, G. B.: Dermatite herpétiforme de Dühring symétrique et localisée aux genoux et aux coudes. Ann. Derm. Syph. (Paris) *82:* 285–286 (1955).

(9) CULLMANN, B., R. DENK und H. HOLZMANN: Zur Häufung von Farbensinnstörungen bei der Porphyria cutanea tarda (Waldenström). Albrecht v. Graefes Arch. Ophthal. *170:* 201–208 (1966).

(10) DEGOS, R., R. TOURAINE, B. KALIS, J. DELORT et D. BONVALET: Porphyrie cutanée tardive après prise prolongée de contraceptifs oraux. Ann. Derm. Syph. (Paris) *96:* 5–14 (1969).

(11) DENK, R.: Elektrokardiographische Untersuchungen bei Hautkranken. Arch. Kreisl.-Forsch. *60:* 33–114 (1969).

(12) DENK, R., und H. HOLZMANN: Paraneoplastische Porphyria cutanea tarda. Med. Welt *20* (N. F.): 1446–1447 (1969).

(13) DICK, H. M., N. G. FRASER and D. MURRAY: Immunofluorescent antibody studies in dermatitis herpetiformis. Brit. J. Derm. *81:* 692–696 (1969).

(14) DONALDSON, E. M., A. J. McCALL, I. A. MAGNUS, J. R. SIMPSON, R. A. CALDWELL and T. HARGREAVES: Erythropoietic protoporphyria: two deaths from hepatic cirrhosis. Brit. J. Derm. *84:* 14–24 (1971).

(15) EHLERS, G., I. GOLDSCHALD und W. KRAUSE: Ichthyosis linearis circumflexa Comèl mit bullöser Variation. Z.

Haut- u. Geschl.-Kr. *44:* [129]–[134] (1969).

(16) EISEN, A. Z.: Human skin collagenase: relationship to the pathogenesis of epidermolysis bullosa dystrophica. J. invest. Derm. *52:* 449–453 (1969).

(17) FRASER, N. G., D. MURRAY and J. O. D. ALEXANDER: Structure and function of the small intestine in dermatitis herpetiformis. Brit. J. Derm. *79:* 509–518 (1967).

(18) HEILMEYER, L.: Porphyria congenita (Günthersche Krankheit). Dtsch. med. Wschr. *88:* 2476–2478 (1963).

(19) HEITE, H.-J., M. IHL und M. WEBER: Zur Abgrenzung des Syndroma mucocutaneo-oculare acutum Fuchs vom Erythema exsudativum multiforme. Arch. klin. exp. Derm. *207:* 354–376 (1958).

(20) HOLUBAR, K.: Zur Bedeutung der Immunfluoreszenz in der Dermatologie. Z. Haut- u. Geschl.-Kr. *45:* 113–120 (1970).

(21) HUNTER, J. A. A., S. A. KHAN, E. HOPE, A. D. BEATTIE, G. W. BEVERIDGE, A. W. M. SMITH and A. GOLDBERG: Hereditary coproporphyria. Photosensitivity, jaundice and neuropsychiatric manifestations associated with pregnancy. Brit. J. Derm. *84:* 301–310 (1971).

(22) IPPEN, H.: Porphyria cutanea tarda. Arch. klin. exp. Derm. *208:* 223–259 (1959).

(23) JABLONSKA, S., und T. CHORZELSKI: Kann das histologische Bild die Grundlage zur Differenzierung des Morbus Duhring mit dem Pemphigoid und Erythema multiforme darstellen ? Derm. Wschr. *146:* 590–603 (1962).

(24) JABLONSKA, S., T. CHORZELSKI, E. H. BEUTNER and M. BLASZCZYK: Juvenile dermatitis herpetiformis in the light of immunofluorescence studies. Brit. J. Derm. *85:* 307–313 (1971).

(25) KALKOFF, K. W.: Zur Nosologie und Ätiologie des Syndrom muco-cutaneo-oculare acutum Fuchs. In: Haut- und innere Krankheiten. Symposium d. Schweiz. Akad. d. Med. Wiss. S. 427–440. Schwabe, Basel, Stuttgart 1968.

(26) KEINING, E., und H. WOHNLICH: Epidermolysis bullosa hereditaria hyperplastica. Derm. Wschr. *127:* 418–426 (1953).

(27) KLUNKER, W.: Zur nosologischen Stellung der Epidermolysis bullosa hereditaria letalis Herlitz (mit Kasuistik). Arch. klin. exp. Derm. *216:* 74–100 (1963).

(28) KORTING, G. W.: Zur Kenntnis der sog. rezidivierenden Blasen-Eruption an den Füßen bei heißem Wetter (Weber-Cockayne). Z. Haut- u. Geschl.-Kr. *17:* 36–40 (1954).

(29) KORTING, G. W.: Über Oesophagusstenosen bei Epidermolysis bullosa. Z. Haut- u. Geschl.-Kr. *22:* 282–285 (1957).

(30) KORTING, G. W., und H. HOLZMANN: Universelle Epidermolysis acuta toxica. Arch. klin. exp. Derm. *210:* 1–13 (1960).

(31) KRAPP, R.: Morbus Darier mit bullösem Exanthem und exogener Psychose. Med. Welt *21* (N. F.): 250–251 (1970).

(32) KRESBACH, H., und A. HARTWAGNER: Zur Differentialdiagnose zwischen Dermatitis herpetiformis Duhring und bullösem Pemphigoid. Z. Haut- u. Geschl.-Kr. *43:* 165–176 (1968).

(33) KÚTA, A., und E. NEUMANN: Porohyperkeratosis bullosa. Dermatologica (Basel) *122:* 90–102 (1961).

(34) LANGHOF, H., H. MÜLLER und L. RIETSCHEL: Untersuchungen zur familiären, protoporphyrinämischen Lichturticaria. Arch. klin. exp. Derm. *212:* 506–518 (1961).

(35) LANGHOF, H., und L. RIETSCHEL: Zur Pathogenese der Melanodermitis toxica. Derm. Wschr. *146:* 481–484 (1962).

(36) LAPIÈRE, S.: Les génodermatoses hyperkératosiques de type bulleux. Ann. Derm. Syph. (Paris) *80:* 597–614 (1953).

(37) LAPIÈRE, S.: »Bullous pemphigoid« de Lever et dermatite herpétiforme de Dühring-Brocq. Dermatologica (Basel) *135:* 46–53 (1967).

(38) LAPIÈRE, S., S. CASTERMANS-ELIAS und H. FIRKET: Elektronenmikroskopische Untersuchungen über die Ultrastruktur der Epidermolysis bullosa letalis bei einem Säugling mit familiärer Belastung. Hautarzt *15:* 30–33 (1964).

(39) LEVER, W. F.: Differentialdiagnose zwischen Pemphigus vulgaris, bullösem Pemphigoid und Dermatitis herpetiformis. Med. Klin. *62:* 1173–1176 (1967).

(40) LOEWENTHAL, L. J. A.: Localized dermatitis herpetiformis (Cottini type). Minerva derm. *34:* 300–301 (1959).

(41) LUNDER, M.: Epidermolysis bullosa »acquisita«. Hautarzt *21:* 553–554 (1970).

(42) LYELL, A.: Toxic epidermal necrolysis: an eruption resembling scalding of the skin. Brit. J. Derm. *68:* 355–361 (1956).

(43) MENDES DA COSTA, S., und J. W. VAN DER VALK: Typus maculatus der bullösen hereditären Dystrophie. Arch. Derm. Syph. (Wien, Leipzig) *91:* 1–8 (1908).

(44) MISGELD, V.: Immunfluorescenzuntersuchungen in der klinischen und experimentellen Dermatologie. »Atypische« blasenbildende Dermatosen. Arch. Derm. Forsch. *242:* 55–69 (1971).

(45) NASEMANN, T.: Die Infektionen durch das Herpes simplex-Virus. Fischer, Jena 1965.

(46) NIEDERLE, J.: Akute toxische Epidermolyse (Lyell-Syndrom). Dtsch. med. Wschr. *93:* 1005–1013 (1968).

(47) ORFANOS, C. E., H. GARTMANN und G. MAHRLE: Zur Pathogenese des Pemphigus erythematosus. Übergang eines chronischen discoiden Erythematodes in einen Pemphigus erythematosus (Senear-Usher). Arch. Derm. Forsch. *240:* 317–333 (1971).

(48) PIÉRARD, J., and I. WHIMSTER: The histological diagnosis of dermatitis herpetiformis, bullous pemphigoid and erythema multiforme. Brit. J. Derm. *73:* 253–266 (1961).

(49) PÖHLER, H.: Ein Fall von benignem Schleimhautpemphigoid mit Hautbeteiligung. Z. Haut- u. Geschl.-Kr. *45:* 207–214 (1970).

(50) PRAKKEN, J. R., and M. J. WOERDEMAN: »Pemphigoid« (Para-Pemphigus): its relationship to other bullous dermatoses. Brit. J. Derm. *67:* 92–97 (1955).

(51) RAAB, W.: Diagnose der Porphyrinstoffwechselstörungen. Med. Klin. *64:* 1993–1999 (1969).

(52) ROENIGK, H. H., and M. E. GOTTLOB: Estrogen-induced Porphyria cutanea tarda. Arch. Derm. (Chic.) *102:* 260–266 (1970).

(53) ROENIGK, H. H., J. G. RYAN and W. F. BERGFELD: Epidermolysis bullosa acquisita. Report of three cases and review of all published cases. Arch. Derm. (Chic.) *103:* 1–10 (1971).

(54) SCHIMPF, A.: Dermatitis herpetiformis (Duhring), zeitweise mit isoliertem Schleimhautbefall. Arch. klin. exp. Derm. *220:* 250–260 (1964).

(55) SCHNYDER, U. W., und D. EICHHOFF:
Zur Klinik und Genetik der dominant-
dystrophischen Epidermolysis bullosa
hereditaria. Arch. klin. exp. Derm. *218:*
62–90 (1964).

(56) SHKLAR, G., and PH. L. MCCARTHY:
Oral lesions of mucous membrane pemphigoid. Arch. Otolaryngol. (Chic.) *93:*
354–364 (1971).

(57) STICH, W., H. J. KARL, D. SCHMIDT,
L. RAITH und D. HUHN: Porphyria
erythropoetica lenta. Eine neue Form
der Porphyrie mit hämolytischer Anämie. Schweiz. med. Wschr. *98:* 1687–
1690 (1968).

(58) SUURMOND, D., J. VAN STEVENINCK and
L. N. WENT: Some clinical and fundamental aspects of erythropoietic protoporphyria. Brit. J. Derm. *82:* 323–328
(1970).

(59) TAPPEINER, J., und K. WOLFF: Zoster.
Fischer, Jena 1968.

(60) TAUGNER, M., U. W. SCHNYDER und
J. ROSSBACH: Jodid-Reagibilität der
Haut und Bromthalein-Retention bei
der Dermatitis herpetiformis Duhring.
Dermatologica (Basel) *139:* 260–265
(1969).

(61) VOGEL, A., und U. W. SCHNYDER: Fein-
strukturelle Untersuchungen an Rezes-
siv-Dystrophischer Epidermolysis Bullosa Hereditaria. Dermatologica (Basel)
135: 149–172 (1967).

(62) WALDENSTRÖM, J., und B. HAEGER-
ARONSEN: Das klinische und biochemische Bild bei den verschiedenen Porphyrien. Münch. med. Wschr. *106:* 1333–
1342 (1964).

(63) WESENER, G.: Beitrag zur Kenntnis der
sogenannten rezidivierenden Blasen-
eruption an den Füßen bei heißem Wetter (Weber-Cockayne) (Summer eruption of the feet), Epidermolysis bullosa
tarda (Epidermolysis bullosa pedum et
manuum aestivalis), Epidermolysis bullosa Weber-Cockayne. Derm. Wschr.
136: 1133–1137 (1957).

(64) WEY, W.: Über Ösophagusstenosen bei
der Epidermolysis bullosa hereditaria
dystrophica s. polydysplastica. Pract.
Oto-rhino-laryng. (Basel) *26:* 29–39
(1964).

(65) WOENCKHAUS, J. W., und D. KLEMM:
Muskuläre Beteiligung beim Erythema
exsudativum multiforme majus (Stevens-Johnson-Syndrom). Med. Klin. *61:*
1423–1424 (1966).

(66) WOERDEMAN, M. J.: Dystrophia bullosa
hereditaria, typus maculatus. Acta
Dermato-venereol., Proc. 11. internat.
Congr. Dermat. *1957:* Vol. III, S. 678–
686.

B. Dermatoses Forming Blisters Secondarily

In this chapter we will discuss those dermatoses in which single lesions only rarely or exceptionally change into blisters.

1. The blister formation of the usually papular or urticarial insect-bite reaction is a very common event. In general, **bullous culicosis** is present on the legs in the form of one or a few tensely filled blisters (Fig. 451). Since a common erythema may be absent, the uninitiated may take this eruption for chronic pemphigus vulgaris.

2. Blisters without accompanying erythema are found occasionally on the legs and feet of **diabetic patients.** These blisters develop intraepidermally, but without signs of acantholysis. Although these diabetics usually suffer at the same time from diabetic neuropathy, the blisters do not originate from an unnoticed mechanical irritation.[1, 3, 16]

3. The bullous variant of **lichen planus** develops, according to our own observations, either from already present typical lichen planus papules or on a previously unaffected site (Fig. 452). In the latter case the question of a more or less coincidental association of lichen planus with a genuine blistering dermatosis such as, most commonly, dermatitis herpetiformis or chronic pemphigus vulgaris may arise. Even the Nikolsky sign in such lichen planus

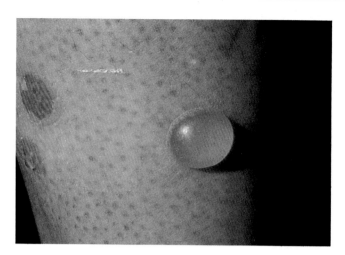

Fig. 451. Bullous culicosis.

patients may be positive near the blister. On the feet and toes bullous lichen planus tends toward more ulcerated destruction, whereas on the scalp, as in the Graham-Little syndrome, cicatricial alopecia may result. Bullous lichen planus is seldom found on the mucous membranes. Only if typical cutaneous and mucosal lesions are present on other sites is a correct diagnosis possible. Since blisters in this location tear open after a short while, one often sees only the usually multiple,

Fig. 452. Bullous lichen planus.

Fig. 453. Lichen sclerosus et atrophicus: rare bullous variety.

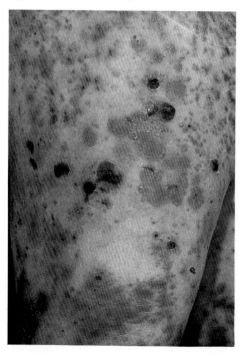

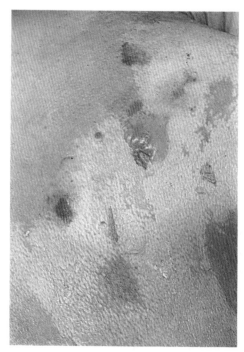

Fig. 454. Eosinophilic reticular hyperplasia with blister formation.

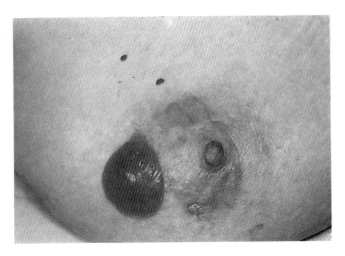

superficial ulcerations (see also Chapter 33, D19 and Chapter 35, B4). Histologically, we are dealing in general with subepidermal blister formation with suffusion in some places of the papillary body with eosinophils, although rather often even acantholysis or ballooning cells have been reported. Of practical importance in bullous lichen planus is the search for additional factors in the sense of a paraneoplastic syndrome, since according to recent observations malignant kidney, adrenal, or pituitary tumors may be present simultaneously.[5,10, 17, 19, 24]

4. Facultative blister formation in circumscribed scleroderma can be explained as increased edema. Such **bullous** or **pemphigoid morphea** occurs most frequently on the lower extremities and is more common in women than in men. Here again, ulcerations may develop. In so-called pseudobullous scleroderma distinct bullous blisters are missing as well as the clinical honeycomblike change due to the absence of subepidermal cleavage. Genuine and sometimes large epidermal bullae may also appear in the lesions of **lichen sclerosus et atrophicus,** but the basic disorder can always be diagnosed from the characteristic findings of porcelain-white, lentil-sized cutaneous indurations (Fig. 453).[8, 22]

5. Among the dermatoses with superimposed blisters **bullous urticaria** must be mentioned; this, however, is doubtless extremely rare. In **urticaria pigmentosa,** transitory bullous changes also occur. This is valid for generalized as well as solitary mastocytosis.[18, 21]

6. In unexplained blistering eruptions, a hematologic examination should be undertaken, since, particularly in chronic lymphatic **leukemia,** hemorrhagic-bullous lesions may be present. This may even happen in the aleukemic stage. In general, subepidermal as well as intraepidermal blisters favor the legs. Histologically, any leukocytic infiltration may be absent even in close proximity to blisters. Reports on bullous stages in reticulogranulomatoses (*mycosis fungoides* and malignant lymphogranulomatosis) are rare. Figure 454 shows blister formation in eosinophilic reticular hyperplasia. Since such blisters originate mostly from an infiltrated base, they may suggest bullous lesions of primary cutaneous **amyloidosis.** The diagnosis can be ascertained by the evidence of amyloid in the diseased skin. Since we are dealing with a localized form of amyloidosis, the inner organs remain completely uninvolved and a rectal biopsy is unnecessary.[4, 6, 9, 12, 20, 23]

7. Pemphigoid manifestations, including a positive Nikolsky sign, are found in **pellagra,** among the avitaminoses. According to our own observations we are dealing here mainly with superficially situated, subcorneal epidermal cleavage, but subepidermal blister formations also occur. In such cases there are changes of the keratohyaline layer with loosening of small pieces of coarse keratohyaline.[15]

8. The Guinea or **Medina worm,** the nematode *Dracunculus medinensis,* causes pemphigoid blisters of about 2 to 3 cm in diameter at the site of penetration (ankles, arms, scrotum, buttocks, and backs of water-carriers). Some constitutional signs such as nausea, fever, and urticaria also occur. The blisters soon rupture and leave flat ulcerations, which result in edematization of the surrounding skin. Occasionally, one can palpate the (female) adult worm as a bandlike thickening. If not removed,

Fig. 455. Barbiturate intoxication: bullous toxic eruption.

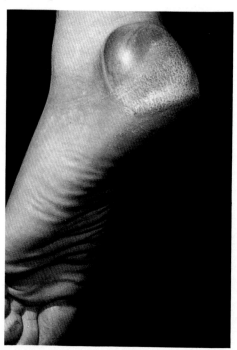

it can lead to chronic pustulation, cyst formation, or calcification (see also Chapter 14, B13).

9. Characteristic also are the blister formations following **barbiturate poisoning.** In most cases the eruption appears 24 to 48 hours after the onset of the poisoning, but the first skin manifestations may become visible as late as eight days afterward. They are not primarily blisters but begin with bluish-red, sometimes elevated infiltrations which may become as large as the palm of the hand (Fig. 455). The number of these eruptions is small, and one rarely encounters more than five or six. Before the blister swells, dark cyanosis of the center of the lesion appears. Locations on the trunk and the extremities are common, whereas the head almost always remains free. Since the generalized signs are so much more important, the blisters rarely attract attention; prolonged bed rest or secondary infections, therefore, may lead to deep ulcerations, which will heal only after many weeks.

Bullous reactions of intolerance may occur after ingestion of *nalidixic acid.* These reactions are brown-red erythemas with large central blisters (Fig. 456) which heal with hyperpigmentations and scar formation. It is characteristic that the blisters occur principally on the exposed parts of the body such as the arms, legs, face, and neck. When asking the patient his history, it should be kept in mind that nalidixic acid may have been ingested several weeks previously.[2]

Blisters may also occur in **carbon monoxide intoxication.** Furthermore, in brain disorders caused by disturbed circulation, as in paresis, bullous skin changes can also occur.[7, 11]

10. With the onset of more intense exposure to sunlight in the spring, children and adolescents may experience the

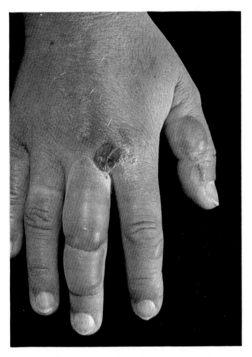

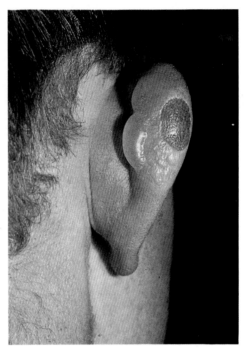

Fig. 456. Blisterous skin changes after taking nalidixic acid.

Fig. 457. Spring perniosis.

development of blisters on the rim of the auricle of the ear. These are the so-called **spring pernioses,** which belong to the group of polymorphous light eruptions. Besides light, cold probably plays a certain etiologic role. The rather characteristic blisters on the rim of one or both helices are surrounded by a distinct basal erythema (Fig. 457). In addition, edematously suffused erythemas and papules of various sizes may be present on the face, neck, and the backs of the hands. Increased porphyrin excretion in the urine or stool or increased intraerythrocytic porphyrin concentrations are absent. Likewise, antinuclear factors as well as immune fluorescent serologic phenomena in the basal membrane zone are not present. In the differential diagnosis second degree frostbite is ruled out without difficulty. In contrast to spring perniosis, no increased light sensitivity can be proved in frostbite. With regard to the localization on the concha, one may have to consider the extremely rare bullous *chronic discoid lupus erythematosus.* This diagnosis must be confirmed histologically.[13, 14]

(1) ALLEN, E. G., and D. R. HADDEN: Bullous lesions of the skin in diabetes. Brit. J. Derm. *82:* 216–220 (1970).

(2) BREHM, G., und G. W. KORTING: Bullöse Hautreaktion auf Nalidixinsäure. Med. Welt *21* (N. F.): 423–426 (1970).

(3) CANTWELL, A. R., and W. MARTZ: Idiopathic bullae in diabetics. Arch. Derm. (Chic.) *96:* 42–44 (1967).

(4) CHOW, C., and R. E. BURNS: Bullous Amyloidosis. Arch. Derm (Chic.) *95:* 622–625 (1967).

(5) CRAM, D. L., R. R. KIERLAND and R. K. WINKELMANN: Ulcerative lichen planus of the feet. Arch. Derm. (Chic.) *93:* 692–701 (1966).

(6) DEGOS, R., E. LORTAT-JACOB et J. DURAND: Leucémie lymphoïde chronique. Manifestations bulleuses atypiques. Bull. Soc. franç. Derm. Syph. *61:* 121–122 (1954).

(7) FRANKL, J., und E. KÖRNYEY: Blasen als trophische Hautveränderungen bei kreislaufbedingten Hirnveränderungen. Hautarzt *16:* 172–174 (1965).

(8) GARB, J., and CH. F. SIMS: Scleroderma with bullous lesions. Dermatologica (Basel) *119:* 341–359 (1959).

(9) GARB, J., and F. WISE: Mycosis fungoides with bullous lesion: Report of a case resistant to roentgen and arsenical therapy: Effects of empiric therapy, partly based on laboratory investigations. Arch. Derm. Syph. (Chic.) *48:* 359–368 (1943).

(10) GRÜNEBERG, T.: Das Lichen-ruber-Pemphigoid. Derm. Wschr. *136:* 1238–1242 (1957).

(11) HOLTEN, C.: Cutaneous phenomena in acute barbiturate poisoning. Acta derm.-venereol. (Stockh.) *32,* Suppl. *29:* 162–168 (1952).

(12) HURIEZ, C., F. DESMONS, P. AGACHE, M. BENOIT et M. BONBART: Manifestation bulleuse au cours d'une leucémie lymphoïde. Bull. Soc. franç. Derm. Syph. *68:* 287–290 (1961).

(13) KEINING, E.: Die »Frühlingsperniosis« zum Unterschied von der Herbstperniosis. Derm. Wschr. *110:* 20–35 (1940).

(14) KOGOJ, F.: Über eine blasige Abart des Erythematodes discoides. Dermatologica (Basel) *117:* 325–335 (1958).

(15) KORTING, G. W.: Pemphigoide Pellagra mit Hautnervenveränderungen. Arch. klin. exp. Derm. *208:* 81–92 (1958).

(16) KORTING, G. W.: Lokalisierte pemphigoide Reaktion im Unterschenkelbereich bei Diabetes mellitus gravis. Pseudo-Klinefelter-Syndrom. Derm. Wschr. *139:* 474 (1959).

(17) MAGNUSSON, B.: Lichen ruber bullosus and tumours in internal organs. Dermatologica (Basel) *134:* 166–172 (1967).

(18) VAN DER MEIREN, L., et G. ACHTEN: Étude clinique et histiologique de l'urticaire bulleuse. Ann. Derm. Syph. (Paris) *82:* 267–276 (1955).

(19) MIDANA, A., et G. ZINA: Lichen ruber pemphigoïdes: manifestation para-néoplasique? Dermatologica (Basel) *140:* 36–44 (1970).

(20) NORTHOVER, J. M., J. D. PICKARD, I. M. MURRAY-LYON, D. G. PRESBURY, R. HASKELL and D. A. KEITH: Bullous lesions of the skin and mucous membranes in primary amyloidosis. Postgrad. med. J. *48:* 351–353 (1972).

(21) ORKIN, M., R. A. GOOD, C. C. CLAWSON, I. FISHER and D. B. WINDHORST: Bullous mastocytosis. Arch. Derm. (Chic.) *101:* 547–564 (1970).

(22) POIARES BAPTISTA, A., A. BASTOS ARAUJO et J. CORTESAO: Sclérodermie bulleuse en plaques. Ann. Derm. Syph. (Paris) *95:* 29–38 (1968).

(23) ROENIGK, H. H., and A. J. CASTROVINCI: Mycosis fungoides bullosa. Arch. Derm. (Chic.) *104:* 402–406 (1971).

(24) SHKLAR, G.: Lichen planus as an oral ulcerative disease. Oral Surg. (St. Louis) *33:* 376–388 (1972).

26. Pustular Dermatoses

A. Pustular Psoriasis

Pustular exanthems occurring with infectious diseases are discussed in Chapter 18, C. Manifestations of psoriasis not of the vulgaris type will be discussed with the several forms of pustular psoriasis. Even psoriasis vulgaris shows a pustular element histologically as an intraepidermal neutrophilic (Munro) abscess. **Generalized pustular psoriasis** in most cases develops from common but often atypical psoriasis. Although the tendency to scaling diminishes, there is an increase of the exudative character with the development of at first sterile pustules in exanthematic distribution. These eruptions often start with or are accompanied by an increase in body temperature (see also Chapter 1, C1). On the trunk and the proximal part of the extremities, pustules may appear within a few hours and soon become confluent (Fig. 1). Some patients show pustular and febrile attacks with a certain rhythmic character, while other patients during the course of the disease finally develop continuous fever with erythroderma and cachexia. Although cytostatic drugs and corticosteroids bring the temperature down to normal, antibiotics have no effect because of the abacterial genesis of pustular psoriasis.[1, 9]

However, if there is a condition of pustulation caused by local irritation following and depending on therapeutic trials, one speaks of **psoriasis with formation of pustules.** In such cases, which are usually without universal spread, the early pustules may no longer be sterile.

Impetigo herpetiformis (pustular psoriasis during pregnancy) consists of groups of pustules on an inflammatory, edematous base with formation of annular or serpiginous figures. Pustular erythroderma does not develop, but the pustules remain localized, appearing as multiple individual areas. The oral mucosa or vulva is frequently involved in the clinical picture. This type of pustular psoriasis can be observed also in nonpregnant women, while, on the other hand, during pregnancy psoriasis vulgaris can change at any time into generalized pustular psoriasis. In our opinion, impetigo herpetiformis is neither a typical dermatosis of pregnancy nor does the hormonal change play a decisive role in its genesis. Although hypocalcemia is often considered a diagnostic factor, it is an irregular finding; it is seen with the same frequency with other pustular variants of psoriasis. Histologically, there is no difference between impetigo herpetiformis and pustular psoriasis.

The differential diagnosis must consider (in the absence of a history or typical lesions of psoriasis vulgaris in addition to the pustular manifestations) extensive moniliasis, bacterids, and follicular pyodermas of exogenous origin. Herpes gestationis, the variant of dermatitis herpetiformis that occurs during pregnancy, however, is principally a polymorphous, almost always papulovesicular, and seldom purely pustular dermatosis; it frequently begins as pruritus without cutaneous manifestations. The important differentiation from subcorneal pustulosis will be discussed later in Section G.[1, 8]

A psoriatic with pustules confined to palms or soles has **pustular palmar and plantar psoriasis** (Fig. 458). This diagnosis requires the presence of other psoriatic lesions, the primarily sterile contents of pustules, and the histologic finding of a spongiform pustule. If these criteria are not present, one should speak only of palmar and plantar pustulosis. Like generalized pustular psoriasis, but restricted to the locations just mentioned (palms and soles), preexisting psoriatic erythemas may show pustules within a short time. Except for local sensations, general signs are always lacking. The thenar eminences and

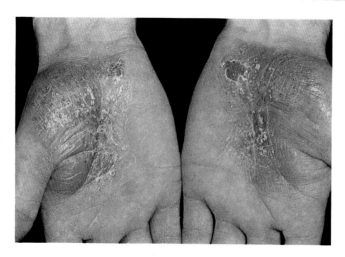

Fig. 458. Pustular psoriasis of the palms.

terminal phalanges of the fingers are typical locations for pustules, whereas an extension to the backs of the hands should raise doubts about the diagnosis and suggest a secondary bacterial or fungal infection. However, if the tips of the fingers or, more rarely, of the toes present pustules, a diagnosis of **acrodermatitis continua suppurativa** (Hallopeau) should be entertained. The primary lesion of this distinctly characteristic acropustulosis consists of a strictly subcorneal pustular vesicle, which according to the observation of the patient develops "spontaneously" with burning and stinging. Subsequently, new pustules appear in crops again and again on the terminal phalanges of other fingers and toes. Furthermore, the continuous attacks of pustular outbreaks result in exhaustion of the regenerative powers of the affected cutaneous areas, which appear subacutely erythematous and thinned out. In addition, local osseous atrophy of the terminal phalanges may develop. Such atrophy does not justify, in our opinion, a decisive difference between acrodermatitis continua and pustular psoriasis palmaris and plantaris. We believe that acrodermatitis continua is the acral type of a palmoplantar pustular psoriasis. In addition, the so-called spongiform pustule (the spongelike net of swollen

epithelial cells and sometimes also of the stratum corneum with deposits of neutrophilic leukocytes) is seen with acrodermatitis continua, pustular palmar and plantar psoriasis, generalized pustular psoriasis, impetigo herpetiformis, and Reiter's disease; therefore, this spongiform pustule is simply a special form of Munro's abscess of psoriasis vulgaris.[2, 7]

(1) BAKER, H., and T. J. RYAN: Generalized pustular psoriasis; a clinical and epidemiological study of 104 cases. Brit. J. Derm. *80:* 771–793 (1968).

(2) BARBER, H. W.: Acrodermatitis continua vel perstans (Dermatitis repens) and psoriasis pustulosa. Brit. J. Derm. *42:* 500–518 (1930).

(3) EISENMAN, H. T., and G. R. MIKHAIL: Pustular psoriasis of the scalp. Arch. Derm. (Chic.) *100:* 598–600 (1969).

(4) ENFORS, W., and L. MOLIN: Pustulosis palmaris et plantaris; a follow-up study of a ten-year material. Acta derm.-venereol. (Stockh.) *51:* 289–294 (1971).

(5) HELLGREN, L., and H. MOBACKEN: Pustulosis palmaris et plantaris; prevalence, clinical observations and prognosis. Acta derm.-venereol. (Stockh.) *51:* 284–288 (1971).

(6) HORNSTEIN, O. P.: Pustulöse Zustände an Handtellern und Fußsohlen, ihre Differentialdiagnose und Therapie. Fort-

schr. der prakt. Derm. und Venerol. Bd. VI, S. 156–167. Springer, Berlin, New York, Heidelberg 1970.

(7) KEINING, E., und H. JUNG-GRIMM: Über Akrodermatitis continua suppurativa Hallopeau inversa. Derm. Wschr. *136:* 900–909 (1957).

(8) SOLTERMANN, W.: Familiäre Psoriasis pustulosa unter dem Bilde der Impetigo herpetiformis. Dermatologica (Basel) *116:* 313–330 (1958).

(9) ZAUN, H.: Psoriasis pustulosa vom Typ Zumbusch. Arch. klin. exp. Derm. *221:* 85–96 (1964).

B. Pustular Bacterid (Palmoplantar Pustulosis)

Pustular bacterid is the name given to pustular eruptions of the volar aspects of the hands and soles without manifestations of psoriasis and with no lesions at the tips of the fingers and toes. However, as with pustular psoriasis the primary pustule must be sterile. Characteristically resisting any therapy, the closely adjacent pustules develop simultaneously on an erythematous base and symmetrically on the palms and soles. During the eruptive phase a few vesicles may appear in addition to the pustules. The difference in location makes possible a clear distinction from acrodermatitis continua. In addition to the numerous vesicles or pustules and brown spots ("honeycomblike structure of the epidermis") of the pustular bacterid, there is a faintly saturated, lacquer-red basic erythema. The disease progresses in chronically recurrent crops, without preference for either sex; practically all patients belong to the middle age group. Frequently, foci of infection can be found within the ear, nose, and throat region or around the teeth. However, the removal of such foci has no influence on the course of the disease. Histologically, one sees mostly unicameral, deeply situated, intraepidermal pustular spaces surrounded by epithelium on all sides; these spaces are not only conspicuous by their uncommon size but also by the almost complete absence of inflammatory reaction of the adjoining tissue. Spongiform pustules are lacking.[1–5]

(1) ANDREWS, G. C., F. W. BIRKMAN and R. J. KELLY: Recalcitrant pustular eruptions of the palms and soles. Arch. Derm. Syph. (Chic.) *29:* 548–563 (1934).

(2) ENFORS, W., and L. MOLIN: Pustulosis palmaris et plantaris; a follow-up study of a ten-year material. Acta Derm.-Venereol. (Stockh.) *51:* 289–294 (1971).

(3) HELLGREN, L., and H. MOBACKEN: Pustulosis palmaris et plantaris; prevalence, clinical observations and prognosis. Acta Derm.-Venereol. (Stockh.) *51:* 284–288 (1971).

(4) HORNSTEIN, O. P.: Pustulöse Zustände an Handtellern und Fußsohlen, ihre Differentialdiagnose und Therapie. Fortschr. der prakt. Derm. und Venerol. Bd. VI, S. 156–167. Springer, Berlin, New York, Heidelberg 1970.

(5) VELTMAN, G., und H. SCHUERMANN: Das Bakteriid von Andrews. Arch. klin. exp. Derm. *215:* 326–361 (1962).

C. Dyshidrosis

The differential diagnosis of the previously mentioned pustular dermatoses of palms and soles must include mycoses, dermatophytids, or **dyshidrosis** (cheiropompholyx). The dyshidrosiform eruptions occur as grouped vesicles (Fig. 459), less often as pustules (bacterial superinfection) within an erythematous base. The multicameral vesicles appear at first as firm globules deeply located in the epidermis; they are slightly transparent, pinhead- to matchhead-sized elevations that typically begin along the sides of the fingers with definite sensations of tenseness and pruritus. After the originally clear watery vesicles of dyshidrosis begin to dry

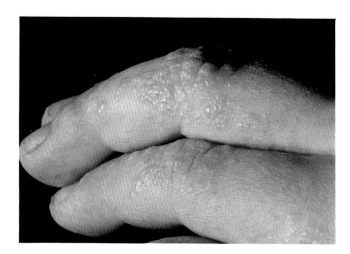

Fig. 459. Dyshidrosis.

up, a dry, rufflike, circular, small, scaly lesion results, called dyshidrosis lamellosa sicca. Clinically characteristic of a vesiculo-pustular dermatophytid, however, is the fact that in fresh groups of vesicles the borders of the lesions are pronounced and have a tendency to central involution, whereas in a fresh outbreak of a pustular bacterid the central portions are more conspicuous. Seasonally, vesiculopustular dermatophytids will be seen mostly during hot humid weather. However, the same is true for dyshidrosiform eruptions also. Quite often there is an obvious connection between a primary fungal focus, as for instance an intertriginous or interdigital tinea infection. In contrast to the primary area of mycosis, the vesicles of a dermato-phytid practically never show any fungi. The primary lesion of dyshidrosis corre-sponds to the papulovesicle of an acute common eczema; however, the erythem-atous eczematous component recedes while the vesicular element becomes more prominent. This vesiculation is due in the main to the peculiar location (thick horny layer at the sides of the fingers). In addi-tion to the more frequent intradermal types of vesicles, primary vesicular forms occur also at acrosyringeal locations. Etio-logically the dyshidrotic syndrome at first appears to have a causal relationship with

dermatomycosis. After the latter has been excluded one has to consider the possi-bility of an acute common eczema of dys-hidrosiform character, a hematogenous eczematous eruption, or the influence of inhalent allergens, gastrointestinal dis-orders, or neurovegetative lability.[1]

(1) KORTING, G. W.: Zur Genese dyshidrosi-former Exantheme, insbesondere der genuinen Dyshidrosis. Berufsdermatosen *3:* 139–143 (1955).

D. Herpes Zoster, Chickenpox, Herpes Simplex

Herpes zoster lesions of the palm occur along the pathways of distribution of nerves from the posterior ganglia C6 to C8 (Fig. 460), and lesions of the sole are found along the distribution of L5 and S1. Morphologically, development of a unilat-eral group of vesicles preceded by an ery-thematous, edematous patch indicates herpes zoster. Radicular neurologic pain can precede, occur simultaneously with, or follow healing of the lesions. The virus of chickenpox is identical with that of herpes zoster; the varicella virus in its exanthematic spread does not involve the

Fig. 460. Herpes zoster of the palm.

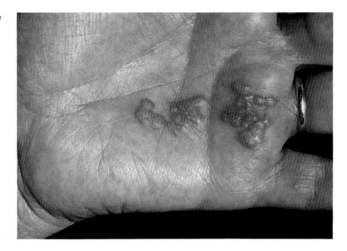

hands and feet. Areas of herpes simplex (Fig. 461) do not usually present segmental distribution and are not accompanied by neurologic pain; herpes simplex has a special tendency to recur (see also Chapter 25, A13). All three of these virus diseases produce primary vesicles which later become pustules.

E. Acrodermatitis Enteropathica

If **acrodermatitis enteropathica** shows a tendency to erythroderma it may sometimes resemble the universally generalized form of pustular psoriasis or acrodermatitis continua. The intestinal signs resembling celiac disease do not coincide at all with the cutaneous changes. Children of both sexes in the first few years of life are principally affected, sometimes at the time breast-feeding stops. The bilateral involvement of the acral parts of the extremities is conspicuous, as is the involvement of the vicinity of all body orifices. Quite often the erythematous areas are interspersed with many vesiculopustular elements.

In addition, pustular paronychias, dystrophies of the nails, and alopecias are present simultaneously. Less frequent is

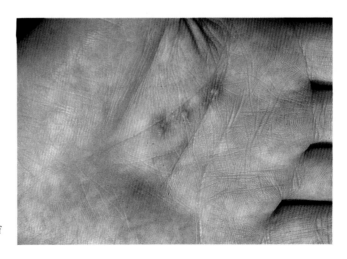

Fig. 461. Herpes simplex of the palm.

blepharoconjunctivitis with light sensitivity. The presence of *Candida albicans* on
all diseased areas and in the intestinal
tract is characteristic. The diagnosis of
this otherwise rather refractory and
prognostically serious disease can also be
made by a therapeutic trial with diiodo-
hydroxyquin.

There are further similarities between
acrodermatitis enteropathica, generalized
primary candidiasis, and impetiginous
generalized bacterial seborrheic eczema.
At some point the changes of palms and
soles consisting of hyperkeratotic, desquamating, and fissured erythemas may
resemble psoriasis. Also, quite often
disturbances in the growth of nails
(thickening, separation of nails, subungual
pustules) occur.[1-3]

(1) DANBOLT, N., und K. CLOSS: Akrodermatitis enteropathica. Acta derm.-venereol.
(Stockh.) *23:* 127–169 (1943).

(2) HEITE, H.-J., und R. ODY: Die Acrodermatitis enteropathica im Lichte der
Häufigkeitsanalyse. Hautarzt *16:* 529
bis 534 (1965).

(3) ROHDE, B., und M. JÄNNER: Zur Differentialdiagnose der Akrodermatitis enteropathica Danbolt-Closs. Derm. Wschr.
147: 196–205 (1963).

F. Reiter's Syndrome

Especially characteristic of **Reiter's
syndrome** are the hyperkera   changes
of the glans penis and the   taneous
squamous lesions of sole and   . These
"blenorrhagic keratoses" start initially
with circumscribed erythemas or papules
and soon change into exudative psoriasiform lesions arranged in groups. Some
plantar areas resemble a pigmented corn.
The appearance of pustules may make it
difficult to separate the condition from
pustular palmar and plantar psoriasis,
especially when the nails are frequently
involved at the same time (thickened,
friable nailplates with longitudinal ridges
and subungual horny masses causing
onycholysis) (see also Chapter 7, B2).

G. Subcorneal Pustulosis

Subcorneal pustulosis requires separation
from generalized pustular psoriasis. The
head, scalp, soles, and palms almost always
remain uninvolved, so that the most
extensive cutaneous changes are found
almost exclusively on the trunk and
intertriginous areas. Another peculiarity
of subcorneal pustulosis is in many cases

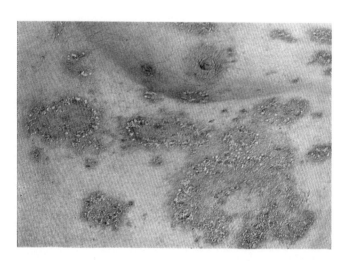

Fig. 462. Subcorneal pustulosis; polycyclic erythematous areas with superficial
pustules.

Fig. 463. Subcorneal pustulosis: subcorneal pustule.
HE stain, 100×.

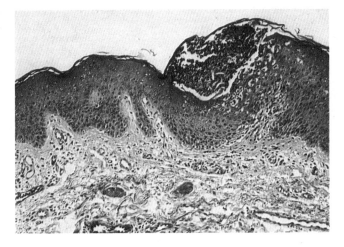

the craniocaudal course of the eruption. Single lesions at the time of the acute eruptive phase are primarily groups of vesicles or pustules which have a tendency to confluence and transformation into circinate, squamous-crusted areas (Figs. 462, 463). Like generalized pustular psoriasis, subcorneal pustulosis produces steeply rising temperatures at the time of a fresh pustular outbreak. A smear of fresh pustules shows many neutrophils, and, more rarely, eosinophils; the absence of bacterial or fungal elements is especially noteworthy. Examination of subcorneal pustulosis with indirect immunofluores-

cence has so far failed to show the typical pattern of fluorescence; this observation can be used to separate subcorneal pustulosis from pemphigoid or chronic pemphigus. Some areas of subcorneal pustulosis may resemble pemphigus foliaceus or seborrheic pemphigus; this may lead to certain differential diagnostic difficulties. Possibilities for differentiation are provided by the negative Nikolsky sign, the absence of mucous membrane involvement, and the histologic appearance. Seborrheic pemphigus favors cutaneous areas that have an abundant secretion of sweat and those that are exposed to light.[1-3]

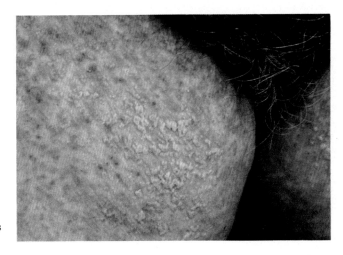

Fig. 464. Pustular Darier's
disease.

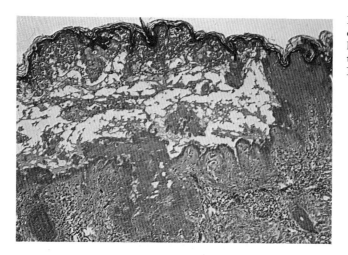

Fig. 465. Pustular Darier's disease: increased acantholytic cleft formation with transformation to blister. HE stain, 63 ×.

(1) KORTING, G. W., und R. DENK: Subkorneale pustulöse Dermatose bei einem Patienten mit ektopischem Pankreasgewebe im Magen. Med. Welt *17* (N. F.): 2256–2257 (1966).

(2) SCHIEFERSTEIN, G.: Zum Krankheitsbild der subcornealen pustulösen Dermatose (Sneddon-Wilkinson). Z. Haut- u. Geschl.-Kr. *44:* 45–56 (1969).

(3) WOLFF, K.: Ein Beitrag zur Nosologie der subcornealen pustulösen Dermatose (Sneddon-Wilkinson). Arch. klin. exp. Derm. *224:* 248–267 (1966).

Fig. 466. Pustular pyodermic scabies of the sole in a child.

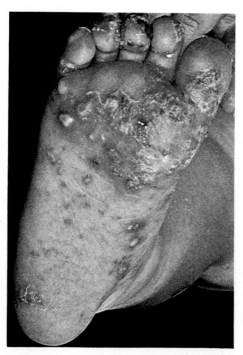

H. Dyskeratosis Follicularis (Darier's Disease)

At certain stages **dyskeratosis follicularis** may have a pronounced pustular aspect. The pustules favor the lower part of the abdomen and the intertriginous areas, where maceration and rapid bacterial dissemination can occur (Fig. 464, 465). This disposition to blister formation is easily understood if one considers the histomorphologic substrate of dyskeratosis and acantholysis in dyskeratosis follicularis. But in these cases it is always a question of pustular change in only a few lesions, so that the diagnosis is still evident from the remaining typical lesions (see also Chapter 29, A3).

(1) KRAPP, R.: Verlaufweise bullöser Morbus Darier mit exogener Psychose. Med. Welt *21* (N. F.): 250–251 (1970).

I. Scabies

Pustules of the palms or soles in small children suggests **scabies** (Fig.466), especially if the eruption is accompanied by violent itching. If one then examines the typical lesions in the interdigital spaces, axillae, and genitals, the diagnosis is not difficult (see also Chapter 2, G1).

K. Variola

Generalized monomorphous pustules with typical central umbilication occur in the suppurative stage of *variola vera* or generalized *eczema vaccinatum*. For more details see Chapter 1, E3 and Chapter 18, C2 and C3.[1]

(1) EHRENGUT, W.: Diagnostik der Pocken. Münch. med. Wschr. *115:* 10–12.(1973).

27. Ichthyoses

A diffuse keratosis should be called an ichthyosis only if, in addition to abnormally dry skin, scaling (possibly platelike or rhombic) is present. Hereditary and acquired types of ichthyosis must be distinguished. Hereditary ichthyosis can be subdivided into several types, which differ from each other. This classification is feasible because of the macro- and micromorphologic characteristic features.

A. Hereditary Ichthyoses

1. In autosomal recessive **ichthyosis congenita** cutaneous changes are present at birth or manifest themselves at the latest within the first months of life. According to the degree of ichthyosis and the chances of survival of the infant one distinguishes ichthyosis congenita, gravis, nitida, or tarda. A large number of patients have a more or less developed erythema, covered by scales like those of a fish. The sites of predilection of these keratoses are the flexor sides of the joints, the trunk, the neck, and, in most cases, also the face (Figs.467, 468). Palms and soles also show hyperkeratoses but the degree of their involvement differs greatly. The keratoses themselves may become so

exaggerated that their dirty gray to almost black color almost completely covers the basic erythema. Deep cracks and a bulging appearance contribute to the picture of crocodile skin. Simultaneously, articular contractures and the development of ectropion on the lips, lids, and

Fig. 467. Ichthyosis congenita.

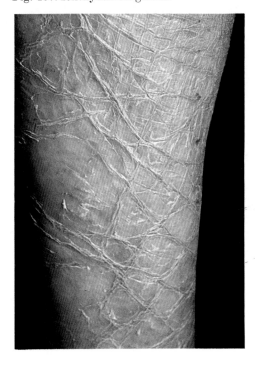

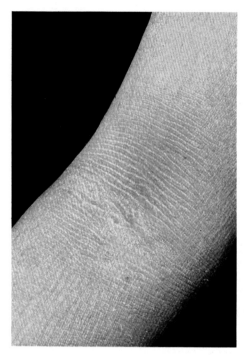

Fig. 468. Ichthyosis congenita: the flexor aspects of the joints are included in the disturbed keratinization.

labia set in. On the other hand, the keratoses may be very thinly lamellar – in which case the erythema becomes distinctly visible. Hairs and nails tend to grow luxuriously, but patients with hypotrichia have also been observed. In addition, there are many associated malformations such as microcephaly, oligophrenia, syndactylia, cardiac defects, small stature, and microphthalmia. Deeper lying corneal cloudiness, however, is always missing, thereby permitting a safe differentiation from X-chromosomal recessive ichthyosis.

Histologically, ichthyosis congenita is characterized by proliferative hyperkeratosis. The stratum corneum is irregularly widened and interspersed with island-forming parakeratoses. The stratum granulosum is normal or somewhat widened. Here one can recognize (most distinctly in follicular areas) perinuclear clearings and

irregularly enlarged keratohyaline granules. The cells, however, do not become loosened as in bullous congenital ichthyosiform erythroderma.

The differential diagnosis must include, above all, bullous ichthyosiform congenital erythroderma and ichthyosis vulgaris. In the former, the demonstration of blisters alone is not sufficient, since blisters may also be present in ichthyosis congenita; the histologic findings must also be evaluated (see also Chapter 22, A2). Ichthyosis vulgaris is easily diagnosed from the noninvolvement of the flexor sides of the joints.[1, 12, 22]

2. A variant of ichthyosis congenita is the so-called **collodion baby.** For the clinical findings and the phenocopies of this disease, see Chapter 22, A1.

3. Clinically and histologically, there are no differences in cutaneous changes between ichthyosis congenita and the **Sjögren-Larsson syndrome.** In the course of the first year disturbances of the pyramidal tracts appear and result in spasticity of all extremities, especially the legs. In addition, some patients show macular degeneration and exudative enteropathy. The transmission is autosomal recessive as in ichthyosis congenita.[15, 17, 29]

4. It has not yet been decided with certainty whether the autosomal recessive **Rud syndrome** is a disease entity. The dermatologic manifestations are similar to those of ichthyosis congenita. The clinical picture is supplemented by cerebral fits, hypogonadism, and mental and physical retardation.[8, 37]

5. In **X-chromosomal recessive ichthyosis** the clinical dermatologic picture is not unequivocal, but sometimes it simulates ichthyosis congenita and other times ichthyosis vulgaris, so that the criterion of noninvolvement or involvement of the flexor aspects of the joints does not help in arriving at a diagnosis. In rare instances a less pronounced collodion skin may even be present at birth. Palms and soles, however, remain uninvolved, in contrast to other forms of ichthyosis. Likewise missing are follicular keratoses, which almost always accompany ichthyosis vulgaris on the arms, buttocks, and thighs, although with variable expression. Malformations of the ears, teeth, and skeleton, and mental retardation are absent in X-chromosomal recessive ichthyosis. On the other hand, almost all patients who manifest the disorder as well as latent carriers show evidence of deep-seated corneal cloudiness. Histologically, X-chromosomal recessive ichthyosis differs from (dominant) ichthyosis vulgaris by the presence of an intermediate zone, a well-preserved granular layer and a distinctly pronounced papillomatosis. Electron-microscopically, in contrast to ichthyosis vulgaris only normally developed keratohyaline granules and tonofibrils are present.[2, 25, 26, 27, 33, 35, 36]

6. Autosomal dominant **bullous congenital ichthyosiform erythroderma** may occasionally offer differential diagnostic difficulties with ichthyosis congenita. For details consult paragraph A1 of this chapter and Chapter 22, A2. Especially in older children, in whom one finds not blister formation but massive hyperkeratoses, the mode of inheritance must be ascertained and acanthokeratolysis must be proved (Fig. 469).[3, 31]

Similar histologic findings of acanthokeratolysis are observed in some linear hystrixlike nevi (Fig. 470) and a few verrucous tumors (so-called solitary epidermolytic acanthoma).[4, 10, 21, 28, 34]

7. The most frequent type of ichthyosis is doubtless dominant **ichthyosis vulgaris.** Noninvolvement of the flexor aspects of the joints and the presence of follicular keratoses on the proximal parts of the extremities, buttocks, and shoulders (Figs. 471, 472) are characteristic, as is hyperkeratotic scaling. In many instances the skin of the palms and soles is thickened and split. The clinical extent of this form of ichthyosis is extremely variable and may range from scaling, which does not amount to more than some roughness, to massive blackish-gray hyperkeratoses. In contrast to ichthyosis congenita and X-chromosomal recessive ichthyosis, the first cutaneous changes appear in the second year of life and are under no

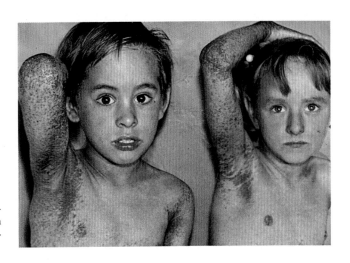

Fig. 469. Hystrixlike hyperkeratoses in siblings with bullous congenital ichthyosiform erythroderma.

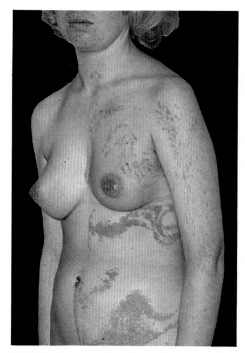

Fig. 470. Systematized linear hyperkeratotic nevus.

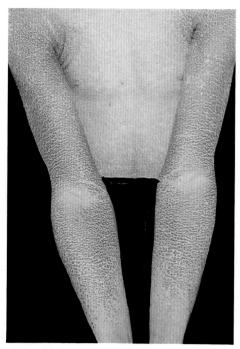

Fig. 471. Ichthyosis vulgaris: the flexor aspects of the joints are uninvolved.

circumstances present at birth. Accompanying signs may be anomalies of the teeth, superficial corneal opacities, and malformations of the ear. Ichthyosis vulgaris represents a retention hyperkeratosis with diminished epidermopoiesis. The granular layer is missing to a large extent, as can be proved by the electron-microscopic evidence of only a few keratohyaline granules. The tonofibrils are clumped together with these remaining keratohyaline granules.

The tendency to reduction of the granular layer in ichthyosis vulgaris differs also from the ichthyosiform cutaneous condition of many patients with atopic dermatitis, in whom such a reduction of the granular layer is missing. The magnesium content of the erythrocytes is significantly reduced in patients with ichthyosis vulgaris, whereas it is normal in atopic dermatitis. On the other hand, patients with ichthyosis vulgaris show the same slowing-down of the neutralization of

alkali and the same decrease in the alkaline resistance as do patients with ichthyosiform atopic dermatitis.[2, 7, 9, 12, 18, 20, 25, 35, 36]

8. Ichthyosis vulgaris-like cutaneous changes with variable and often only vague expression are also characteristic of the dermatologic findings in **Refsum's syndrome,** heredopathia atactica polyneuritiformis. This is a lipid storage disease, in which alpha-hydroxylation of phytanic acid is absent. Neurologic signs are most important, among them night blindness, tapetoretinal degeneration, chronic polyneuropathy with distally accentuated paresis of the extremities, and cerebral ataxia. The disease begins in some cases as early as childhood. Just as often, there is a distinct increase of albumin in the cerebrospinal fluid with a normal number of cells. About as frequent as the cutaneous changes are various pathologic electro-

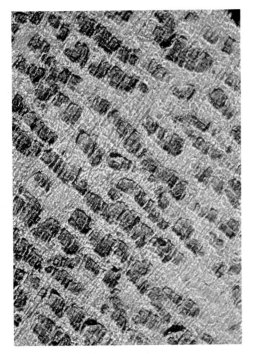

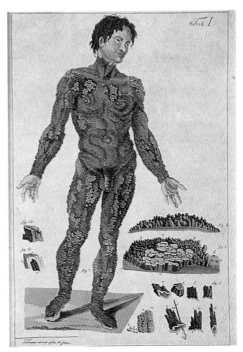

Fig. 472. Ichthyosis vulgaris.

Fig. 473. Ichthyosis hystrix gravior of the Lambert family.

cardiographic findings, but definite cardiac involvement cannot be determined. The Refsum syndrome is transmitted as an autosomal recessive trait.[11, 13, 19, 24, 30]

9. Ichthyosis hystrix gravior shows massive, somewhat spurlike, blackish-brown hyperkeratoses (Fig. 473). In the cases observed so far, the face, palms, and soles have been free of hyperkeratotic lesions. On the other hand, the flexor surfaces are not spared as in ichthyosis vulgaris. Since erythrodermic early stages and blister formations are absent, no certain relationship to congenital ichthyosiform erythroderma can be construed, although the two disorders definitely show an autosomal dominant mode of heredity.[23, 31]

10. The various forms of **ectodermal dysplasia** may also manifest ichthyosis vulgaris-like skin changes. The same can

be said about congenital deafness associated with goiter.[5, 16, 38]

11. So-called **ichthyosis linearis circumflexa** represents a constantly changing, congenital, circinate dermatosis, which at present belongs nosologically less to the ichthyosis group than to the variable squamous erythrokeratodermas. It is usually observed on the trunk and extensor and flexor aspects of the extremities. (On the latter there are also lichenifications similar to those of atopic dermatitis.) It appears as polycyclic, serpiginous, elevated hyperkeratoses which have small erythematous margins and are slowly progressive peripherally and occasionally sharply edged. When these signs regress rather similar changes may recur. Occasionally, two parallel edges appear, and closed annular lesions are absent. In the course of this disorder blister formation may be observed at times. These are either small, rapidly

Table 6. Clinical-genetic Classification of Ichthyoses (according to SCHNYDER et al.[26])

	Manifestation in the First Year of Life	Clinical Type		Follicular Keratoses	Retention Hyperkeratosis	Proliferation Hyperkeratosis	Histology
		Ichthyosis Congenita	Ichthyosis Vulgaris				
I Autosomal dominant							
1. Ichthyosis vulgaris	−		+	+	+		Stratum corneum widened; intermediary zone is absent; stratum granulosum varies between normal and to absent
2. Congenital ichthyosiform bullous erythroderma	+	+					Stratum corneum widened; acanthokeratolysis
3. Ichthyosis hystrix gravior	+	+		?	?	?	?
II Autosomal recessive							
1. Ichthyosis congenita	+	+		+		+	Stratum corneum widened; stratum granulosum has at least two rows; pregranular degeneration
2. Sjögren-Larsson syndrome	+	+				+	Stratum corneum widened; stratum granulosum has at least two rows
3. Rud syndrome	+	+			+	+	
4. Refsum's syndrome	−	+					
III X-chromosomal recessive ichthyosis	+/−	+/−	+/−	−		+	Stratum corneum widened; intermediary zone present; stratum granulosum always present

drying, subcorneal blisters within the serpiginous lesions or larger, flaccid blisters. For a description of **Netherton's syndrome** see Chapter 21, D3.[6, 14]

(1) ANTON-LAMPRECHT, I.: Zur Ultrastruktur hereditärer Verhornungsstörungen. I. Ichthyosis congenita. Arch. Derm. Forsch. *243:* 88–100 (1972).

(2) ANTON-LAMPRECHT, I., and M. HOFBAUER: Ultrastructural distinction of autosomal dominant ichthyosis vulgaris and x-linked recessive ichthyosis. Humangenetik *15:* 261–264 (1972).

(3) BLOOM, D., and M. S. GOODFRIED: Lamellar ichthyosis of the newborn. Arch. Derm. (Chic.) *86:* 336–342 (1962).

(4) DEGOS, R., J. CIVATTE, S. BELAICH et G. TSOITIS: Image histologique particulière de certains naevi verruqueux systématisés. Ann. Derm. Syph. (Paris) *96:* 361–374 (1969).

(5) DERAEMAEKER, R.: Congenital deafness and goiter. Amer. J. hum. Genet. *8:* 253–256 (1956).

(6) DIMITROWA, J., und S. GEORGIEWA: Ichthyosis linearis circumflexa mit subkornealen Bläschen. Derm. Wschr. *144:* 1041–1046 (1961).

(7) ERICKSON, L., and G. KAHN: The granular layer thickness in atopy and ichthyosis vulgaris. J. invest. Derm. *54:* 11–12 (1970).

(8) EWING, J. A.: The association of oligophrenia and dyskeratoses, a clinical investigation and an inquiry into its implications. Amer. J. ment. Defic. *60:* 575–581 (1956).

(9) GEBHARDT, R.: Ohr- und Zahnanomalien als Randsymptom bei Ichthyosis vulgaris. Z. Haut- u. Geschl.-Kr. *41:* 465–467 (1966).

(10) GEBHART, W., und R. L. KIDD: Das solitäre epidermolytische Akanthom. Z. Haut- u. Geschl.-Kr. *47:* [1–4] (1972).

(11) GORDON, N., and R. E. V. HUDSON: Refsum's syndrome. Heredopathia atactica polyneuritiformis. A report of three cases, including a study of the cardiac pathology. Brain *82:* 41–55 (1959).

(12) GREITHER, A.: Zur Klassifikation der Ichthyosis-Gruppe. Dermatologica (Basel) *128:* 464–482 (1964).

(13) HARDERS, H., und H. DIECKMANN: Heredopathica atactica polyneuritiformis. Klinik und Diagnostik des Refsum-Syndroms. Dtsch. med. Wschr. *89:* 248–254 (1964).

(14) HERSLE, K.: Netherton's disease and ichthyosis linearis circumflexa. Report of a case and review of the literature. Acta derm.-venereol. (Stockh.) *52:* 298–302 (1972).

(15) HOOFT, C., J. KRIEKEMANS, K. VAN ACKER, E. DEVOS, S. TRAEN and G. VERDONK: Sjögren-Larsson syndrome with exudative enteropathy. Influence of medium-chain triglycerides on the symptomatology. Helv. paediat. Acta *22:* 447–458 (1967).

(16) JUNG, E. G., und M. VOGEL: Anhidrotische Ektodermaldysplasie mit Hornhautdystrophie. Schweiz. med. Wschr. *96:* 1477–1483 (1966).

(17) KOLLMANNSBERGER, A., und F. MITTELBACH: Sjögren-Larsson-Syndrom. Zur Differentialdiagnose der Ichthyosis mit neurologischen Erscheinungen. Münch. med. Wschr. *110:* 2347–2350 (1968).

(18) KORTING, G. W., H. HOLZMANN und B. MORSCHES: Über einen Unterschied des Magnesium-Gehalts der Erythrocyten von endogenen Ekzematikern und Kranken mit Ichthyosis vulgaris. Arch. klin. exp. Derm. *229:* 126–130 (1967).

(19) KREMER, G. J.: Organlipoiduntersuchungen bei einem Kind mit Refsum-Syndrom. Klin. Wschr. *44:* 1089–1092 (1966).

(20) MORSCHES, B., H. HOLZMANN und R. DENK: Zum Mg-Gehalt von Serum und Erythrocyten bei Kranken mit Ichthyosis vulgaris. Klin. Wschr. *45:* 316 (1967).

(21) NICOLAU, ST. GH., und L. BALUS: Über die Identität der histologischen Veränderungen bei Erythrodermia ichthyosiformis congenita bullosa und der systematisierten hyperkeratotischen Naevi. Derm. Wschr. *143:* 462–469 (1961).

(22) NIX, T. E., H. W. KLOEPFER and V. J. DERBES: Ichthyosis-lamellar exfoliative type. Derm. trop. *2:* 142–152 (1963).

(23) PENROSE, L. S., and C. STERN: Reconsideration of the Lambert pedigree (ichthyosis hystrix gravior). Ann. hum. Genet. *22:* 258–283 (1958).

(24) Ribadeau Dumas, J.-L.: La maladie de Refsum. Presse méd. 77: 2085–2090 (1969).

(25) Schnyder, U. W., und B. Konrád: Zur Histogenetik der Ichthyosen. Hautarzt 18: 445–450 (1967).

(26) Schnyder, U. W., B. Konrád, K. Schreier, P. Nerz und W. Crefeld: Über Ichthyosen. Dtsch. med. Wschr. 93: 423–428 (1968).

(27) Sever, R. J., Ph. Frost and G. Weinstein: Eye changes in ichthyosis. J. Amer. med. Ass. 206: 2283–2286 (1968).

(28) Shapiro, L., and Ch. S. Baraf: Isolated epidermolytic acanthoma. A solitary tumor showing granular degeneration. Arch. Derm. (Chic.) 101: 220–223 (1970).

(29) Sjögren, T., and T. Larsson: Oligophrenia in combination with congenital ichthyosis and spastic disorders; a clinical and genetic study. Acta psychiat. neur. scand. 32 (Suppl. 113) 1957.

(30) Steinberg, D., J. H. Herndon Jr., B. W. Uhlendorf, Ch. E. Mize, J. Avigan and G. W. A. Milne: Refsum's disease: nature of the enzyme defect. Science 156: 1740–1742 (1967).

(31) Stevanovic, D. V., and R. L. Pavic: Dyskeratosis ichthyosiformis congenita migrans; a variant of congenital ichthyosiform erythroderma. Arch. Derm. (Chic.) 78: 625–629 (1958).

(32) Tilesius, W. G.: Ausführliche Beschreibung und Abbildung der beiden sogenannten Stachelschweinmenschen aus der bekannten englischen Familie Lambert oder The Porcupine-Man. Literarischer Comtoir: Altenburg 1802.

(33) Virbans, U., and J. E. Altwein: An X-linked recessive variety of ichthyosis vulgaris different from the X-linked ichthyosis of Wells and Kerr. Clin. Genet. 1: 304–309 (1970).

(34) Weidner, F., und O. P. Hornstein: Bilateraler systematisierter hyperkeratotischer Naevus mit »granulöser Degeneration«. Z. Haut- u. Geschl.-Kr. 47: 63–69 (1972).

(35) Wells, R. S., and C. B. Kerr: Genetic classification of ichthyosis. Arch. Derm. (Chic.) 92: 1–6 (1965).

(36) Woźniak, L., und A. Omulecki: Unterscheidungsmerkmale der x-chromosomalen rezessiven und der autosomalen dominanten Ichthyosis vulgaris. Derm. Mschr. 156: 503–513 (1970).

(37) York-Moore, M. E., and A. T. Rundle: Rud's syndrome. J. ment. Defic. Res. 6: 108–118 (1962).

(38) Zeligman, I., and T. L. Fleisher: Ichthyosis follicularis. Arch. Derm. (Chic.) 80: 413–420 (1959).

B. Secondary (Acquired) Ichthyoses

1. These ichthyosiform skin changes demand additional differential diagnostic considerations, since they accompany, as "dermatoses monitrices," several other dermatoses such as the previously mentioned atopic dermatitis, malignant lymphogranulomatosis, mycosis fungoides, or the reticuloses. **Paraneoplastic ichthyosis** may also occur in combination with visceral carcinomas.[1-5]

2. More familiar is the almost physiologic "ichthyosis simplex" of older people, **senile pityriasis,** or ichthyosis in *starvation cachexia, vitamin-A deficiency,* or *hypothyroidism.* In the last, however, xeroderma may eventually develop from a vitamin-A deficit due to the lack of activation of the carotenes by thyroxin. After some *infectious diseases,* especially typhus, ichthyotic skin conditions may also occur.

(1) Balabanov, K., und V. Ch. Andreev: Ichthyosis acquisita bei Morbus Hodgkin. Hautarzt 17: 252–256 (1966).

(2) Degos, R., J. Civatte et R. Touraine: État ichtyosique circonscrit sur érythème prémycosique. Bull. Soc. franç. Derm. Syph. 67: 191–192 (1960).

(3) Degos, R., E. Lortat-Jacob et J.-F. Tinthoin: Ichtyose tardive diffuse avec réticulo-sarcome ganglionnaire. Bull. Soc. franç. Derm. Syph. 69: 596–597 (1962).

(4) Kuske, H.: Acquirierte Ichthyosen und Keratosen bei Reticulose und Karzinom. In: Cutane paraneoplastische Syndrome. Hrsg. J. J. Herzberg. S. 26–30. Fischer, Stuttgart 1971.

(5) Stevanovic, D. V.: Hodgkin's disease of the skin. Acquired ichthyosis preceeding tumoral and ulcerating lesions for seven years. Arch. Derm. (Chic.) 82: 96–99 (1960).

28. Palmoplantar Keratoses

The differential diagnosis of palmoplantar keratoses depends first of all on whether or not we are dealing with one of the hereditary palmoplantar keratoses, accompanying signs of other hereditary disturbances of keratinization, or hyperkeratoses of a different cause in this location.

A. Hereditary, Diffuse Palmoplantar Keratoses

The hereditary palmoplantar keratoses have different hyperkeratoses, modes of heredity, and regularly associated signs.[10, 19]

1. The autosomal dominant **diffuse circumscribed palmoplantar keratosis** is probably the most frequent hereditary form. In general, the first cutaneous changes are noticed between the fifth and fifteenth year of life but may be present even at birth. In the beginning the palms and soles show sharply demarcated areas of keratosis with a distinct erythematous border (Fig. 474). In abortive cases only an erythema – erythema palmoplantare hereditarium (see also Chapter 18, E2) – without keratotic thickening may be present. The hyperkeratoses themselves are shaped like cobblestones and show fissured lichenification or (rarely) a delled pattern. Palmoplantar hyperhidrosis, which bothers the patient greatly, is pronounced. In general, the keratoses are sharply limited at the edges of the hands and feet, but rather often the eruption extends to the Achilles tendon. Small aberrant keratotic lesions are in exceptional cases present on the dorsa of the hands and feet. Associated changes of the nails (onychogryphoses) and oral mucosa are rare, and the teeth and hairs almost always remain unaffected.[17]

2. Keratosis palmoplantaris mutilans is presumably also transmitted in an autosomal dominant fashion. This palmoplantar keratosis shows, in addition to diffuse, wartlike, single, closely aggregated lesions, circumscribed hyperkeratoses on the backs of the hands, elbows, and knees. More important, however, are the slowly developing constricting furrows, which eventually lead to self-amputation of the proxi-

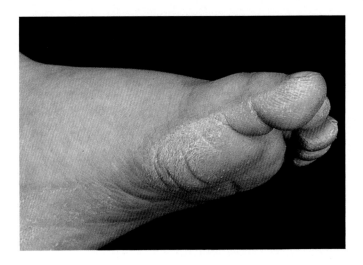

Fig. 474. Beginning diffuse palmoplantar keratosis with a distinctly red border.

mal phalanges (see also Chapter 16, A7). Some of these patients also suffer from deafness of the inner ear (see also Chapter 9, 4).[6, 14, 15]

3. Extensive hyperkeratoses are part of the clinical picture of **palmoplantar keratosis** with **esophageal carcinoma.** The mode of transmission is presumably auto-somal dominant, and the formation of the hyperkeratoses starts relatively late (around the fourteenth year of life). The male sex is affected primarily. Keratoses may be confined to the soles and tend to be accompanied by distinct hyperhidrosis. In the later course of the disease a high percentage of patients develop deeply situated esophageal carcinómas.[3]

4. Keratosis extremitatum hereditaria transgrediens et progrediens was first observed on the island of Mljet (Meleda). The onset of the disorder is the same as that of diffuse circumscribed palmoplantar keratosis, i. e., soon after birth, but in any case it occurs before the fifteenth year of life. The disorder is most probably trans-mitted as an autosomal recessive charac-teristic. In the beginning only flat kerato-ses limited to the palms and soles develop. They are not regularly surrounded by a red border. With advancing age fissured, dirty gray-brown, thick hyperkeratoses develop, which extend continuously to-ward the periphery so that finally the backs of the hands and feet and the flexor sides of the forearms are included. Due to the increased keratinization dermatog-enous contractures and even mutilations of the fingers occur. The hyperhidrosis sur-passes that of circumscribed diffuse palmo-plantar keratosis considerably and may lead to foul-smelling macerations. Besides the transgredient keratoses of the palms and soles there are occasionally single lesions over the ankles, knees, sacrum, and elbows. Associated changes of the hairs

and teeth are absent but the nails occasion-ally show subungual hyperkeratoses.[12, 18]

5. It is still undecided whether the **dominant form of keratosis extremitatum hereditaria transgrediens et progrediens** constitutes a separate entity. Except for the established autosomal dominant mode of heredity it strongly simulates keratosis extremitatum hereditaria transgrediens et progrediens, but after the fortieth year of life a distinct tendency to regression of the hyperkeratoses is discernible.[8, 16]

6. Extended transgredient palmoplantar keratoses are characteristic also of the **Papillon-Lefèvre syndrome** (palmoplantar keratosis with periodontopathy). Hyper-hidrosis as well as the formation of kerato-ses is much milder than those of keratosis extremitatum hereditaria progrediens et transgrediens. The most important char-acteristic is the lack of a tendency to progress. There is even distinct regression at an advanced age. At times the keratoses assume a higher degree of intensity (Fig.476), which coincides with inflamma-tory changes of the periodontal apparatus of the teeth. When these inflammations regress, the keratosis always improves. The Papillon-Lefèvre syndrome as an entity, however, implies the accompanying loss of teeth. The teeth have a normal "anlage," break through normally, and remain unchanged themselves. But soon after the breakthrough of the first and second dentition, periodontitis with pro-gressive inflammatory and pustular des-truction of the periodontium sets in. The alveoli are completely resorbed, and finally the teeth are held only by connec-tive tissue. Normal use will result in com-plete loss (Fig.475). After the loss of the teeth the inflammatory process comes to a halt. Palmoplantar kera-toses and loss of teeth are essential signs, which do not occur separately in individual patients. Another relatively frequent asso-

Fig. 475.   Papillon-Lefèvre
syndrome: complete loss of
teeth.

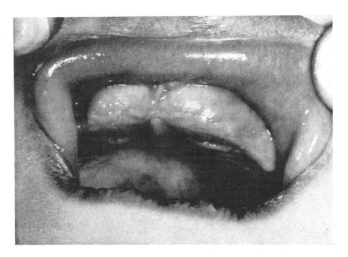

ciated sign is calcification of the dura. The
mode of transmission is unequivocally
autosomal recessive.[7, 9]

7. The differential diagnosis of hereditary
or congenital diffuse palmoplantar keratoses requires the study of a number of
pathologic signs, which until now have
been observed in only a few patients; they
will be mentioned only briefly here. In
**palmoplantar keratosis with granular de-
generation** acanthokeratolysis is histologically evident. Cobblestonelike keratoses
appear in early childhood and do not
progress further; they remain limited to

the palms and soles. The mode of transmission is probably dominant. In some
families there are also patients with
bullous congenital ichthyosiform erythroderma – thus a mutual etiology of both
disorders can be assumed. Another probably autosomal recessive palmoplantar
keratosis, which is confluent but does not
extend beyond the palms and soles, is
**palmoplantar keratosis with watch-glass
nails** and osseous changes. It results in
diminution of the cortices of the long hollow
bones and spatulalike deformities of the
distal phalanges. **Palmoplantar keratosis
with hypotrichosis** is also accompanied by

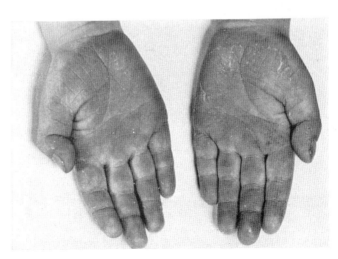

Fig. 476.   Papillon-Lefèvre
syndrome: palmar keratoses.

Table 7. Hereditary Palmoplantar Keratoses with Associated Signs (modified after SCHNYDER et al.[18])

	Keratosis Extremitatum Hereditaria Transgrediens et Progrediens	Keratosis Extremitatum Hereditaria Transgrediens et Progrediens Dominant	Papillon-Lefèvre Syndrome	Richner-Hanhart Syndrome	Pachyonychia Congenita Syndrome
Palmoplantar keratosis					
diffuse	+	+	+	−	+
small lesions	−	−	−	+	+
Extension to backs of hands and feet	+	+	+	−	−
Progression	+	At first +, later regression	−	−	−
Keratoses at other locations	(+)	+	−		+
Hypohidrosis	+	+	(+)	+	+
Nail changes	(+)	−	+	+	+
Loss of teeth	−	−	+	−	−
Dystrophic keratitis	−	−	−	+	−
Short terminal phalanges	+	−	−	+	−
Dural calcifications	−	−	+	−	−
Mental retardation	−	−	−	+	−
Mode of inheritance	Autosomal recessive	Autosomal dominant	Autosomal recessive	Autosomal recessive	Autosomal dominant

+ present, − absent, ( ) facultative

diffuse, widespread hyperkeratoses and hyperhidrosis of the palms and soles. The hypotrichosis is congenital. In addition, there may be subungual hyperkeratoses.[1, 4, 11, 13, 20, 21]

Accompanying extensive palmoplantar keratoses in generalized disturbances of keratinization occur in *ichthyosis congenita*, *ichthyosis vulgaris*, *hidrotic ectodermal dysplasia*, *bullous congenital ichthyosi-*

form erythroderma, incontinentia pigmenti (Franceschetti-Jadassohn type), *erythrokeratodermas*, and *epidermolysis bullosa hereditaria simplex*.[*, 2, 5]

(1) BUREAU, Y., H. BARRIÈRE et M. THOMAS: Hippocratisme digital congénital avec hyperkératose palmo-plantaire et troubles osseux. Ann. Derm. Syph. (Paris) *86:* 611–622 (1959).

(2) CALDWELL, I.: Epidermolysis bullosa simplex with tylosis plantaris. Brit. J. Derm. *67:* 315 (1955).

(3) CLARKE, C. A., A. W. HOWEL-EVANS and R. B. McCONNELL: Carcinoma of oesophagus associated with tylosis. Brit. med. J. *1957/I:* 945.

(4) FISCHER, E., und U. W. SCHNYDER: Keratodermia palmo-plantaris mit Hypotrichose und subungualen Keratosen. Dermatologica (Basel) *116:* 364–365 (1958).

(5) FRANCESCHETTI, A., et W. JADASSOHN: A propos de l'»Incontinentia pigmenti« délimitation de deux syndromes différents figurant sous le même terme. Dermatologica (Basel) *108:* 1–28 (1954).

(6) GIBBS, R. C., and S. B. FRANK: Keratoma hereditaria mutilans (Vohwinkel). Arch. Derm. (Chic.) *94:* 619–625 (1966).

(7) GORLIN, R. J., H. SEDANO and V. E. ANDERSON: The syndrome of palmar-plantar hyperkeratosis and premature periodontal destruction of the teeth. A clinical and genetic analysis of the Papillon-Lefèvre syndrome. J. Pediat. *65:* 895–908 (1964).

(8) GREITHER, A.: Keratosis extremitatum hereditaria progrediens mit dominantem Erbgang. Hautarzt *3:* 198–203 (1952).

(9) GREITHER, A.: Keratosis palmo-plantaris mit Periodontopathie (Papillon-Lefèvre). Dermatologica (Basel) *119:* 248–263 (1959).

(10) GREITHER, A.: Systemische Keratosen. In: Handbuch der Haut- und Geschlechtskrankheiten von J. JADASSOHN. Ergänzungswerk III/2, S. 1–306. Springer, Berlin, Heidelberg, New York 1969.

(11) HEDSTRAND, H., G. BERGLUND and I. WERNER: Keratodermia palmaris et plantaris with clubbing and skeletal deformity of the terminal phalanges of the hands and feet. Acta derm.-venereol. (Stockh.) *52:* 278–280 (1972).

(12) HOEDE, K.: Die Meleda-Krankheit (Keratosis hereditaria palmo-plantaris transgrediens). Arch. Derm. Syph. (Berl.) *182:* 383–395 (1942).

(13) KLAUS, S., G. D. WEINSTEIN and P. FROST: Localized epidermolytic hyperkeratosis. A form of keratoderma of the palms and soles. Arch. Derm. (Chic.) *101:* 272–275 (1970).

(14) KORTING, G. W.: Zur Klinik der atypischen Palmo-Plantar-Keratosen. Z. Haut- u. Geschl.-Kr. *11:* 149–152 (1951).

(15) NOCKEMANN, P. F.: Erbliche Hornhautverdickung mit Schnürfurchen an Fingern und Zehen mit Innenohrschwerhörigkeit. Med. Welt (Stuttg.) *1961:* 1894–1900.

(16) ŠALOMON, T.: Über einige Fälle von Keratosis extremitatum hereditaria progrediens mit dominantem Erbgang (Greither). Z. Haut- u. Geschl.-Kr. *29:* 289–298 (1960).

(17) SCHIRREN, C., und R. DINGER: Untersuchungen bei Keratosis hereditaria palmo-plantaris diffusa. Arch. klin. exp. Derm. *220:* 266–282 (1964).

(18) SCHNYDER, U. W., A. TH. FRANCESCHETTI, B. CESZAROVIC et J. SEGEDIN: La maladie de Meleda autochtone. Ann. Derm. Syph. (Paris) *96:* 517–530 (1969).

(19) SCHNYDER, U. W., und W. KLUNKER: Erbliche Verhornungsstörungen der Haut. In: Handbuch der Haut- und Geschlechtskrankheiten von J. JADASSOHN. Ergänzungswerk VII, S. 861–961. Springer, Berlin, Heidelberg, New York 1966.

(20) VÖRNER, H.: Zur Kenntnis des Keratoma hereditarium palmare et plantare. Arch. Derm. Syph. (Wien, Leipzig) *56:* 3–31 (1901).

(21) WILGRAM, G. F., and J. B. CAULFIELD: An electron microscopic study of epidermolytic hyperkeratosis. Arch. Derm. (Chic.) *94:* 127–143 (1966).

B. Acquired Macular Palmar and Plantar Keratoses

These palmar or plantar hyperkeratoses are acquired together with either a localized

---

* And in malignant and sometimes benign acanthosis nigricans. (Tr.)

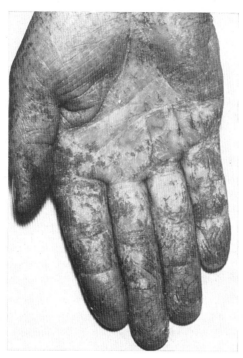

Fig. 477. Extensive hyperkeratosis from contact with paraformaldehyde.

or a generalized skin disease. As a rule they lack the pronounced symmetry of the hereditary palmoplantar keratoses, and the palms and soles are not equally affected. Observation of the complete cutaneous picture will usually permit a quick distinction from the hereditary types. On the other hand, the distinction between the various acquired types themselves may be difficult.

1. At first sight a **tylotic (common) eczema** may simulate palmoplantar keratoderma very closely. However, differences can be found in the duration of the disease itself; on the one hand, the manifestation of a tylotic eczema in childhood would be most unusual, while, on the other hand, such an eczema would not be present continuously for years without appropriate exposure. Pruritus, exacerbation after renewed contact with offending substances, and irregular spread to the extremities are further indications of an external cause.

The presence of papulovesicular lesions at the edges of the affected areas and positive skin tests will verify the diagnosis. A typical example of such tylotic palmoplantar keratoses is the cutaneous changes observed after contact with paraformaldehyde used in the manufacture of rubber and synthetic fibers (Fib. 477).[3]

2. Difficulties may inevitably arise in distinguishing a **hyperkeratotic tinea** infection of the hands and feet, due to the fact that regular washing of the hands may make it impossible to discover fungi, and also a tylotic eczema of the hands may become infected secondarily with fungi. In spite of these facts the finding of pathogenic fungi by culture is of decisive diagnostic importance. Clinically, a pronounced, peripheral, walled zone with a tendency toward central healing indicates mycosis. Pruritus is the same in mycosis as in tylotic eczema. The distinction between hyperkeratotic tinea and the hereditary palmoplantar keratoses requires the same considerations as outlined before with tylotic eczema.

3. Psoriasis vulgaris of the palms can be recognized by its basal, sharply circumscribed erythema and its multilayered, silvery white scaling. The presence of typical psoriatic lesions on the body simplifies the diagnosis. In addition, nail changes showing psoriatic pitting, oily spots, and friability will help in establishing the diagnosis.

4. The volar aspects of the hands in **secondary syphilis** may show lesions of psoriasiform character. However, lenticular lesions predominate and only seldom are macular hyperkeratotic areas observed.

Other syphilitic changes of skin and mucous membranes are also found. The classic seroreactions as well as the treponema antibody tests will definitely be positive.

5. Keratoderma climactericum starts as a small, symmetrical palmoplantar keratosis; soon, however, eczematous changes are superimposed, resulting in the simulation of an extensive disturbance of cornification. This condition is seen almost exclusively in women in menopause and only occasionally in older men. Similar cutaneous changes can be seen during pregnancy or with hypothyroidism. At first, the formation of keratoses favors the center of the palms and does not involve the thenar or hypothenar eminences; usually there is severe pruritus. The relationship with concomitant signs such as adiposity, hypertonia, or arthritis is uncertain. The differential diagnosis has to exclude tylotic eczema, fungus infection of the hands, and the inverted type of psoriasis.[1, 4]

6. The first dermatologic sign of **syringomyelia** may be relatively slightly elevated, light yellow macular hyperkeratoses. They

Fig. 478. Papular palmoplantar keratosis.

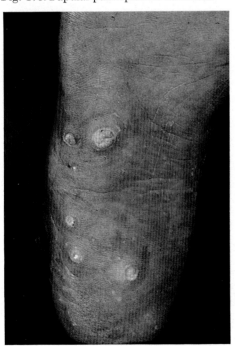

appear with no inflammatory phenomena; the edges of these lesions are indefinite and blend imperceptibly with the normal skin. Only later when dissociated anesthesia has taken place do cutaneous manifestations follow, caused by the absence of perception of pain and temperature (see also Chapter 5, A4).[2]

7. Chronic **lymphedema** may be accompanied occasionally by pronounced papillomatous plantar hyperkeratoses with special involvement of the anterior metatarsal region and the heels. Similar cutaneous manifestations can be seen on other pressure points of the feet. As a rule the diagnosis depends on the visible evidence of lymphostasis of long duration.

(1) HAXTHAUSEN, H.: Keratoderma climactericum. Brit. J. Derm. *46:* 161–167 (1934).
(2) SCHIRNER, G.: Hyperkeratosen der Handteller als Früherscheinung bei Syringomyelie. Arch. Derm. Syph. (Berl.) *173:* 27–33 (1936).
(3) WEBER, G., und R. BARNISKE: Paraform-Hyperkeratosen nach Art des Keratoma palmare et plantare. Berufsdermatosen *8:* 306–312 (1960).
(4) WOLF, J.: Keratoderma climactericum (Haxthausen). Arch. Derm. Syph. (Chic.) *43:* 731–732 (1941).

C. Hereditary Circumscribed Small Palmoplantar Keratoses

Here again one has to distinguish between small-sized keratoses of the palms and soles with and without associated signs.

1. Since there are no associated signs in autosomal dominant **papular palmoplantar keratosis,** we are dealing only with symmetrical palmar and plantar disturbances of keratinization. The lesions are isolated and only rarely confluent, pinhead- to lentil-

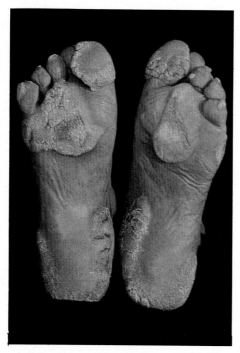

Fig. 479. Keratosis palmoplantaris varians.

after a short while. The lesions first become visible between the fifteenth and thirtieth years of life. This is substantially later than the age of manifestation of the diffuse keratodermas. In contrast to other keratoses, distinct hyperhidrosis is also absent. The most important differential diagnosis is that from multiple arsenical keratoses (see following section D5).[7, 10]

2. Keratosis palmoplantaris varians has more possibilities for morphologic variation. The term comprises autosomal dominant palmoplantar keratoses in the form of islands or stripes. They may occur alternately in affected families. The first cutaneous changes are usually observed before the tenth year of life; this is distinctly earlier than in papular palmoplantar keratosis. On the inner sides of the hands there are groups of keratoses consisting of multiple small hyperkeratoses, which extend in streaks from the palms to the flexor sides of the fingers. The individual hyperkeratoses may occasionally occur so densely that they give the impression of a diffuse confluent keratosis. The isolated keratoses may be replaced by paperlike keratosis membranacea. The eponychium of the fingernails is as a rule thickened and fissured. In some patients

sized, horny papules with a verrucous surface (Fig. 478). The papules occasionally have a central pit. After removal of the small horny cone, a dimple-like depression remains. The hyperkeratosis, however, grows back unchanged in the same place

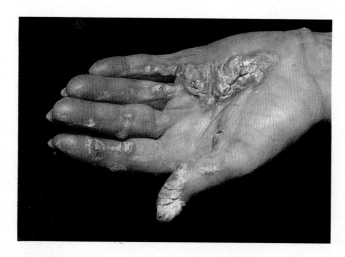

Fig. 480. Pachyonychia congenita: disseminated keratomas of the palm.

Fig. 481. Pachyonychia congenita: scleronychia.

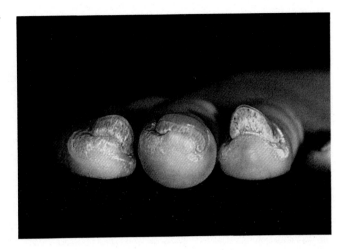

subungual keratoses develop. Only rarely
are scattered keratotic lesions present on
the backs of the fingers, elbows, or knees.
On the soles the hyperkeratoses simulate
clavi. If one considers them alone, without
reference to the rest of the body, one
would have difficulty distinguishing them
from clavi or warts of the soles (Fig. 479).
Hyperhidrosis is almost always present.
Hair on the helix of the ear seems to be
the only accompanying sign.[2–4, 10]

3. Palmoplantar keratoses with small
lesions are also present in the **Richner-
Hanhart syndrome.** But equally important

are the herpetiform corneal erosions and
superficial corneal opacities. Some patients
in addition show mental retardation,
brachytelephalangia, and multiple lipomas.
The hyperkeratoses remain limited to the
palms and soles and are accompanied by
hyperhidrosis. Occasionally, patients have
subungual hyperkeratoses.[5, 6, 12]

4. The **pachyonychia congenita syndrome**
shows keratinizing anomalies which extend
far beyond the palmoplantar area. According to the associated signs the following
subtypes are distinguished, illustrating the
wide range of the original syndrome: the

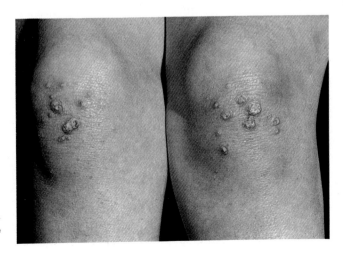

Fig. 482. Pachyonychia congenita: keratomas on the
knees in the form of islands.

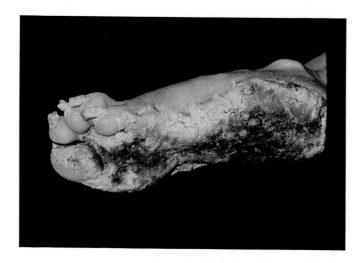

Fig. 483. Pachyonychia congenita: diffuse keratomas on the sole.

Fischer syndrome, the Brünauer syndrome, the Schäfer syndrome, and the Spanlang-Tappeiner syndrome. The mode of heredity is in all cases autosomal dominant. The important sign is pachyonychia. Although the speed of growth of the nails is normal and the lunula is well visible, the nails are monstrously thickened. Their compact horny substance is in general unusually hard (Fig. 481). These changes of the nailplate are almost always associated with subungual hyperkeratoses. In exceptional cases pachyonychia may occur as an isolated phenomenon, but usually, palmoplantar keratoses occur with the same frequency. Limited to the palms and soles, the keratoses themselves are isolated, or, much less frequently, they are diffuse, and in exceptional cases, striated (Figs. 480, 483). Usually distinct hyperhidrosis is also present. Additional isolated keratotic lesions are present on the elbows and knees (Fig. 482), but they do not occur as frequently as the hyperkeratoses of the body (which have a predilection for the buttocks). The third, also almost constant, sign is extensive leukokeratosis of the lips, tongue, and buccal mucosa (see also Chapter 34, B1). Similar changes may also occur on the pharynx and the nasal mucosa. If the disorder lasts several years,

one should always be aware of a possible malignant degeneration of ocular lesions. Rare associated signs are hypotrichias, corneal dystrophies, malformations of the teeth, and mental and physical retardation. Of all these signs only pachyonychia is present in infancy, whereas the other signs become manifest not earlier than the third year of life.[1, 8, 11]

(1) ÅKESSON, H. O.: Pachyonychia congenita in six generations. Hereditas (Lund) 58: 103–110 (1967).
(2) BREHM, G.: Ungewöhnliche striäre Palmar- und Plantarkeratose mit dorsalen Hyperkeratosen. Derm. Wschr. 134: 1173–1178 (1956).
(3) BOLOGA, E. I.: Ein Fall von plantarer, inselförmiger Keratose in 5 Generationen mit dominantem Erbgang. Hautarzt 16: 231–234 (1965).
(4) FRANCESCHETTI, A., und U. W. SCHNYDER: Versuch einer klinisch-genetischen Klassifikation der hereditären Palmoplantarkeratosen unter Berücksichtigung assoziierter Symptome. Dermatologica (Basel) 120: 154–178 (1960).
(5) FRANCESCHETTI, A., und C. J. THIER: Über Hornhautdystrophien bei Genodermatosen unter besonderer Berücksichtigung der Palmoplantarkeratosen. Albrecht v. Graefes Arch. Ophthal. 162: 610–670 (1961).
(6) HANHART, E.: Neue Sonderformen von Keratosis palmoplantaris, u. a. eine regelmäßig-dominante mit systemati-

sierten Lipomen, ferner zwei einfach-rezessive mit Schwachsinn und z. T. Hornhautveränderungen des Auges (Ektodermalsyndrom). Dermatologica (Basel) *94:* 286–308 (1947).

(7) Heierli-Forrer, E.: Zur Klinik und Genetik der hereditären papulösen Palmo-Plantarkeratosen. Dermatologica (Basel) *119:* 303–327 (1959).

(8) Jannasch, G., und A. Wiskemann: Keratosis multiformis idiopathica Siemens (Pachyonychia congenita Jadassohn-Lewandowsky). Arch. klin. exp. Derm. *212:* 275–281 (1961).

(9) Schirren, C., und R. Dinger: Untersuchungen bei Keratosis palmoplantaris papulosa. Arch. klin. exp. Derm. *221:* 481–495 (1965).

(10) Sutton-Williams, G. D.: Keratosis palmo-plantaris varians mit Helicotrichie. Arch. klin. exp. Derm. *236:* 97–106 (1969).

(11) Thompson, H.: Hereditary dystrophy of the nails. J. Amer. med. Ass. *91:* 1547 (1928).

(12) Žmegač, Z. J., and M. V. Sarajlić: A rare form of an inheritable palmar and plantar keratosis. Dermatologica (Basel) *130:* 40–52 (1964).

D. Symptomatic Circumscribed Palmoplantar Keratoses with Small Lesions

The first rule is to differentiate point-sized palmoplantar keratoses from similar findings that occasionally occur in other hereditary diseases.

1. It should be mentioned in this connection that, at least in a high percentage of blacks, **idiopathic dimples** occur on palms and soles. These dimples are 1 to 3 mm wide and favor the soles, particularly the lateral edges of the feet. It is important, of course, to rule out intake of arsenic, as well as syphilis and other disorders that are accompanied by disturbances of keratinization.

2. Poriform losses of substance on the palms and soles may be caused by the small papules of **follicular dyskeratosis.** This condition gives rise to the typical interruptions of the papillary line pattern, which are valuable for the diagnosis.

Similar cutaneous changes occur occasionally in patients with **chronic benign familial pemphigus.** Since both disorders have several nosologic factors in common, such findings are not surprising.[13]

3. Indentations of the size of a needle prick and dimplelike holes on the palms and soles accompany the **basal cell nevus syndrome.** In general, these cutaneous changes are observed after the appearance of multiple nevoid basal cell carcinomas, but in exceptional cases they may precede the tumors. An extension of the dimplelike holes to the sides and extensor surfaces of

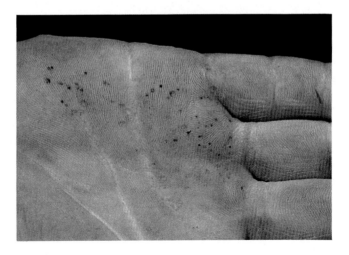

Fig. 484. Pitted keratolysis.

the fingers is not uncommon. In contrast to arsenical keratoses, no circumscribed hardening is palpable. Histologically, the dimples indicate a circumscribed loss of the stratum corneum and a slightly smaller rete malpighi, in which the basal cells are extraordinarily increased and show vacuoles.[5, 8, 14]

4. Dimplelike keratolyses ("pitted keratolyses") are predominantly limited to the soles. They may be caused by infections with fungi or bacteria, as for instance *Dermatophilus congolensis* or Corynebacteria. The dimples are closely aggregated at the sites of pressure. The individual lesion has a diameter of 1 to 3 mm, and its bases may be darkly discolored (Fig.484). Proof of pathogenic organisms within the small lesions is best obtained from a histologic specimen for a biopsy.[11, 12, 15]

5. Arsenical keratoses are of practical importance in the differential diagnosis of papular palmoplantar keratosis. Their favorite location is again the main pressure points of the soles and hands. The individual keratoses vary from the size of a pinhead to that of a lentil bean (Fig.485). The larger keratoses have a rough and warty surface; the smaller ones have a

smooth surface and can be found only by palpation. The size and number of the arsenical keratoses are directly dependent on the quantity of the arsenic consumed. Isolated arsenical keratoses are occasionally found also at other areas of the extremities and on the trunk. An isolated lesion is macroscopically not different from a common wart. The simultaneous presence of epitheliomas of the trunk (Bowen's disease or pagetoid basal cell epitheliomas) or diffuse melanoses suggests, even with a negative history, the etiologic role of arsenic in such a papular palmoplantar keratoderma. Histologically, the individual arsenical warts are characterized above all by manifestations similar to those of Bowen's disease and by spinaliomalike features. This makes them precancerous. In addition, the presence of an arsenical keratosis demands an examination for a neoplasm of the inner organs (especially of the lungs and larynx) and continuous observation for the possible early discovery of malignant tumors (Table 8). It should be noted that the incidence of multiple carcinomas in one patient is above the average.[1–4, 10]

6. In palmar, plantar, and disseminated porokeratosis the palms and soles are extensively affected. The palmoplantar skin changes consist of polycyclically

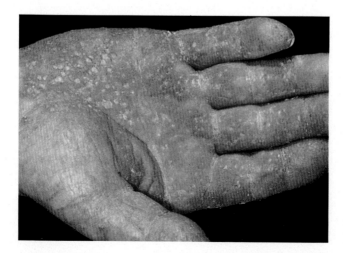

Fig. 485. Arsenical hyperkeratoses in a psoriatic treated years ago with arsenic.

Fig. 486: Secondary syphilis: maculopapulosquamous lesions of the palm.

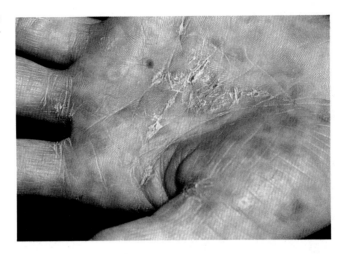

Table 8. Arsenic-induced* Carcinomas in Vintners of the Moselle. Organ Distribution in 101 Autopsies.

Organ	Number of Tumors
Larynx	3
Lungs	65
Stomach	2
Pancreas	2
Skin	29

* Arsenic is no longer used in Germany as a pesticide. (Tr.)

formed, 3 to 5 mm wide, shallow dimples with a low horny wall at the border. Here again, the sites of increased pressure are affected most. Other similar multiple lesions extend as far as the extremities and the trunk, but the face always remains unaffected. In the disseminated form there is no distinct dependence on light, a fact which is already clear from the onset of disease on the palms and soles. For the histologic description see the chapter on follicular keratoses (Chapter 29, B1).[7]

7. So-called "clavi syphilitici" occasionally occur in the course of **secondary**

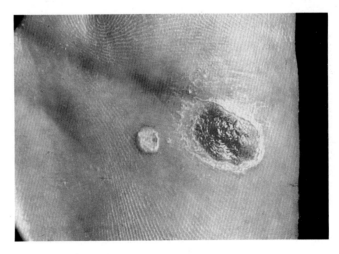

Fig. 487. Bowen's disease of the palm; adjacent to it are arsenical hyperkeratoses.

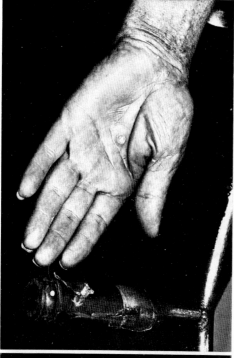

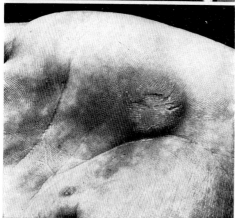

Fig. 488. Clavus from pressure.

syphilis as lenticular or lichenoid elements on the palms and soles (Fig. 486). The individual copper-brownish papule has a slightly scaling and barely keratotic surface. Moreover, the lesions are only transiently present. If pressed with a probe many patients note distinct pain.*

---

* This is the Buschke-Ollendorff sign. (Tr.)

The diagnosis is decided by additional characteristic skin changes and positive seroreactions.

8. The so-called gonorrheic palmoplantar keratoses are often large and polymorphous and intermixed with vesicular pustules. They usually are manifestations of **Reiter's disease.** Only rarely are explicitly clavuslike formations with red borders present, together with more exudative parakeratotic lesions. Here again, only the evaluation of all the signs of the disorder allows us to arrive at a definite diagnosis (see also Chapter 7, B2).

9. Unilateral circumscribed keratotic lesions, if they have been present for a long time, must be examined histologically to rule out the possibility of a malignant tumor lying underneath. This is especially valid for hyperkeratotic **Bowen's disease** located in the palmoplantar area which may have originated from an arsenical wart (Fig. 487).[9]

10. It is especially difficult to differentiate **clavi** (corns) from palmoplantar common warts, which are viral acanthomas (papova group) with subsequent hyperkeratosis. Both thorny warts and corns develop at prominent areas exposed to pressure (Fig. 488) and are highly painful. In contrast to the evenly developed hyperkeratotic **callum** (callosity) one finds in the clavus (for instance, after it has been planed) a single central horny plug. This alone, however, cannot be considered the cause of the special sensitivity of such a modified hyperkeratosis, especially since underneath the developing clavus, a polymorphous morphologic substrate of neural tissue is evident. Etiologically, the development of clavi above the terminal heads of the metatarsal bones or the joints of the toes above exostoses, or in anomalies of posture, is conspicuous. Clavi on the palms are often caused by certain instruments, for instance, those of barbers, jewelers, and many others.

(1) BEAN, S. F., E. G. FOXLEY and R. M. FUSARO: Palmar keratoses and internal malignancy. Arch. Derm. (Chic.) *97:* 528–532 (1968).

(2) DENK, R., H. HOLZMANN, H.-J. LANGE und D. GREVE: Über Arsenspätschäden bei obduzierten Moselwinzern. Med. Welt *20* (N. F.): 557–567 (1969).

(3) DOBSON, R. L., M. R. YOUNG and J. S. PINTO: Palmar keratoses and cancer. Arch. Derm. (Chic.) *92:* 553–556 (1965).

(4) FIERZ, U.: Katamnestische Untersuchungen über die Nebenwirkungen der Therapie mit anorganischem Arsen bei Hautkrankheiten. Dermatologica Basel) *131:* 41–58 (1965).

(5) GERBER, N. J.: Zur Pathologie und Genetik des Basalzell-Naevus-Syndroms. Humangenetik *1:* 354–373 (1965).

(6) GIBBS, R. C., und R. ANDRADE: Punktförmige Grübchen an den Füßen und Handflächen bei Negern. Hautarzt *21:* 306–308 (1970).

(7) GUSS, ST. B., R. A. OSBOURN and M. A. LUTZNER: Porokeratosis plantaris, palmaris et disseminata. A third type of porokeratosis. Arch. Derm. (Chic.) *104:* 365–373 (1971).

(8) HOWELL, J. B., and A. H. MEHREGAN: Pursuit of the pits in the nevoid basal cell carcinome syndrome. Arch. Derm. (Chic.) *102:* 586–597 (1970).

(9) MICHAELIDES, P., and A. B. HYMAN: Bowen's disease of the palm. Dermatologica (Basel) *128:* 239–244 (1964).

(10) PETRES, J., K. SCHMID-ULLRICH und U. WOLF: Chromosomenaberrationen an menschlichen Lymphozyten bei chronischen Arsenschäden. Dtsch. med. Wschr. *95:* 79–80 (1970).

(11) RUBEL, L. R.: Pitted keratolysis and dermatophilus congolensis. Arch. Derm. (Chic.) *105:* 584–586 (1972).

(12) TAPLIN, D., and N. ZAIAS: The etiology of pitted keratolysis. In: XIII. Congressus Internationalis Dermatologiae, München 1967. Bd. 1, S. 593–595. Springer, Berlin, Heidelberg, New York 1968.

(13) VERROV, J. L.: Palmar lesions in familial benign pemphigus. Brit. J. Derm. *81:* 77 (1969).

(14) WARD, W. H.: Nevoid basal celled carcinoma associated with a dyskeratosis of the palms and soles: A new entity. Austral. J. Derm. *5:* 204–208 (1960).

(15) ZAIAS, N., D. TAPLIN and G. REBELL: Pitted keratolysis. Arch. Derm. (Chic.) *92:* 151–154 (1965).

29. Follicular Keratoses

A. Hereditary Follicular Keratoses

This group of hereditary follicular keratoses at present comprises lichen albus,* ulerythema ophryogenes, *keratosis follicularis spinulosa decalvans* (see also Chapter 11, E3), the follicular keratoses of the *pachyonychia congenita syndrome* (keratosis follicularis acneiformis) (see also Chapter 28, C4), the follicular keratoses of *ichthyosis vulgaris* (see also Chapter 27, A7), the follicular keratoses of the monilethrix syndrome (see also Chapter 11, A18), *pityriasis rubra pilaris* (see also Chapter 19, B and Chapter 22, C14), and dyskeratosis follicularis (Darier's disease). The majority of these diseases have been discussed in other chapters; only three additional follicular keratoses will be discussed here.

---

* Also known as lichen sclerosus et atrophicus. (Tr.)

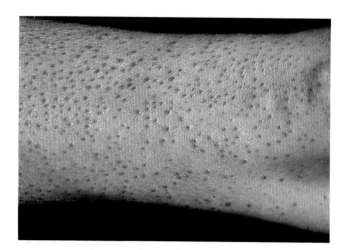

Fig. 489. Lichen pilaris.

1. Lichen pilaris (albus et ruber) usually manifests itself at or near the time of puberty in both sexes with the same frequency. Because considerable regression takes place during early adulthood, lichen pilaris in older people is seen rather rarely. The "anlage" of this disturbance of cornification is most likely inherited as an autosomal dominant trait. The sites of predilection – extensor aspects of the upper arms and thighs, shoulders, and buttocks – show isolated hyperkeratoses arising out of dilated follicular openings shaped like tulip cups. The facial skin remains unaffected to a large extent. Because the keratoses occur close together, they give the impression of a nutmeg-grater. As a rule, the follicular corny plugs barely reach the size of a pinhead. The immediate vicinity of such a papule may show either a bluish-red cyanosis or a distinct fading of color; the result simulates the white or red variety of lichen pilaris (Fig.489). The hairs of the affected follicles either remain within the follicular funnel or disappear completely. In contrast to the follicular keratoses of ichthyosis vulgaris the disturbance of cornification in lichen pilaris remains restricted to the follicular opening and does not affect the entire follicle; also lacking are the obstructions of secretions and the inflammations that are commonly seen in ulerythema ophryogenes.

In some cases lichen pilaris may be accompanied by formation of cornified spinous material (lichen spinulosus). The lesions are raised a few millimeters above the papule proper. Since the addition of such excrescences to "common" lichen pilaris does not result in further differences, it is doubtful whether keratosis follicularis spinulosa congenita is a separate entity. In any case, it is necessary to establish a distinction from the secondary forms of spinulosism; they will be discussed later in Section C.[10, 13]

2. Although **ulerythema ophryogenes** is an autosomal dominant trait showing a disturbance of cornification of the upper third of the hair follicle, the development of the entire clinical picture requires additional exogenous factors (possibly, invasion of staphylococci). Among the affected individuals many possess light hair. The disease usually begins either in childhood or in early adulthood with persistent symmetrical facial erythema; favorite sites are the lateral frontal hair line, the lateral parts of the eyebrows, and the cheeks. Later, follicular hyperkeratoses appear within the erythematous areas;

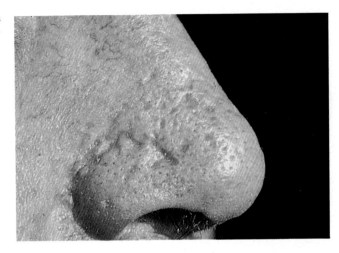

Fig. 490. Vermicular scars following ulcerating serpiginous folliculitis of the nose.

they fill out each follicle completely and result in complete destruction of the hair bulb. In addition to the two leading signs of erythema and follicular keratosis, the formation of comedones and pustules of variable extension and severity completes the clinical picture. If the presence of comedones is predominant, one uses the term acneiform ulerythema; if pustules are more prominent, the term sycosiform ulerythema is preferred (Fig. 490). Each affected area is sharply circumscribed at the edge. Although the central portion heals with a smooth scar, the periphery often shows wall-like elevations interspersed with numerous pustules. In many patients a later residual condition appears, so-called atrophoderma vermiculata (see also Chapter 17, C4), and, above all, an irreversible loss of hair (see also Chapter 11, E2).

The erythematous stage in children requires, from a differential diagnostic point of view, separation from granulosis rubra nasi. However, the latter condition lacks follicular hyperkeratoses – above all, the tendency to heal with scar formation – and moreover, lacks the additional lesions outside the nasal region. The presence of areas of vermicular atrophoderma and also comedones and pustules rules out pseudopélade Brocq, which is restricted to the scalp. Chronic discoid lupus erythematosus does not show comedones and pustules; however, single lesions show definite hyperesthesia. Also, the hyperkeratosis of lupus erythematosus is not conical but has a firmly attached scale (like a carpet tack); when in doubt, a histologic analysis will result in

Fig. 491. Darier's disease: grayish-brown, hyperkeratotic papules on the trunk.

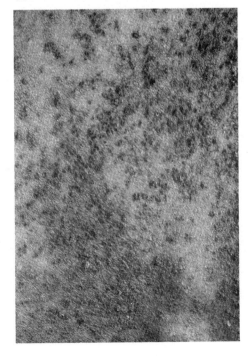

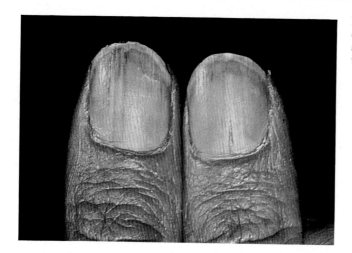

Fig. 492. Darier's disease: increased longitudinal streaks and longitudinal ridging of the nails.

a definite diagnosis. In any case, the succulent walled edge of sycosiform ulerythema lesions requires exclusion of deep trichophytosis; this can be easily accomplished by proving the presence of fungi.[8, 9, 11]

3. Dyskeratosis follicularis (Darier's disease) may resemble follicular keratosis, although the individual papules are not connected with follicles. The mode of inheritance is autosomal dominant without preference to either sex. The first manifestation of this disease may extend over a wide range of time; there have been

observations of this disease in early infancy and also after the age of 50. A certain peak of frequency is seen at prepuberty. The primary lesions consist of pinhead-sized, isolated, reddish papules; they are soon covered by brown, firmly attached keratoses creating a rough, warty surface (Fig. 491). The individual papules show a definite tendency toward grouping and frequently coalesce into verrucous, fetid, macerated patches. Definitely favored is the so-called seborrheic localization, i. e., the scalp, nasolabial folds, anterior and posterior midline regions of the trunk,

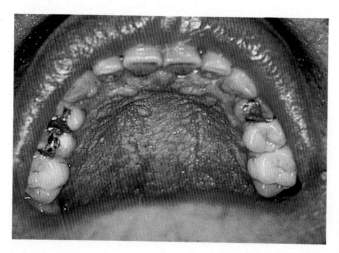

Fig. 493. Darier's disease: mucous membrane of the palate.

and also the anogenital area. The legs may develop especially hypertrophic verrucous and also partly ulcerated vegetations. Formations of vesicles and pustules seldom predominate (see also Chapter 26, H). Characteristic are the interruptions of the papillary ridges of the palms and soles (see also Chapter 28, D2). In addition, the buccal mucous membrane, more frequently the palate (Fig. 493) and the mucosa of the esophagus, rectum, and genitals sometimes show typical, somewhat leukoplakialike papules. The nails show conspicuous longitudinal ridges and the free edges have a sawtooth appearance (Fig. 492). The cystic changes of the bones that are found occasionally in Darier's disease most likely represent an additional sign. Psychic schizoid or epileptic changes may be pathognomonic for this disease.[1, 3, 6, 7]

In the initial stage of development the previously mentioned predilection for the seborrheic or intertriginous cutaneous regions and the presence of white spots on the back are important for the differential diagnosis (see also Chapter 24, A6).

Histologically, Darier's disease presents hyperkeratosis, acanthosis, and dyskeratotic elements ("corps ronds," "grains") as well as the formation of suprabasal lacunae and clefts within the epidermis. Benign chronic familiar pemphigus, however, usually shows acantholytic cells still in loose connection with their intercellular bridges.[2, 4]

Degenerative dyskeratotic forms can also be observed in isolated tumors, i. e., as an atypical form similar to Darier's disease in *senile keratoma*, but above all they are found in warty dyskeratomas as in *isolated follicular dyskeratosis* (Fig. 494), *epithelioma spinocellulare segregans*, and *dyskeratoma lymphadenoides*.[5, 12]

(1) BORUP SVENDSEN, I., and B. ALBRECT-SEN: The prevalence of dyskeratosis follicularis (Darier's disease) in Denmark. Acta derm-venereol. (Stockh.) *39:* 256–269 (1959).

Fig. 494. Warty dyskeratoma (dyskeratosis segregans): macroscopic and microscopic views.

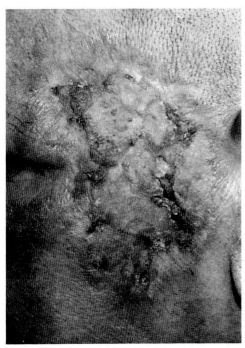
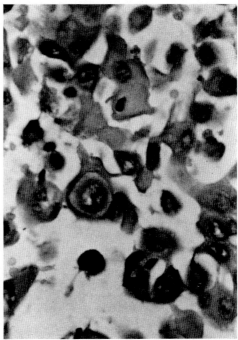

(2) FORSSMANN, W. G., H. HOLZMANN und
N. HOEDE: Elektronenmikroskopische
Untersuchungen der Haut beim Morbus
Darier. II. Der stufenweise Ablauf der
Dyskeratose und die Degeneration der
pathologischen Zellformen. Z. Haut- u.
Geschl.-Kr. *42:* 211–228 (1967).

(3) HALTER, K.: Röntgenologisch und
endoskopisch erfaßbare Speiseröhren-
veränderungen bei Morbus Darier und
Morbus Pringle. Z. Haut- u. Geschl.-Kr.
6: 228–229 (1949).

(4) HOEDE, N., W. G. FORSSMANN und
H. HOLZMANN: Elektronenmikroskopische Untersuchungen der Haut beim
Morbus Darier: I. Die Anfangsstadien
der Akantholyse. Z. Haut- u. Geschl.-Kr.
42: 175–184 (1967).

(5) KORTING, G. W.: Dyskeratoma lymphadenoides. Derm. Wschr. *146:* 534–543
(1962).

(6) KORTING, G. W., und R. DENK: Kno-
chenzysten bei Morbus Darier. Med.
Welt *20* (N. F.): 215–216 (1969).

(7) KRINITZ, K.: Tumoröse Veränderungen
bei Morbus Darier. Hautarzt *17:* 445–
450 (1966).

(8) MARX, W.: Beitrag zur Histologie des
Ulerythema ophryogenes. Arch. Derm.
Syph. (Berl.) *163:* 6–17 (1931).

(9) MASCHKILLEISSON, L. N.: Über Ulerythema sycosiforme Unna (Sycosis lupo-
ides Brocq).Acta derm.-venereol. (Stockholm) *12:* 115–128 (1931).

(10) MEYER, D., A. STOLP und A. KNAPP:
Über eine Familie mit Keratosis follicularis spinulosa bei vermutlich dominantem Erbgang. Derm. Wschr. *151:*
201–206 (1965).

(11) STEPPERT, A.: Terramycin beim Ulerythema sycosiforme. Hautarzt *6:* 504–
505 (1955).

(12) TANAY, A., and A. H. MEHREGAN:
Warty dyskeratoma. Dermatologica
(Basel) *138:* 155–164 (1969).

(13) TOURAINE, A.: Essai de classification
des kératoses congénitales. Ann. Derm.
Syph. (Paris) *85:* 257–266 (1958).

B. Probably Nonhereditary Follicular Keratoses

Some of the dermatoses to be discussed
next have already been described in other
chapters, such as *hyperkeratosis follicularis*
et parafollicularis in cutem penetrans
(Chapter 19, D), *elastosis perforans serpiginosa* (Chapter 19, D), and *hyperkeratosis
lenticularis perstans* (Chapter 19, E).

1. Porokeratosis occurs only rarely as an
isolated lesion but is more often observed
as **disseminated porokeratosis.** It originates
mainly on skin that is continuously exposed
to light, such as the face, backs of the
hands, and the legs. The involvement of
palms and soles is discussed in Chapter 28,
D. However, lesions on the trunk, transitional mucous membranes, and mucous
membranes are not exceptional. Males
suffer from the disease twice as often as
females. The age of the patient with
manifestations varies greatly, and definite
statements with regard to the presumably
autosomal dominant mode of heredity are
not yet possible. The tendency toward
characteristic ringlike extension and the
typical histologic picture are best explained at the present time by presuming
that latent epidermal cell clones are responsible; the growth of these clones is
induced by rays which act as a trigger.
The primary lesion is a smooth, later
slightly verruciform papule with a punched-out, comedolike center. Such singular
lesions form after a growth phase in which
peripheral, closed polycyclic rings with
hard, keratotic borders that are elevated
over the normal skin have formed; these
separate a suggestively atrophic, dark, and
sunken-in center from the neighboring
skin (Fig. 495). Histologically, the disorder
shows a sharply demarcated parakeratotic
strip with reactions of acanthosis and
hyperkeratosis. Occasionally, a certain
dyskeratosis is present. Primary changes
of sweat glands and follicles are absent.

The differential diagnosis of the macroscopic lesion must consider elastosis
perforans serpiginosa, which, however,
produces much coarser papules, and
annular lichen planus; but chronic discoid
lupus erythematosus can be eliminated
(usually it has a different location and is

also serpiginous, yet with strictly follicular hyperkeratosis and follicular atrophy).[1, 4, 5, 8, 9, 11]

2. A **reactive perforating collagenosis** is occasionally seen in children.* In it collagenous material is eliminated transepidermally. There is a connection with a preceding trauma – thus a positive Köbner phenomenon is not surprising. Clinically, this condition appears with brownish-red, rice-corn- to lentil-sized papules, which are present mainly on the legs. The center of the papule contains a tough mass which can be lifted up without bleeding, so that the papule subsequently shows a pit. After removal of the collagenous plug the papules heal with superficial scar formation. A definite diagnosis can be made only from the histologic findings, in which plug-like parakeratosis in the center of the papule is the dominant feature. In the differential diagnosis hyperkeratosis follicularis et parafollicularis in cutem penetrans (see also Chapter 19, D) and perforating folliculitis should be ruled out first.[2, 7, 12]

3. The preceding reactive perforating collagenosis and hyperkeratosis follicularis et parafollicularis in cutem penetrans must be differentiated from **perforating folliculitis**. This dermatosis consists of nodules which are strictly limited to the follicles. They occur mainly on the more hairy extensor aspects of the extremities. The individual lesion is a slightly elevated papule, 2 to 5 mm in diameter, with a central horny plug. In contrast to reactive perforating collagenosis, however, this plug is relatively firmly attached, and can be removed only by causing some minor bleeding. The patients in general do not report any subjective sensations. The histologic picture is characteristic of one showing dilated hair follicles. The affected hair

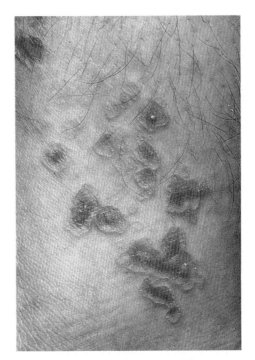

Fig. 495. Disseminated porokeratosis.

follicles are filled with orthokeratotic and parakeratotic hyperkeratosis, and the epithelium of the follicle shows numerous perforations. Through these perforating gaps connective tissue that is partly necrotic and interspersed with inflamed areas intrudes into the follicle. The proximal part of the hair shaft is often found wedged into such a perforation, and it may be assumed that the perforation itself was caused by mechanical irritation of the broken hair in the follicle.[6]

Pinhead-sized, either hyperkeratotic or umbilicated papules are occasionally also present on the edges of the fingers or hands in patients who show typical granuloma annulare at other sites. Histologically, the individual papule represents a highly situated, palisading granuloma, whose central necrobiosis perforates the epidermis. In analogy to the disorder just described, this transepithelial elimination is called **granuloma annulare perforans**.[3, 10]

---

* And adults. (Tr.)

(1) BAZEX, A., et A. DUPRÉ: Porokératose
de Mibelli zoniforme avec dégénéres-
cence. Présentation de deux observations. Ann. Derm. Syph. (Paris) *95:*
361–374 (1968).

(2) BOVENMYER, D. A.: Reactive perforating collagenosis. Experimental production of the lesion. Arch. Derm. (Chic.)
102: 313–317 (1970).

(3) CALNAN, C. D.: Granuloma annulare.
Brit. J. Derm. *66:* 254 (1954).

(4) CHERNOSKY, M. E., and D. E. ANDER-
SON: Disseminated superficial actinic
porokeratosis: Clinical studies and experimental production of lesions. Arch.
Derm. (Chic.) *99:* 401–407 (1969).

(5) GUSS, ST. B., R. A. OSBOURN and
M. A. LUTZNER: Porokeratosis plantaris, palmaris et disseminata. A third type
of porokeratosis. Arch. Derm. (Chic.)
104: 366–373 (1971).

(6) MEHREGAN, A. H., and R. J. COSKEY:
Perforating folliculitis. Arch. Derm.
(Chic.) *97:* 394–399 (1968).

(7) MEHREGAN, A. H., O. D. SCHWARTZ and
C. S. LIVINGOOD: Reactive perforating
collagenosis. Arch. Derm. (Chic.). *96:*
277–282 (1967).

(8) MIESCHER, G.: Über »Porokeratosis
Mibelli«. Arch. Derm. Syph. (Berl.) *181:*
532–548 (1941).

(9) MIKHAIL, G. R., and F. W. WERTHEI-
MER: Clinical variants of porokeratosis
(Mibelli). Arch. Derm. (Chic.) *98:*
124–131 (1968).

(10) OWENS, D. W., and R. G. FREEMAN:
Perforating granuloma annulare. Arch.
Derm. (Chic.) *103:* 64–67 (1971).

(11) REED, R. J., and PH. LEONE: Porokeratosis – a mutant clonal keratosis of
the epidermis I. Histogenesis. Arch.
Derm. (Chic.) *101:* 340–347 (1970).

(12) WORINGER, F., und P. LAUGIER: Collagenoma perforans verruciforme. Derm.
Wschr. *147:* 64–68 (1963).

C. Secondary Follicular Keratoses

1. Keratosis follicularis is etiologically
not a uniform disorder. This form of
disturbed keratinization includes follicular-lichenoid disturbances of superordinate
dermatoses (i. e., monilethrix and lichen
pilaris) as well as "id" reactions in
syphilis (lichen syphiliticus), tuberculosis
(lichen scrofulosorum), mycoses (lichen
trichophyticus), as well as follicular keratoses (see also Chapter 31, A3). The
disease consists of papules which are at the
most pinhead-sized with central hyperkeratosis and are limited to the follicles.
The lesions have a striking tendency
toward grouping (Fig. 496). According
to site, spinulosism is more or less
distinct. In some papules the central
hyperkeratosis is blackened like a comedo;
the black center, however, cannot be
removed by pressure as in an acne lesion.
Exogenous causes that irritate the follicles

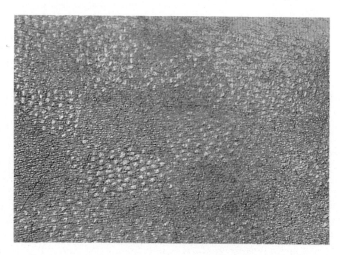

Fig. 496. Keratosis follicularis spinulosa.

lead, in our experience, less to follicular-lichenoid or follicular-spinulous than to acneiform keratoses. Known examples are keratoses following contact with paraffin, vaseline, or lubricating oil.

2. Follicular keratoses also occur in various **vitamin deficiencies.** In such cases, however, the striking group formation of the keratotic papules found in keratosis follicularis is absent. The follicular-lichenoid keratoses in vitamin-A deficiency (phrynoderma) occur mostly at the base of the flourdustlike, strangely ashy-gray skin and are accompanied by diminished activity of the sweat and sebaceous glands. Early signs are photophobia, night blindness, and retarded adaptation to the dark. In contrast, the nutmeg grater- or goose-fleshlike follicular keratoses of avitaminosis-C are characterized by pointlike bleeding spots distributed in a checkerboard pattern and located mainly on the legs. In severe cases further confluent bleeding spots may occur in areas of special muscular strain, or in children subperiosteally, and also as swellings of the interdental papillae with loosening and loss of teeth. Follicular-spinulous hyperkeratoses of ariboflavinosis, i. e., vitamin-B_2 deficiency, are located mainly in the nasolabial area. They are complemented by additional signs of lactoflavin deficiency (perlèche, dysphagia, scrotal dermatitis, koilonychia, keratitis, retrobulbar neuritis, and others).

3. Follicular mucinosis (alopecia mucinosa) also produces circumscribed areas with spinulosislike changes. The clinical appearance is that of lichenoid-follicular, plaquelike papules, which are located on infiltrated patches, or else of grouped papules alone; these are somewhat larger than pinheadsize and follicular.

The plaquelike changes occur typically in the eyebrow area, on the neck, and on the scalp, where they become noticeable early because of the accompanying loss of hair (see also Chapter 11, D10). In the large majority of cases only one or two separate lesions exist, although occasionally multiple extension of infiltrates occurs on the trunk and extremities. Such plaques develop step by step, so that in the beginning only the papules are present; later the plaquelike infiltrates develop. Plaquelike cutaneous changes are almost entirely limited to adults, whereas disseminated follicular manifestations predominate in children.

It should be possible to distinguish between idiopathic and symptomatic follicular mucinosis. After a variable period of time, the former is permanently arrested, at least in children and when the cutaneous changes are limited to a few single lesions. After regression of the infiltrate and the follicular papules, normal hair growth is again restored. Elderly patients who have multiple lesions in addition must be suspected of suffering from the secondary form and must receive regular follow-up care. As the infiltrates constantly increase, these patients may develop mycosis fungoides, lymphogranulomatosis, or chronic lymphadenosis after a few months.

The diagnosis of follicular mucinosis can be only suspected macroscopically and needs histologic confirmation in every case. The histologic findings are so characteristic that they cannot be mistaken for any other disease. The primary action of the disease takes place at the hair-sebaceous gland unit and is characterized by degeneration of the follicular epithelium together with storage of mucin in the follicle. In the beginning the mucinous deposit between the cells of the sheath of the hair root may be inconspicuous. The deposits, however, are distinctly metachromatic and almost always PAS-negative. Even if the mucinous deposits assume greater proportions, they are always, in contrast to other disorders with increased mucinous deposits (such as lichen myxedematosus or circumscribed myxedema), limited to the follicles and their sebaceous glands. In more pronounced cases cysts filled with mucin may form within the outer sheath of the hair root. The amount of stored mucin does not correspond at all to the perifollicular infiltrate. This may be absent or only slightly developed; it may, on the other hand, have a great many cells, invade the follicle, and lead to dermatitic changes of the surrounding epidermis. In idiopathic follicular mucinosis the infiltrate consists predominantly of lymphocytes, numerous histiocytes, and eosinophils. Atypical cells are lacking. However, the secondary form shows atypical cells and an increased rate of mitoses, even if the infiltrate is thin. The presence of Pautrier's microabscesses and invasion of the infiltrate into the epidermis indicate a transition into mycosis fungoides.[3, 4, 7, 10]

Secondary mucus accumulation in the follicles occasionally occurs in chronic discoid lupus erythematosus and hyperkeratotic lichenifications, as well as in mycosis fungoides, which sometimes reveals even macroscopically a distinct follicular papulosis.[1, 2, 8, 9]

Important for the differential diagnosis of follicular mucinosis are keratosis follicularis, lichen pilaris, and perhaps also pityriasis rubra pilaris; if the disease occurs on the scalp, chronic discoid lupus erythematosus and ulerythema ophryogenes must be differentiated.

4. Whether or not **disseminated – recurrent infundibulum folliculitis** represents a special disease entity is still debatable. Over months or years it produces small papules which are strictly limited to the follicle. Single lesions grow no bigger than the size of a pinhead. Because no tendency to confluence exists, the skin has the appearance of gooseflesh. Formation of pustules or blisters is always lacking. Although the trunk is the favored site, the same papules can occur on the extremities

and occasionally also on the face. Preceding or accompanying general signs are not present. In spite of the involvement of the hair follicle, growth of hair is undisturbed; thus, circumscribed areas of hair loss as in follicular mucinosis are never observed. Histologically, an uncharacteristic edema with loose lymphocytic infiltration of the follicular infundibulum is present. In the differential diagnosis, in addition to follicular mucinosis one must rule out follicular keratosis (tendency to grouping), lichen pilaris (the trunk usually remains uninvolved), and pityriasis rubra pilaris.[5, 6, 11]

(1) BERGGREEN, P.: Verlaufsweisen der Mycosis fungoides (unter Berücksichtigung der Atypien). Arch. Derm. Syph. (Berl.) *178:* 501–549 (1939).

(2) CABRÉ, J., und G. W. KORTING: Zum symptomatischen Charakter der »Mucinosis follicularis«; Ihr Vorkommen beim Lupus erythematodes chronicus. Derm. Wschr. *149:* 513–518 (1964).

(3) COSKEY, R. J., and A. H. MEHREGAN: Alopecia mucinosa. A follow-up study. Arch. Derm. (Chic.) *102:* 193–194 (1970).

(4) EMMERSON, R. W.: Follicular mucinosis. A study of 47 patients. Brit. J. Derm. *81:* 395–413 (1969).

(5) HITCH, J. M., and H. Z. LUND: Disseminate and recurrent infundibulo-folliculitis. Arch. Derm. (Chic.) *105:* 580–583 (1972).

(6) KAIDBEY, K. H., F. S. FARAH and M. T. MATTA: Disseminate and recurrent infundibulo-folliculitis. Report of two cases. Dermatologica (Basel) *143:* 29–35 (1971).

(7) KIM, R., and R. K. WINKELMANN: Follicular mucinosis (alopecia mucinosa). Arch. Derm. (Chic.) *85:* 490–498 (1962).

(8) KORTING, G. W.: Mykosis fungoides. Derm. Wschr. *135:* 569–570 (1957).

(9) PINKUS, H.: Differentialdiagnose Mycosis fungoidesverdächtiger Hauterscheinungen. Fortschr. der prakt. Derm. und Venerol. Bd. V, S. 1–9. Springer, Berlin, New York, Heidelberg 1965.

(10) Tappeiner, J., L. Pfleger und H. Holzner: Zur Mucinosis follicularis (Alopecia mucinosa Pinkus). Arch. klin. exp. Derm. *215*: 209–222 (1962).

(11) Thew, M. A., and M. Gray Wood: Disseminate and recurrent infundibulo-folliculitis. Report of a second case. Arch. Derm. (Chic.) *100*: 728–733 (1969).

30. Acneiform Dermatoses

A. Acne Vulgaris

1. In practice the most important and most common disorder of the sebaceous glands is **acne vulgaris.** In addition to a hereditary predisposition, excessive cornification of the follicular openings and increased lipolysis (excessive liberation of free fatty acids from the triglycerides of cutaneous sebum) are basic factors. These two factors bring about a rupture of the follicle and transport of free fatty acids into the surrounding tissue, resulting in an inflammatory response. Additional bacterial growth increases the inflammation to the point of suppuration. Acne vulgaris is a disease of adolescents and young adults; after the thirtieth year of life it is observed much less frequently. The height of frequency is around puberty, although younger children may regularly show a few comedones. There is no definite predilection for either sex. In some young girls or women there may be either a premenstrual exacerbation of a preexisting acne or an eruption of acne only at this time. In the latter case, however, localized infiltrates are observed mainly on the chin and cheeks. Cutaneous regions with an abundance of sebaceous glands such as the face, back, chest, and, less frequently, the proximal extensor aspects of the upper arms first develop blackish keratoses of the follicular openings (comedones) with subsequent retention of sebum. Depending on the degree of activity of acne vulgaris, papular and papulopustular elements will appear. Deeply situated suppurating infiltrates may coalesce subepidermally, producing cylindrical or plaquelike protuber-ances (Fig. 497). Almost always polymorphous types of acne are present simultaneously, with the result that pure forms such as comedonal, papular, pustular, or indurated acne are hardly ever seen. After the secretion has stopped and the infiltrates have become absorbed, retracted, funnel-like, partly varioliform scars will remain. In exceptional cases multiple pinhead-sized areas of ossification remain as a residue of healed acne vulgaris.

Whenever acne papules are firmly squeezed, pressed, or excoriated by the patient, the traumatized lesion will hide the true character of the disease; such a

Fig. 497. Acne vulgaris.

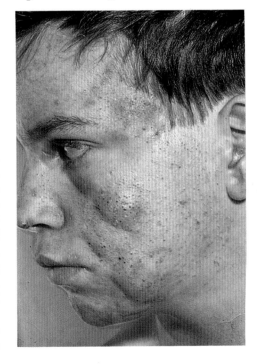

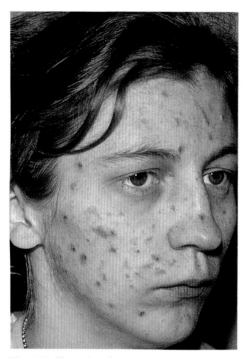

Fig. 498. Excoriated acne.

Fig. 499. Nevus comedonicus.

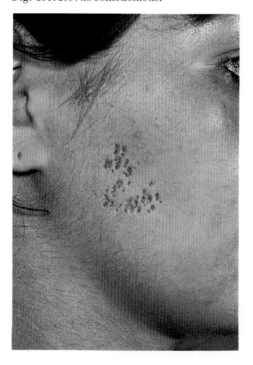

condition is called excoriated acne (Fig. 498). However, this name does not describe a specific form of acne.[3, 4, 7, 19]

Acneiform eruptions may also be seen in rare instances as **acne neonatorum** in the newborn or in infants. The cutaneous changes are virtually confined to the facial region; the lesions may be either grouped comedones or papulopustular infiltrates. Acne of the newborn depends on hormonal factors (progesterone of the mother). In infants the exogenous influence of skin creams and of prophylactic doses of vitamin D_2 against rickets administered in large divided doses should not be overlooked. In rare cases infants may have a Candida infection that simulates acne neonatorum or acne infantum; if such an eruption becomes persistent the contents of the pustules should be inoculated on culture media.[10, 11]

2. Nevus comedonicus is characterized by groups of comedones present since birth or childhood. In this disease the pilosebaceous follicles are dilated with comedo-like plugs; however, there is no connection with acne vulgaris. At first inspection the areas of nevus comedonicus show sharply circumscribed, cuplike, more or less shallow depressions with central comedolike formations. In contrast to acne vulgaris, this nevus shows only follicular keratoses without involvement of the sebaceous glands (Figs. 499, 500). Inflammatory changes are always absent. Such a nevus may be found on any cutaneous region with no preference as to site. Lately a syntropy of a unilateral nevus comedonicus with a homolateral cataract has been reported. The differential diagnosis must consider, besides acne vulgaris (differs in duration and dredominance of inflammatory infiltrates, and is not confined to small circumscribed areas), ulerythema ophryogenes (occurs in conjunction with inflammatory phenomena, is progressive, and is marked by basal erythema).[12, 18]

3. A circumscribed area with comedones and sebaceous retention cysts restricted to the retroauricular area could be due to the lather of shaving soap. Most of the patients are men who do not remove the lather behind the ears carefully enough.[20]

4. Trichostasis spinulosa can be differentiated from acne vulgaris without difficulty. Trichostasis also shows dilated and blackish follicular openings, which are caused, not by ordinary hyperkeratosis but by the retention of bundles of lanugo hairs (Fig. 501). Such pseudocomedones are seen almost always in older people in the region of the nose, forehead, back of the neck, and lower abdomen. When in doubt, such a follicle can be expressed and the contents examined directly under the microscope. Bundles of lanugo hairs can be seen especially well with polarized light, although histologically, only the roots of the hairs can be demonstrated.[8, 14, 15]

5. Nodular elastosis (elastéidose cutanéenodulaire avec kystes et comédons) involves the development of comedones in the periorbital region of older persons; it is discussed in Chapter 17, A1.

6. Acne conglobata requires differential diagnostic separation from acne vulgaris.

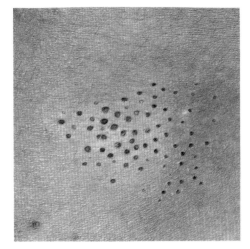

Fig. 500. Nevus comedonicus.

Acne conglobata is not confined to a certain period of life; it favors males* and extends considerably beyond the usual localization of acne vulgaris (Fig. 502). A leading diagnostic clue is the involvement of the entire back, and sometimes also of the buttocks and the anogenital region. The perineal region and the groin of

---

* Nodulocystic acne has been noted in males of abnormal height with an XYY genotype (Tr.)

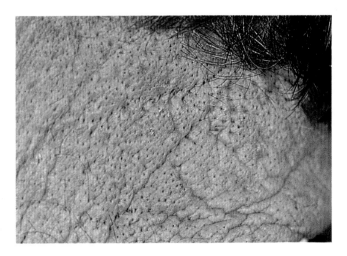

Fig. 501. Trichostasis spinulosa.

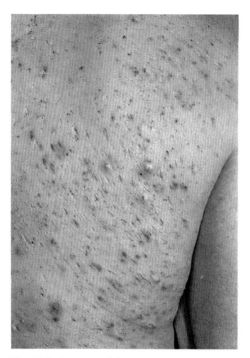

Fig. 502. Acne conglobata.

differentiation from acne vulgaris. Only acne conglobata has numerous groups of comedones or giant comedones in addition to subcutaneous necroses, subsequent torpid ulcerations with undermined edges, and fistulous ducts (Fig. 503). Healing takes place with formation of somewhat retracted, atrophic scars (so-called pressure atrophy scars) or with hypertrophic scars that form bridges and lobes (Fig. 504). Isolated attacks involving the perineum-buttock region may result in extensive fistulation (see also Chapter 14, B11). Occasionally, exacerbation of acne conglobata may be accompanied by polyarthralgias and increased temperature (see also Chapter 1, O1).[5, 13]

almost every patient with acne conglobata show some comedones and inflammatory infiltrates. In addition to the topographical signs that are helpful in arriving at a diagnosis of acne conglobata, examination of the individual lesions will confirm the

7. Some secondary types of acne also have to be separated from acne vulgaris. So-called **steroid acne** has extensive monomorphous papular or papulopustular lesions which, however, are found in the same location as acne vulgaris (Fig. 505). Comedones and marked inflammatory infiltrates are lacking, as are necrotizing abscesses of the infiltrates. Steroid acne may be caused either by hyperfunction of the adrenal cortex or by a basophilic adenoma of the hypophysis, and it occurs above all after treatment with ACTH and cortisone.

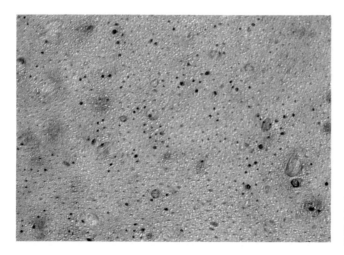

Fig. 503. Acne conglobata: giant and grouped comedones and pressure atrophies.

Treatment with corticosteroid ointments results in development of steroid acne confined to the site of application. There is no morphological difference between steroid acne and acneiform cutaneous eruptions caused by INH and vitamin D_2.[11]

Another type of secondary acne is *trade or occupational acne*. Among these is *oil acne*, caused by cutting oils and industrial oils which result in black follicular hyperkeratoses and follicular inflammations on the region of the skin that is in constant contact with the oil, especially the extensor aspects of the forearms and thighs. In contrast to chloracne, follicular cysts do not develop. The cutaneous changes of *coal tar acne* correspond to those of oil acne. However, *chloracne* [perna disease (*perchlornaphthalene*)] differs distinctly from oil and tar acne. Weeks and months after exposure to tetrachlordiphenylendioxide, multiple comedones and follicular hyperkeratoses appear on the entire body (Fig. 506). In mild cases most of the lesions are on the face, sparing the nose. The flexural parts of the joints and also the hands and feet are almost always noninvolved. The presence of follicular cysts is diagnostically important; occasionally on first inspection they are overlooked because they are quite small (pinhead-sized) and skin-colored.

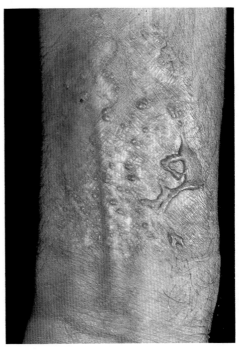

Fig. 504. Acne conglobata: pressure atrophies and bridging scars.

Without the presence of such cysts the diagnosis of chloracne should not be made.

Chloracne lacks inflammatory changes; if present, they are much less pronounced than those in oil or tar acne. Frequently chloracne is accompanied by extensive

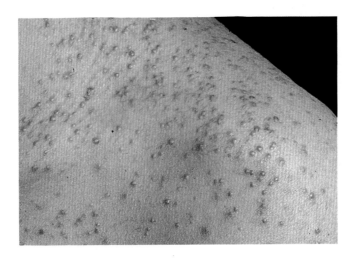

Fig. 505. Steroid acne.

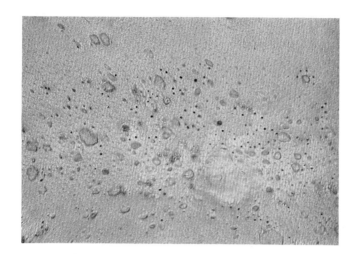

Fig. 506. Cloracne.

hyperpigmentations, especially on the fingers and toes. In addition to these cutaneous changes one should search for simultaneous damage to the liver, which will become evident after a long latent period. Some patients have permanent psycho-organic damage with labile affectivity, mild mental disintegration, and loss of libido suggestive of premature senility.[1, 2, 6, 9]

Occasionally acne lesions may appear within fields of radiation **after x-ray therapy.** In addition to comedones, multiple, flesh-colored, follicular cysts similar to chloracne occur; they may be as large as rice grains. The differential diagnosis must consider the presence of small nodular cutaneous metastases, but the separation from other types of acne is not important.[16, 17]

(1) BRAUN, W.: Chlorakne. Editio Cantor, Aulendorf 1955

(2) CROW, K. D.: Chloracne. A critical review including a comparison of two series of cases of acne from chlornaphthalene and pitch fumes. Trans. St. John's Hosp. Derm. Soc. (Lond.) *56:* 79–99 (1970).

(3) CUNLIFFE, W. J.: The relationship between surface lipid composition and acne vulgaris. Brit. J. Derm. *85:* 86–89 (1971).

(4) DENK, R., B. KNICK und K. LINDE: Intravenöse Tolbutamid-Belastung, Serum-Insulinaktivität (ILA) und Tolbutamid-stimulierte Insulinreserve bei Akne-vulgaris-Kranken. Z. Haut- u. Geschl.-Kr. *41:* 429–434 (1966).

(5) FISCHER, H., und I. KÄPPEL: Zur Pathogenese der Acne conglobata. Arch. klin. exp. Derm. *207:* 377–396 (1958).

(6) GOLDMANN, P. J.: Schwerste akute Chlorakne durch Trichlorphenol-Zersetzungsprodukte. Beitrag zum Perna-Problem. Arbeitsmed., Sozialmed., Arbeitshyg. *7:* 12–18 (1972).

(7) HALTER, K.: Multiple cutane Verknöcherungsherde nach Akne vulgaris. Aesthet. Med. *14:* 58–63 (1965).

(8) ISHIKAWA, K.: Trichostasis spinulosa. Hautarzt *20:* 367–369 (1969).

(9) KLEU, G., und R. GÖLTZ: Spät- und Dauerschäden nach chronisch-gewerblicher Einwirkung von Chlorphenolverbindungen. Katamnestische neurologisch-psychiatrische und psychologische Untersuchungen. Med. Klin. *66:* 53–58 (1971).

(10) KLOSTERMANN, G. F., und M. NIETZKI: Candida-Infektion unter dem klinischen Bilde der Acne neonatorum. Arch. klin. exp. Derm. *221:* 611–621 (1965).

(11) KORTING, G. W., und D. K. MIOWSKI: Akne vulgaris als Nebenerscheinung der Vitamin D_2-Therapie. Z. Haut- u. Geschl.-Kr. *8:* 85–91 (1950).

(12) NABAI, H., and A. H. MEHREGAN: Nevus comedonicus. A review of the literature and report of twelve cases. Acta derm.-venereol. (Stockh.) *53:* 71–74 (1973).

(13) NÜRNBERGER, F.: Zur Kenntnis der Akne conglobata im Damm-Gesäßbereich. Z. Haut- u. Geschl.-Kr. *38:* 188–197 (1965).

(14) POSCHACHER, A.: Über Trichostasis spinulosa. Acta derm.-venereol. (Stockholm) *6:* 107–117 (1925).

(15) SARKANY, I., and P. M. GAYLARDE: Trichostasis spinulosa and its management. Brit. J. Derm. *84:* 311–315 (1971).

(16) STEIN, K. M., J. J. LEYDEN and H. GOLDSCHMIDT: Localized acneiform eruption following cobalt irradiation. Brit. J. Derm. *87:* 274–279 (1972).

(17) SWIFT, S.: Localized acne following deep x-ray therapy. Arch. Derm. Syph. (Chic.) *74:* 97–98 (1956).

(18) WHYTE, H. J.: Unilateral comedo nevus and cataract. Arch. Derm. (Chic.) *97:* 533–535 (1968).

(19) WRONG, N. M.: Excoriated acne of young females. Arch. Derm. Syph. (Chic.) *70:* 576–582 (1954).

(20) WULF, K., und F. FEGELER: Komedonen und Talgcysten hinter den Ohren durch Seifenschaum. Hautarzt *4:* 371–373 (1953).

B. Rosacea

1. Unlike the various forms of acne, **rosacea** is not a disorder of the follicles and sebaceous glands. Its etiology and pathogenesis are still unclear, although the increased incidence in seborrheic patients remains conspicuous. Definite connections with gastrointestinal disturbances, focal infections, hormonal factors, or influence of light cannot be proved. Rosacea occurs less often in men than in women. Most of the manifestations occur between the fourth and fifth decades of life. Rosacea has a butterfly distribution on the face, but there may be a special accentuation of the forehead or chin. The eyelids and upper lip are usually spared, but this is not a safe differential diagnostic criterion versus lupus miliaris disseminatus faciei. Extension of rosacea to the neck and chest is not as rare as is still

assumed (Fig. 507). The disorder usually starts with facial redness, which in the beginning occurs in the form of attacks; later, as it persists, it is interspersed with telangiectases. This is the reason why confusion with climacteric erythema or with beginning lupus erythematosus easily occurs (see also Chapter 18, F5). In most of the cases erythematous rosacea develops into papular or pustular rosacea. On the erythematous base various large nodules, which may show a central pustule, develop (Fig. 508). These infiltrates are not bound to the follicle, but develop on any area in the upper layers of the corium. In contrast to acne vulgaris, comedones are always lacking and the pustular breakdowns are in a distinctly higher location, so that deep subepidermal necrotic areas do not occur. From a rosacea nodule, moreover, sebaceous matter cannot be expressed. In so-called lupoid rosacea the nodules easily reach rice-corn size and, under dias-

Fig. 507. Rosacea with extrafacial localization.

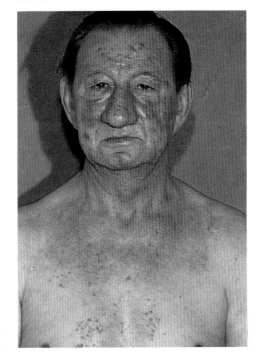

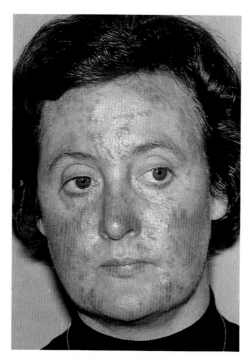

Fig. 508. Rosacea.

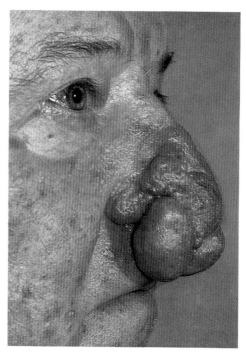

Fig. 509. Rhinophyma.

copy, brownish infiltrates become visible. In addition, the histologic picture may show tuberculoid structures, but no conclusions of a connection with tuberculosis should be drawn from this. However, it can be seen how necessary it is to definitely rule out lupus miliaris disseminatus faciei (see later, Section 3).

The most important complication of rosacea is the involvement of the eyes. This may be simple conjunctivitis, but more important is so-called rosacea keratitis, which may eventually lead to ulcerations. Involvement of the sclera and iris is rare.[1, 2, 6, 11]

Rhinophyma is not an inevitable sequela of erythematous or papulopustular rosacea, but has often been observed in connection with rosacea or distinct seborrhea. Moreover, rhinophyma is mainly a disorder of men in the sixth and seventh decades of life. Sometimes it has more fibrous features, or a pronounced angi-

ectatic or glandular-hyperplastic aspect. In the differential diagnosis the nodular and tuberous, almost always distinctly seboglandular character of rhinophyma (Fig. 509) should not be difficult to recognize. Lupus perniosarcoidosis, on the other hand, is distinctly dark blue, smooth, and without hyperplasia of the sebaceous glands.

2. The most important disorder to be differentiated from rosacea is at present the so-called **perioral rosacealike dermatitis** of the face. Since neither etiologic nor morphologic differences that are constant and definite can be cited, the assumption that this is only a variant of rosacea is justified. The age of patients with rosacealike dermatitis, however, is definitely younger than that of patients with rosacea. The high proportion of women is even more distinct than in rosacea. Etiologically, endocrine factors can be blamed as little as microbial-toxic disturbances or intolerance of detergents, cosmetics, or drugs. Morphologically, the disorder appears as pinhead-sized, firm, red to brown-red papules, often with a central pustule. The papules have a distinct tendency toward grouping, and they are located on a pale, yellow-red, slightly scaling erythema (Fig. 510). As in rosacea, telangiectases are present. Seborrhea is always present. The location is always the medial part of the face, including the chin area; a small perioral zone, however, is almost always free. A similar "free zone" occurs in rosacea and in many infectious diseases (e.g., scarlet fever). In the histologic picture, the differences between rosacealike dermatitis and rosacea vary by only gradual degrees (see also Chapter 18, F6).[4, 10]

2. Lupus miliaris disseminatus faciei is no longer considered to be tuberculous but instead is classed as one of the tuberculids of the skin. It indeed prefers young adults, but, in contrast to rosacea, there is a distinctly higher proportion of men. The individual lesions are pinhead- to rice-corn-sized, semispherical, brown-red papules. They are always isolated and do not spare the upper lip and eyelids (Fig. 511). Under diascopy, the typical, light-brown lupoid infiltrates become visible. They are distinctly fragile if pressed by a probe. The individual papules develop relatively rapidly and remain essentially unchanged for several months, in rare cases for years. Pustules and fistulae do not occur. Healing leaves tender and atrophic scars. Histologically, lupus miliaris disseminatus shows the distinct picture of a tubercular granuloma (epithelioid cell tubercle with giant cells of the Langhans' type, peripheral accumulation of lymphocytes, and great central caseation) known in all forms of cutaneous tuberculosis or tuberculids.

Compared to acne vulgaris the absent comedones and pustules seem to be important. Rosacea is characterized by the simultaneous presence of erythema and telangiectases in young women.* In the histologic examination of so-called lupoid rosacea, central caseations are always lacking. In addition, many cells with segmented nuclei are present in the infiltrate. Papular secondary syphilis does not remain limited to the face and is accompanied by other secondary cutaneous changes. The classical and the specific seroreactions are positive. Some difficulties may arise in the differentiation from small-nodular sarcoidosis (Fig. 512). Considera-

---

* Rosacea occurs mainly in the fourth and fifth decades of life. (Tr.)

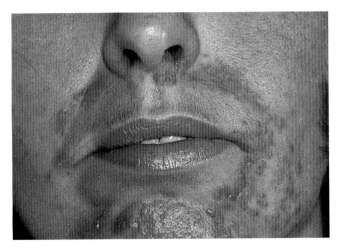

Fig. 510. Perioral rosacealike dermatitis.

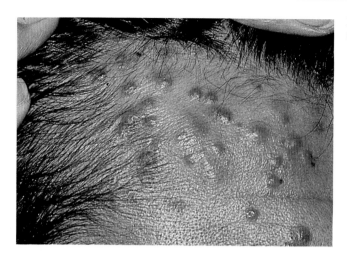

Fig. 511. Lupus miliaris disseminatus faciei.

tion of the involvement of other organs (hilar lymph nodes, liver [to be ascertained by liver biopsy], and others) and of the histologic findings is helpful. In the facial region disseminated nodular (as pustules or comedones are absent, the appearance is not especially acneiform) hypertrophies of the sebaceous glands from cortisone or INH should be considered in the differential diagnosis.

4. Rosacealike cutaneous changes are also present in **granulosis rubra nasi.** This disorder is seen exclusively in children and

Fig. 512. Sarcoidosis with small nodes.

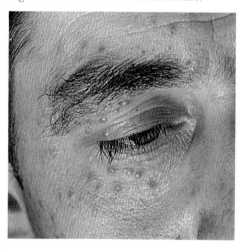

with a certain frequency in families. The main sign is hyperhidrosis limited to the nose. Only after this hyperhidrosis has lasted some time do small erythematous spots appear on the nose. From these erythemas a few more dark red nodules emerge; they are hardly ever larger than the size of a pinhead. The relatively pointed nodules are grouped together but do not show confluence. Comedones and pustules are absent, but occasionally small vesicles may occur. Only in exceptional cases do the cutaneous changes affect the neighboring cheeks and the upper lip.[5, 8, 12]

5. In the **Haber syndrome** a persistent, diffuse facial erythema covered by discrete scaling appears at an early age. On the forehead, nose, and chin the erythema is especially noticeable, owing to numerous telangiectases. Moreover, the similarity with rosacea is increased by the numerous red papules limited to the follicles, but pustules never develop. In addition to formation of erythema and papules, dimplelike, keratin-filled follicular openings are present. After exposure to sunlight, patients complain of an increased sensation of tension of the facial skin. A sex preference is not present in this probably autosomal dominant disorder.

Histologically, increased and dilated superficial vessels with perivascular inflammatory infiltrates, superficial lymphedema, and fibrosis of the corium are present. The epidermis is characterized by acanthosis, increased mitotic activity, and, in places, spongiosis and parakeratosis. Proliferations of the sebaceous glands and unusual intraepidermal epitheliomas are important. The epitheliomas may show bowenoid features on the one hand, or assume the aspect of clear cell acanthomas on the other.

6. Intake of halogens (bromines and iodides) in anorganic form may lead to an acutely inflammatory exacerbation of an already existing acne vulgaris. This is caused by excretion of the halogens through the sebaceous glands. Morphologic differences from acne vulgaris do not exist. On the other hand, doses of these halogens alone may cause primary **bromine** or **iodide acne** (Figs. 513, 514). Dusky red, papulopustular infiltrates develop on the face and on the back; comedones are absent.

(1) DENK, R., F. NÜRNBERGER und H. FASSL: Häufigkeit morphologischer Veränderungen der Magenschleimhaut bei Rosacea-Kranken. Klin. Wschr. *46:* 1112–1113 (1968).

(2) KLINGMÜLLER, G.: Über lupoide Rosacea. Derm. Wschr. *130:* 1058-1064 (1954).

(3) KORTING, G. W.: Kleinknotige disseminierte Talgdrüsenhypertrophie durch INH. Z. Haut- u. Geschl.-Kr. *37:* 158 – 162 (1964).

(4) MILBRADT, R.: Die rosaceaartige Dermatitis des Gesichts. Klinik, Histologie und Pathogenese. Lehmann, München 1972.

(5) RITTER, H.: Zur Ätiologie der Granulosis rubra nasi. Derm. Wschr. *72:* 366–370 (1921).

(6) RÖCKL, H., F. SCHRÖPL und M. SCHERER: Rosacea mit extrafacialer Lokalisation. Hautarzt *20:* 348–351 (1969).

Fig. 513. Bromine acne.

Fig. 514. Iodide acne.

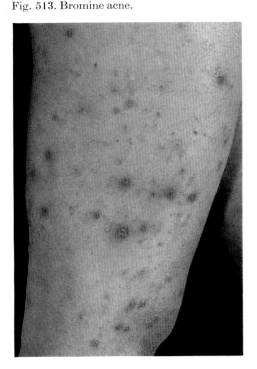

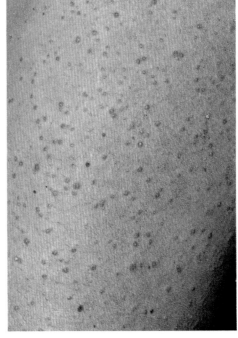

(7) SANDERSON, K. V., and H. T. H. WIL-
son: Haber's syndrome. Familial rosacealike eruption with intraepidermal
epithelioma. Brit. J. Derm. 77: 1–8
(1965).

(8) SCHILLER, E. A.: Granulosis rubra nasi.
Arch. Derm. Syph. (Chic.) 65: 365 (1952).

(9) SEIJI, M., and N. OTAKI: Haber's syndrome. Familial rosacealike dermatosis
with keratotic plaques and pitted scars.
Arch. Derm. (Chic.) 103: 452–455 (1971).

(10) STEIGLEDER, G. K., und A. STREMPEL:
Rosaceaartige Dermatitis des Gesichts.
»Periorale Dermatitis«. Hautarzt 19:
492–494 (1968).

(11) TRIEBENSTEIN, O.: Die Rosazeaerkran-
kungen des Auges. Klin. Mbl. Augenheilk. 68: 3–36 (1922).

(12) VELTMAN, G.: Über das familiäre Vorkommen der Granulosis rubra nasi.
Arch. Derm. Syph. (Berl.) 188: 188–196
(1949).

31. Lichenoid Eruptions

The term lichen in its usual sense describes a small area composed of closely
adjacent nodules; ordinarily they do not
develop into a more advanced morphologic
entity (an exception is lichen planus
pemphigoides, for instance). They heal
without scar formation, but with occasional residual pigmentation. The form of
the lichenoid elements is extremely variable. When especially small these nodules
are seen as glistening minute facets.

The basic nodule of lichen planus (at
least, those of a certain size) has a polygonal outline with a flat surface; the
eczematous nodule is a round lesion with
a diffuse border and a semispherical protuberance, whereas the lichenoid elements
of lichen simplex chronicus can be characterized as round and flat. Moreover, nodules in follicular arrangement have, in
general, round borders; they have a conical or pointed elevation, in the center of
which one can sometimes visualize a
pointlike follicular opening with either a
hair or a dark pluglet. When such follicular
papules are arranged closely together and
regularly disseminated they produce a
gooseskinlike appearance (cutis anserina).
Further details about follicular keratoses
were discussed in Chapter 29. Larger,
blunt, or flattened papules are called

obtuse; however, this term does not indicate a nosologic relationship of such
papular elements to lichen planus, chronic
lichen simplex, or to one of the forms of
prurigo. However, the term acuminated
papules refers exclusively to otherwise
mostly follicularly oriented lichen planus
papules.

A. Lichen Planus

1. The differential diagnosis of a typical
case of **lichen planus** with its characteristic
primary lesion is easily made. The primary
elements are generally seen on the flexor
aspects of the wrists and forearms, the
sides of the trunk, the lower lumbar region,
and the extensor sides of the legs. On these
sites plaquelike areas show a verrucous
character. In addition, lichen planus involves concomitant pruritus (see also Chapter 2, E1) and a tendency to formation of
isomorphic lesions (Koebner's phenomenon). The individual lesions are plane, polygonal papules of about rice-corn size when
fully developed. When the lesions are still
small, they appear rounded, but when
larger, they may have more angular borders
(Figs. 241, 515). The color of fresh papules
is a light red, although a steel blue color
develops after some time, in spite of the

term lichen "ruber" planus [used in Germany]. Even without the polish caused by scratching, indurated lichen planus papules have a waxlike sheen. The surface of larger lenticular papules may show grayish-white points and streaks. These Weyl-Wickham's striae form a network on the surface of the papule; the streaks become more visible if the horny layers are rendered transparent by application of oil or xylol. In addition to typical lichen planus papules, pointed spinular nodules are seen occasionally; they are called lichen planopilaris. Such follicular types of lichen planus are coupled, apparently more than coincidentally, with pseudo-peiade-like conditions of the scalp, and to a lesser extent of the axillae or pubic region (Graham-Little syndrome; see also Chapter 11, E6). Like cicatricial alopecia, lichen planus may cause disturbances of the nails, such as micaceous splintering of the nailplate (which is of normal thickness), formation of clefts and fissures of the distal part of the nail, and ridgelike elevations. Pronounced involvement of the nail's matrix may result in complete atrophy of the nail.

Further variations of the usual clinical appearance of lichen planus can be substantiated by histopathologic examination. The differential diagnosis of lichen

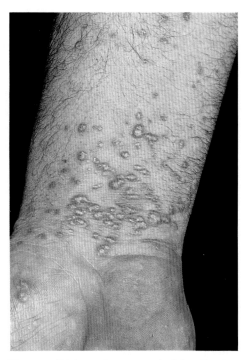

Fig. 515. Lichen planus: typical localization on the wrist.

verrucosus will be discussed in Chapter 21, E. Lichen planus bullosus has been previously considered in Chapter 25, B3, and its ulcerous after-effects will be elucidated again in Chapter 33, D19 and in Chapter 35, B4.

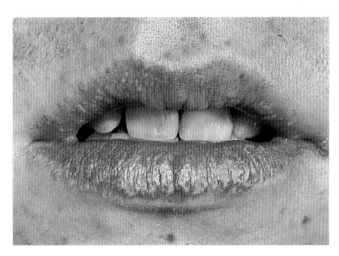

Fig. 516. Lichen planus of the vermilion border.

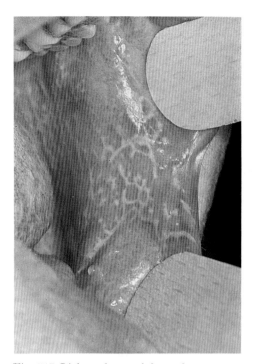

Fig. 517. Lichen planus of the oral mucosa.

Changes in the mucous membranes of the mouth and genitals are typical of lichen planus and are generally observed in the majority of cases. In these regions there are white and somewhat linear designs forming ringlike or netlike patterns. Unless a bullous variant is present the surface remains closed. When located on the tongue the white lesions are often so close together that they simulate a uniform bluish-white membrane (Figs. 516, 517). Erosive mucous membrane changes of lichen planus should be watched carefully for possible malignant degeneration. It is sometimes possible to arrive at a differential diagnostic distinction between candidiasis and leukoplakia by inspection. Otherwise it will be necessary to examine the patient for the presence of fungi and to perform a biopsy. However, systemic lupus erythematosus may also show net-like white linear designs on the mucous membranes. The simultaneous presence of pointlike bleeding dots speaks more in favor of systemic lupus. In general, the presence of other cutaneous changes allows a correct diagnosis of the mucous membrane condition.

Histologically, the lichen planus nodule in a typical case consists of an epidermocutaneous papule. The epidermal changes include orthohyperkeratosis, irregular widening of the granular layer, and an arcadelike course of the borderline between the dermis and the epidermis. Sometimes a separation of the epidermis from the corium may occur (as for instance at the onset of lichen planus bullosus). Moreover, immediately below the epidermal-dermal junction one may find circumscribed homogenization or colloidal globules and lumps. The dermal changes of lichen planus consist of a bandlike infiltrate with a sharp lower border. The infiltrate is generally confined to the upper papillary border; it consists primarily of lymphocytes, and sometimes also of plasma cells and a few mast cells. Multinuclear giant cells, perhaps responding to necrosis of the basal cell line ("liquefaction necrosis") are seen more rarely, whereas pigment-carrying melanophages are found regularly. In addition, fibrinous deposits occur within the infiltrates and also form the nucleus of the colloidal globules. The atrophic senile skin shows less epidermal involvement of the lichen planus papule, so that the infiltrate of the corium becomes more prominent. This explains the well-known lupoid brownish hue of the lichen planus of "old people." Generally, local hyperkeratosis is apparently responsible for the rarity of excoriations of lichen planus areas, aside from the fact that the patient with lichen planus, in spite of his rebellious pruritus, will soon refrain from scratching because the lichen planus lesions are unusually painful. The widening of the granular layer is visible clinically owing to the Weyl-Wickham's striae and the reticulated figures of the mucous membrane.

Table 9 Drugs Capable of Eliciting Lichen Planus-like Eruptions

Amiphenazole	PAS
Arsenic	Penicillin
Quinine	Phenothiazine derivatives
Chloral hydrate	Mercury
Chloroquine	Salicylates
Chlorothiazide	Thiouracil
Demethylchlor-tetracycline	
Gold	Tolbutamide
Mepacrine	Triprolidine
Methyldopa	Bismuth

Color film developer (paraphenylenediamine)

Our knowledge of the etiology of lichen planus extends no further than conjecture. About the only definitely established fact is that the primary manifestation of the disease starts in the basal cells. It is also established that some drugs (Table 9) and substances present in color film developers may give rise to lichen planus-like eruptions. However, histologically, such lichen planus manifestations sometimes show less bandlike but rather perivascular lymphocytic infiltrates; they also show parakeratosis instead of the hyperkeratosis that is so typical of genuine lichen planus.

Only the lichenoid **Atabrine dermatitis** of the second world war (New Guinea lichen planus, tropical lichen) shows certain clinical peculiarities which can be explained on the basis of previous functional arrest of perspiration by Atabrine, producing miliaria or anhidrosis. The underlying lichenoid character of the Atabrine dermatitis is probably responsible for the residual atrophic or alopecic permanent conditions.

Lichen sclerosus et atrophicus is not difficult to distinguish from lichen planus (see also Chapter 16, A2). Macroscopically it is recognizable by its porcelain white, punctiform, depressed lesions lying within the level of the surrounding skin, and above all by its focal hyperkeratosis. Histologically it has small subepidermal areas with sparse nuclei, interspersed with horny plugs, homogeneous connective tissue sclerosis, and shrinkage of the elastica. These findings are different from the small macular variant of circumscribed scleroderma on the one hand, and from lichen planus on the other. Differentiating unusual variants of lichen planus from lupus erythematosus is not at all simple, as the histologic and macroscopic findings may differ markedly. Macroscopically, patients with lichen sclerosus show round or oval lesions with accentuated borders; these lesions may occur on the palms or the backs of the hands, but also on other places, appearing as slightly indurated or succulent, sometimes ulcerated, scaly, silver-white grouped areas without any special presence of follicular keratoses. Lichen planus eruptions, one should remember, may terminate as poikiloderma-like "anonymous" conditions. Special difficulties may arise when lichen planus occurs in combination with another dermatosis, for instance, the previously mentioned lupus erythematosus or psoriasis. Experience shows how difficult it sometimes is to diagnose a single area of lichen planus. For instance, one may encounter solitary keratotic changes on sun-exposed cutaneous areas which clinically correspond mostly to actinic or seborrheic keratoses, but surprisingly on histologic examination turn out to show the character of lichen planus.[1-5, 7-13, 15]

2. Lichen nitidus in the final analysis is only a subspecies of lichen planus (Fig. 518). The lesions of lichen nitidus are pinhead-sized, yellow-brownish, round, single efflorescences with no central depression. The Koebner phenomenon is lacking. There are certain sites of predilection, for instance, the shaft of the penis and its glans. Lacking also are the annular figures so typical of lichen planus of the

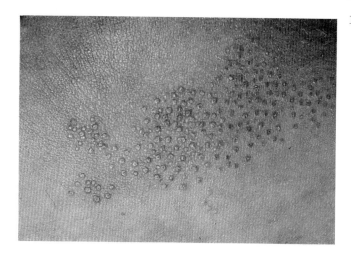

Fig. 518. Lichen nitidus.

penile area; pruritus, if present at all, is only moderate. The reason for assuming that lichen nitidus is a subspecies of lichen planus lies in the fact that, in the beginning, exanthematic-eruptive lichen planus shows the same roundish, miliary type of nodule as lichen nitidus. Histologically, lichen nitidus differs distinctly from lichen planus because it has a typical tuberculoid granuloma, which is attached like a swallow's nest beneath the epidermis (Fig. 519). Suggestions of such a structure are visible, at least in the very early stages, in a lichen planus nodule. An additional difference from fully developed lichen planus is the parakeratotic cover of the lichen nitidus papule.[6, 14]

3. Lichen scrofulosorum (Fig. 520) may occur on the sides of the trunk and may be difficult to differentiate from an exanthematic type of the lichen nitidus variety of lichen planus, especially because histologically lichen nitidus shows a typical tubercle. Lichen nitidus and lichen scrofulosorum are equally rare eruptions that occur mainly on the sides of the thorax in children or young adults. The two diseases

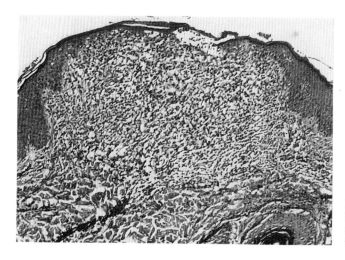

Fig. 519. Lichen nitidus: tuberculoid granuloma adjacent to the epidermis. Hematoxylin and eosin, 75 ×.

Fig. 520. Lichen scrofulosorum.

cause few subjective complaints and usually heal in time more or less by themselves. However, in contrast to lichen nitidus, the male genitals are not a favorite location of lichen scrofulosorum. In addition, the duration of lichen scrofulosorum is much shorter. As a rule, the lichenoid tuberculoid appears almost unnoticed in sudden crops; the single lesions, which may give a somewhat spinous appearance, are arranged in follicular or perifollicular groups. This may be similar to the small papular (nonpruritic) lichenoid syphilid and to the spinulism of some special forms of many dermatophytids *(lichen trichophyticus)*. On the other hand, lichen scrofulosorum may show only inconspicuous small nodular lesions which may suggest a common superficial, finely scaling plaque of eczema. As a rule, a diagnosis of lichen scrofulosorum should be made only if a young individual (up to the age of puberty) shows a barely visible phlyctenular reaction on the sides of the trunk as well as a focus of visceral tuberculosis; the same cutaneous reaction may follow a Moro test.

4. The so-called **lichen scorbuticus** is a distinctly follicular disseminated keratosis with a nutmeg grater-like or gooseflesh-like appearance. The single nodule may

have a markedly hard consistency (Fig. 521). In places the extensor aspects of the extremities show acneiform and hemorrhagic lesions that soon raise the possibility of scurvy or prescurvy (see also Chapter 29, C2).

Fig. 521. Lichen scorbuticus.

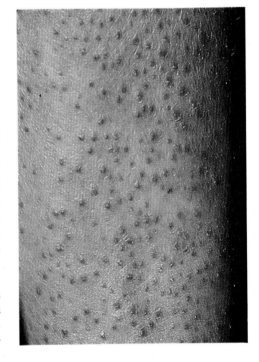

5. The single elements of **parakeratosis variegata** may be similar to the papules of lichen planus, especially in the beginning. However, in such cases the nodules are mainly roundish, and sometimes have a waxlike sheen similar to that of the classic papule of lichen planus. In contrast to the latter, the lesions of parakeratosis variegata have a tendency to form reticulated areas rapidly. These areas become atrophic in a short time while retaining the characteristic streak arrangement. In contrast to lichen planus, parakeratosis variegata lacks pronounced infiltration, the verrucous aspect of the lesions, and mucous membrane changes, unless transition to mycosis fungoides has already taken place. In addition, the patient with parakeratosis variegata hardly ever suffers from pruritus. The histologic changes of parakeratosis variegata remain insignificant in contrast to the distinct changes of lichen planus (see also Chapter 20, C).

6. Pityriasis rubra pilaris is discussed in Chapter 22, C14.

(1) BLACK, M. M.: The pathogenesis of lichen planus. Brit. J. Derm. *86:* 302–305 (1972).

(2) COPEMAN, P. W. M., A. L. SCHROETER and R. R. KIERLAND: An unusual variant of lupus erythematosus or lichen planus. Brit. J. Derm. *83:* 269–272 (1970).

(3) DOSTROVSKY, A., and F. SAGHER: Lichen planus in subtropical countries. Arch. Derm. Syph. (Chic.) *59:* 308–328 (1949).

(4) EBNER, H., und D. KRAFT: Fibrinablagerungen beim Lichen ruber planus. Eine licht-, immunfluorescenz- und elektronenmikroskopische Studie. Arch. Derm. Forsch. *243:* 305–317 (1972).

(5) EL-LABBAN, N. G.: Light and electron microscopic studies of colloid bodies in lichen planus. J. Periodont. Res. (Kopenhagen) *5:* 315–324 (1970).

(6) FRITSCH, P.: Der Lichen nitidus (Pinkus). Z. Haut- u. Geschl.-Kr. *42:* 649–666 (1967).

(7) GOUGEROT, H., et A. CIVATTE: Oscillations entre le lupus érythémateux, le lichen plan, et la poïkilodermie. Ann. Derm. Syph. (Paris) *1943:* 233–245.

(8) KOBERG, W., D. SCHETTLER und G. SELLE: Zur Frage der Karzinomentstehung auf dem Boden eines Lichen ruber planus der Mundschleimhaut. Münch. med. Wschr. *107:* 463–466 (1965).

(9) KRAMER, I. R., R. B. LUCAS, N. EL-LABBAN and L. LISTER: A computer-aided study on the tissue changes in oral keratoses and lichen planus, and an analysis of case groupings by subjective and objective criteria. Brit. J. Cancer *24:* 407–426 (1970).

(10) LUMPKIN, M. L. R., and E. B. HELWIG: Solitary lichen planus. Arch. Derm. (Chic.) *93:* 54–55 (1966).

(11) MALE, O.: Über Nagelveränderungen beim Lichen ruber planus. Hautarzt *21:* 445–454 (1970).

(12) PETZOLDT, D., und H.-J. VOGT: Lichen ruber-ähnliche Kontaktdermatitis durch einen Farbfilmentwickler. Hautarzt *21:* 281–283 (1970).

(13) SHAPIRO, L., and A. B. ACKERMAN: Solitary lichen planus-like keratosis. Dermatologica (Basel) *132:* 386–392 (1966).

(14) TAPPEINER, S.: Zur Stellung des Lichen nitidus im System der Hautkrankheiten. Dermatologica (Basel) *107:* 1–12 (1953).

(15) ZAIAS, N.: The nail in lichen planus. Arch. Derm. (Chic.) *101:* 264–271 (1970).

B. Lichen Myxedematosus

1. Slightly shiny, pale, skin-colored, predominantly semispherical papules are characteristic of **lichen myxedematosus.** The individual papules develop rather rapidly within a few days and are only rarely accompanied by itching. In the beginning they remain isolated or are grouped into a bizarre, stringlike pattern (Fig. 522).

This is in any case an extremely monomorphic disorder, which first becomes manifest after the fortieth year of life. Simultaneously occurring disorders of the inner organs, especially disturbances of thyroid activity, are not present. In the later course of the disease some patients show a close aggregation of individual papules accompanied by dense thickening and formation of gross cutaneous folds, i.e., transition into scleromyxedema. At this stage mucin may be deposited in the brain, heart, and esophagus.

The histologic picture of both forms of the disease is characterized by massive deposits of acid mucopolysaccharides in the upper corium. Within the zones of the deposits star-shaped connective tissue cells ("mucoblasts") can be found, as well as typical fibroblasts. Lichen myxedematosus as well as scleromyxedema is considered today to be a paraproteinemic reticulosis. In both diseases paraproteins of types IgG or IgM are present. In some cases a plasmacytoma or Waldenström's macroglobulinemia has been observed simultaneously. Since the ESR and electrophoresis may be normal, an immunoelectrophoretic decision should be sought.[1-3, 5-8]

2. With regard to the previously mentioned chainlike or net-shaped distribution of the papules in lichen myxedematosus it should be mentioned that so-called **lichen moniliformis,** although showing a special similarity to lichen myxedematosus, is supposed to be histologically mucinfree. It has not yet been definitely decided if cases of this disease are misdiagnosed or beginning instances of lichen myxedematosus. In any case, however, there are no clinical or histological similarities to lichen planus.[4, 9]

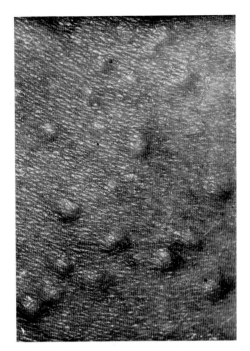

Fig. 522. Lichen myxedematosus.

(1) DALTON, J. E., B. H. BOOTH, H. R. GRAY and P. V. EVANS: Lichen myxedematosus (papular mucinosis). Arch. Derm. (Chic.) *83:* 230–240 (1961).

(2) DELACRÉTAZ, J., G.-F. MAILLARD, M. EMCH et M. P. GLAUSER: Paraprotéinémie familiale et lichen myxoedémateux. Ire partie: Etude clinique. Schweiz. med. Wschr. *100:* 626–630 (1970).

(3) DENK, R.: Elektrokardiographische Untersuchungen bei Hautkranken. Arch. Kreisl.-Forsch. *60:* 33–114 (1969).

(4) FEUERMAN, E. J.: Zur nosologischen Stellung des Morbus moniliformis. Z. Haut- u. Geschl.-Kr. *45:* [19]–[22] (1970).

(5) GLAUSER, M. P., G.-F. MAILLARD, M. EMCH et J. DELACRÉTAZ: Paraprotéinémie familiale et lichen myxoedemateux. IIe partie: Etude immunologique. Schweiz. med. Wschr. *100:* 666–671 (1970).

(6) HARDMEIER, TH., und A. VOGEL: Elektronenmikroskopische Befunde beim Skleromyxödem Arndt-Gottron. Arch. klin. exp. Derm. *237:* 722–736 (1970).

(7) HUTH, K., G. EHLERS, W. KNOTH, K. KUNZE, H. LÖFFLER, G. MÄHR und D. PETZOLDT: Lichen myxoedematosus bei Makroglobulinämie Waldenström mit Polyneuropathie und Carpaltunnel-Syndrom. Dtsch. med. Wschr. *97:* 152–159 (1972).

(8) RUDNER, E. J., A. MEHREGAN and H. PINKUS: Scleromyxedema; a variant of lichen myxedematosus. Arch. Derm. (Chic.) *93:* 3–12 (1966).

(9) WISE, F., and C. R. REIN: Lichen ruber moniliformis (morbus moniliformis lichenoides). Arch. Derm. Syph. (Chic.) *34:* 830–849 (1936).

C. Eczema Group

In complete contrast to the typical primary polygonal lesion of lichen planus, the eczema nodule, although also an epidermal papule, extends somewhat deeper than the lichen planus nodule, has a round dome shape, and is diffusely limited. Furthermore, whereas the lichen planus papule represents a stable nodule which can hardly be scratched open, the eczema nodule is somewhat frail owing to its exudative pathologic substrate, or, in other word, its spongiosis. Therefore, the papulovesicle is really the primary lesion representing common eczema. Both the serous-spongy infiltration and the parakeratosis, which skips the keratohyalin-developmental phase, contribute to the moderate pointlike destruction of the eczematous substrate (for example, by scratching).

1. Lichen simplex chronicus (neurodermatitis circumscripta) shows an almost skin-colored or gray-reddish, flat but also roundish, pinhead-sized papule as the primary lesion. In the center of the affected area these papules are confluent, so that the inner part seems to have rough and thickened skin markings, i.e., they appear lichenified. On the third outer zone a washed out, dirty brownish pigmentation develops. On the other hand, in the center of especially long-existing areas, vitiligolike depigmentations may be present. In other cases, however, the isolated character of the nodule persists against the otherwise typical confluent lichenification of the individual lesions.

Instead of macular, shagreen leatherlike skin, the surface assumes the appearance of a netlike or mosaiclike, quadrilated mesh, a thickly compressed system of small, dull, adjacent squares without the typical three zones. Even more lightly dispersed and without confluence and lichenification are the usually larger lichen simplex nodules partly mixed with urticarial lesions that are seen in lichen Vidal urticatus. With regard to itching see Chapter 2, D4, and for the differential diagnosis see Chapter 21, E1.

2. The single element of **lichen amyloidosus** is again a firm, variable brown, semispherical nodule that is verrucous-rough on the surface. The eruption of these nodules is rather often preceded by itching (see Chapter 2, D5). Occasionally these lichen amyloidosus nodules, which tend to occur on the extensor surfaces of the extremities in groups, do not remain isolated, and this confluence, especially on the legs, produces areas reminiscent of lichen simplex chronicus. If, however, the single nodules of lichen amyloidosus have polygonal borders and a dull sheen, there may be a certain similarity to lichen planus of the legs. Decisive for the diagnosis is the evidence of amyloid deposits in the areas affected by the disease. Since this is a primary amyloidosis limited to the skin, involvement of other organs is lacking. (See also Chapter 21, E3.)[1-3]

3. A definite morphologic contrast to the just described lichen simplex chronicus area is presented by the transient lichen simplex-like reaction of **atopic dermatitis** (neurodermatitis disseminata, endogenous eczema), which is characterized by a mixture of lichen simplex-like and common eczematous reactions in irregular relationship to each other. Moreover, atopic dermatitis differs from lichen simplex by its familial involvement, its initial development as "infantile eczema," its more than coincidental involvement with bronchial asthma and hay fever, and the different ages of the patients. For further details see Chapter 2, D3 and Chapter 21, D1.

(1) Brownstein, M. H., and E. B. Helwig: The cutaneous amyloidoses. I. Localized forms. Arch. Derm. (Chic.) *102:* 8–19 (1970).

(2) Saltzer, E. I., L. G. Cranmer and J. W. Wilson: Lichen amyloidosus and the nature of amyloid. Arch. Derm. (Chic.) *98:* 331–335 (1968).

(3) Schneider, W., und H. P. Missmahl: Lichen amyloidosus als Beispiel der peri-kollagenen, primären, hautbeschränkten und vorwiegend umschriebenen Amylo-idose. Arch. klin. exp. Derm. *224:* 235–247 (1966).

32. Xanthomas and Xanthomalike Cutaneous Changes

Xanthomas develop from deposits of lipids in circumscribed conglomerations of reticuloendothelial cells. It remains an open question whether or not in the individual case this development is caused by inordinate deviations of the fat metabolism or solely by local tissue factors favoring the storage of fat. In the differential diagnosis as xanthomatous, or better, as xantheloid tumors, all tumors or plano-tuberous protuberances, which because of their form or their yellow-brownish color resemble typical xanthomas, should eventually be considered.

A. Xanthomatoses

First, pronounced multiple development of xanthomas is observed in **primary and secondary hyperlipoproteinemias.** Formerly, not least for prognostic considerations, only hypercholesterinemia and hyperlipemia were differentiated in this connection, but today primary hyper-lipoproteinemias are divided into five types for biochemical reasons. An unequivocal distinction is not possible from the dermatologic findings. In the hypercholes-terinemic xanthomatoses, deleterious involvement of the cardiovascular system (stenoses, aneurysms of the walls, and infarcts) occurs frequently. In the hyper-triglyceridemic xanthomatoses, vascular diseases, although not as distinct, also occur more than coincidentally.

1. As mentioned before, since the clinical manifestations do not permit a satisfactory classification of the individual types, this classification must be carried out according to analyses of the serum fat. A preliminary, approximate clinical differentiation is possible by inspection of the blood serum, which may be clear or milky-cloudy. A milky-creamy cloudiness of the serum which clears after standing (with the exception of the overlying chylo-micron layer) is characteristic of hyper-chylomicronemia (fat-induced hypertri-glyceridemia) **(type I).** The serum fat analysis shows a distinct increase in the triglycerides and chylomicrons, whereas the cholesterol fraction is usually normal or, in exceptional cases, slightly increased. Furthermore, postheparin-lipolytic activity is distinctly lowered. This results in distinct chylomicronemia in patients who have a daily fat intake of only 10 gm. This type of hyperlipoproteinemia is inherited as an autosomal recessive trait. It mani-

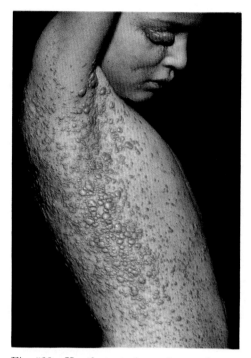

Fig. 523. Xanthomatosis: primary hyperlipoproteinemia type II.

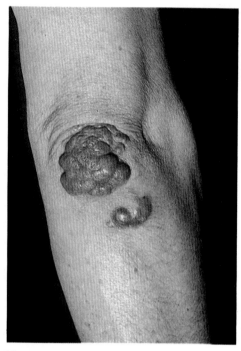

Fig. 524. Tuberous xanthomas in primary
hyperlipoproteinemia type II.

fests itself in childhood at about the tenth year of life. In addition to multiple eruptive xanthomas and retinal lipemia, recurrent colics of the upper abdomen are the predominant signs. It is remarkable that no predisposition to arteriosclerosis exists.[3, 6, 9, 10, 12, 20]

2. Essential hypercholesterolemia (hy-per-beta-lipoproteinemia, **type II**) is char-acterized by clear serum with an exces-sive increase in cholesterol and cholesterol esters, whereas the other serum fat frac-tions, with the exception of the likewise increased lipoproteins, are normal. Here-dity is probably incompletely autosomal dominant. Clinically, tuberous xanthomas of the tendon sheaths and xanthelasmas (Fig. 523) are present most often. The development of xanthomas is apparently parallel to the increase and duration of

the cholesterol level in the serum. Eruptive* xanthomas and streaky palmar xanthomas do not occur. Tuberous xan-thomas are present especially on the knees and elbows (Fig. 524) but also on pro-tuberances of the bones and tendons. Arcus lipoides of the cornea and coronary disturbances of the blood supply are as-sociated with these xanthomatous forma-tions, often even in early childhood. If these patients remain untreated, they die early of sudden cardiac arrest, which is usually caused by the acute closure of a coronary artery. Often mitral or aortic defects are present also, caused by deposits of cholesterol in and on the valves.[3, 6, 9, 10, 20]

3. In **type III** of the hyperlipoprotein-emias (a disorder with wide beta bands) the serum is either milky-dull or clear,

---

* As in an exanthematous eruption. (Tr.)

depending on whether increases of the triglycerides or cholesterols predominate. In any case, both parameters are increased, and are even higher owing to the increase of pre-beta-lipoproteins. In contrast to the earlier described types I and II, type III also shows a lower glucose tolerance threshold. The diagnosis is made possible by the evidence of beta-lipoproteins of very low density after ultracentrifugation and electrophoretic separation. The recessive inheritance of type III is questionable. Clinically, xanthelasmas and tuberous and tendonous xanthomas as in type II are present, as well as eruptive xanthomas and, above all, lipoid deposits along the volar aspects of the hands (Fig. 525). Coronary sclerosis and disturbances of peripheral arterial circulation become manifest in combination with the xanthomas around the forty-fifth year of life. Occasionally, the patients complain of pain in the upper abdomen and show hepatosplenomegaly and hyperuricemia. 3, 9, 10, 12, 20

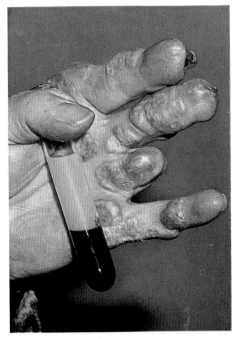

Fig. 525. Primary hyperlipoproteinemia type III, milky-dull serum.

4. Among the laboratory findings in **type IV** (hyper-pre-beta-lipoproteinemia, endogenous hypertriglyceridemia) is a distinct increase in the pre-beta- (= alpha 2–) lipoproteins and the triglycerides, and

to a lesser extent in cholesterols, with reduced glucose tolerance. Here again the serum may be clear or milky-dull. Many patients are obese and suffer from prematurely beginning arteriosclerosis with disturbances of peripheral circulation and coronary insufficiency. Tuberous xan-

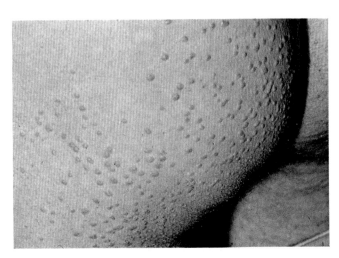

Fig. 526. Eruptive xanthomas in primary hyperlipoproteinemia type IV.

Table 10 Differential Diagnosis of the Hyperlipoproteinemias (according to Berg et al. 1970[4])

Type	I	II	III	IV	V
	Hyperchylo-micronemia	Hyper-beta-lipoproteinemia = Essential Hypercholes-terinemia	Disorder with Broad Beta-disease	Hyperpre-beta-lipoproteinemia	Hyperpre-beta-lipoprotein-emia plus Hyperchylomi-cronemia
A. Primary Hyperlipoproteinemias					
Laboratory findings					
PHLA (post-heparin lipoly-tic activity)	*Low*	Normal	Normal	Normal	*Low* or normal
Triglycerides	*Considerably increased*	Normal	*Increased*	*Increased*	*Increased*
Cholesterin	Normal or slightly increased	*Increased*	*Increased* (trigl: chol. ∼ 1:1)	Slightly increased (trigl: chol. ∼ 5:1)	Slightly increased
Chylomicrons	*Considerably increased*	–	–	–	*Increased*
Pre-beta (=alpha$_2$-) lipoprotein	Normal	Normal	*Increased*	*Increased*	*Increased*
Beta-lipo-proteins	Normal	*Increased*	*Increased*	Normal or slightly increased	Normal or slightly increased
Glucose tolerance	Normal	Normal	Reduced	Reduced	Reduced
Ultracen-trifugation	Unnecessary	Unnecessary	Uncondition-ally necessary	Unnecessary	Unnecessary
Diet tests					
Fat tolerance test	Pathologic	–	Only rarely pathologic	Occasionally pathologic	Pathologic
Carbohydrate tolerance test	–	–	Pathologic	Pathologic	Pathologic in most cases
B. Secondary Hyperlipoproteinemias					
	Diabetes mellitus, acute pancreatitis, alcoholism	Nephrotic syndrome, hypothyroid-ism, plasma-cytoma, macro-globulinemia, cholestatic hepatopathy	Pancreatitis, chronic alcoholism, Tangier disease, dys-globulinemia	Diabetes mellitus, pancreatitis, chronic alcoholism, plasmacytoma, glycogenoses, hypothyroid-ism, pregnancy, inhibitor of ovulation	Diabetes mellitus, pancreatitis, nephrotic syndrome, chronic alcoholism, acute alcoholism, dysglobulin-emia

thomas and xanthomas of the tendon sheaths as well as xanthelasmas are relatively rare. However, multiple papular xanthomas, most frequently on the buttocks and flexor sides of the thighs, are rather characteristic (Fig. 526). Another characteristic of papular xanthomas is their astoundingly rapid onset. As in type III, streaky xanthomas occur along the lines of the hands.[3, 6, 9, 10, 12, 20]

5. Type V represents, according to serum lipid analysis, a mixed form of types I and IV (mixed endogenous-exogenous hyperlipemia). The serum is dull when taken and does not clear even after long standing. However, after standing, the supernatant chylomicron layer becomes visible. In addition to the distinctly increased triglyceride fraction, cholesterol is also increased. With lipid electrophoresis, widened bands of chylomicrons and pre-beta-lipoprotein are present. As in type I the patients complain of coliclike pains in the upper abdomen; however, these first become manifest in adulthood. The same can be said for the eruptive xanthomas, which do not occur regularly. They are found on the buttocks, knees, and elbows. In addition, hepatomegaly and retinal lipemia may be present. The usually obese patients also have a lowered glucose tolerance.[3, 9, 10, 12, 20]

Histologically, xanthomas represent areas of accumulated histiocytes or monocytic cells containing lipids. Formation of foam cells and, more important, deposits of lipids are preceded by proliferation of these lymphoid or histiocytic cells. This is especially evident in the lipoid granulomas. In addition to this growth of large round cells, the formation of giant cells, among which the so-called Touton type occurs especially often, is cytologically characteristic of the xanthomas. Touton giant cells, however, are also present in other skin diseases such as lepromatous leprosy, in the walls of degenerated sebaceous cysts, and in certain tumors such as pseudosarcomatous

xanthofibromas. Although in certain types of xanthomas Touton cells seem to predominate and, on the other hand, lipid deposition (as in the eruptive papular xanthomas) seems to be greater than in the tuberous xanthomas, an absolutely certain classification of the xanthomas without consideration of the remaining clinical and biochemical findings is not possible. The basic individual elements of the xanthoma, i.e., the lymphoid and histiocytic, foam and Touton giant cells, correspond to macrophages of the tissue. Occasionally a remarkable mixture with mast cells occurs. The prevalence of eosinophils suggests an eosinophilic granuloma, and the presence of hemorrhage suggests the existence of Hand-Schüller-Christian disease. In both cases, however, both cellular proliferation and a granuloma as a basic or storage center for subsequent deposits should be present.[11]

6. Distinct from these primary hyperlipoproteinemias are the **secondary hyperlipoproteinemias** in diabetes mellitus, the nephrotic syndrome, myxedema, disorders of the pancreas, alcoholism, primary biliary liver cirrhosis, and disturbances of glycogen metabolism (see Table 10). Correlated cutaneous changes, i.e., xanthomas, occur irregularly in these secondary forms and do not follow any special distribution pattern.[7]

7. Outside of the hyperlipoproteinemic xanthomatoses, normolipoproteinemic xanthomatoses rarely occur. In **generalized xanthelasma** the first cutaneous changes begin in adulthood, usually around the fiftieth year of life. In the beginning the patients notice only the formation of xanthelasmas on the lids, but in the later course of the disease there are eruptions in other locations. Xanthelasmas then occur mostly on the neck, trunk, and extremities. The flexor aspects of the joints are not affected, and the mucous membranes are always free; these are differentiating criteria from xanthoma disseminatum. Most of the affected areas remain very flat and attract attention only by their light yellow color. Lipoprotein electrophoresis may show low values for alpha- and beta-lipoproteins, whereas the remaining fat status of the serum is normal. Histologically these areas show foam cells situated perivascularly for the most part, but also lying diffusely in the corium. Giant cells and granulomas are absent. Such striking perivascularly oriented foam cell formations are also observed only in primary biliary liver cirrhosis, Tangier disease (an alpha-lipoproteinemia), and Wolman's disease (primary familial xanthomatosis). At the present time no involvement of internal organs is known to occur in generalized xanthelasma. In particular, neither diabetes insipidus, exophthalmos, nor osseous lesions exist even transiently.[2, 17]

8. Disseminated xanthoma, which is also normolipoproteinemic, either greatly resembles histiocytosis X or represents its abortive form. The disease appears in adults as orange-colored to red-brown, isolated confluent papules on the flexor aspects of the large joints and intertriginous spaces. Similar deposits occur in the oral cavity, pharynx, and upper airways. Lipid deposits may also occur on the conjunctiva and cornea. Histologically, proliferation of histiocytic cells without striking cellular polymorphism or increased mitotic activity is present. The primary changes are similar to those of a histiocytoma. The storage of lipids within histiocytes and giant Touton cells is a secondary phenomenon. In addition, there are often iron deposits. In spite of these signs the histologic differentiation from a nevoxanthoendothelioma or a histiocytoma may be impossible at certain stages. It is, therefore, essential to recognize diabetes insipidus, which is often only transient. Part of the cutaneous changes may regress spontaneously. In spite of many similarities, transition into genuine Hand-Schüller-Christian disease has not yet been observed.[1, 13]

9. Hand-Schüller-Christian disease usually develops in childhood. Disseminated or tuberous xanthomas appear on dry and pale brownish skin with no specific location in the intertriginous areas and flexor aspects of the joints as would be seen in disseminated xanthoma. Here the xanthomas occur on the neck, axillae, sides of the trunk, face, and above all on the eyelids. The mucous membranes of the oral cavity, airways, and genitals often show lipid deposits. Exophthalmos of one or both eyes is another characteristic sign. It is caused by the narrowing of the orbital space. Other typical signs of the disorder are diabetes insipidus and multiple osseous defects (osteoporotic lacanae) of the skull. Histologically, a reticulohistiocytic granulation tissue composed of histiocytes, giant cells, plasma cells, lymphocytes, eosinophilic granulocytes, and Langerhans' cells is present. The occurrence of foam cells is essential and is probably caused by intracellular disturbed lipid decomposition.[22]

In other systemic diseases such as *plasmacytoma, Waldenström's macroglobulinemia, eosinophilic reticulocytosis, acrodermatitis chronica atrophicans,* and many *erythrodermas,* plane xanthomas without hyperlipoproteinemia may occur.[5, 8, 18, 21, 24, 26]

10. Because **multiple nevoxanthoendotheliomas** also occur primarily in childhood, they may be mistaken for Hand-Schüller-Christian disease. Further details are discussed in Section B 1 of this chapter.

11. Wolman's disease is also a generalized xanthomatosis without hyperlipoproteinemia. Since the children die a few weeks after the onset of the disease, a visible formation of xanthomas on the skin does not develop, although in histologic examination perivascular and periadnexal foam cells are present. There may be in addition extracellular free lipid deposits between the collagen fibers of the corium. Clinical manifestations begin with developmental disturbances, vomiting, distinct signs of malabsorption, and hepatosplenomegaly. Radiologically, calcifications of the adrenals can be observed early. Infants generally die in the first half year of life. In the beginning the plasma alpha-lipoproteins are diminished and later they are no longer present. Triglycerides and cholesterol-storing cells are present not only in the skin but also in the liver, bone marrow, small intestines, lymph nodes, and adrenals. In contrast to Niemann-Pick's disease (storage of phospholipids), the central nervous system always remains unaffected. The intracellular storage of lipids results from a lack of acid lipase, so that the decomposition of triglycerides and cholesterol esters cannot proceed normally.[19, 27, 28]

12. Aggregations of cutaneous, perivascular foam cells combined with deposits of cholesterol esters also occur in **Tangier disease** (an alpha-lipoproteinemia). Only in exceptional cases do the cell aggregates lead to visible cutaneous changes in the form of reddish-brown pinhead-sized papules. The main clinical sign is the hyperplastically enlarged tonsils with orange-yellow saturation. These discolorations, caused by cholesterol deposits, can extend to parts of the pharynx. With the rectoscope a grayish-yellowish marbleizing of the mucous membrane is visible. Some patients suffer also from a purely motoric polyneuropathy and hepatosplenomegaly. The eyes show central spotty corneal opacities. The previously mentioned foam cells are also evident in the liver, spleen, lymph nodes, and bone marrow, as well as the skin. The diagnosis is confirmed if, in addition to the clinical

findings, hypercholesterinemia and a high-grade diminution or complete lack of alpha 1-lipoproteins (lipoproteins with great density) are present. Heredity is probably autosomal recessive.[14, 15, 16, 23]

13. Xanthomas also occur in **dystrophia dermochondrocornealis familiaris** (Francois' disease). Modern analyses of the serum lipids of patients have not been made, and one can state only that no hypercholesterinemia and no milky-dull serum exist. Particularly important are the extensive osseous defects of the carpal bones of the hands and feet with resulting subluxations and contractures. The forearms appear too short owing to the compressed bones of the hands. Corneal opacities, which are subepithelial and centrally degenerative, appear early. The corneal parenchyma and Descemet's membrane remain clear. The etiology of this very rare disease is still not known.[25]

14. Xanthelasmas have no connection with a lipoid thesaurismosis. They remain confined to the eyelids (Fig. 527), occurring only very rarely on the conjunctivae and sclerae, and usually not before the fourth decade. In spite of this, a xanthelasma of the lid indicates the need for an examination of the serum lipid fractions and suggests the possible presence of diabetes mellitus and hypertonia. The more or less flat, ivory- to lemon yellow-colored xanthelasmas develop from the inner angle of the eye toward the upper lid. The lower lid is rarely involved. This development usually proceeds slowly and symmetrically, until it becomes stationary. Spontaneous involution even of part of the area occurs very rarely. In older persons xanthelasmas of the lids may be interspersed with comedones or cysts; this is understandable as the periorbital region tends to develop grouped late comedones. In women, especially if there are multiple xanthelasmas on the eyelids associated

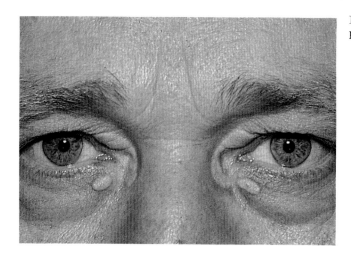

Fig. 527. Xanthelasma palpebrarum.

with itching and icterus of varying intensity, biliary liver cirrhosis may have to
be considered. Normal values of fat in the
serum, however, rule out primary biliary
liver cirrhosis.

(1) ALTMAN, J., and R. K. WINKELMANN:
Xanthoma disseminatum. Arch. Derm.
(Chic.) *86:* 582–596 (1962).

(2) ALTMAN, J., and R. K. WINKELMANN:
Diffuse normolipemic plane xanthoma;
generalized xanthelasma. Arch. Derm.
(Chic.) *85:* 633–640 (1962).

(3) BAES, H., M. K. POLANO, C. PRIES and
C. M. VAN GENT: Distribution of various
forms of xanthomata in three types of
primary hyperlipoproteinemia. Dermatologica (Basel) *136:* 300–303 (1968).

(4) BERG, G., D. BERGNER, W. GRABNER
und F. MATZKIES: Praktische Hinweise
zur Diagnostik von Hyperlipidämien.
Fortschr. Med. *88:* 938–940 (1970).

(5) CRAMER, H. J.: Normolipämische Xanthome bei Akrodermatitis chronica atrophicans Herxheimer. Derm. Wschr. *154:*
1177–1182 (1968).

(6) DENK, R.: Elektrokardiographische
Untersuchungen bei Hautkranken. Arch.
Kreisl.-Forsch. *60:* 33–114 (1969).

(7) FALK, I.: Die primär biliäre Leberzirrhose. (Beziehung zu den Kollagen-
krankheiten). Med. Welt (Stuttg.) *1964:*
244–249.

(8) FEIWEL, M.: Xanthomatosis in cryo-
globulinaemia and other paraproteinae-
mias with report of a case. Brit. J.
Derm. *80:* 719–729 (1968).

(9) FUHRMANN, W.: Erbliche Anomalien
der Plasmalipoide. Humangenetik *2:*
1–20 (1966.)

(10) GRETEN, H.: Diagnose und Differenzierung von Hyperlipoproteinämien. Klin.
Wschr. *47:* 893–896 (1969).

(11) HOEDE, N., und G. W. KORTING: Pseudosarkomatöses Xanthofibrom. Arch.
klin. exp. Derm. *232:* 119–126 (1968).

(12) KAHLKE, W., G. SCHETTLER und
G. SCHLIERF: Die essentiellen Hyper-
lipämien (primäre Hyperlipoproteinämien). Dtsch. med. J. *19:* 258–264
(1968).

(13) KALZ, F., M. M. HOFFMAN and A. LA-
FRANCE: Xanthoma disseminatum.
Clinical and laboratory observations
over a ten year period. Dermatologica
(Basel) *140:* 129–141 (1970).

(14) KRACHT, J., K. HUTH, W. SCHOENBORN
und W. FUHRMANN: Hypo-α-Lipopro-
teinämie (Tangier disease). Verh. dtsch.
Ges. Path. *54:* 355–360 (1970).

(15) KUMMER, H., J. LAISSUE, H. SPIESS,
R. PFLUGSHAUPT und U. BUCHER:
Familiäre Analphalipoproteinämie
(Tangier-Krankheit). Schweiz. med.
Wschr. *98:* 406–412 (1968).

(16) LAISSUE, J., H. KUMMER und J. HOD-
LER: Speicherzellen bei An-alpha₁-
Lipoproteinämie. Virchows Arch. path.
Anat. Abt. A. *344:* 119–124 (1968).

(17) LINDESKOG, G. R., A. GUSTAFSON and
L. ENERBÄCK: Serum lipoprotein deficiency in diffuse "normolipemic" plane
xanthoma. Arch. Derm. (Chic.) *106:*
529–532 (1972).

(18) MOSCHELLA, S. L.: Plane xanthomatosis associated with myelomatosis. Arch.
Derm. (Chic.) *101:* 683–687 (1970).

(19) PATRICK, A. D., and B. D. LAKE: Deficiency of an acid lipase in Wolman's
disease. Nature (Lond.) *222:* 1067–1068
(1969).

(20) POLANO, M. K., H. BAES, H. A. M.
HULSMANS, A. QUERIDO, C. PRIES and
C. M. VAN GENT: Xanthomata in
primary hyperlipoproteinemia. A classification based on the lipoprotein pattern
of the blood. Arch. Derm. (Chic.) *100:*
387–400 (1969).

(21) RABBIOSI, G., e C. BERNASCONI: Xanto-
matosi cutanea plana generalizzata nor-
mocolesteremica in una paziente affetta
da linforeticulosi macroglobulinemica
di Waldenström. Minerva derm. *42:*
666–667 (1967).

(22) TREBBIN, H.: Die Lipoidgranulomatose.
Med. Welt *20* (N.F.): 587–590 (1969).

(23) WALDORF, D. S., R. I. LEVY and
D. S. FREDRICKSON: Cutaneous chole-
sterol ester deposition in Tangier disease.
Arch. Derm. (Chic.) *95:* 161–165 (1967).

(24) WALKER, A. E., and I. B. SNEDDON:
Skin xanthoma following erythroderma.
Brit. J. Derm. *80:* 580–587 (1968).

(25) WIEDEMANN, H. R.: Zur François'schen
Krankheit; dystrophia dermo-chondro-
cornealis familiaris. Ärztl. Wschr. *13:*
905–909 (1958).

(26) WINKELMANN, R. K., und W. R. WEL-
BORN: Xanthome und maligne Retikulosen. Hautarzt *20:* 550–555 (1969).

(27) WOLMAN, M., V. V. STERK, S. GATT and
M. FRENKEL: Primary familial xanthomatosis with involvement and calcification of the adrenals. Report of two
more cases in siblings of a previously
described infant. Pediatrics *28:* 742–757
(1961).

(28) YOUNG, E. P., and A. D. PATRICK:
Deficiency of acid esterase activity in
Wolman's disease. Arch. Dis. Child. *45:*
664–668 (1970).

B. Xanthomalike Cutaneous Changes

1. In children who have a few xanthoma-
like tumors a **nevoxanthoendothelioma**
should be considered first. The lesions occur mainly in multiples and only seldom
remain solitary; they are yellowish-red,
as a rule quite hard, semispherical nodes
(Fig. 528). Sometimes the tumors are
present at birth and the nodes may be
surrounded by an erythematous border;
when more elevated, telangiectases will be
noticed. Spontaneous regression almost
always occurs; however, it may extend
over several years. During the regressive
phase the nodes sometimes show central
depressions and are covered by crusts;
finally only a flabby anetodermalike scar
remains. In rare instances the disease may
have a systemic character with involvement of internal organs by the same type
of nodes (eyes, intestinal tract, lungs,
heart, and testes). The inexperienced may

Fig. 528. Typical semispherical nevoxanthoendotheliomas.

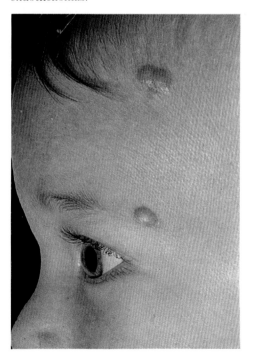

in such cases suspect metastases of a malignant tumor, thereby causing unnecessary surgical intervention. Histopathologically, the nevoxanthoendothelioma is considered today to be a histiocytoma that stores lipids. Giant cells are almost always seen only in the tumorous part near the epidermis. The foam cells in most cases remain smaller than those in a xanthoma.

The differential diagnosis must consider primarily Hand-Schüller-Christian disease. However, the nevoxanthoendothelioma lacks involvement of the mucosa, skeletal changes, exophthalmos, and diabetes insipidus. Hand-Schüller-Christian disease is a progressive affliction which frequently has a lethal ending, whereas multiple nevoxanthoendotheliomas show spontaneous regression. Furthermore, the individual lesions require the exclusion of a solitary mast cell tumor. Such a tumor, usually found on the trunk (shoulders, gluteal region), is a brownish-yellow, round lesion which either itches spontaneously or produces an urticarial response upon rubbing. Urticaria pigmentosa (xanthelasmoidea), when its reddish-brown color is receding, may also assume an appearance simulating xanthoma or nevoxanthoendothelioma. A biopsy may be necessary if the clinical picture, for instance, simultaneous formation of bullae or the presence of areas with typical color and swelling after intensive rubbing, makes differentiation impossible (see also Chapter 24, E 12).[6, 12, 19, 29, 33, 35]

2. Pseudoxanthoma elasticum (Grönblad-Strandberg syndrome) represents a systemic, metabolic, dysplastic elastosis which is most likely inherited recessively. The cardinal signs usually appear in the first or second decade but in rare instances may be present earlier. The ivory-white to lemon-yellow, striated or somewhat reticular, grouped formations of nodules are located primarily on the sides of the neck (Fig. 529), the axillae, the folds of the

large joints, and occasionally on the inner aspects of the thighs and the genitocrural folds. Not infrequently the lesions show thin telangiectases. In addition, in some patients the skin has a marked flabbiness in the vicinity of the affected areas. Sometimes changes similar to those observed on the skin are found in the gastrointestinal tract. Above all, an important additional sign of this systemic elastorrhexis is the tendency to calcification, which perhaps has a genetic basis (Fig. 530). Increasing rigidity of the peripheral arteries with markedly diminished flow can be observed early. Even at a youthful age patients have "essential" hypertension and sometimes complain of angina pectoris. Pseudoxanthoma elasticum must be ruled out from a medical point of view in the presence of etiologically obscure hemorrhages of the gastrointestinal tract or the bladder, especially in connection with early hypertension. Rare but not merely accidental syntropies occur in Paget's disease of the bones, familial hyperphosphatemias, and sickle cell anemia. The ocular fundus shows pigmented glistening streaks of the retina, known as "angioid streaks" (Fig. 531).

The differential diagnosis must consider some phenocopies of pseudoxanthoma elasticum; for instance, similar suggestive changes of the sides of the neck are occasionally seen these days after prolonged therapy with corticosteroids ("stippled skin"). Changes that faintly resemble those in pseudoxanthoma elasticum are the colloidal cicatricial degenerations formerly seen after healed tuberculosis of the skin or, to a lesser extent, the atrophic changes observed after tuberoserpiginous tertiary syphilids have regressed. This is perhaps understandable because in genuine pseudoxanthoma elasticum, collagenous accompanying components can be easily seen either by humoral means or by electronmicroscopy. Cutis rhomboidalis nuchae, as the term implies, shows senile degeneration of the back of the neck and not of its

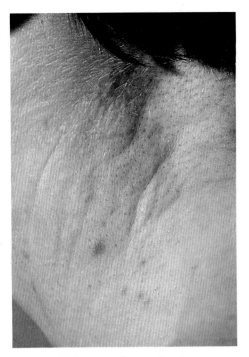

Fig. 529. Pseudoxanthoma elasticum: pseudoxanthomas at the side of the neck.

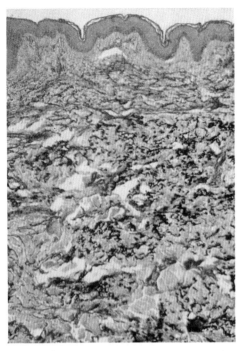

Fig. 530: Pseudoxanthoma elasticum: elastorrhexis with calcification of the elastic fibers. Elastica von Kossa stain, 63 × .

sides. Primary papules are lacking, although they may be imitated by furrows and diamond-shaped squares. The senile skin of the face and neck may also have somewhat thickened, yellow-whitish to yellow-brownish structural changes which produce a xanthelasmatoid appearance owing to their color (see also Chapter 17, A 1).[1, 5, 6, 10, 15, 23, 32]

3. Sebaceous nevi are seen even in children; they consist in most cases of typical multiple or circumscribed, usually striated, yellow-reddish or straw yellow, papillomatous areas. They occur most frequently on the scalp, the pre- and post-auricular areas, the temples, and the cheeks (Fig. 532). These nevi may be observed even at birth as hamartomas but may develop as late as the second or third decade of life. In contrast to its prejudicial name, histologic examination of sebaceous

nevi shows that often other cutaneous appendages take part in its structure. Although the decisive factor in a sebaceous

Fig. 531. Pseudoxanthoma elasticum: fundus with angioid streaks.

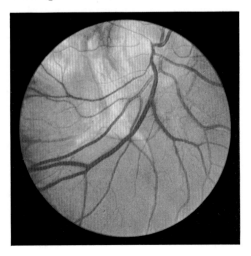

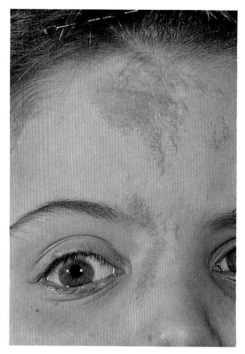

Fig. 532. Nevus sebaceus.

connective tissue, and plasma cell infiltration. A sebaceous nevus and a nevus
syringocystadenomatosus may occur within the same area or closely adjacent to
each other; moreover, frequently basalomas or basaloid or other pseudoepitheliomatous proliferations may occur in the
same neighborhood.[38]

Although a solitary sebaceous nevus is
in general seen without corresponding
internal involvement of other organs,
when systematic spreading occurs, consideration should be given to the presence
of the *Schimmelpenning syndrome*. Such
patients show ocular malformations, for
instance, dermoid cysts (Fig. 533), colobomas, changes of the cranial bones, and
cerebral epileptic attacks, often with
definite mental retardation. Similar associations have been observed, although
much less frequently, with nevus syringocystadenomatosus papilliferus.[7, 22, 24]

Yellow, subconjunctival lipomas are
part of the *Goldenhar's syndrome* (oculo-
auriculovertebral dysplasia), consisting of
auricular appendages, auricular fistulas,
malformation of the auricles, and unilateral facial dysplasia (Fig. 534), as well as
part of the *Wildervanck syndrome*, which
mostly affects females (acoustic labyrinth
deafness, congenital paresis of the ab-

nevus is the presence of grapelike clusters
of sebaceous glands, a nevus syringocystadenomatosus papilliferus shows dilated sweat gland systems with two
layers of cylindrical epithelium, villiferous

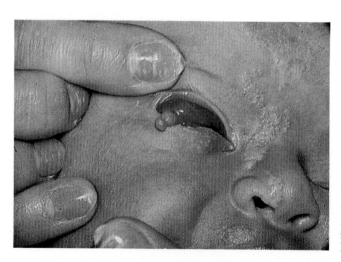

Fig. 533. The Schimmelpenning syndrome [systematized
extension of nevus sebaceus
with ocular malformations
and cerebral fits (Tr.)]. Dermoid cyst on the right upper
lid.

Fig. 534. Goldenhar syndrome: subconjunctival lipoma.

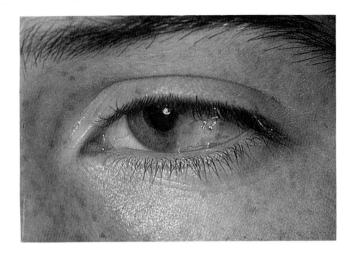

ducens nerve, unilateral facial hypoplasia, auricular appendages).[13, 37]

4. Nevus lipomatosus cutaneus superficialis distinctly favors the gluteal region as well as the lumbosacral region and the proximal parts of the thighs. This nevus almost always shows grouped nodules with a turbid, dirty yellow color and sometimes a reddish sheen; they may be as large as peas. These nodules consist of soft papules which can easily be invaginated by pressure with a finger; their soft consistency is definitely different from that of the hard and more yellowish-red or carrot-colored xanthomas. Histologically, the nevus lipomatosus cutaneus superficialis is characterized by masses of fat cells in the upper corium extending up to the epidermis. There is hardly any difference histologically between the isolated fat cell nevus and *focal dermal hypoplasia*, unless one wishes to emphasize the extreme thinning of the collagen in the latter.[14, 20, 28]

5. In addition, larger sebaceous retention cysts may have a xanthomatous color (Fig. 535). Sites of predilection of such **sebocystomatoses** are the scrotum, labia majora, and the middle of the back, regions with especially large and multilobu-

lated formations of sebaceous glands. In addition to the characteristic location and in contrast to tuberous xanthomas, sebaceous cysts are spherical and when punctured show a viscous or tallowy-crumbly content. On the surface of these retention

Fig. 535. Sebocystomatosis of the scrotum.

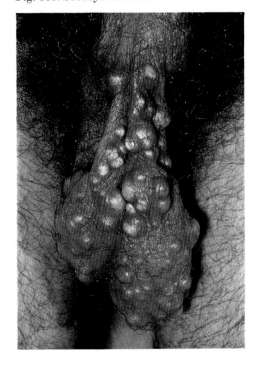

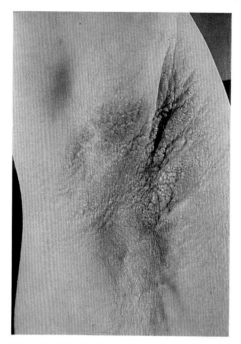

Fig. 536. Hyalinosis cutis et mucosae of the axillary region.

cysts the former follicular openings can be seen as small blackish dots. Although this disease has an autosomal dominant mode of inheritance, individual sebaceous cysts first develop after puberty, and sometimes not until the third decade of life.[11,16,31]

6. Hyalinosis cutis et mucosae (lipoid proteinosis) is discovered in early childhood by hoarseness, which regularly initiates the disorder. The most important dermatologic signs are the yellowish-white nodular deposits at the margins of the upper and lower eyelids and lips, and along the sides of the fingers, elbows, and armpits (Figs. 536, 537). The individual nodules are about twice the size of a pinhead and later become confluent, forming plaquelike firm areas whose surface may assume verrucous features. In particular, the papillomatous-verrucous areas in the axillae occasionally assume a brown color; this may lead to a mistaken diagnosis of acanthosis nigricans. The densely aggregated deposits make the face look relatively rigid. As in porphyria cutanea tarda, blisters and flat ulcerations develop even after minor injuries. They heal with slightly sunken, smallpoxlike scar formation. Either the growth of hair and nails is delayed, or the hyaline deposits cause permanent loss of hair (eyelashes). Aplasia or hypoplasia of the upper lateral incisors is rather typical. Before the cutaneous changes, as early as the onset of hoarseness, the oral mucosal manifestations become visible. Pale white to whitish-yellow, usually distinctly prominent deposits appear pri-

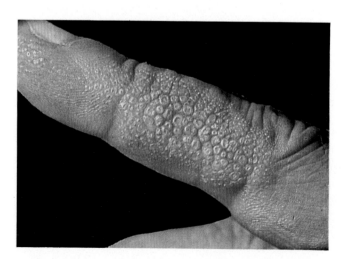

Fig. 537. Hyalinosis cutis et mucosae: hyaline deposits along the sides of the finger.

marily on the buccal mucosa, pharynx, tonsils, and larynx (vocal cords, epiglottis). Owing to the encroachment on the parotid duct, very painful recurrent swellings of the parotid gland occur. The tongue gradually increases in size and loses its normal flexibility at the same time (Fig. 538). Often it cannot be protruded at all. The frenulum of the tongue also thickens and becomes indurated owing to the deposits. In addition to the mucous membranes of the oral cavity and pharyngeal space, those of the esophagus, stomach, rectum, and vagina also have similar leukoplakialike changes.

Another characteristic sign of hyalinosis cutis et mucosae is the presence of intracranial symmetrical parasellar calcifications. They may be present in the pallidum, nucleus caudatus, corpus amygdaloideum, or oral part of the gyrus hippocampus, and they are always associated with epileptic attacks. These wing-shaped intracranial calcifications are so typical that they alone furnish the diagnosis. On the other hand, there are no laboratory examinations leading to the diagnosis. It is striking, however, that many patients show a diabetic metabolism and hyperproteinemia or dysproteinemia. Analysis of the serum fat shows normal values.

Histologically, in the corium between the fibers there are cell-free hyaline masses which have distinct connections with the vessels and the sweat glands. Tests for evidence of amyloid give negative results. Chemical analysis of the stored hyaline shows that it contains less lipoids than normal skin. Electronmicroscopically, it represents a disorderly woven pattern of filaments of 40–60 Å thickness.

The diagnosis of hyalinosis cutis et mucosae is easy to make from the signs of hoarseness beginning in childhood, intracranial calcifications, and cutaneous and mucosal changes. Morphologically, hyaline deposits occurring in erythropoietic protoporphyria may simulate hyalinosis cutis et mucosae very closely, but in the former they remain limited to light-exposed skin areas. There are additional differences in the analysis of porphyrin (see also Chapter 25, A10). If any doubt exists, amyloidosis should be ruled out by a rectal biopsy. Erythropoietic protoporphyria also lacks the typical onset characterized by hoarseness. A mistaken diagnosis of progressive scleroderma may result from the whitish sclerosis of the frenulum of the tongue, but the other clinical signs have nothing in common. An extensive colloid milium of the face may

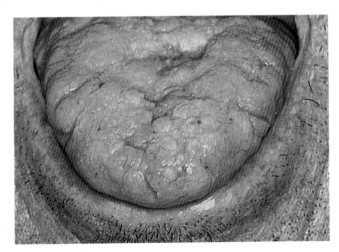

Fig. 538. Hyalinosis cutis et mucosae: enlarged tongue with coarsened surface.

simulate hyalinosis cutis et mucosae (see also Chapter 17, A2), but the patient's age, the time when manifestations occur, and the involvement of the mucosa permit a final decision.[4, 8, 17, 18, 21, 26, 27]

7. The group of **amyloidoses** includes various disorders that differ clinically or microscopically and are in part associated with cutaneous changes. Amyloid itself is an extracellularly located glycoprotein with a fibrillar ultrastructure. Moreover, lack of the amino acids hydroxylysine and hydroxyproline is characteristic. A rough distinction can be made by separating the localized from the systemic amyloidoses. Localized amyloidoses include lichen amyloidosus, macular amyloidosis, tumor-forming amyloidosis, blister-forming amyloidosis, and poikilodermic amyloidosis. These disorders usually do not show involvement of inner organs, which occurs only in exceptional cases. These disorders are discussed in the chapters dealing with their manifestations.

Systemic amyloidoses are subdivided into hereditary amyloidoses (familial Mediterranean fever, familial amyloid neuropathy, familial cardiac amyloidosis, and familial amyloidosis with urticaria and deafness); accompanying amyloidoses (chronic infections, chronic inflammatory disorders, malignant neoplasms without paraproteinemias); accompanying amyloidoses in paraproteinemias and plasmacytomas; and idiopathic systemic amyloidosis (old age amyloidosis and primary systemic amyloidosis). Of these systemic amyloidoses, only the accompanying amyloidoses in paraproteinemias and plasmacytoma and the primary systemic amyloidosis are associated with relatively typical visible skin changes. Using methods of histologic examination (optic polarization after staining with Congo red, the Congo red modification according to *Puchtler*, optic fluorescence after staining with thioflavine T), small amounts of amyloid deposits in the skin can also be demonstrated in other systemic amyloidoses. The diagnosis of amyloidosis should never be based on the clinical picture alone but should always include an evaluation of the histologic findings of a rectal or cutaneous biopsy (Fig. 541).

Early signs of **primary systemic amyloidosis** are increasing weakness, loss of weight, pains in the back and abdomen, cough, and diarrhea alternating with obstipation. The patients often complain also of drawing pains in the extremities, and difficulties in swallowing and speak-

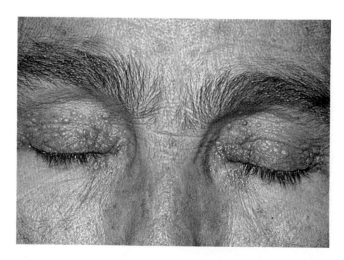

Fig. 539. Systemic amyloidosis: multiple skin-colored nodules on the upper eyelids.

Fig. 540. Systemic amy-
loidosis: subcutaneous
amyloid deposits on
the fingertips.

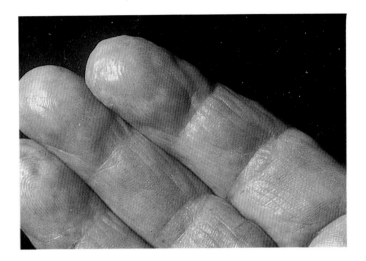

ing. Edema of the legs is an early sign. The liver may be found to be enlarged on palpation. Later, a cardiac insufficiency that is refractory to treatment sets in. Another frequent finding is polyneuropathy. Macroglossia, which was emphasized formerly, escapes clinical observation for a long time and becomes evident chiefly by disturbances in articulation. In addition to these generally indicative findings, the cutaneous changes especially point to the basic disorder. This is especially true of papular and flat deposits in the area of the eyelids, oral cavity, anogenital region, and the tips of the fingers (Figs. 539, 540). The epidermis remains unchanged except for some point-sized bleedings in the area of the deposits, but through it glassy or white to yellow-white scleroses can be felt or seen. At times the semitransparent nodules resemble taut swollen vesicles, especially when they occur on the sides of the tongue and the mucous membranes of the cheeks. The small amyloid papules usually appear in close proximity. In addition, larger, hematomalike suggillations exist in the periorbital region and on the mucous membranes. Larger plaquelike, cordlike, or

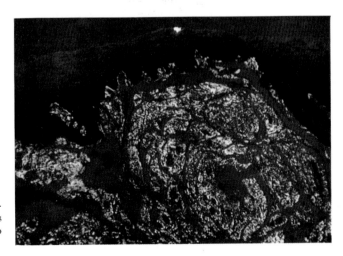

Fig. 541. Evidence of subepidermal amyloid deposits
with polarized light (Congo
red stain).

nodular infiltrates are usually localized irregularly. If the course of the disease is exceptionally long, a diffuse scleroderma-like or myxedematous cutaneous change finally develops. In this event, the infiltrated lip area and the anogenital region in particular tend to develop fissures. A differential diagnosis from hyalinosis cutis et mucosae or lichen myxedematosus may become necessary. Laboratory methods can provide no certain confirmation of the clinically suspected diagnosis apart from general signs such as anemia or dysproteinemia and an increase in gamma-globulin. This is also true of the results of immunoelectrophoresis, with the exception of the paraproteinemic combination with a plasmacytoma or macroglobulinemia.

If macroglossia is the most important symptom, a diffusely infiltrated carcinoma of the tongue, glossitis granulomatosa, or syphilitic glossitis interstitialis profunda must be considered. They, however, lack the previously mentioned interspersion of small nodules and bleeding areas on the surface.[2, 3, 9, 25, 30, 34, 36]

(1) ÅLINDER, I., and H. BOSTRÖM: Clinical studies on a Swedish material of pseudoxanthoma elasticum. Acta med. scand. (Stockh.) *191:* 273–282 (1972).

(2) BRAUN, H. J.: Eigenschaften und Vorstellungen über die Pathogenese des Amyloids. Med. Klin. *67:* 1267–1270 (1972).

(3) BROWNSTEIN, M. H., and E. B. HELWIG: The cutaneous amyloidoses. II. Systemic forms. Arch. Derm. (Chic.) *102:* 20–28 (1970).

(4) CAPLAN, R. M.: Visceral involvement in lipid proteinosis. Arch. Derm. (Chic.) *95:* 149–155 (1967).

(5) COCCO, A. E., D. I. GRAYER, B. A. WALKER and L. J. MARTYN: The stomach in pseudoxanthoma elasticum. J. Amer. Med. Ass. *210:* 2381–2382 (1969).

(6) DENK, R.: Elektrokardiographische Untersuchungen bei Hautkranken. Arch. Kreisl.-Forsch. *60:* 33–114 (1969).

(7) DENK. R.: Schimmelpenning-Syndrom. Naevus sebaceus mit Augenfehlbildungen, Anfallsleiden und geistiger Retardierung. Med. Welt *22* (N. F.): 666–668 (1971).

(8) EBERHARTINGER, C., und F. REINHARDT: Das Serumeiweißbild bei Lipoidproteinose Urbach-Wiethe (Hyalinosis cutis et mucosae). Hautarzt *9:* 503–507 (1958).

(9) EBNER, H.: Licht- und elektronenmikroskopische Untersuchungen über das Amyloid der Haut. Z. Haut- u. Geschl.-Kr. *43:* 833–852 (1968).

(10) EDDY, D. D., and E. M. FARBER: Pseudoxanthoma elasticum. Arch. Derm. (Chic.) *86:* 729–740 (1962).

(11) ENGEL, S., und B. PINZER: Über die Kombinationsmöglichkeiten von Sebozystomatosis Günther mit anderen Erkrankungen. Derm. Mschr. *155:* 687–699 (1969).

(12) GARTMANN, H., und H. TRITSCH: Klein- und großknotiges Naevoxanthoendotheliom. Arch. klin. exp. Derm. *215:* 409–421 (1963).

(13) GOLDENHAR, M.: Association malformatives de l'oeil et de l'oreille. J. Génét. hum. *1:* 243–282 (1952).

(14) GOLTZ, R. W., R. R. HENDERSON, J. M. HITCH and J. E. OTT: Focal dermal hypoplasia syndrome. Arch. Derm. (Chic.) *101:* 1–11 (1970).

(15) GOODMAN, R. M., E. W. SMITH, D. PATON, R. A. BERGMAN, C. L. SIEGEL, O. E. OTTESEN, W. M. SHELLEY, A. L. PUSCH and V. A. MCKUSICK: Pseudoxanthoma elasticum: a clinical and histopathological study. Medicine (Baltimore) *42:* 297–334 (1963).

(16) GRIMMER, H.: Erkrankungen des äußeren weiblichen Genitale. Epidermale Cysten. 1. Comedomen, 2. Milien, 3. Retentionscysten, 4. Epidermoid- und Dermoidcysten. Z. Haut- u. Geschl.-Kr. *46:* [25]–[32] (1971).

(17) GROSFELD, J. C. M., J. SPAAS, W. J. B. M. VAN DE STAAK and A. M. STADHOUDERS: Hyalinosis cutis et mucosae (Lipoidproteinosis Urbach-Wiethe). Dermatologica (Basel) *130:* 239–266 (1965).

(18) HASHIMOTO, K., G. KLINGMÜLLER and O. E. RODERMUND: Hyalinosis cutis et mucosae. An electron microscopic study. Acta derm.-venereol. (Stockh.) *52:* 179–195 (1972).

(19) HASSENPFLUG, K.: Naevoxanthoendo-theliom oder jugendliches Histiozytom. Derm. Wschr. *136:* 1345–1351 (1957).

(20) HOLTZ, K. H.: Beitrag zur Histologie des Naevus lipomatodes cutaneus super-ficialis (Hoffmann - Zurhelle). Arch. Derm. Syph. (Berl.) *199:* 275–286 (1955).

(21) HOLTZ, K. H., und W. SCHULZE: Bei-trag zur Klinik und Pathogenese der Hyalinosis cutis et mucosae (Lipoid-Proteinose Urbach-Wiethe).Arch.Derm. Syph. (Berl.) *192:* 206–237 (1950).

(22) JANCAR, J.: Naevus syringocystade-nomatosus papilliferus with skull and brain lesions, hemiparesis, epilepsy and mental retardation. Brit. J. Derm. *82:* 402–405 (1970).

(23) KORTING, G. W., und H. HOLZMANN: Zur Frage humoraler Kollagen-Begleit-komponenten beim Pseudoxanthoma elasticum. Arch. klin. exp. Derm. *231:* 408–414 (1968).

(24) LANTIS, S., M. THEW and C. HEATON: Nevus sebaceus of Jadassohn. Part of a new neurocutaneous syndrome? Arch. Derm. (Chic.) *98:* 117–123 (1968).

(25) MISSMAHL, H. P.: Rektumbiopsie zum Nachweis der Amyloidose. Dtsch. med. Wschr. *88:* 1783–1785 (1963).

(26) NEUTSCH, W. D., und H. J. CRAMER: Typische intrakranielle Verkalkungen bei Hyalinosis cutis et mucosae (Lipoid-proteinose). Fortschr. Röntgenstr. *107:* 131–134 (1967).

(27) NEWTON, F. H., R. N. ROSENBERG, P. W. LAMPERT and J. S. O'BRIEN: Neurologic involvement in Urbach-Wiethe's disease (lipoid proteinosis). A clinical, ultrastructural, and chemical study. Neurology (Minneap.) *21:* 1205–1213 (1971).

(28) NIKOLOWSKI, W.: Über Naevus lipo-matodes cutaneus superficialis (Hoff-mann-Zurhelle). Derm. Wschr. *122:* 735 741 (1950).

(29) NÖDL, F.: Systematisierte großknotige Naevoxanthoendotheliome. Arch. klin. exp. Derm. *208:* 601–615 (1959).

(30) NÖDL, F., und H. ZAUN: Zur Klinik und Histologie der systematisierten Haut-Muskel-Par-amyloidose. Arch. klin. exp. Derm. *220:* 393–416 (1964).

(31) OYAL, H., und W. NIKOLOWSKI: Sebo-cystomatosen. Arch. klin. exp. Derm. *204:* 361–373 (1957).

(32) PIÈRARD, J., et A. KINT: Le pseudo-xanthome élastique. Ann. Derm. Syph. (Paris) *97:* 481–492 (1970).

(33) SCHMID, A. H., und M. USENER: Groß-knotiges Naevoxanthoendotheliom mit Lungenbeteiligung. Arch. klin. exp. Derm. *228:* 239–248 (1967).

(34) SENN, H. J., H. J. HEINIGER, H. BÜRKI und U. RIEDER: Zur klinischen Dia-gnose der Amyloidose. Schweiz. med. Wschr. *96:* 1363–1374 (1966).

(35) WEBSTER, S. B., H. C. REISTER and L. E. HARMAN: Juvenile xanthogranu-loma with extracutaneous lesions. A case report and review of the literature. Arch. Derm. (Chic.) *93:* 71–76 (1966).

(36) WESTERMARK, P., and B. STENKVIST: Diagnosis of secondary generalized amyloidosis by fine needle biopsy of the skin. Acta med. scand. (Stockh.) *190:* 453–454 (1971).

(37) WILDERVANCK, L. S.: Een cervico-oculo-acusticus-syndrom. Med. T. Ge-neesk. *104:* 2600–2605 (1960).

(38) WILSON JONES, E., and T. HEYL: Nae-vus sebaceus. A report of 140 cases with special regard to the development of secondary malignant tumours. Brit. J. Derm. *82:* 99–117 (1970).

33. Ulcers

We will discuss here as ulcers those defects of the cutaneous substance that extend to the papillary body and in general show necrosis. They are subdivided not according to their etiology but from a topographic viewpoint; they will be discussed each time under the site that is most frequently affected.

A. Head

1. Among the tumors leading to ulcerations on the face the **basaloma** (basal cell cancer) as the so-called **rodent ulcer** (Figs. 542, 543) must be considered first. It develops somewhat more frequently in men than in women and shows a distinct preference for the upper two-thirds of the face, chiefly the nasal region, cheeks, and temporal area. Special attention should

Fig. 542. Basal cell epithelioma (rodent ulcer).

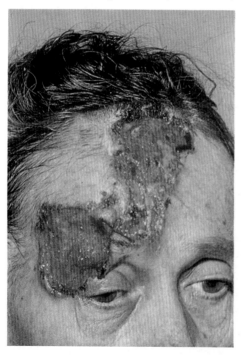

be directed to the retroauricular area, since at this location there are likely to be ulcerating basalomas growing inside the cartilage (Fig. 544) owing to the closely attached skin. The rodent ulcer usually begins as a small, nodular, slightly elevated lesion, which, however, ulcerates in the center very rapidly. The continuously spreading ulceration lacks the pearly border typical of a basaloma. The ulcerated tumor is hard and can be grasped like a plaque as long as it is still movable. Only its firm border rises slightly above the normal level of the skin; the ulcerous base with its poor blood supply lies deeper. Since the rodent ulcer is covered at an early stage by a serous-pustular and sometimes fibrinous crust, it is necessary to remove this crust carefully to evaluate the tissue lying below. This removal is almost always possible without causing any serious bleeding. To ascertain the histologic diagnosis, a smear from the cells of the base of the ulcer can be made, but a biopsy would be preferable and more reliable. Differential diagnostic difficulties of a macromorphologic nature may arise from Bowen's disease, which is also superficially eroded and therefore indistinguishable from a rodent ulcer. In these cases the microscopic examination leads to the correct diagnosis, which is important not only as a matter of form but also because of the tendency to metastases of Bowen's disease, as opposed to the only locally destructive growth, with rare exceptions, of a rodent ulcer.

Whereas the rodent ulcer is one of the slowly growing forms of basaloma, **ulcus terebrans** represents an especially fast and deeply destructive basaloma of the midface (Fig. 545). The progression of this tumor is evident on the skin surface only by a peripheral, thin, hard infiltrate with a raised border. The depth of the skin is soon penetrated and the tumorous tissue attacks the cartilage and bone, finally de-

Fig. 543. Basal cell epithelioma (rodent ulcer) with
pearly border.

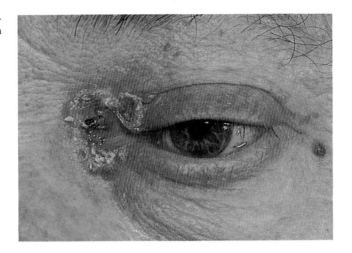

stroying the nose and opening the maxillary cavities and the orbits. For practical
purposes, the only important point here is
the boundless local destruction, which may
be followed by secondary infections, vascu-

lar erosions, meningitis from erosions, or
other sequelae. This type of basaloma generally progresses without metastases but at
some point it runs wild, i.e., a squamous
cell cancer develops. Histologically, ulcus

Fig. 544. Ulcerated basal cell epithelioma of
the auricle.

Fig. 545. Basal cell epithelioma (ulcus terebrans).

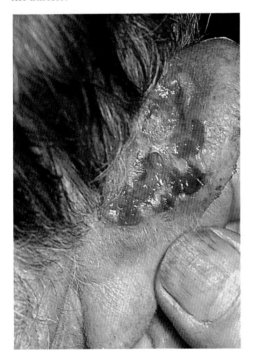

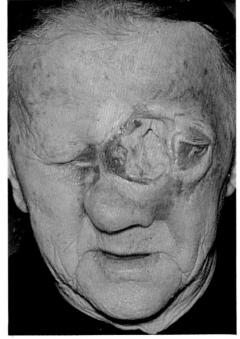

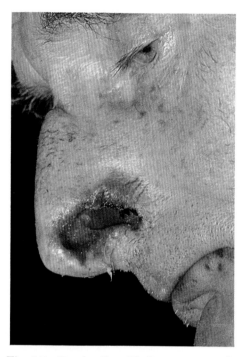

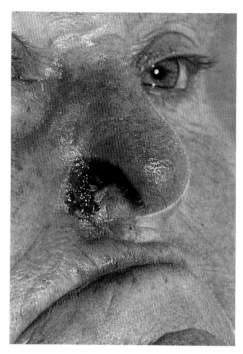

Fig. 546. Basal cell epithelioma ot the ala nasi.

Fig. 547. Trophoneurotic ulceration of the ala nasi following electrocoagulation of the gasserian ganglion.

terebrans appears to be only a basaloma, and no histologic pecularities explain these special growth tendencies.[11, 13]

2. As mentioned earlier, a rodent ulcer often develops in the nasal region and can lead to a slowly progressive destruction of the ala nasi (Fig. 546). Scrupulous inspection of the margin of such an ulcer will reveal without difficulty a basaloma as the cause. Rather similar looking defects of the alae nasi, however, may develop in the course of trophic disturbances. Such **trophoneurotic ulcers of the alae nasi** are known to occur after operative procedures on the *trigeminal nerve* or the *semilunar ganglion*. Occasionally, many years after coagulation of the ganglion, a unilateral "ointment" face may first occur, or a unilateral anesthesia or paresthesia, or limited itching with unilateral nasal dis-

charge from irritation; these are then followed by characteristic sickle-shaped loss of tissue (Fig. 547). At these spots sometimes only stubborn dermatitides or vitiligolike depigmentation exists. Much more seldom, the *Wallenberg syndrome*, i.e., a lesion of the lateral medulla oblongata following a vascular disease, an embolus, or a tumor, may be responsible for this picture. Also, in *Parkinsonism* following encephalitis lethargica, ulcerations of the ala nasi may occur, but because the ulceration tends to be larger, perforations of the nasal septum and the palate may develop in addition.[7, 9, 12, 17]

3. Signs similar to those of ulcus terebrans occur in the midface in **midline lethal granuloma** (granuloma gangraenescens). In the beginning only an unspecific purulent hemorrhagic cold or infection of the upper airways is present; this, however, is soon followed by an edema of the nose with necrosis of the alae nasi and the nasal septum. Extensive necroses and gangrene combined with destruction of cartilage and bone finally lead to bleeding by erosion or septicopyemic complications. At the stage of manifestations irregular attacks of fever often occur, but the general health is still good at that time (see also Chapter 1, K15). The ESR is markedly increased, in the peripheral blood smear a certain shift to the left may be present, and the immune globulins of all fractions may be slightly or distinctly increased. In any case, these data do not point to a specific diagnosis. Histologically, a necrotizing granulation tissue of lympho-histiocytic cell elements and polymorpho-nuclear neutrophils, eosinophils, and plasma cells is present. Endothelial swellings and proliferations lead to closed vessels, but no vasculitis is present as in panarteritis. Although no manifestations in other organs are noted, the patients die within a few months either from generalized cachexia or complications of the locally destructive granulomatous growth.[1, 2, 8, 19]

4. Destructive granulomas of the nose, pharynx, and larynx that are similar to granuloma gangraenescens also occur in a high percentage of patients with **Wegener's granulomatosis.** This is essentially a systematized giant cell granulomatous angiitis in the areas of the nose, sinuses, lungs, spleen, and above all, the kidneys. It affects mainly the male sex in the third to fifth decades of life. In addition to the ulcerating and easily bleeding cutaneous and mucosal changes of the face (nose, palate, middle ear, and eyes), hemorrhagically mixed, eventually ulcerating, macular or nodose changes are also present on the extremities. The diagnosis results from the triad: (1) necrotizing inflammations in the nasopharyngeal region, (2) multiple granulomas in the lungs or other internal organs, and (3) areas of granulomatous glomerulonephritis. The diagnosis is, how-

ever, rarely made during (the patient's) lifetime. For an early diagnosis, biopsies of the nose or kidneys should be performed. The disease usually progresses with attacks of high fever (see also Chapter 1, K5), distinctly elevated ESR, leukocytosis, eosinophilia, and severe anemia. The patients usually die during the terminal loss of kidney function. Histologically, the formation of tuberculoid granulomas interspersed with lymphocytes, plasma cells, eosinophils, and giant cells is notable. It is important for the diagnosis to prove the presence of angiitic vascular changes within the granulomas, which show an especially dense cellular infiltration of the intima. In the differential diagnosis in the early stages a granuloma gangraenescens or a reticulosarcoma arising from the palate must be excluded. In the later phases of the disease a similarity with panarteritis nodosa may exist; this, however, can be distinguished because of the absence of granulomas.[4, 14, 15, 18, 21]

5. Involvement of large areas and striking loss of tissue from fulminant progression in the facial area are suspicious of a fusotreponematosis, called in the facial area nosocomial gangrene or **noma.** The rapidly spreading lesion begins with a brownish-red spot and develops in a few hours to a rapidly gangrenous tissue defect, which leads to complete exposure of the underlying facial bones. In spite of the rapid destruction of the tissue, distinct local inflammatory signs are missing. The body temperature also increases only insignificantly. The overwhelming number of patients are undernourished or severely weakened from other underlying diseases. Without specific antibiotic treatment they die within a few days.[5, 24]

6. Anthrax of the skin starts on uncovered sites after an incubation time of two to three days or less. It begins as a moderately itching red spot and may be

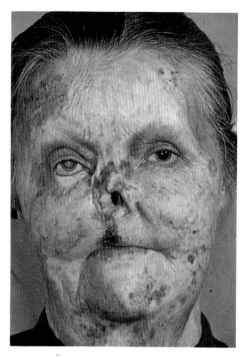

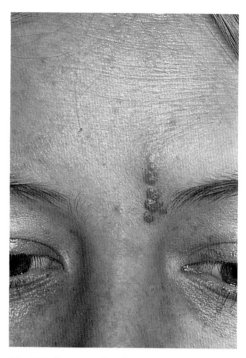

Fig. 548. Lupus vulgaris with mutilations and taut-atrophic scars. Numerous, partly ulcerated basal cell epitheliomas.

Fig. 549. Lupus vulgaris.

located in the center of the face or on the eyelid (see also Chapter 1, F3). This edematous, usually sharply circumscribed erythema then becomes vesicular and pustular and progresses to a character- istic blackish scab (Fig. 3). The crusted area finally reaches an extent of several centimeters but hardly the size and never the depth of noma. In contrast to noma the crusted area is surrounded

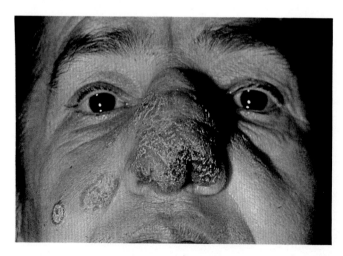

Fig. 550. Lupus vulgaris.

by an inflammatory margin. In any case, to establish the diagnosis, especially in cases with little fever or an atypical appearance, a bacteriologic smear is necessary, followed by culture and animal testing.[6]

7. Among the chronic infectious diseases of the skin, **lupus vulgaris** (tuberculosis cutis luposa) before the era of tuberculosis-inhibiting drugs frequently led to ulcerous mutilating destruction of the face (Fig. 548). Starting with a small brown-red spot, it was eventually followed after years or decades by the loss of the nose, ears, or even whole parts of the extremities. The primary lupus lesion is only rarely recognized as tuberculosis, since only under diascopy will the light brown, relatively sharply circumscribed infiltrate become visible. Although at this time the epidermis is still completely uninvolved, a probe easily breaks through it into the corium and leads to mild hemorrhaging. In the course of the disease the lupoid lesion becomes larger by apposition of additional granulomas. Finally it is raised above the level of the surrounding skin (Fig. 549). The pressure of the granulation tissue from the corium finally affects the epidermis so that scales and crusts (Fig. 550) and eventually also ulcerations

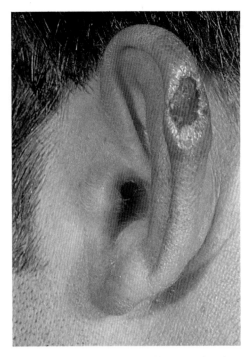

Fig. 551. Centrally ulcerated lupus vulgaris.

(Fig. 551) become visible. The ulcers have sharp and irregular borders and usually dirty base coverings. The diagnosis is based on the light brown infiltrates at the margin, the positive probe phenomenon, the histologic findings, and the presence

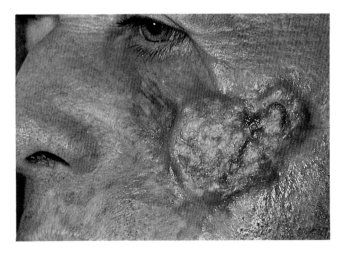

Fig. 552. Carcinoma in lupus.

of tubercle bacilli in the culture or in animal experiments.[22]

Ulcerations in old, tautly atrophic lupoid scars may be caused either by localized recurrence or malignant degeneration. Previously irradiated lupoid lesions especially show increased malignant degeneration, but even without preceding irradiation carcinomas develop in the taut cicatricial regions of patients with lupus more frequently and at an earlier age than they do in other patients. The differential diagnosis between recurrent lupus and carcinoma should always be decided by a biopsy. So-called *lupus carcinoma* is not different histologically from other squamous cell carcinomas; it is characterized clinically by relatively fast growth and a distinct tendency to central necrosis (Fig. 552).

8. Like lupus vulgaris, **leishmaniasis cutis** of the Mediterranean starts with a small erythematous macule. This lesion develops a few weeks or months after the sting of a sandfly (*Phlebotomus papatasii* and similar species). This insect becomes a vector of *Leishmania tropica* by feeding on reservoir hosts such as dogs and small rodents and then infecting human beings. The development of the various species of Phlebotomus is absolutely dependent on a warm climate, and as a rule they do not thrive in the temperate zone, in the northern latitudes, or in the southern high mountains (Fig. 553). Leishmaniasis cutis occurs in 80 per cent of the cases on exposed skin areas. The macular early stage is observed only rarely; from it a hard, lentil-sized papule with a brownish-red or livid brown color develops. Diascopy reveals a brownish infiltrate; however, in contrast to lupus vulgaris, it is difficult to penetrate the lesion with a probe. This papule soon shows small erosions on its surface covered with a firmly attached white scale. In its subsequent course the papule enlarges into a nodule surrounded usually by an ill-defined livid red border. The white scale may become quite thick; when it is removed an underlying ulceration is visible. The undersurface of the scale shows fingerlike horny plugs similar to the "carpet tacks" observed in the scales of discoid lupus erythematosus; however, the leishmaniasic plugs are considerably larger. Healing finally takes place with formation of a maplike, flat,

Fig. 553. Distribution of tropical leishmaniasis around the Mediterranean.

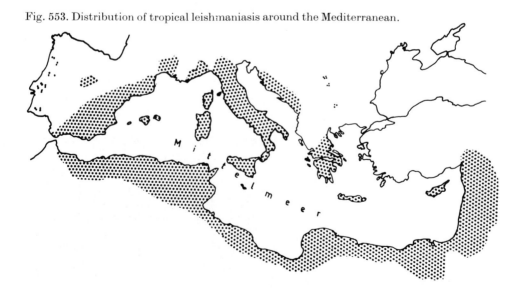

depressed scar. The diagnosis is established by finding the causative organism in Giemsa-stained smears obtained from the edge of the ulcer or in excised material (fixed by mercury bichloride alcohol). The organism can also be grown in cultures. The differential diagnosis must exclude chronic vegetating pyoderma, lupus vulgaris, tuberculosis verrucosa cutis, discoid lupus erythematosus, tertiary syphilis, keratoacanthoma, and squamous cell cancer.[16, 23, 25]

9. The differential diagnosis of facial lesions (especially of the nasolabial region) must include, besides tuberculosis, tertiary **syphilis.** In contrast to tuberculosis, which favors the cartilage, syphilis almost always attacks the bone. However, a mutilating appearance in the sense of a "lupus syphiliticus" is a great rarity, whereas a perforated palate is found more frequently with ulcerogummatous syphilis. Although in most cases numerous plasma cells will be seen together with a tuberculoid structure in the histologic examination, the diagnosis should be verified by performing the treponema immobilization test.*

10. Tertiary frambesia (yaws), also known as gangosa or rhinopharyngitis mutilans, can also cause severe destruction and mutilating scar formation, again especially of the midface region. Sometimes only perforations of the palate and, in more advanced cases, mutilations of the nose and upper lip are observed. However, the clinical picture by itself will provide a diagnostic answer only with due consideration of the epidemiologic aspects. It may be very difficult to differentiate frambesia from ulcerogummatous syphilis; the classical serology of syphilis or the treponema immobilization test do not permit a definite distinction between the two diagnostic possibilities.

---

* Or the FTA absorption test. (Tr.)

11. South American blastomycosis may show midface destruction caused by localized fungal granulomas; the infection begins with an intraoral primary lesion. As the disease progresses, the lips, perioral region, and nasal mucosa become involved. At the same time the cervical lymph nodes break down, forming fistulous ducts; the causative organism, *Paracoccidioides brasiliensis*, can be found in the sputum and mucous membrane smears but more easily in the secretion from the lymph nodes (direct smear, culture, or guinea pig inoculation). If there is in the beginning only an erosive-ulcerating or mulberry-like vegetating stomatitis, the differential diagnosis must also include mucous membrane pemphigus.

Coccidioidomycosis shows bronchopulmonary involvement that resembles grippe clinically; the nasolabial region is the chief site of the manifestations, which are blackish, warty, vegetating papules.

The primary lesion of **sporotrichosis,** when located on the lips or on other perioral sites, may look very much like a syphilitic chancre; in the differential diagnosis of gummatous sporotrichosis one must exclude mainly cancer and tuberculosis.

12. The clinical signs of **temporal arteritis** have already been discussed in Chapter 1, K2 and Chapter 5, B11. Here attention will be called to the ulcerations located mainly in the temporal region or in the midline of the skull; the diagnosis of these ulcerations of course depends on the correct recognition of the underlying condition. Because these ulcerations result from the blockage of a blood vessel, they develop relatively rapidly – within a few days. The tongue may become involved in the course of this disease also, frequently not only with circumscribed erythemas and vesiculations but also with gangrenous formations. Clinically difficult cases may require histologic examination of the temporal vessels; one can expect to find

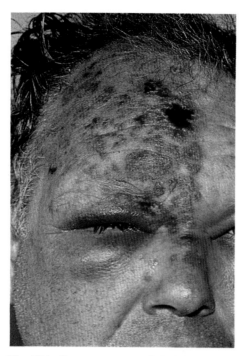

Fig. 554. Gangrenescent ophthalmic herpes zoster.

obliterative thickening of the intima, degeneration of the elastica interna, fibrinoid necrosis, and extensive proliferation of histiocytes with many giant cells.[3, 10, 20, 26]

13. Rather deep ulcerations of the head region may also be seen in **herpes zoster;** their favorite site is the first branch of the trigeminal nerve, and they are mostly seen in older or marasmic patients with an underlying systemic disease (Fig. 554). The diagnosis depends on the appropriate history and the segmental distribution (see also Chapter 1, E2, Chapter 5, B1, Chapter 15, A14, and Chapter 18, H1.

(1) ALEXANDER, B. R.: Idiopathic lethal granulomas of the midline facial tissues. Arch Derm. (Chic.) 79: 390–394 (1959).

(2) ALTENBURGER, K., und K. PFEIFFER: Beitrag zum Krankheitsbild Granuloma gangraenescens. Med. Klin. 57: 1940–1946 (1962).

(3) BAREFOOT, S. W., and H. Z. LUND: Temporal (giant-cell) arteritis associated with ulcerations of scalp. Arch. Derm. (Chic.) 93: 79–83 (1966).

(4) BECK, D., und W. SIEGENTHALER: Wegenersche Granulomatose. Dtsch. med. Wschr. 92: 111–115 (1967).

(5) BOULNOIS et RABEDAORO: Le noma de Madagascar. Étude clinique, pathogénique, étiologique et thérapeutique. Sem. Hôp. Paris 26: 517–528 (1950).

(6) FLECK, F.: Das Oedema malignum, seine Erkennung und derzeitige Behandlung. Derm. Mschr. 155: 673–686 (1969).

(7) FREEMAN, A. G.: Neurotrophic ulceration of the face with erosion of the ala nasi in vascular disorders of the brainstem. Brit. J. Derm. 78: 322–331 (1966).

(8) GERTLER, W., A. SCHIMPF und K. PFEIFFER: Zum Granuloma gangraenescens der Nase. Derm. Wschr. 134: 1125–1135 (1956).

(9) HAENSCH, R.: Neurotrophic ulcer associated with the Wallenberg syndrome. Acta derm.-venereol. (Stockh.) 48: 622–629 (1968).

(10) HITCH, J. M.: Dermatologic manifestations of giant cell (temporal, cranial) arteritis. Arch. Derm. (Chic.) 101: 409–415 (1970).

(11) JACOB, A.: An ulcer of peculiar character which attacks the eye-lids and other parts of the face. Dubl. Hosp. Rep. 4: 232–239 (1827).

(12) JAEGER, H.: Un type nouveau d'ulcère neurotrophique de l'aile du nez après neurotomie rétrogassérienne. Dermatologica (Basel) 100: 201–206 (1950).

(13) KLEEMANN, W.: Zur morphologischen Wertigkeit des Ulcus terebrans innerhalb der Basaliome. Derm. Wschr. 154: 1203–1211 (1968).

(14) KNOTH, W., G. BENEKE und E. KUNTZ: Zur Kenntnis der Wegenerschen Granulomatose. Hautarzt 16: 289–294 (1965).

(15) KORTING, G. W., und H. LACHNER: Arteriolitis hyperergica als Hauterscheinungsbild bei Wegenerscher Granulomatose. Med. Welt 19 (N. F.): 2115–2116 (1968).

(16) KRAMPITZ, H. E., W. SCHOPP und H. KILLIG: Zur Diagnose und Epidemiologie der mediterranen Hautleishmaniase. Münch. med. Wschr. 115: 13–19 (1973).

(17) KREBS, A., und H. KUSKE: Trophische Störungen der Haut bei Läsion des Nervus trigeminus. Schweiz. med. Wschr. 93: 1687–1692 (1963).

(18) MAAS, D., W. HAMANN, H. NOETZEL, G. KIMPEL und H. SCHUBOTHE: Wegenersche Granulomatose. Schweiz. med. Wschr. *101:* 141–148 (1971).

(19) NOSKO, L.: Granuloma gangraenescens der Haut. Z. Haut- u. Geschl.-Kr. *17:* 1–7 (1954).

(20) PAULLEY, J. W., and J. P. HUGHES: Giant-cell arteritis or arteritis of the aged. Brit. Med. J. *1960:* 1562–1567.

(21) REED, W. B., A. K. JENSEN, B. E. KONWALER and D. HUNTER: The cutaneous manifestations in Wegener's granulomatosis. Acta derm.-venereol. (Stockh.) *43:* 250–264 (1963).

(22) SCHMITZ, R.: »Lupus« der mittleren Gesichtsanteile. Medizinische *1958:* 1905–1910.

(23) SCHWARZ, K. J.: Zur Diagnose und Differentialdiagnose der kutanen Leishmaniose. An Hand von 7 in Zürich beobachteten Fällen. Schweiz. med. Wschr. *100:* 2073–2078 (1970).

(24) SIROL, J., J. VEDY et A. SABRIÉ: Le noma ou la laideur oubliée. Étude clinique et essai pathogénique à propos de six cas observés à Fort-Lamy (Tchad). Ann. Derm. Syph. (Paris) *99:* 511–516 (1972).

(25) STEIGLEDER, G. K., und J. SCHULZ: Kutane Leishmaniose in Deutschland. Med. Welt *15* (N. F.): 1889–1895 (1964).

(26) WAGNER, A., J. ANNWEILER und E. KRAUS: Klinische Beobachtungen bei Patienten mit Riesenzellarteriitis. Arteriitis temporalis. Med. Welt *23* (N. F.): 641–645 (1972).

B. Oral Cavity and Lips

1. Flat and crusted ulcerations, which generally do not grow beyond fingernail size, when they occur on the transitional mucosal surfaces suggest first ulcerated **herpes simplex.** Following preceding subjective symptoms such as a feeling of tension, among others, densely grouped, pinheadsized vesicles appear and are soon filled with leukocytes. Because of the thin blisterous covering on the lips, blisters or pustules remain intact for only a short while. Then erosions, which in the beginning are vividly red and later are covered by a somewhat dirty exudate, appear; they are almost always polycyclically outlined or cloverleaf-shaped. Occasionally, because of the superinfection, regionally tender lymph node swellings are palpable. The tendency of herpes simplex to recur is especially pronounced and may gradually lead to circumscribed swelling (see also Chapter 10, A4). In patients who are being treated with immunosuppressive drugs or who suffer from a basic disorder that impairs the immunologic system, herpes simplex of the lips can in the beginning assume vegetating features, extending itself continuously in the neighborhood of the mouth, and finally breaking down in a hemorrhagic-ulcerous fashion (Fig. 555).

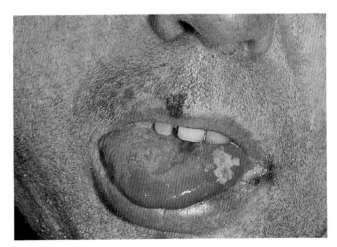

Fig. 555. Multilocular, vegetating herpes simplex.

The diagnosis of ulcerated herpes simplex is made chiefly by the local findings and attention to the course of the disease. At the blistering stage one should try to find proof of herpes simplex virus, i.e., of type I. The small extent of the infection, however, does not generally lead to a proven increase in the antibody titer of the serum. Labial carcinomas take a much longer time for development, arise from an atrophic vermilion border, and do not appear as periodical recurrences. If any doubt remains, a histologic examination definitely resolves it.[9]

2. Ulcerations developing from an induration in the region of the lips, tongue, and tonsils may suggest a primary **syphilitic** lesion. In syphilis a labial primary lesion is the most frequent of all extragenital primary lesions. It may be papular, erosive, or crusted. The crusts as a secondary phenomenon may completely hide the underlying bowl-like induration with its elevated borders. Occasionally only an indurated edema of the entire labial region is present. An important accompanying sign of the syphilitic primary lesion of the lips is the unilaterally protuberant, large and hard lymph node enlargement, which in secondary mixed infections may become painful. On the gingiva the syphilitic primary lesion may assume the aspect of a typical erosive sclerosis or only of an unspecific gingival ulceration. On the tongue the primary lesion is generally situated on the dorsum of the anterior third, i.e., especially on the tip of the tongue. Here also it appears as an erosive or ulcerated induration, in whose ulcerated part there is a granular base or coating.

Deep-lying ulcerations in the region of the soft palate or pharyngeal wall may also represent a syphilitic primary lesion, which, even if deeply ulcerated, may not be accompanied by submaxillary, preauricular, or nuchal lymph node enlargement. If, however, an accompanying lymph node enlargement is present, it is not necessarily indolent in all cases, since, as mentioned earlier, in superinfections and mixed infections syphilitic scleradenitis may be painful. If such a finding is unilateral, it definitely indicates a primary lesion; if both sides are affected, it indicates specific tonsillitis. The latter may be preceded by macular, dusky red enanthe-

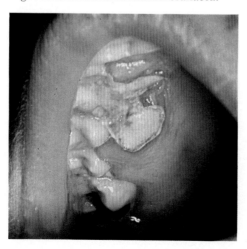

Fig. 556. Stomatitis ulceromembranacea.

Fig. 557. *Borrelia vincentii* and *Fusobacterium fusiforme* in smear from angina ulceromembranacea. Gram's stain, 1000 × .

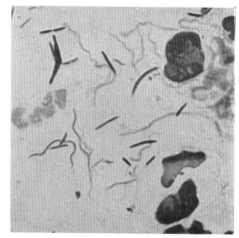

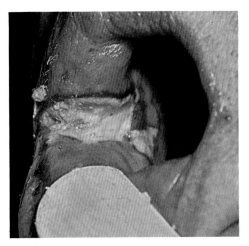

Fig. 558. Acute paramyeloblastic leukemia: ulceration of the oral mucosa.

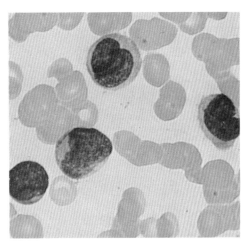

Fig. 559. Acute paramyeloblastic leukemia: peripheral blood smear. May-Grünwald stain, 1000×.

mas, which later become opaline or erosive. A clinical sign in favor of specific tonsillitis is simultaneous or subsequent specific laryngitis (hoarseness).

Any ulceration with a surprisingly hard wall or an accompanying indurative edema in the labial, oral, or genital regions must raise the suspicion of a primary lesion. For a definite diagnosis at this stage, demonstration of *Treponema pallidum* from the secretion is absolutely necessary. This is especially difficult in the oral cavity because the danger of confusion with other treponemas is particularly great; with the darkfield examination not only the form but also the type of locomotion has to be carefully observed. Serologic tests are negative at the early stage of a primary lesion, with the exception of the fluorescent treponema antibody (FTA) test, which may become positive as early as 14 days after the infection. Ulcerations of the tongue with positive serology for syphilis, however, always need exclusion of a malignant tumor, since such a carcinoma of the tongue may develop on the basis of a deep syphilitic interstitial glossitis.[7]

3. At the onset of **stomatitis ulceromembranacea** white-grayish coatings of the interdental papillae or other areas of the gingiva appear with distinct general signs (fever, sore throat, lymphocytosis, and loss of appetite). Transformation into gray-greenish pseudomembranous areas, which easily bleed when touched (Fig. 556), rapidly follows. If the coverings are carefully removed, shallow, extremely painful ulcerations become visible. Through contact large ulcerations develop on the buccal mucosa or the sides of the tongue. At the examination, moreover, a highly disagreeable, foul-smelling fetor ex ore is noticed. The patients themselves are bothered by disagreeable salivation and severely handicapped in eating and drinking by great pain. A similar process occurs in **angina ulceromembranacea** on the tonsils. Such an angina may occur alone or in close chronologic association with the stomatitis. Both forms of the disease are accompanied by considerable regional lymph node enlargements. In smears from the ulcerous mucosal changes a symbiosis of *Borrelia vincentii* and *Fusobacterium fusiforme* is predominant, but there is no proven etiologic significance to these bacteria (Fig. 557).

In the differential diagnosis ulcerous mucosal defects in acute *hemoblastoses*

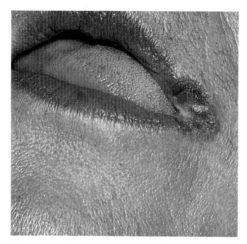

Fig. 560. Ulceration at the angle of the mouth in agranulocytosis.

(Figs. 558, 559), *panmyelophthisis*, and *agranulocytosis* (Fig. 560) have to be considered first. The same is true for perlèche-like reactions, which develop quickly with a febrile general condition and progress with an unusually erosive and ulcerating course.[6]

4. Also extremely painful are the ulcerations of mucosal tuberculosis. These are evident in **primary mucosal** (or cutaneous) **tuberculosis.** It starts with a soft blue-red nodule, which changes relatively rapidly into an ulcer with undermined border and a base covered with a dirty exudate. After some time via regional lymphangitis and lymphadenitis, the primary complex is established. The diagnosis can only be assumed from the clinical findings but can be confirmed by the presence of tubercle bacilli from the ulcer.

Furthermore, **lupus vulgaris of the mucosa** may break down and form a tuberculous ulcer. In this case, however, usually small lupoid infiltrates remain at the border as an indication of the original lupus vulgaris (Fig. 561). An attempt to find tubercle bacilli in the smear from the ulcer never succeeds. Proof of the diagnosis therefore requires a histologic examination of a biopsy and animal inoculation.

Tuberculosis miliaris ulcerosa mucosae is an overwhelming infection on the mucous membranes and transitional mucous membranes in patients with far advanced organ tuberculosis. The infection ascends via the larynx, palate, sides of the tongue, cheeks, and lips. In addition to small nodules and verrucous infiltrates, shallow ulcerations of varying size predominate. Ulcerations develop by necrotic disintegration and confluence of single miliary

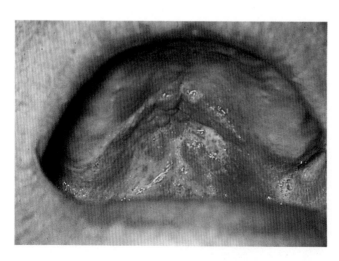

Fig. 561. Lupus vulgaris of the palate.

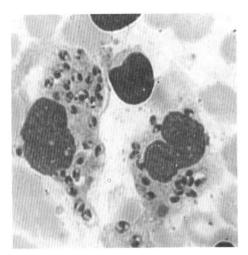

Fig. 562. Brazilian leishmaniasis: peripheral blood smear. Intracellularly situated stages of leishmania. May-Grünwald stain, 1000 ×.

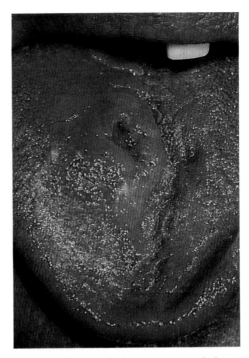

Fig. 563. Leishmaniasis cutis: unusual ulcerative changes of the tongue.

tubercles. The borders of the ulcer are undermined, whereas the base has either flaccid granulations or dirty coatings which, in contrast to stomatitis ulceromembranacea, are not foul-smelling. Demonstration of the tubercle bacilli from the ulcerations is a simple matter. Histologically, unspecific miliary abscess formation is present, whereas tuberculoid structures are hardly noticeable.

5. In exceptional cases such miliary necroses in jaggedly circumscribed ulcerations may hide **syphilis miliaris ulcerosa mucosae.** In complete contrast to patients with tuberculous mucosal ulcerations, it affects only persons in the best of health. This is not a deeply extensive and therefore gummatous process, but a kind of tuberoserpiginous, high-lying, tertiary mucosal syphilid. The demonstration of tubercle bacilli remains negative; the serology, however, is positive for syphilis, and under treatment with penicillin complete cure is achieved. Macroscopically and from the histologic picture differentiation from tuberculosis miliaris ulcerosa mucosae is impossible.[3]

6. Of the diseases caused by protozoa, South American leishmaniasis or **mucocutaneous leishmaniasis** (causative organism: *Leishmania brasiliensis*) should be mentioned. It not only lasts longer than Mediterranean leishmaniasis cutis but affects the mucous membranes to a much greater degree. Areas in the middle of the face may be destroyed not only from the skin side but also from the mucosal side. In this process the nose, lips, and palate are the chief sites of nodose-vegetating and even necrotizing ulcerations. Demonstration of leishmania should be attempted above all from "fresh" areas, therefore especially from the sides of the ulcer (Fig. 562). The leishmania (Montenegro) test is reported to be positive in 90 per cent of cases. Only exceptionally does *leishmaniasis cutis* (causative organism: *Leishmania tropica*) show ulcerous mucosal changes (Figs. 563, 564).[4, 5]

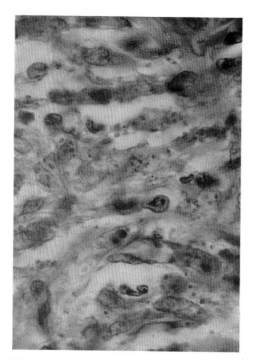

Fig. 564. Leishmaniasis cutis: intracellularly located Leishman-Donovan bodies. Giemsa stain, 1000×.

by irregularly placed teeth (Fig. 567). After correction of the dental misplacement they heal in a very short time. Other mechanical injuries can cause sharply limited, fissured ulcerations with firm fibrinous pseudomembranes on the oral mucosa. Ulcers from the pressure of ill-fitting prostheses present no diagnostic difficulties.

9. Periadenitis mucosa necrotica recurrens also leads to deep ulcerations of the oral mucosa. They are difficult to differentiate clinically from a neoplasm. Since these mucosal ulcers occur exclusively in patients with chronic recurrent aphthae, they will be discussed more thoroughly in Chapter 35, B1.

10. Recurrent ulcerations of the oral mucosa may be a partial manifestation of **regional enteritis.** The histologic findings are the same as those of the perianal ulcerations occurring in this disorder (see this chapter, Section C17 and Chapter 14, B9.[10, 11]

7. Relatively slightly tender, sharply punched-out ulcerations within a tumorous increase in volume of the tonsils or palate should be examined for the presence of a **reticulosarcoma** (Fig. 565). The **ulcerating eosinophilic granuloma** (Fig. 566), in spite of its crater-shaped appearance, can also be diagnosed with certainty only from histologic studies. This form of granuloma is not at all an eosinophilic granuloma as a partial manifestation of histiocytosis X but instead perhaps a mucosal manifestation of a benign tissue hyperplasia in the sense of an eosinophilic facial granuloma.[1, 2, 8]

8. An example of a common **traumatic mucosal ulcer** is the ulcer of the frenulum of the tongue in children with *whooping cough.* Other ulcers on the sides of the tongue and buccal mucosa are decubitus ulcers (so-called Bednar's aphthae), caused

(1) GOSEPATH, P., und K. H. HASSENPFLUG: Tumorförmiges ulcerierendes eosinophiles Granulom der Zungenunterseite. Z. Haut- u. Geschl.-Kr. *33:* 118–123 (1962).
(2) HJORTING-HANSEN, E., and H. SCHMIDT: Ulcerated granuloma eosinophilicum diutinum of the tongue. Acta. derm.-venereol. (Stockh.) *41:* 235–239 (1961).
(3) KEINING, E.: Zum Krankheitsbild der Lues miliaris ulcerosa mucosae (G. Arndt). Derm. Wschr. *136:* 985–989 (1957).
(4) KORTING, G. W., und N. HOEDE: Ulceröses Leishmania-Granulom der Zunge. Arch. Derm. Forsch. *247:* 111–116 (1973).
(5) KRAMPITZ, H. E., W. SCHOPP und H. KILLIG: Zur Diagnose und Epidemiologie der mediterranen Hautleishmaniase. Münch. med. Wschr. *115:* 13–19 (1973).
(6) LUHR, H.-G., und W.-J. HÖLTJE: Mundschleimhautveränderungen bei Erkrankungen des leukopoetischen Systems. Dtsch. zahnärztl. Z. *25:* 1108–1113 (1970).

Fig. 565. Reticulosarcoma of the oral cavity.

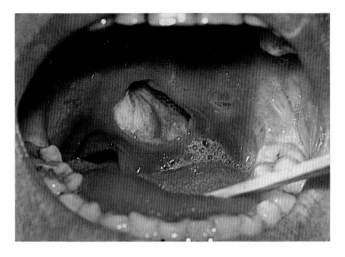

Fig. 566. Eosinophilic granuloma of the tongue.

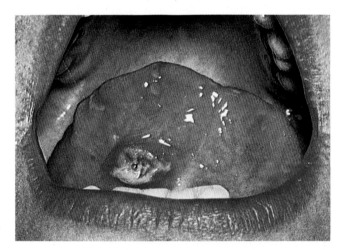

Fig. 567. Decubital ulcer of the tongue.

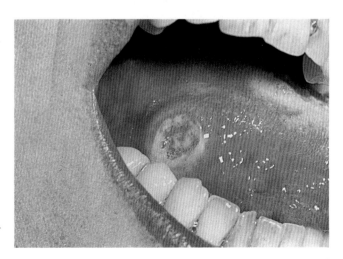

(7) MEYER-ROHN, J.: Die Bedeutung des FTA-Tests für die Primärsyphilis. Z. Haut- u. Geschl.-Kr. *42:* 309–312 (1967).

(8) SCHIRREN, C. G.: Das sogenannte eosinophile Granulom der Schleimhaut. Arch. klin. exp. Derm. *216:* 402–411 (1963).

(9) SCHNEWEIS, K. E.: Die Typen 1 und 2 des Herpes-simplex-Virus bei verschiedenen Krankheitsbildern. Dtsch. med. Wschr. *92:* 2313–2314 (1967).

(10) STANKLER, L., S. W. B. EWEN and N. W. KERR: Crohn's disease of the mouth. Brit. J. Derm. *87:* 501–504 (1972).

(11) VERBOV, J.: Crohn's disease with mouth and lip involvement. Brit. J. Derm. *88:* 517 (1973).

C. Anogenital Region

1. In spite of sometimes rather unspecific early development a genital ulceration should always be suspected of being a **syphilitic primary lesion.** The typical case

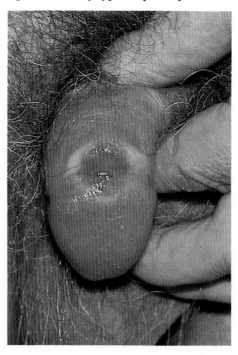

Fig. 568. Primary syphilis: primary lesion.

shows an extremely hard, oval, meaty-colored, moist, finely granular, and painless ulcer, which develops from a closed papule (Fig. 568). The typical aspect of a primary lesion is complemented by the appearance of a regional and at first unilateral indolent lymphadenopathy (see also Chapter 13, A1). Further attributes of such a primary lesion are its induration – more pronounced in the male than in the female – and its clear serum which will exude after adequate local abrasion, permitting darkfield examination for the presence of *Treponema pallidum*. In men most of the primary lesions are located on the inner foreskin, especially in the coronary sulcus of the glans penis. An intraurethral chancre, a possibility which should not be overlooked, shows a seropurulent or hemorrhagic urethral discharge but not the greenish-yellow secretion of gonorrhea; in most cases a cylindrical or spherical induration can be palpated close to the urethral opening. In women a conspicuous indurative edema of one labium should initiate a search for a sometimes insignificant rhagadiform primary lesion. Because of the anatomical difference women show smaller imprintlike chancres of the external genitalia more frequently than men. Primary lesions within the vagina (shallow, perhaps slightly depressed, dark brown-red tissue defects) are seen more rarely than painless, erosive, or ulcerated indurated lesions of the cervix that are sometimes covered with a greasy smear.

The differential diagnosis of lesions of the cervix must include, besides secondary or tertiary syphilitic lesions, the extremely rare tuberculosis of the mucous membrane (peripheral undermined areas with gray-yellowish nodules), and above all the possibility of a cervical cancer (contact bleeding, blood-tinged watery vaginal discharge, nodular, crumbly, sanguineous lesions on the vaginal portion of the cervix. The absence of *Treponema pallidum* and a persistent negative serology require an early biopsy. The location of the primary lesion on the external genitalia, or even more within the vagina or on the cervix, may make it difficult or impossible to palpate enlarged superficial or deep inguinal lymph nodes; in the main the iliac lymph nodes are enlarged. However, the lymph vessels of the lower part of the vagina drain into superficial groups of lymph nodes. Patients often claim that genital primary lesions are traumatic erosions, but it is always important to exclude a syphilitic chancre regardless of an unusual location.*

2. Herpes progenitalis is very important from a differential diagnostic point of view; as recurrent herpes progenitalis it is seen primarily on the prepuce, coronary

* Such as a chancre of the big toe in a homosexual, observed by the translators. (Tr.)

sulcus, and glans penis. In contrast to the syphilitic chancre with its indurated oval eroded lesion, herpes shows polycyclic erosions. The patient himself has quite often observed their rapid development after an initial burning sensation from the small vesicles, which will soon rupture. Herpes progenitalis shows minute miliary and superficial erosions with hardly any regional lymphadenopathy (Fig. 569). Nevertheless, such a herpes simplex area can become important as a portal of entry for *Treponema pallidum;* subsequent observation may therefore detect induration and require a search for spirochetes (see also this chapter, Section B1).

3. Chancroid (soft chancre, ulcus molle) develops three to eight days after an infection with the Ducrey bacillus. The disease starts with a painless macule or small nodule which develops into a short-

Fig. 569. Herpes simplex of the prepuce.

Fig. 570 Ulcera mollia. Additional findings: hirsutoid papillomas of penis.

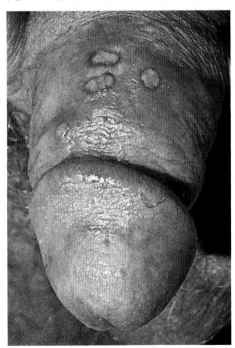

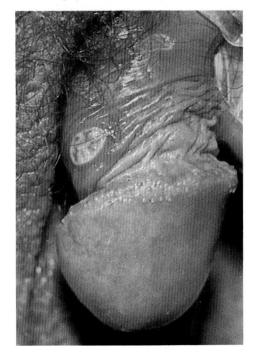

lived pustule; the latter then ruptures and within one to four weeks, either simultaneously or subsequently, several separate ulcers will form close together (Fig. 570). These lesions are covered with pus but have no infiltration at all. The ulcers may have widely undermined edges, and it is noteworthy that their bases may be quite painful. For the involvement of the regional lymph nodes see Chapter 13, A4. The causative organism can be found in smears obtained from the overhanging edges of the ulcer and examined with Giemsa's stain. If the search for the Ducrey bacillus from the genital ulcerations is not successful one can make use of the easy transmissibility of this organism. The abdominal skin of the patient is disinfected and scarified, then pus from an ulcer is rubbed in. The area is covered with a watchglass held in place by a bandage; in a positive case a papulopustule will develop within 24 to 72 hours, and it will then be easy to demonstrate Ducrey bacilli. The papulopustule caused by inoculation will soon change into a typical chancroid. Clinically, a syphilitic chancre can be diagnosed by its considerable induration and its absence of pain, as well as by additional ulceration (which is not invariable). Further differences are the result of the duration of the different periods of incubation. In both cases the diagnosis should be verified by finding the respective organism. In order not to overlook a double infection a control of the seroreactions or, better, the Treponema immobilization test should be undertaken before starting treatment and again after four to six weeks.

4. Gonococcal ulcerations, which are extremely rare, may occur either as primary or secondary lesions, especially on the glans or on the penile skin or, in women, near the urethra or in the vicinity of the ducts of Bartholin's glands. Because such ulcerations look rather unspecific clinically, a diagnosis should be made only if by scraping the deeper parts of the ulcer

gonococci can be grown in culture (in most cases gonorrhea of the urethra is present at the same time). The possibility of gonococcic ulcerations should be entertained in general only if other efforts to find gonococci are fruitless and a smear obtained from tissue of the ulcer shows intracellular gram negative diplococci.[7]

5. Granuloma inguinale (venereum) affects the genital and anal region and its vicinity (groins). In the tropics it causes the development of large, vegetating, frequently greasy yellowish, fetid granulations.* These conditions are preceded by small vesiculopustules. The inguinal or anogenital areas may also develop ulcerations, but the hypertrophic-verrucous, cicatrizing, vegetating granulations containing many crypts are characteristic of the disease. It should be emphasized in this connection that other cutaneous regions may be affected by metastases and also that extracutaneous lesions may be seen in the liver and bones. The causative organism *(Calymmatobacterium granulomatis* or *Donovania granulomatis)* is best found by taking a smear from a biopsy of the tissue at the edge of the affected cutaneous areas. The histologic preparation stained with Giemsa will show inclusion bodies within the histiocytes (so-called Donovan bodies). In cases of granuloma inguinale the possibility of coexisting syphilis should be kept in mind.

6. Tuberculosis of the external genitalia of men and women, which is seldom seen today, is generally spread by the lymphatics or blood vessels and hardly ever appears as a primary exogenous infection. One usually encounters ulcerated manifestations without special clinical characteristics, and in most cases a definite

---

* In the southern United States, the lesions are locally destructive, progressive, indolent, and only slightly elevated serpiginous ulcerations. (Tr.)

detailed classification is not possible. The diagnosis cannot be made on histologic grounds alone; it is necessary to look for tubercle bacilli in smears and cultures and by means of animal inoculation; atypical mycobacteria should also be considered. Should ulcerations of the glans penis show only tuberculoid changes on histologic examination, one may be dealing with an isolated ulcerous tuberculid (Fig. 571). In such cases it is always necessary to exclude tuberogummatous syphilids.[5, 10]

7. Gangrenous ulcer (acute ulcerating gangrene of the genitals) has a clinically well defined, dramatic, foudroyant, febrile course from the beginning. Such an explosive septic-pyemic course may start so to speak overnight without other premonitory signs. Locally severe pain accompanies intense redness and swelling of a genital area which at the edges rapidly develops yellowish blue-black infarcts. Following sequestration accompanied by massive exudation and intense fetor, a large ulcer finally appears; if, for instance the scrotum is involved the ulcer may extend down to the testicles. After the necrotic sequestrum has become detached, it is surprising how soon general and local improvement takes place, followed by a striking tendency to quick healing of the wound. Gangrenous ulcers are seen much more rarely in the female. Apparently no specific microorganism can be identified as the sole etiologic factor of the acute gangrene of the genitals.[14, 16]

In addition to gangrene of the genitals already mentioned there exists a *gangrenous balanitis;* it shows milder general signs and is confined to the glans penis. Etiologically it must be considered a fusospirochetosis in most cases.

8. Ulcus vulvae acutum usually starts with burning pains on urination caused by localized ulcerations of the vulva and perigenital regions. These ulcers may be single or multiple, sharply circumscribed,

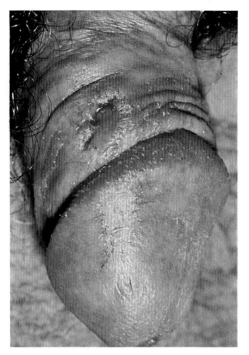

Fig. 571. Ulcerated tuberculid of the preputium. Additional findings: hirsutoid papillomas of penis.

and have a firmly attached white-yellow coating. The entire ulcer is surrounded by an erythematous halo. Over half of the cases occur before the twenty-fifth year of life. The cause of ulcus vulvae acutum is heterogeneous and the diagnosis does not depend on finding *Bacillus crassus.* Febrile episodes similar to those of typhoid, primary atypical pneumonias, and an increase in cold agglutinins raise the possibility of a viral infection. The rare gangrenous types may be caused by a fusospirochetosis corresponding to gangrenous balanitis or stomatitis ulceromembranacea. Finally, ulcus vulvae acutum may be a partial manifestation of Behçet's syndrome, which is even more probable if oral aphthae and erythema nodosum are present simultaneously.[3, 8]

9. Erythema multiforme of the penis or vulva almost always shows multiple, oc-

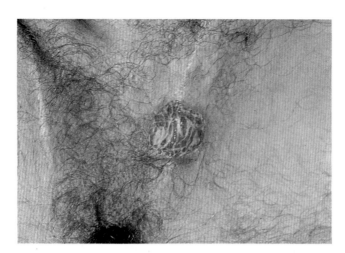

Fig. 572. Behçet's syndrome: ulceration of the perineum.

casionally confluent, polycyclic areas that appear as dirty greasy érosions. In most cases there are concomitant lesions on the oral mucosa; less frequently there are also cutaneous changes with inverted locations. Vesiculoerosive "toxic-allergic" drug eruptions, especially after administration of

Fig. 573. Carcinoma of the penis.

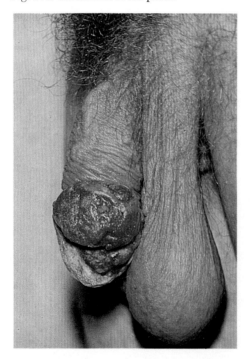

antipyrine or phenolphthalein, may also resemble erythema multiforme with a genital location.

10. Dequalinium or Dequalinium chloride (1,1'-decamethylenebis [4-aminoquinaldinium chloride]) is a quaternary ammonium compound which is used as a local disinfectant (NFN Dequalonum, in England Dequadin). After prolonged application to intertriginous areas or to the previously mentioned genital locations, small and superficial, white necrotic areas surrounded by a thin erythematous halo will appear. If the cause is not recognized, larger confluent polycyclic necroses will develop; they are covered with a white or brownish crust. Such deep necroses will cause considerable cicatricial distortion after healing. * 17, 18

11. In **Behçet's syndrome** ulcers of the genital region are the cardinal sign; they are shallow oval ulcerations without definite infiltration or other inflammatory signs. The borders are sharply circumscribed and not undermined (Fig. 572).

---

* Similar necroses have been observed also after application of other cationic quaternary ammonium compounds. (Tr.)

Favorite locations are the scrotal skin, the root of the penis, and the labia majora. Because these genital ulcers quite often are the first signs of the disease, it is difficult to evaluate them diagnostically until further signs become evident. However, even at this time one observes an unspecific cutaneous hyperreactivity, as shown by a small infiltrate or pustule which appears after an injection of physiological saline. For further manifestations of Behcet's syndrome see Chapter 7, A3 and Chapter 36, A6.[4, 11]

12. Cancer of the penis may appear as a papillomatous, tuberous, nonpapillary ulcer or as a carcinomatous ulcer (Fig. 573). Most penile cancers appear in men between the ages of 50 and 70; apparently phimosis or retention of smegma favors such a development. A prelude to cancer of the genitals is the stenotic shrinkage effect usually known as kraurosis vulvae or kraurosis penis. Such a final stage of shrinkage can be the result of different underlying diseases, although lichen sclerosus et atrophicus is the chief cause. Penile cancer, like the syphilitic primary lesion, usually begins in the coronary sulcus. The cancer spreads either by diffuse infiltration or by exophytic vegetating growth while at the same time extending into the deeper tissue. In the first case one sometimes sees widespread thickening and induration. The second type at first shows lesions that resemble condylomata acuminata. The two chief types, the infiltrating penile cancer and the vegetating cancer, may show ulcerating decay; however, the ulcerous appearance as such may not always take precedence. Histologically, squamous cell carcinomas of the penis are for the most part highly differentiated cancers with varying degrees of keratinization and only a small degree of mitotic activity, although there is also some variation with this type of tumor. Although the inguinal lymph nodes in general become involved rather late, these nodes

are always the first ones to show cancerous changes. In any case, a biopsy should be performed to substantiate the diagnosis; if the pathological report is negative, additional biopsies may be necessary.[1, 9, 12]

Bowen's disease (erythroplasia) of the glans penis should be considered a preinvasive carcinoma (see also Chapter 38, H1); its further growth leads to nodular or papillomatous tumors and only rarely to definite ulcerations. The surface of such a lesion of Bowen's disease located in the genital mucosa lies at the level of the surrounding skin and has a fine velvety granular surface. Sometimes small erosions are present. The color remains red and will not be interspersed by brown lines as with balanitis chronica plasmacellularis (see also Chapter 21, A4).

Paget's disease of the penis is extremely rare; its behavior corresponds clinically and histopathologically to that of the *in situ* cancer of the nipple. In other words,

Fig. 574. Fenestrating condylomata acuminata.

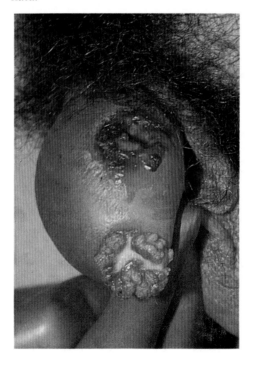

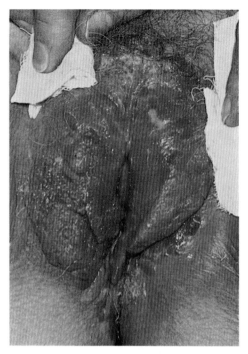

Fig. 575. Carcinoma of the vulva.

we find here on the genitals the same erythematous, eczematoid changes that remain circumscribed for a long time.*

---

* These changes, however, may not be associated with an underlying cancer. (Tr.)

13. The differential diagnosis of **condylomata acuminata** as opposed to penile cancer requires special comment because of the frequency and importance of the former condition. In contrast to cancer of the penis, condylomata as a rule lack early ulceration or rapid necrotic disintegration. But in spite of the histologically unequivocal benign aspect of these fibroepitheliomas, from a clinical point of view they cannot be considered benign without exception. This is especially true when we are dealing not with "vulgar" venereal warts but with a special giant type that perforates into the urethra or fenestrates into the prepuce, a condition known as the **Buschke-Loewenstein tumor** (Fig. 574). Criteria such as the mostly firm infiltrating broad base of the cancer or the lack of condylomata acuminata of the glans penis do not permit a definite decision. In any case it is today undeniable that venereal warts of many years' duration that are repeatedly irritated by treatment may form the basis for the development of a penile cancer.[2, 6]

14. Cancer of the vulva, like the genital cancer of men, consists of diffuse infiltrating or irregular ulcerated growths. Almost half of such vegetative tumors are found on the external labia, and another 20 per cent

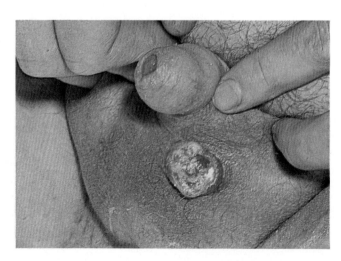

Fig. 576. Carcinoma of the scrotum.

occur on the inner aspect of the labia and the clitoris (Fig. 575). Histologically, practically all cancers of the vulva are squamous cell carcinomas, with the exception of some classified as Bowen's disease.

15. Ulcerations in the scrotal region that show no tendency to heal must in the beginning be suspect of a **scrotal carcinoma** (Fig. 576). The diagnosis should be verified by an early biopsy, especially if the patient might have been exposed to irritants in his occupation. Formerly chimneysweeps frequently developed scrotal cancers, but this is no longer true owing to improved hygiene; today workers in contact with paraffin, cutting oil, and other hydrocarbons may develop carcinomas of the scrotum.[13, 15]

16. Inflammatory changes of the glans penis are given the name balanitis, but this term does not give any information about the etiology. Erosive balanitis following herpes simplex infection or Bowen's disease and the dequalinium necrosis have been discussed before.

Balanitis erosiva circinata shows a few polycyclic erosions located mostly in the coronary sulcus but hardly ever deeper. Each erosion develops as a red spot surrounded by a white border. The lesions of the coronary sulcus extend to the glans penis and the inner foreskin. If the etiology is unknown, balanitis due to *Candida albicans* must be excluded (diabetes).

Balanitis parakeratotica circinata, which is part of Reiter's disease, does not cause erosions. The festooned or droplike erythemas are covered by a thin parakeratotic laminated scale, which also forms a frame. The diagnosis is based on the mucosal findings and other signs of the disease as described in Chapter 7, B 2.

In **balanitis "specifica"** there are more infiltrated brownish or reddish-gray syphilitic papules, which are almost always soon eroded on the glans penis or the prepuce but do not show deeper ulceration.

In association with other secondary syphilitic skin and mucous membrane manifestations this "specific" balanitis can be grouped with syphilis with no hesitation.

17. Ulcerations located in the immediate vicinity of the anus that are also interspersed with single fistulating ducts can be observed in **regional enteritis** (see also Chapter 14, B9).

18. Ulcerations within the perianal region may also be caused by **tuberculosis miliaris ulcerosa cutis;** they are found in patients who have an almost complete lack of resistance owing to miliary tuberculosis. For the signs and verification of the diagnosis see Chapter 14, B10 and Chapter 33, B4.

(1) BAUER, K. M., und H. C. FRIEDERICH: Peniscarcinom auf dem Boden vorbehandelter Condylomata acuminata. Z. Haut- u. Geschl.-Kr. *39:* 150–163 (1965).
(2) BECKER, F. T., H. J. WALDER and D. M. LARSON: Giant condylomata acuminata; Buschke-Loewenstein Tumor. Arch. Derm. (Chic.) *100:* 184–186 (1969).
(3) BERLIN, C.: The pathogenesis of the so-called ulcus vulvae acutum. Acta derm.-venereol. (Stockh.) *45:* 221–222 (1965).
(4) CABRÉ, J., und G. BREHM: Histologische und immunbiologische Untersuchungen zum Behçet-Syndrom. Derm. Wschr. *150:* 566–576 (1964).
(5) EISSNER, H.: Ulceröser Lupus vulgaris des Penis. Z. Haut- u. Geschl.-Kr. *35:* 173–182 (1963).
(6) GILBERT, CH. F.: Giant condyloma acuminatum (Buschke-Loewensteintumor). Arch. Derm. (Chic.) *93:* 714–717 (1966).
(7) GLICKSMAN, J. M., D. H. SHORT, J. M. KNOX and R. G. FREEMAN: Gonococcal skin lesions. Arch. Derm. (Chic.) *96:* 74–76 (1967).
(8) HAMMERSCHMIDT, E., und G. W. KORTING: Ein Beitrag zur Pathogenese des Ulcus vulvae acutum. Dermatologica (Basel) *99:* 362–371 (1949).
(9) HANASH, K. A., W. L. FURLOW, D. C. UTZ and E. G. HARRISON: Carcinoma of the penis: a clinicopathologic study. J. Urol. *104:* 291–297 (1970).

(10) HELLERSTRÖM, S.: Papulo-nekrotische Tuberkulide mit Lokalisation an der Glans penis. Acta derm.-venereol. (Stockh.) *23:* 170–184 (1943).

(11) JENSEN, T.: Sur les ulcérations aphteuses de la muqueuse de la bouche et de la peau génitale combinées avec les symptômes oculaires. (= Syndrome Behçet.) Acta derm.-venereol. (Stockh.) *22:* 64–79 (1941).

(12) LANGKOPF, B., und G. PAUL: Zur Klinik des Peniskarzinoms. Dtsch. Gesundh.-Wes. *23:* 415–420 (1968).

(13) LARKIN, J. C., W. T. MURDOCK and S. PHILIPS: Carcinoma of the scrotum in a tire recap worker. Arch. Derm. (Chic.) *89:* 247–249 (1964).

(14) MELCZER, N.: Die fulminante Gangrän der äußeren Geschlechtsorgane. Acta derm.-venereol. (Stockh.) *25:* 338–349 (1945).

(15) PETRES, J., und M. HUNDEIKER: Berufsbedingte Scrotalcarcinome bei Automatendrehern. Z. Haut- u. Geschl.-Kr. *40:* 230–236 (1966).

(16) SCHIEFERSTEIN, G., und Z. FOURAD: Hodenatrophie nach akuter Gangrän des Genitale. Med. Welt *21* (N. F.): 964–967 (1970).

(17) TILSLEY, D. A., and D. S. WILKINSON: Necrosis and dequalinium. II. Vulval and extra-genital ulceration. Trans. St. John's Hosp. Derm. Soc. (Lond.) *51:* 49–54 (1965).

(18) WILKINSON, D. S.: Durch Dequalinium hervorgerufene Hautnekrosen. Hautarzt *21:* 114–116 (1970).

D. Extremities

For practical purposes the differential diagnosis of leg ulcers is limited by the fact that 90 per cent of these ulcers are of venous origin, 5 per cent have an arterial genesis, and only the remainder depend on rare heterogeneous causes.

1. The clinical appearance provides only indefinite information about the causal factors responsible for the development of a leg ulcer; final evaluation requires a thorough history and methodical investigation.

The **arterial leg ulcer** is almost always a partial manifestation of a generalized incomplete or complete arterial insufficiency. Etiologically important are arteriosclerosis, endangiitis obliterans, diabetes mellitus, embolic closure of a vessel, periarteritis nodosa, ergotamine or arsenic toxicity, and syphilitic vasculitis. The fact that arteriosclerosis is apparently the most frequent cause of arterial leg ulcers explains the development of such tissue defects, which occur mainly in men after the fiftieth year of life. Some patients have suffered for years from intermittent claudication and must lower the position of the affected extremity at night to ease the pain (increasing the arterial pressure gradient). The ulcer itself causes considerable pain, often after a common trauma. Furthermore, the supposedly ingrown toenail is not infrequently the first visible manifestation of an arterial vascular disturbance of circulation. The effect of an embolic closure is so sudden that immediate intervention is required. In contrast, necroses that occur after endangiitis obliterans take months to develop, and the necroses that follow arteriosclerosis quite often require years. The usual sites of the ulcers are the middle of the tibial region, toes, sides of the feet, and heels. The ulcers are sharply outlined and look as if they had been punched out. A tendency to spontaneous formation of granulations is absent; after a long period, firmly attached fibrinous coatings are formed. The evidence of decreased arterial blood flow can be roughly determined by palpation and auscultation of the peripheral vessels. Exact localization of the blockage requires selective arteriography; however, one must remember that leg ulcers may be the result of a high stenosis of the iliac artery (Fig. 577). The differential diagnosis should consider that a slowly developing leg ulcer may in reality be a squamous cell cancer, Bowen's disease, or a basal cell epithelioma.[9, 19, 27, 31]

In contrast to the common ulcerations of the legs, a leg **ulcer due to hypertension** (ulcus cruris hypertonicum) represents a

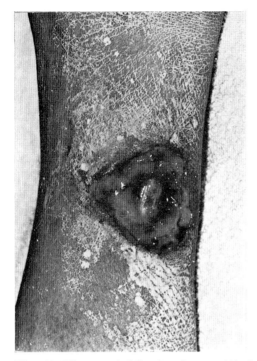 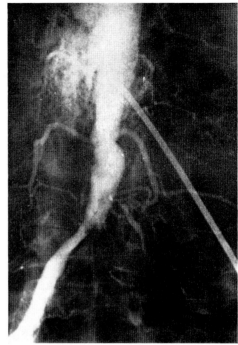

Fig. 577. Ulcus cruris following closure of the left iliac artery.

Fig. 578. Callous ulcus cruris in chronic venous insufficiency.

diagnosis which is doubtless made too often. This latter condition should be diagnosed only in the presence of considerable arterial hypertension and absent closure of the larger vascular trunks. This ulcer is almost always seen in women and is symmetrically located on both legs between the middle and lower thirds. Such leg ulcers begin after a common trauma with a bluish patch which changes quickly into a circumscribed ischemic necrosis; there is no simultaneous venous inflammation, frostbite, or edema. Considerable doubt exists as to whether the leg ulcer due to hypertension really represents a disease entity by itself.[26]

2. A simple varicosity is a consequence of a valvular insufficiency of the great saphenous vein and sometimes also of the small saphenous vein combined with continuing function of the valvular apparatus

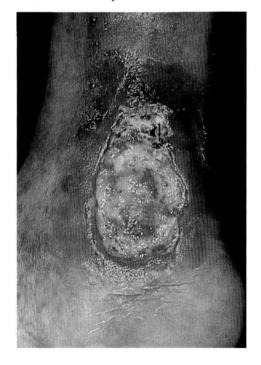

of the venae perforantes of the thigh. If in the course of years these veins also become insufficient, retrograde congestion of the venous blood may bring about chronic venous insufficiency of the lower extremities. Step by step this condition will develop through the intermediate stages of congestive erythema and congestive eczema, finally producing a **venous stasis ulcer.** Quite often a dermatitis venenata will be superimposed on a varicose eczema through contact sensitization to various local medications; in addition, a generalized absorption type of dermatitis may occur. Such stasis ulcers present as small, oval, painful, greasy tissue defects (Fig. 578), in contrast to the more proximal, callous, post-thrombotic ulcers located deep within sclerotic skin. The vicinity of the ulcer is not especially infiltrated or indurated; edema is absent also. The location around the inner malleoli is typical. A further consequence of the chronic retrograde congestion is the development of *atrophia alba (atrophie blanche; capillaritis alba)*, which is located behind the malleoli in most cases. The lesions of this atrophy are characterized by half dollar-sized, polycyclically ragged, tautly atrophic, sometimes speckled pigmented areas with peripheral telangiectases. Sometimes such circumscribed retromalleolar poikilodermas show isolated or aggregated pinhead-sized nodules. Not infrequently such lesions may break down, forming multiple, extremely painful, sharply circumscribed, bizarre ulcers.

Insufficiency of the valves of the superficial veins can be demonstrated by Trendelenburg's test: with the patient in the supine position the leg is raised above the level of the heart, and compression is applied to the junction of the great saphenous vein and the femoral vein just below the inguinal ligament. As soon as the patient gets up, the compression is released; if the veins become distended at once the presence of varicosities and the incompetence of the valves are established.[35]

3. The majority of venous leg ulcers develop within the framework of the post-thrombotic syndrome. A prerequisite for the development of the post-thrombotic syndrome and the **post-thrombotic stasis ulcer** is a thrombosis of a deep vein of a lower extremity which has undergone either partial recanalization or none. Therefore the backflow of the blood must follow the superficial veins and then the perforating veins, emptying into the deep femoral vein. This constantly increasing pressure of the collateral circulation will result secondarily in phlebosclerosis and the formation of varicosities, thereby impairing the retrograde flow of fluid out of the tissue. Chronic edema with increased formation of connective tissue, including small hemorrhages emanating from the overloaded veins, is the result. Finally an ulcer will develop within these areas of disturbed local metabolism. Such a stasis ulcer in most cases will be located between the middle and lower thirds of the leg. The skin around a stasis ulcer is hardened (dermatosclerosis) and becomes hyperpigmented through deposits of hemosiderin. Scar formation around the ulcer can result in dumbbell-like retractions. In contrast to the arterial ulcer, the venous ulcer in general becomes painful only in the presence of severe superinfection. Walking diminishes the pain if the bandage does not rub, whereas standing or lowering the legs either initiates or increases the pain.

To test for sufficient collateral circulation of the deep veins of the lower extremities (Perthes' test) in patients with varicose veins, a bandage is applied to the upper part of the leg below the junction of the saphena parva vein and the popliteal vein – i.e., below the knee; the patient then walks around for about ten minutes. If the varicose veins distal to the compression become tightly filled and pain occurs, it signifies that drainage through the deep veins has become impossible. They are either blocked or insufficiently recanalized.

If the varicosities are evacuated it means that the passageway through the deep veins is free.[35]

4. So-called **summer ulcerations,** located along the sides of the feet and around the malleoli in connection with a vasculitis racemosa, are discussed in Chapter 18, M 2.

The **ulcus cruris postpoliomyeliticum,** a leg ulcer that occurs in the paralyzed lower extremities after polio, must not be considered a trophoneurotic ulceration. These ulcers are really ulcerated perniones, which have a ready tendency to occur in a paralyzed extremity. Such ulcers occur most commonly in young women and are seen almost exclusively on the legs. Typically they appear a long time after the attack of poliomyelitis has subsided, at first presenting themselves as erythematous nodes during the cold season. These nodes disappear with bedrest or when the outside temperature becomes warmer. Compared with the healthy extremity, the ulcer forms earlier on the paralyzed side and reaches a larger size. After repeated recurrences the ulcers persist regardless of outside temperatures.[22, 34]

5. Since **periarteritis nodosa** is a systematized vascular disease, it may be associated with extensive ulcerations (which show a predilection for the extremities) and other signs of disturbed peripheral circulation. The supposedly characteristic palpable nodules, measuring 0.2 to 1.0 cm and located in the subcutis or muscles, are found rather rarely. The existence of vasculitis racemosa is likewise not of decisive importance, because this disease may have many different causes. Some patients show sudden cutaneous or subcutaneous hemorrhages which could be the result of a rupture of diseased arterial segments. Migrating phlebitis (phlebitis saltans) may be the only manifestation of periarteritis nodosa for a long period. About half the patients suffer from irregular febrile episodes and prolonged attacks of tachycardia independent of fever. Involvement

of the kidneys leads to hypertension. In addition, focal defects of the central and peripheral nervous system play an important role. Laboratory tests show leukocytosis (often accompanied by eosinophilia), anemia, and an elevated sedimentation rate. The clinical diagnosis can be made only by evaluating all signs together. It is important to remember that signs affecting various organs may change relatively quickly. Often only a biopsy of the diseased part of a vessel will permit the definite diagnostic classification of periarteritis nodosa.[5, 9b, 11, 16]

6. Systemic lupus erythematosus seldom produces ulcerations, and then only in connection with vasculitis racemosa or cryoglobulinemia. Moreover, these ulcers indicate, by their symmetrical character as distal gangrene or by their multiplicity over bony protuberances, especially of the hand, that they are dependent on the blood vessels. For a discussion of the diagnosis see Chapter 16, D 2.[23, 28]

7. Necrobiosis lipoidica shows exclusively focal ulcerations which betray clinically and histologically their causal dependence on obliterative vascular changes. The clinical diagnosis can be made easily in every case by the presence of residual areas with the typical aspect of necrobiosis lipoidica (see also Chapter 16, A 8).

8. Whereas the ulcers of necrobiosis lipoidica generally are located on the extensor sides of the legs, similar punched-out ulcerations on the sides of the calf will suggest **erythema induratum.** The clinical signs and differential diagnosis were discussed in Chapter 18, G 4.

9. The diagnosis of **tertiary syphilis** should be considered in the presence of a solitary, sharply circumscribed ulcer suggestive of a disintegrating gumma. A bluish-brown, spherically protuberant,

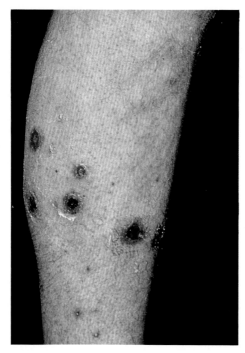

Fig. 579. Multiple ecthymas.

sions which subsequently attain a characteristic kidney shape. Such syphilitic gummas may at first exactly resemble a furuncle or an abscess; when submandibular, they suggest cutaneous actinomycosis or scrofuloderma, and on the legs they may be confused with an ulcer of different origin.

10. Ecthyma has no clinical connection with the vascular or follicular apparatus; it is characterized by bacterial inflammatory lesions on the legs that become ulcerated. After a vesicular pustule appears in the beginning stage of (streptococcal) *ecthyma simplex*, it later develops a flat crust which covers an ulcer. The ecthymatous ulceration has a sharp and ragged border with a more or less greasy, purulent coating. Its diameter hardly ever is more than 2 cm and it has an erythematous livid halo (Fig. 579). It may be associated with further bacterial complications (for instance, lymphangitis) as well as with a simultaneous occurrence of other types of pyodermas. The term *ecthyma gangrenosum* defines an erosive ulcerated pyoderma caused by *Pseudomonas aeruginosa*. This disease is seen in its typical acute form as a pyocyanic infection of the skin in cachectic children. Besides con-

subcutaneous node will show a shrinkage in its consistency, then a slitlike perforation will develop with subsequent discharge of the contents. Ulcerative tertiary syphilis of this type produces punched-out, not undermined, roughly protuberant le-

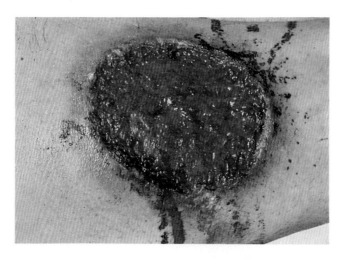

Fig. 580. Pyoderma gangrenosum.

taining the pyocyanic organism, such large, superficial, circinate, ragged ulcerations frequently show small bandlike vesicular elevations at their edges. Further characteristics are satellite groups of soft small-nodular lesions or spongy, tinderlike areas.[17]

11. Pyoderma gangrenosum is also the name given to dermatitis ulcerosa and postoperative progressive gangrene. The etiology is not clear but infections or vascular changes are not etiologically significant. It is, however, more than a coincidence that the disorder occurs in combination with ulcerative colitis and a plasmacytoma.* Paraproteinemias of the IgM or IgA type are observed in almost all patients, but deficient immunoglobulins occur considerably less often. One or more lesions exist, usually on the extremities. In principle, however, pyoderma gangrenosum can occur at any site. The fully developed picture is rather typical, and only the early stages present diagnostic difficulties. The first lesions are mostly blisters, pustules, or papules, which extend rapidly by apposition of new lesions. The whole disease process, with a few exceptions, remains limited to the skin and subcutaneous fat tissue, resulting in extended, flat, but not very deep ulcerations. The ulceration itself consists of torpid granulation tissue and has no cover. Characteristic signs, however, are located at the margin. It is elevated like a wall, has a dusky blue-red color, and is interspersed with multiple tiny abscesses. The ulcer's borders are very sensitive and are often undermined for several millimeters (Fig. 580). Peripherally, there is a light red, ill-defined erythematous ring. The bacterial invasion is extremely variable and no diagnostic conclusions can be drawn from it. The same can be said of the histo-

logic findings, so that besides the macroscopic findings, the diagnosis depends on evidence of paraproteinemia or one of the two previously mentioned disorders. Patients with proven paraproteinemia should receive regular follow-up care to insure early recognition of a plasmocytoma, if present.[6, 18, 30]

12. Coumarin necroses are discussed because of their similarity to pyoderma gangrenosum. They appear two to ten days after anticoagulative treatment with coumarin or indandione has been started. Cessation or continuance of the drug does not bring a change in the course of the disease. Signs of an overdosage of the anticoagulants cannot be found. Preferred locations of the necroses are again the extremities, thighs, buttocks, and also the breast. In the beginning, circumscribed blue-red spots form within a few hours, and these by confluence constitute a raggedly circumscribed area. This red region is firmly infiltrated, warmer than the surrounding skin, and rather tender. Soon the epidermis is raised in blisters and subsequent hemorrhagic necroses of the subcutaneous tissue appear. In exceptional cases deeper lying tissue or even several toes may be included in the necrosis. For the differential diagnosis it is important that the peripheral pulse is maintained and no disturbance of arterial circulation is present. Healing extends over several weeks and leads to deeply shrunken scars.[14, 15, 25]

13. Among the diffuse connective tissue diseases ulcerations of the legs are observed less in **rheumatoid arthritis** than in Felty's syndrome and in Werner's syndrome. In *rheumatoid arthritis* frequently only minimal ulcerations are present clinically, and these therefore respond promptly to treatment. Histologically, the tissue changes vary according to zone; centrally there is fibrinoid necrosis;

---

* Not commonly found in patients with pyoderma gangrenosum in the United States. (Tr.)

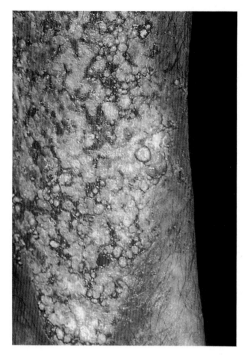

Fig. 581. Vegetating dyskeratosis follicularis of the leg.

next, the adjacent histiocytes and fibroblasts form a palisadelike structure with round cells; and finally at the periphery there is fibrous tissue with numerous disturbed blood vessels.[2]

Felty's syndrome (chronic polyarthritis, splenomegaly, leukopenia with relative lymphocytosis, generalized lymph node swellings, subfebrile temperatures, and dirty brownish erythematous or purpuric cutaneous changes) may likewise be associated with leg ulcers.

They usually are large and deep, drug-resistant ulcers located supramalleolarly or on the extensor and flexor sides of the legs. Pathomechanical disturbances of nutrition or the defense mechanism should be considered as causes.[13, 16]

In **Werner's syndrome** (see also Chapter 16, B9) two-thirds of the patients regularly have torpid trophic ulcerations. They develop in areas of taut atrophies following even minor traumas. Typical sites are the malleolar region, the legs, and the dorsa of the feet, mainly on pressure-exposed places, especially over osseous protuberances.[7]

14. Occasionally patients with **dyskeratosis follicularis** may show macular ulcerations on the legs (Fig. 581). Simultaneously, however, the ulcerations show large hyperkeratotic excrescences. If they are removed, a rough, very tender, and easily bleeding ulcer base becomes visible. Since these tissue defects may exist for years,

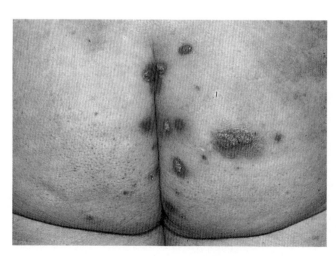

Fig. 582. Papulonecrotic tuberculids.

the possibility of malignant degeneration
must be kept in mind.

15. Ulcerations of the leg in connection
with hematologic disturbances are rare.
They are observed accompanying **familial
hemolytic icterus** and **pernicious anemia.**
The location on the lower third of the leg,
frequently near the ankle, is characteristic,
as is the lack of fresh, "inflammatory"
(e.g., eczematous) changes in the vicinity
of such ulcerations. The surrounding skin
may have a certain bluish color, whereas
the ulcerations themselves present wall-
like, elevated, steep, and firm borders.
There are no definite histologic criteria.
One knows today that similar ulcerations
also occur in **Mediterranean anemia, sickle
cell anemia,** and **elliptocytoses,** that is,
hemoglobinopathies of various types.
Pathomechanically, an inadequate supply
of oxygen to the tissue has been blamed
because of the altered hemoglobin conditions. [1, 3, 4, 24, 29, 33]

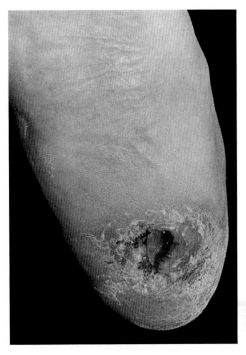

Fig. 583. Malum perforans pedis in tabes
dorsalis.

16. The tendency of **tuberculosis cutis
papulonecrotica** to ulcerations can be
especially pronounced on the lower extremities. The disorder affects mainly
adolescent girls and young adults, who may
have had recurrent attacks of the disease
for a long time. On the lower half of the
trunk and on the extremities pinhead- to
pea-sized blue-red nodules appear; after
several weeks they break down centrally
and heal with slightly atrophic scars
(Fig. 582). If they are grouped more
closely, fingernail-sized shallow ulcerations
occur; these have been described as ulcerous tuberculids. Histologically, necroses
with surrounding infiltrates of neutrophilic
granulocytes, lymphocytes, epithelioid
cells, fibroblasts, and single giant cells
are observed in close connection with the
vessels. The vessels are closed by thrombi
and proliferations of the intima. The
typical structure of a tuberculoid granulo-
mâ is missing, as are tubercle bacilli. In

testing, high-grade tuberculin sensitivity
is present.[12]

17. Frequently, badly infected ulcerations that lack specific characteristics
occur on the backs of the hands and the
arms, following unskilled injections in **drug
addicts.** They are conspicuous by their
location along the veins. In connection
with nodular infiltrates, abscesses, scar
formations, and hyperpigmentations an
artificial origin must always be considered.
For a discussion of possible accompanying
edemas see Chapter 10, B10. [10, 39]

18. On the soles, besides endangiitic
necroses of the tips of the toes or gangrenous ulcerations, **malum perforans pedis** is
most important and should in every case
lead to an investigation of the neural
cause. It may be caused by trophangió-
neuroses in *tabes dorsalis* (Fig. 583), *pseudo-*

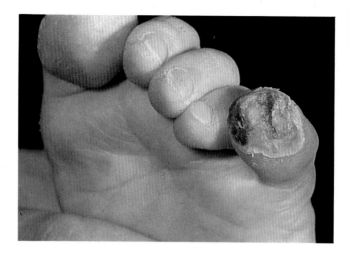

Fig. 584. Trophoneurotic
postpoliomyelitic ulcer of
the fifth toe.

tabes diabetica (frequently in association
with chronic alcoholism and vitamin-B$_1$-
deficiency), *leprosy, syringomyelia, poliomyelitis* (Fig. 584), or, more infrequently,
myelodysplasia or a *lesion in an intervertebral disk.* Malum perforans usually
develops as a single lesion. The triggering
factors are usually only common irritations
(pressure and friction). The typical malum
perforans is frequently preceded by a circumscribed succulent edema and later by
a circumscribed callosity. [32, 34, 37]

Trophic ulcerations on the flexor sides
of the toes or on the balls of the toes
occur in **familial acroosteolysis** (Fig. 585).

They develop from inflammatory preceding stages. For further details of this
disease see Chapter 5, A3 and Chapter 16,
B1. [28]

19. In rare cases **lichen planus** may be
accompanied by extensive ulcerations of
the soles and toes. The typical finding in
these patients at the onset of the disease
is chronic paronychia, which leads to nail
dystrophies and finally to complete loss
of the nail. The ulcerations are preceded
by attacks of blisters, which, however,
may continue simultaneously. Only in
rare cases do the erosive ulcerous changes

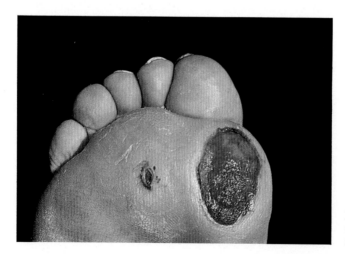

Fig. 585. Acroosteolysis:
trophoneurotic ulcer over
metatarsal of big toe.

extend later to the backs of the feet. It is striking that patients with such ulcerative lichen planus are predestined to a cicatricial loss of hair. The diagnosis can be easily made from the accompanying typical cutaneous and mucosal changes. Difficulties arise only if the ulcerations constitute the first sign. In such cases a biopsy from the border of the ulcer may help, as it will show the characteristic lichen planus histologic picture (see also Chapter 11, E6, Chapter 25, B3, and Chapter 31, A). [8, 20, 21]

(1) ARGÜELLES-CASALS, M. D.: Les ulcères de jambe dans l'anémie a hématies falciformes. Presse méd. *59:* 956–957 (1951).

(2) BENINSON, J., and D. C. ENSIGN: Leg ulcers in rheumatoid arthritis. J. Amer. Med. Ass. *175:* 437–440 (1961).

(3) BERGE, G., E. BREHMER-ANDERSSON and H. RORSMAN: Thalassemia minor and painful ulcers of lower extremities. Acta derm.-venereol. (Stockh.) *50:* 125–128 (1970).

(4) BOETTCHER, W., und W. LINDEMAYR: Unterschenkelgeschwüre als Begleitsymptom des familiären hämolytischen Ikterus. Arch. klin. exp. Derm. *207:* 472–485 (1958).

(5) BORRIE, P.: Cutaneous polyarteritis nodosa. Brit. J. Derm. *87:* 87–95 (1972).

(6) BREHM, G., und R. GEBHARDT: Dermatitis ulcerosa und γA-Mangel. Arch. klin. exp. Derm. *239:* 266–274 (1970).

(7) COHEN, M., and W. B. SHELLEY: Ankle ulcer sign of Werner's syndrome. Arch. Derm. (Chic.) *87:* 86–88 (1963).

(8) CRAM, D. L., R. R. KIERLAND and R. K. WINKELMANN: Ulcerative lichen planus of the feet. Bullous variant with hair and nail lesions. Arch. Derm. (Chic.) *93:* 692–701 (1966).

(9a) DENK, R., und N. HOEDE: Unterschenkelgeschwüre bei hochsitzendem arteriellen Gefäßverschluß. Med. Welt *19* (N. F.): 1257–1258 (1968).

(9b) DENK, R., und G. W. KORTING: Aspekte der Beziehungen von Haut und Herz bei den sog. Kollagenosen. Hautarzt *15:* 211–214 (1964).

(10) DUNNE, J. H., and W. C. JOHNSON: Necrotizing skin lesions in heroin addicts. Arch. Derm. (Chic.) *105:* 544–547 (1972).

(11) FREUND, F.: Apoplexia cutanea – Periarteriitis nodosa. Arch. Derm. Syph. (Berl.) *152:* 158–188 (1926).

(12) HAMMERSCHMIDT, E. E., and G. W. KORTING: Ulcerative tuberculids. Brit. J. Derm. *62:* 361–364 (1950).

(13) HJORTH, N.: Felty's syndrome with varicose ulcer. Acta derm.-venereol. (Stockh.) *35:* 236–238 (1955).

(14) JIPP, P.: Subcutane Fettgewebsnekrosen nach Antikoagulantientherapie. Chirurg *33:* 481–485 (1962).

(15) JOST, P.: Cumarinnekrosen. Schweiz. med. Wschr. *99:* 1069–1077 (1969).

(16) KORTING, G. W.: Über cutane Periarteriitis nodosa unter besonderer Berücksichtigung begleitender Leberstörungen und der sogenannten Thrombophlebitis migrans. Arch. Derm. Syph. (Berl.) *199:* 332–349 (1955).

(17) KORTING, G. W., und W. Adam: Ecthyma gangraenosum adultorum. Arch. Derm. Syph. (Berl.) *199:* 481–495 (1955).

(18) KRESBACH, H.: Ein Beitrag zum Problem der sogenannten Pyodermia ulcerosa. Arch. klin. exp. Derm. *208:* 128–159 (1959).

(19) MAHLER, F., U. BRUNNER und A. BOLLINGER: Das Kompressionssyndrom der Arteria poplitea. Dtsch. med. Wschr. *94:* 786–788 (1969).

(20) MAHRLE, G., H. GARTMANN und C. E. ORFANOS: Ulcerierender Lichen ruber der Füße. Zugleich eine elektronenmikroskopische Studie der »subepidermalen« Blasenbildung beim Lichen ruber bullosus. Arch. Derm. Forsch. *243:* 292–304 (1972).

(21) MALE, O.: Über die ulzerös-atrophisierende Form des Lichen ruber planus. Z. Haut- u. Geschl.-Kr. *45:* 17–28 (1970).

(22) MARTORELL, F., T. ALONSO and V. SALLERAS: Treatment of post-poliomyelitis ulcerations of the legs with lumbar sympathectomy. Angiology *4:* 118–122 (1953).

(23) METZ, G., E. SCHUBERT und J. METZ: Die periphere Erythematodes-Gangrän. Münch. med. Wschr. *113:* 729–734 (1971).

(24) MONTAGNANI, A., M. PISANI und G. ARGENZIANO: Hautschädigungen im Verlaufe von Hämoglobinopathien. Hautarzt *17:* 201–208 (1966).

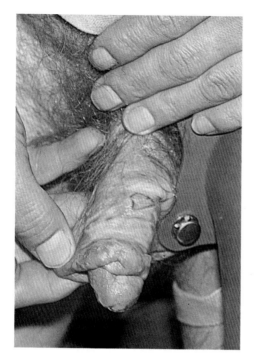

Fig. 586. Decubital ulcer from metal button of a urinal.

Fig. 587. Burn from extinguishing a burning cigarette on the dorsum of the hand.

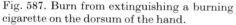

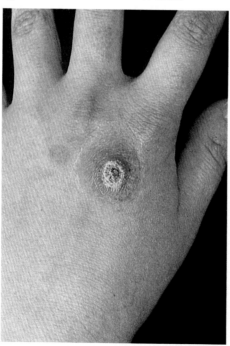

(25) MUELLER-ECKARDT, CHR.: Über lokale Blutungen und Nekrosen der Haut und des subkutanen Gewebes bei der Antikoagulantienbehandlung. Med. Klin. *57:* 2135–2137 (1962).

(26) NITZSCHNER, H.: Zur Problematik des Ulcus Martorell. Z. Haut.- u. Geschl.-Kr. *40:* 188–193 (1966).

(27) OETTEL, H.: Toxische Gefäßschäden und Durchblutungsstörungen. Hippokrates *40:* 285–295 (1969).

(28) PARTSCH, H.: Ulceromutilierende Neuropathien der unteren Extremitäten. Zum Krankheitsbild der »Acropathie ulcéro-mutilante«. Hautarzt *22:* 283–289 (1971).

(29) PASCHER, F., and R. KEEN: Chronic ulcers of the leg associated with blood dyscrasias. Arch. Derm. Syph. (Chic.) *66:* 478–487 (1952).

(30) PIERARD, J., J. DE BERSAQUES et A. KINT: A propos du »Pyoderma gangraenosum« de Brunsting, Goeckerman et O'Leary. Arch. belg. Derm. Syph. *16:* 421–443 (1960).

(31) RATSCHOW, M.: Zur Ätiologie der arteriellen Verschlußkrankheiten. Med. Klin. *58:* 344–346 (1963).

(32) RODER, H., und G. SEBASTIAN: Zur Ätiologie des Malum perforans pedis. Derm. Mschr. *157:* 356–360 (1971).

(33) SAMITZ, M. H., D. S. WALDORF and J. SHRAGER: Leg ulcers in mediterranean anemia. Arch. Derm. (Chic.) *90:* 567–571 (1964).

(34a) SCHMITZ, R.: Zur Klinik der Hypertoniegeschwüre. Derm. Wschr. *131:* 271–277 (1955).

(34b) SCHMITZ, R.: Über einige seltene Formen trophoneurotischer Geschwüre und deren Differentialdiagnose. Arch. klin. exp. Derm. *205:* 497–511 (1958).

(35) SCHNEIDER, W., und H. FISCHER: Die chronisch-venöse Insuffizienz. Enke, Stuttgart 1969.

(36) SCHOCH, E. P.: Ulcers of the leg in Felty's syndrome. Arch. Derm. Syph. (Chic.) *66:* 384–390 (1952).

(37) THIVOLET, J., et H. PERROT: A propos de 32 cas de maux perforants plantaires. Bull. Soc. franç. Derm. Syph. *77:* 453–457 (1970).

(38) TUFFANELLI, D. L., and E. L. DUBOIS: Cutaneous manifestations of systemic lupus erythematosus. Arch. Derm. (Chic.) *90:* 377–386 (1964).

(39) WEIDMAN, A. I., and M. J. FELLNER: Cutaneous manifestations of heroin and other addictive drugs. Study and analysis. N. Y. St. J. Med. *71:* 2643–2646 (1971).

E. Ulcerations Not Referring to Any Specific Body Region

1. Deep ulcerations, especially on the scrotum and the legs, arising from gangrenous and phlegmonous **erysipelas** as well as from **gangrenous vaccinia** are possible. In such processes, which are conspicuous owing to the unusual ulcerations, the causative co-factors are usually immunologic deficiencies (i.e., secondary antibody deficiency syndromes) and resistance-diminishing influences either from cytostatica or immunosuppressive drugs (which were indicated for other therapeutic reasons), or from basic diseases (lymphogranulomatosis). [1, 2]

2. Decubital ulcers after **carbon monoxide** or **barbiturate poisoning** develop from the stages of blistering and exudation from necrosis. They are presumably caused by additional peripheral circulatory disturbances. Because barbiturates are eliminated by sweat, the increased local concentration of barbiturates in the sweat glands and their ducts must be considered

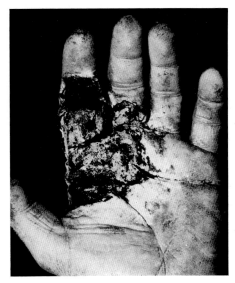

Fig. 588. Acute necrosis from x-rays.

a direct harmful factor. As expected, in such barbiturate poisoning the specific sedative can be found in the contents of the blister. [7, 8]

Other signs of **decubital ulcers** ("pressure sores," "bed sores") are rapid development within a few days and preferred locations on the coccyx, buttocks, hips, and heels, as well as initially circumscribed erythemas (Fig. 586). Osteomyelitis or at least periostitis may develop as a possible adjacent reaction of such decubital ulcers.

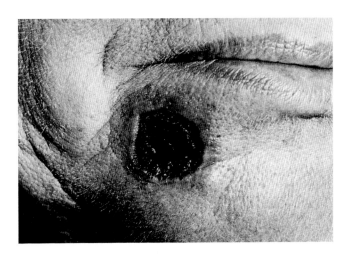

Fig. 589. Necrosis from microwave irradiation.

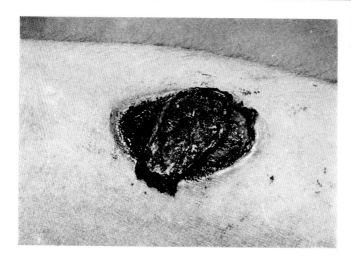

Fig. 590. Necrosis from para-venous infusion of Hyper-tensin.

3. Acute ulcerations caused by **chemical** or **physical agents** (Fig. 587) are not necessarily limited to a definite location. Ulcers resulting from all caustic substances become visible only after removal of the crust. Determination of the responsible agent may be difficult only in unconscious persons. The color of the caustic crust (sulfuric acid, black; nitric acid, yellow; carbolic acid, yellow-brown) may suggest the noxious substance.

Chronic ulcerations **caused by x-rays** are conspicuously round or square according to the shape of the cone and appear as deep and sharply demarcated defects (Fig. 588). Poikilodermic remnants may still be present, at least at the margin. The surrounding skin near the ulceration is often indurated and very tender owing to secondary infections. If the ulcerations are present for a long time and show no tendency to heal, a biopsy is indicated to exclude malignant degeneration. [4, 6]

Similar tissue defects may also be caused by the faulty application of **short** or **microwaves** (Fig. 589), whereas the end-pieces of medical electric equipment such as cardiac fibrillators or instruments that arouse patients suffering from enuresis usually show only contact burns and no deep loss of tissue. [5, 6]

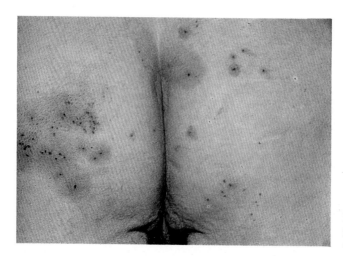

Fig. 591. Necroses from potassium permanganate crystals.

The puncture site for **infusions** may turn into an ulceration. This is usually the result of paravenously penetrating drugs with vasoconstrictive or cytotoxic effects (Fig. 590).[3]

4. Punctiform violet-black loss of tissue was formerly known as **tissue necrosis due to ink pencil.** These are characterized by poor healing of the stab wounds, subsequent serous secretion from fistulas, and a progressive course with mild tenderness.

If **potassium permanganate** is mistakenly too highly concentrated or is incompletely dissolved, multiple necroses caused by penetrating crystals may be observed (Fig. 591).

5. **Lime**, cement, or calcium nitrate can cause a blister with a black caustic crust on the top. After removing the blister a circular ulcer becomes visible. Similarly, beryllium granulomas, which occur in workers making fluorescent light tubes, result in necroses or ulcerations that heal with difficulty.

(1) BARTSCHIES, G.-G., und H.-D. JUNG: Das gangränöse und phlegmonöse Erysipel. Z. ärztl. Fortbild. (Jena) *60:* 1261–1264 (1966).

(2) BAUM, P., und K. H. MEYER ZUM BÜSCHENFELDE: Vaccinia gangraenosa et generalisata bei Lymphogranulomatose. Med. Welt *17* (N. F.): 878–881 (1966).

(3) BREHM, G., und I. BREHM: Über flächenhafte Hautnekrosen nach therapeutischen Maßnahmen. Derm. Wschr. *141:* 217–224 (1960).

(4) DREPPER, H., F. EHRING und D. VOJTECH: Die Radionekrose der Haut. Med. Welt *22* (N. F.): 155–162 (1971).

(5) GREAVES, M. W.: Scarring due to enuresis blankets. Brit. J. Derm. *81:* 440–442 (1969).

(6) KORTING, G. W.: Bericht über zwei akute physikalische Schädigungen der Haut. Med. Welt *21* (N. F.): 1359–1360 (1970).

(7) OBERSTE-LEHN, H., und L. KAULEN-BECKER: Nekrosen nach Barbitursäure- und Nodularintoxikation. Z. Haut- u. Geschl.-Kr. *44:* 169–174 (1969).

(8) RAAB, W.: Dekubitalgeschwüre bei Barbituratvergiftung. Derm. Wschr. *146:* 107–115 (1962).

34. Leukoplakias

Leukoplakia is marked by the development of a whitish thickening upon the mucous membrane that is caused by increased cornification. Such white patches cannot be wiped off; this fact alone distinguishes them from a monilia infection

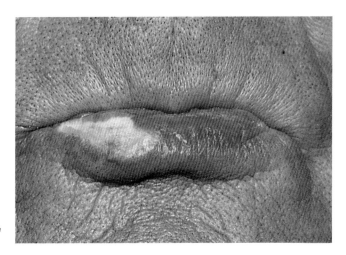

Fig. 592. Leukoplakia of the lower lip.

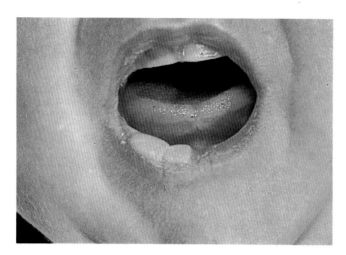

Fig. 593. Swelling from sucking of the lower lip.

or mucous coverings of a different origin. Leukoplakia is a condition that may hide many different diagnoses. These keratotic changes of mucous membranes or muco-cutaneous transitional tissue may occur either as isolated findings or as partial manifestations of a systemic skin disease.

A. Isolated Patches of Leukoplakia

1. An isolated patch of leukoplakia should be considered a callus of the mucous membranes. Such a lesion appears as a superficial enclosed whitish hyperkeratotic epithelial thickening, which stays well below the level of the surrounding tissue (Fig. 592). Only after prolonged continuous irritation will the area occasionally take on a cobblestonelike or villous appearance. Possible causes are chronic irritation caused by poorly fitting dentures and professional stigmas (glassblowers, trumpet players). Small children can develop such calluses by constant sucking (Fig. 593); chewing of tobacco or betelnuts may also give rise to leukoplakia. If removal of the irritating agent does not eliminate the leukoplakia, or if ulcerations and proliferations begin to develop, a biopsy is indicated in order to exclude Bowen's disease or a squamous cell epithelioma.

2. Bowen's disease of the mucous membranes may present as erythroplasia (see Chapter 21, A4) or as an "anonymous" leukoplakia. Macroscopically, the latter type may show hyperplastic, protuberant, or vegetating changes of the mucous membranes. Most of the patients are men in the sixth decade of life or beyond. Histologically, the well-known elements of Bowen's disease are present (dyskeratosis, blocks of acanthotic cells, irregular arrangement of the epidermal structure, parakeratosis, and infiltration of the corium); these changes at first are confined to the epithelium with no penetrating growth. This pre-invasive phase of growth is as a rule much shorter in the mucous membranes than in the epidermis, and therefore, from a therapeutic point of view, ordinary control observations are not sufficient. However, one must remember that sometimes there is an abrupt tendency to rapid invasive growth with early metastasis.[3, 4]

3. Oral florid papillomatosis (papillomatosis mucosae carcinoides) may suggest leukoplakia at first until the later development of multiple plaquelike, whitish-

gray, cauliflowerlike tumors. These vegetations spread not only to the buccal mucosa
but also to the larynx and lips. In exceptional cases the tongue may become
involved also, or the tumors may grow
into the bones and even perforate the
epidermis of the cheek to the outside. In
spite of this cancerlike behavior, the
histologic findings are those of a benign
epithelial hyperplasia which does not
penetrate the basal membrane. [9, 10, 14]

4. At any time the epithelial whitish
surface of a leukoplakia may conceal
an underlying **squamous cell carcinoma**
(Figs. 594, 595). Such a cancer, like
Bowen's disease, can be discovered only
by an early biopsy (see also Chapter 38).

5. Leukokeratosis nicotinica (or stomatitis nicotinica) is located on the part of
the hard palate directly affected by tobacco
smoke, especially in pipe-smokers. This
condition shows small, hard, semispherical
umbilicated papules of grayish-white color
with a central erythematous point; the
lesions apparently arise from the mucous
ducts on both sides of the raphe of the
hard palate.[13]

6. The **white sponge nevus of the mucosa**
(Cannon 1935) is either present at birth

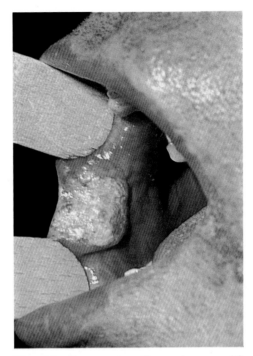

Fig. 594. Squamous cell carcinoma with
leukoplakic surface.

or becomes manifest at the latest by the
fourth year of life. The abnormality is
familial and is an autosomal dominant
trait. Generally, consideration of the
history makes the diagnosis possible without difficulty. Clinically, the affected

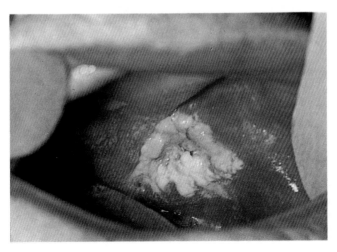

Fig. 595. Squamous cell carcinoma with leukoplakic surface.

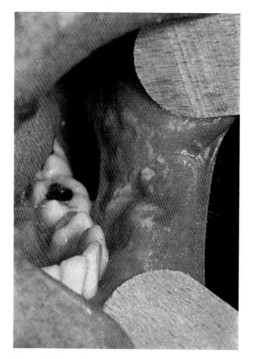

Fig. 596. Morsicatio buccarum (cheek-biting).

Fig. 597. Geographic tongue.

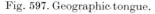

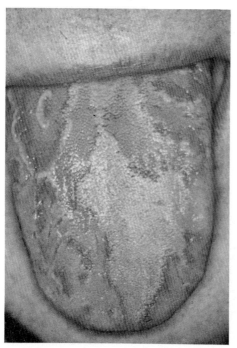

areas show an opal-white, spongy, irregularly folded thickening of the mucous membrane without ulcerations or papillomatous growths. The most frequently affected site is the oral mucosa, including the palate and the edges of the tongue. In addition, similar changes can be observed on the lips and the mucosa of the nose, vagina, and rectum. This nevus may maintain a certain tendency to grow until puberty and then remain constant in its extension (except during pregnancy). Malignant degeneration does not take place. Histologically, the chief findings are spongy, enlarged epithelial cells interspersed through the entire epidermis as well as acanthosis and parahyperkeratosis. [1, 2, 12, 16]

7. Hereditary benign intraepithelial dyskeratosis is also (like Cannon's nevus) inherited as an autosomal dominant trait. Macroscopically, the changes of the oral mucosa do not differ from those of the white sponge nevus. The histologic findings are also identical to a large extent except for the numerous eosinophils and eosinophilic bodies (dyskeratotic nuclear substance ?) that are interspersed in places throughout the epidermis. Important differences are the noninvolvement of the mucosa of the anus and genitals and the evidence of participation of the eye in hereditary benign intraepithelial dyskeratosis. The ocular changes also begin in early infancy with photophobia and constant shedding of tears. The conjunctiva bulbi shows fine, cloudy, gelatinous, proliferating plaques adjacent to the limbus of the cornea; in the spring the cornea may be covered by a form of veil, which may disappear in the fall unless vascularization takes place. [11, 16]

8. Morsicatio buccarum (cheek-biting) produces small, white, cloudy, epithelial spots on the surface of the buccal mucosa (Fig. 596). For details see Chapter 10, A3. [6, 15]

9. Glossitis rhomboidea mediana, which may resemble leukoplakia, is located on the dorsum of the midline of the tongue; it is one of the keratotic conditions. The surface of the tongue is abnormally red, lacquerlike, and rhomboid-shaped with separate nodular protuberances at the site of the tuberculum impar (see also Chapter 38, F3).

10. Geographic tongue produces red exfoliations surrounded by whitish zones resembling a geographic map. The lesions look as if they had been mowed down, and their appearance may change from day to day. In addition, the slightly depressed patches have a curly border medially (Fig. 597). The exfoliation of the patches is caused by desquamation of the filiform papillae. The cause of this anomaly is not known.

11. Syphilitic interstitial glossitis is frequently accompanied by leukoplakic keratoses. This diffuse sclerosing glossitis leads to either a superficial or a deep interstitial increase of connective tissue which results in a hard and plump consistency of the tongue; sometimes the organ looks as if it were divided into lobules or nodules. This type of syphilitic glossitis frequently shows leukoplakic transformations. Because these leukoplakias are precancerous, such patients must remain under strict medical observation even after specific treatment for their syphilis.[3]

12. Oral submucosal fibrosis is a disease almost completely confined to the Indian subcontinent. One of its possible causes is the constant consumption of heavily spiced food. The clinical manifestations may occur on any part of the oral cavity or the pharynx. Initial signs are burning sensations, especially when eating. These are followed by the appearance of vesicles on the gums, buccal mucosa, and lower lip; these lesions soon change into flat and

very painful aphthae. The subsequent course of the disease produces an opal-white discoloration of the mucosa that is very conspicuous compared with the normal pigmentation of the mucosa of East Indians. In addition to the macular cloudy lesions, there are striated figurations which produce a marbled appearance. The final stage shows fibrosis of the uvula, the palatine arches, and the lips, as well as impairment of the movement of the tongue. The endstage is a high degree of microstomia.[7, 8]

13. Obviously superficial coatings of the top layers of the mucosa that can be removed easily are suspicious of a **candida mycosis;** following such removal a dark red, swollen, easily bleeding surface is seen. The diagnosis is verified by staining a smear with methylene blue or by culture. However, a superimposed candidal infection on preexisting leukoplakias is not rare.[5]

(1) BROWNE, W. G., M. M. IZATT and J. H. RENWICK: White sponge naevus of the mucosa: clinical and linkage data. Ann. Hum. Genet. *32:* 271–281 (1969).
(2) CANNON, A. B.: White sponge nevus of the mucosa (naevus spongiosus albus mucosae). Arch. Derm. Syph. (Chic.) *31:* 365–370 (1935).
(3) HAYM, J.: Die Praecancerose in der Mundhöhle. Dtsch. zahnärztl. Z. *16:* 57–70 (1961).
(4) HORNSTEIN, O., und H.-D. PAPE: Morbus Bowen der Mundschleimhaut. Dermatologica (Basel) *131:* 325–342 (1965).
(5) JANSEN, G. TH., C. J. DILLAHA and W. M. HONEYCUTT: Candida cheilitis. Arch. Derm. (Chic.) *88:* 325–329 (1963).
(6) OBERMAYER, M. F.: Cheekbiting (morsicatio buccarum). Arch. Derm. (Chic.) *90:* 185–190 (1964).
(7) PINDBORG, J. J., F. S. MEHTA and D. K. DAFTARY: Occurrence of epithelial atypia in 51 Indian villagers with oral submucous fibrosis. Brit. J. Cancer *24:* 253–257 (1970).
(8) PINDBORG, J. J., and S. M. SIRSAT: Oral submucous fibrosis. Oral Surg. *22:* 764–779 (1966).

(9) RICHTER, G., S. ENGEL und H. JACOBI:
Zum Krankheitsbild der sogenannten
»oral florid papillomatosis«. (Papillomatosis mucosae oris carcinoides). Dermatologica (Basel) *144:* 75–82 (1972).

(10) ROCK, J. A., and E. R. FISHER: Florid
papillomatosis of the oral cavity and
larynx. Arch. Otolaryng. *72:* 593–598
(1960).

(11) v. SALLMANN, L., and D. PATON: Hereditary benign intraepithelial dyskeratosis. I. Ocular manifestations. Arch.
Ophthal. (Chic.) *63:* 421–429 (1960).

(12) STÜTTGEN, G., H. H. BERRES und
W. WILL: Leukoplakische, epitheliale
Naevi der Mundschleimhaut und ihre
Keratinisierungsform. Arch. klin. exp.
Derm. *221:* 433–446 (1965).

(13) TAPPEINER, J.: Zur Klinik und Pathogenese der Leukokeratosis nicotinica
palati. Hautarzt *17:* 152–154 (1966).

(14) TAPPEINER, J., und K. WOLFF: Papillomatosis mucosae carcinoides (»oral florid
papillomatosis«). Hautarzt *20:* 102–108
(1969).

(15) VAKILZADEH, F.: Zur Morsicatio labio-
rum. Z. Haut- u. Geschl.-Kr. *42:* 253–
256 (1967).

(16) WITKOP, JR. C. J., and R. J. GORLIN:
Four hereditary mucosal syndromes.
Arch. Derm. (Chic.) *84:* 762–771 (1961).

B. Secondary Leukoplakias

1. Among the genodermatoses the group
of palmoplantar keratoses should be
mentioned first because some of these
conditions may show leukoplakias. However, with the exception of **pachyonychia
congenita** (also known as Jadassohn-
Lewandowsky syndrome) (Fig. 598), definite diagnostic conclusions cannot be
drawn from such a sign (see also Chapter 28,
C4). Pachyonychia congenita almost always shows leukoplakia of the mucosae
of the mouth and nose. Leukoplakia may
also be present on the anal mucosa as
part of the syndrome. In all these locations
malignant degeneration may develop.

2. Dyskeratosis congenita (see also
Chapter 23, A2) is accompanied even in
early infancy by leukoplakic changes of
the mucosa. Such changes occur not only
on the oral mucosa but also in the rectum
or around the urethra; these leukoplakias
are of precancerous significance.

3. Among the genodermatoses with formation of bullae **epidermolysis bullosa
dystrophica recessiva** (see also Chapter 25,
A9) should be mentioned here because
leukoplakias of the oral cavity and lips
may develop owing to recurrent formation
of bullae. For the same reason cicatricial
adhesions may form simultaneously.

4. In rare instances **dyskeratosis follicularis** may produce whitish-gray papules
on the palate that generally do not exceed
the size of pinheads. Usually they are
sharply circumscribed and only exceptionally do they develop knotty-verrucous
formations.

5. Lichen planus has the greatest differential diagnostic importance in relation

Fig. 598. Leukoplakia in pachyonychia congenita.

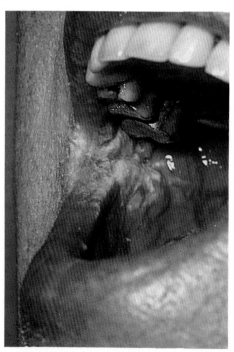

to leukoplakia proper. In a typical case lichen planus of the mucosa does not offer any diagnostic difficulties because it has reticulated or lacelike patterns which resemble spiderwebs or ferns (Fig. 517). The vermilion part of the lips shows similar finely structured cloudy lesions which can be easily differentiated from the coarse, sometimes verrucous areas of leukoplakia and from the equally coarse, hyperkeratotic-erosive lesions of chronic lupus erythematosus. Above all they are different from eczematous-exudative or exfoliative cheilitis. Strangely enough this exquisite papulosis of the skin hardly ever shows nodular elements on the mucosa. Annular patterns of lichen planus of the oral mucosa, however, appear as rounded, occasionally multiple infiltrates on the dorsum of the tongue. [1,2]

6. Chronic lupus erythematosus may also produce annular areas with central atrophy of the papillae; otherwise this disease has lesions which are less reticulated and more striated and also definitely rather erosive;

telangiectases of the vermilion part of the lips are interspersed. Altogether the lesions are more variegated than those seen in lichen planus and leukoplakia. Chronic lupus erythematosus is hardly ever seen in the middle of the buccal mucosa; the latter area is the keratotic domain of lichen planus.

7. Some dermatoses with primary blister formation, for instance, **chronic pemphigus vulgaris** or the **pemphigus of the conjunctivae** (see also Chapter 25, A6) may also show leukoplakialike lesions on the gingival mucosa or on the borderline epithelium of the lips.

(1) HERRMANN, D.: Zur Diagnose und Differentialdiagnose des Lichen ruber planus der Mundschleimhaut. Dtsch. zahnärztl. Z. 25: 977–985 (1970).
(2) KOBERG, W., D. SCHETTLER und G. SELLE: Zur Frage der Karzinomentstehung auf dem Boden eines Lichen ruber planus der Mundschleimhaut. Münch. med. Wschr. 107: 463–466 (1965).

35. Aphthae

Aphthae are round to oval, sharply limited, flat erosions of the mucous membranes. They usually do not become larger than the size of lentils. They are often covered with a gray-white to yellowish coating and have a dusky red hyperemic

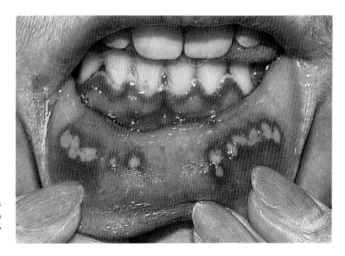

Fig. 599. Gingivostomatitis herpetica: multiple aphthae on the mucosa of the lower lip and marginal gingivitis.

margin. The extremely evanescent vesicular preceding stage is almost never visible. Aphthae may be solitary or multiple.

A. Aphthae in Infectious Diseases

1. Stomatitis aphthosa or gingivostomatitis herpetica is a primary herpes simplex manifestation, which can be observed especially in children and debilitated adults. Accompanied by pronounced general signs such as lassitude, vomiting, and fever, multiple aphthae develop in the oral cavity within a short time. Usually large parts of the oral mucosa including the tongue (Figs. 599, 600) are affected. Simultaneously, easily bleeding gingivitis, increased salivation, a considerable lymphadenopathy, and foul-smelling fetor ex ore are present. In contrast to common herpes simplex, recurrent attacks are extremely rare. Stomatitis aphthosa is to be expected, however, in anergic states – classically, after measles and whooping cough, and also in lymphadenoses, lymphogranulomatosis, or during treatment with immunosuppressive drugs. Gingivostomatitis herpetica may extend, especially under this treatment, to large areas around the mouth and including the nose and cheeks as in **aphthoid Pospischill-Feyrter** (Figs. 601, 602). The diagnosis of gingivostomatitis herpetica is confirmed by an increase of herpes simplex antibodies in the blood.

On the tongue the lesions may look like eruptive chickenpox, but the patients have additional lesions on the trunk and scalp. [12, 13]

Analogous herpes simplex infections may also affect the genital mucosa. This may lead to the picture of **vulvovaginitis herpetica.** Here again the diagnosis is confirmed by an increase in the antibody titer.

2. In the differential diagnosis, **stomatitis epidemica** (foot-and-mouth disease) must be considered, although it is rare in human beings. This viral infection is transmitted to humans chiefly by contact with diseased animals. The sources of infection are mostly ruminants, with the exception of solipeds; dogs and cats transmit the disease only rarely. Occasionally, unpasteurized milk and milk products can transmit the infection. The incubation period is between three and eight days. Prodromal signs are fever, back pain, headache, and dryness and burning of the oral cavity. Still in the fever stage, evanescent, very tender blisters, which rapidly change into aphthoid lesions, appear on the buccal mucosa, tongue, and lips. In some patients blisters as large as lentils and later pustules also occur on the palms and soles, fingers (paronychia), toes and on the breasts. Blisters near the mouth may become confluent and form ulcerations. Changes similar to those on the oral mucosa may also become manifest on the genital mucosa. On the fifth day, at the latest, the fever drops. Blisters and aphthae completely heal in about 8 to 14 days. The whole course may be so mild that the infection is not recognized. In the differential diagnosis, besides stomatitis aphthosa, hand-foot-and-mouth disease and other coxsackievirus or echovirus infections should be ruled out first. This is usually possible only by serologic tests. The virus of foot-and-mouth disease (there are various strains that do not leave cross-immunization) can be proved by intraperitoneal inoculation of the contents or covering of the blisters into baby mice. The complement fixation test also permits demonstration of antibodies, but it must not be forgotten that the titer drops rapidly after healing. [6, 7]

3. Hand-foot-and-mouth disease is an infection with coxsackieviruses of groups A5, A10, and A16. Children are affected predominantly. After an incubation period

Fig. 600. Aphthous glossitis.

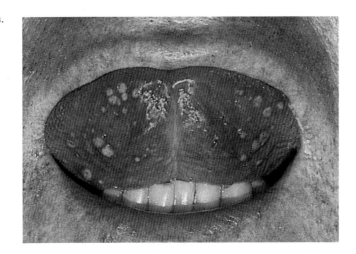

Fig. 601. Aphthoid Pos-
pischill-Feyrter: extensive
hemorrhagic crusts around
the oral and nasal openings.

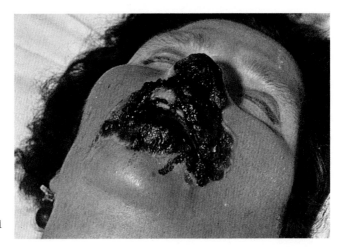

Fig. 602. Aphthoid Pospi-
schill-Feyrter: circinate, pustular borderline.

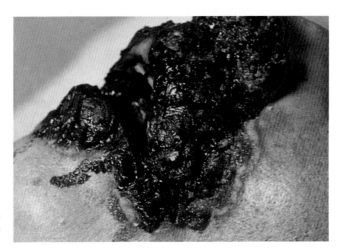

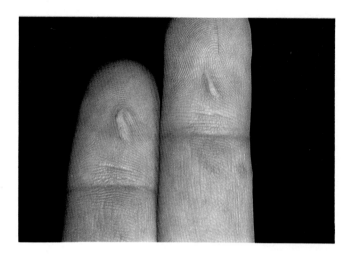

Fig. 603.   Hand-foot-and-mouth disease: typical longitudinal pustules.

of about one week and unspecific preliminary signs lasting about two weeks, small erythematous lesions may appear on the palms and soles. They are followed by first vesicular and then pustular changes with distinctly angular borders (Fig. 603). On the oral mucosa the eruption is definitely aphthoid. Demonstration of the virus can be accomplished from fresh stool specimens or from the contents of the blisters (see also Chapter 1, E 5).[2, 8, 14]

4. Another coxsackievirus infection (groups A 2, A 4, A 6, A 8, A 10, and B 4) with aphthouslike oral lesions is **herpangina.** The incubation period is between two and five days. After this is over, blisters of about pinhead size appear on the soft palate and on both palatinal arches. Concurrent signs and symptoms include an acute rise in temperature, headaches, vomiting, and occasionally meningism. The lesions rapidly change into flat, dirty erosions which are surrounded by a distinctly hyperemic area. An attempt to isolate the coxsackieviruses, preferably by inoculation of baby mice, can be made by using a specimen from the fresh blisters, or from water used for gargling, or from stool.[15]

5. The changes of the oral mucosa in an **echovirus infection** cannot be distinguished clinically from herpangina. This is usually an infection with types 3, 6, or 30 and mainly affects children or adolescents. After the usual prodromal signs of fever, nausea, and headaches, aseptic meningitis or gastrointestinal disturbances appear, but exanthems and enanthems are not among the regular findings. The exanthems may be very diversified and are not diagnostic of this disorder. In addition to rubeoliform, morbilliform, or scarlatiniform eruptions, urticarial, vesicular, and petechial changes may occur. Confirmation of the diagnosis can be obtained by isolation of the virus from gargling water and stools and from the presence of an increase in the antibody titer.[9, 10]

6. Behçet's syndrome, the uveoaphthous syndrome in the sense of a "la grande aphthose," is not a definitely infectious disease and it affects various organ systems (see also Chapter 7, A 3). The course of the disease is characterized by chronic attacks of highly painful, single or multiple, and frequently long-persistent aphthous lesions on the mucous membranes (Fig. 604). Sharply circumscribed ulcerations appear on the genitals; these have already been mentioned in Chapter 33, C 11. Besides these aphthous and ulcerated manifestations, other cutaneous

Fig. 604. Behçet's syndrome: oral aphthae.

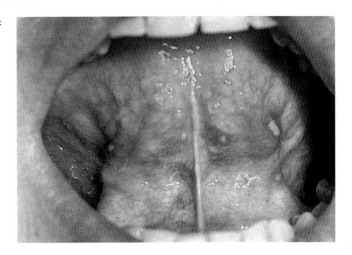

signs in such patients consist of papulo-pustular or erythema nodosum-like changes, which, together with the not too rare thrombophlebitides or deep phlebothromboses, strengthen the concept of a "vasculitis." This impression is aided by other panarteritis nodosa-like appearances, for example, those resembling apoplexia cutanea as well as many other visceral manifestations (pleurisy, spleno-megaly, polymorphonodopathy, subacute polyarticular arthritis, myocarditis, and others). Neurologic involvement may produce signs that correspond to meningo-encephalitis or encephalomyelitis ("neuro-Behçet"). In addition to the cutaneous and mucosal signs, recurrent hypopyon-iritis (Fig. 605) may occur. Ocular involvement develops in 80 per cent of young patients between 15 and 35 years of age, usually relatively late, i.e., after the onset of urogenital changes. There are, however, some cases which start as spontaneous ophthalmia. Other ocular manifestations are ulcerations of the sclera, hemorrhage into the vitreous, or tapetoretinal degenerations. The patient with Behçet's syndrome usually shows diminution of fungiform papillae on the tip of the tongue. Occasionally, these may be completely absent. If one watches for these signs, it may be possible to diagnose

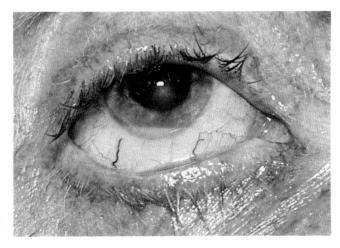

Fig. 605. Behçet's syndrome: hypopyoniritis.

Behçet's syndrome even in the early mono- or oligosymptomatic stages. For nonspecific skin hyper-reactivity, see Chapter 33, C11.

The histologic picture in Behçet's syndrome unquestionably shows the importance of the vascular component with consecutive necrosis in the cutis. Other cutaneous signs such as erythema nodosum-like lesions or an accompanying panniculitis do not show the characteristic histologic features, which would by themselves reveal the correct diagnosis. The differential diagnosis may be difficult if signs such as aphthae, genital ulcerations, erythema nodosum, and hypopyoniritis occur as isolated phenomena. In such cases the nonspecific cutaneous hypersensitivity and the rarefaction of the fungiform lingual papillae may be helpful. The diagnosis, however, will be confirmed first when several signs occur.[1, 3-5, 11]

(1) BECKER, J.: Die Behçetsche Krankheit. Dtsch. med. Wschr. 87: 1903–1906 (1962).

(2) BORN, W.: Das Hand-Fuß-Mund-(Coxsackie A-)Exanthem, eine neue Kinderkrankheit. Klin. Wschr. 45: 953–954 (1967).

(3) CABRÉ, J., und G. BREHM: Histologische und immunbiologische Untersuchungen zum Behçet-Syndrom. Derm. Wschr. 150: 566–576 (1964).

(4) DAVIS, E., and E. MELZER: A new sign in Behçet's syndrome. Scanty fungiform papillae in tongue. Arch. intern. Med. 124: 720–721 (1969).

(5) DENK, R.: Elektrokardiographische Untersuchungen bei Hautkranken. Arch. Kreisl.-Forsch. 60: 33–114 (1969).

(6) EISSNER, G., H. O. BÖHM und E. JÜLICH: Eine Maul- und Klauenseuche-Infektion beim Menschen. Dtsch. med. Wschr. 92: 830–832 (1967).

(7) HEINIG, A., und H. NEUMERKEL: Beitrag zur Maul- und Klauenseuche beim Menschen. Dtsch. Gesundh.-Wes. 19: 485–490 (1964).

(8) HJORTH, N., und H. KOPP: Hand-Foot-Mouth-Disease. Hautarzt 17: 533–537 (1966).

(9) HORNSTEIN, O. P., und V. SEIDL: Zur Klinik und Histologie des ECHO-6-Virusexanthems. Hautarzt 24: 6–11 (1973).

(10) KEUTH, U., I. ESSER, J. WILHELMI und I. WILHELMI: Die »Herpangina«-Epidemie 1967/68 (ECHO 30/6/3). Dtsch. med. Wschr. 94: 1959–1965 (1969).

(11) MONACELLI, M., and P. NAZZARO: Behçet's disease. Karger, Basel, New York 1966.

(12) NASEMANN, TH.: Die Infektionen durch das Herpes simplex-Virus. Fischer, Jena 1965.

(13) NASEMANN, TH.: Virusinfektionen der Mundschleimhaut und aphthöse Erkrankungen mit noch unbekannter Ätiologie. Münch. med. Wschr. 110: 2559–2566 (1968).

(14) OEHLSCHLAEGEL, G., H. MEIER-EWERT und H.-J. VOGT: Diagnose und virologischer Erregernachweis des Hand-Fuß-Mund-Exanthems. Arch. Derm. Forsch. 240: 271–277 (1971).

(15) WINDORFER, A.: Die Coxsackievirusinfektion im Kindesalter. Med. Klin. 58: 1–5 (1963).

B. Aphthae of Noninfectious Origin

1. Habitual or **chronically recurrent aphthae,** which have a distinct familial involvement, are usually observed in gastrolabile, "neuropathic" individuals. In many patients there is also a connection with certain foods (e.g., vanilla or walnuts). In any case, no association with an infectious agent is present. Chronic recurrent aphthae occur in attacks and are limited to a few lesions. They favor adults – children are affected only exceptionally. General signs are always absent and other cutaneous manifestations do not occur. Within a few hours, extremely painful, sharply demarcated, oval erosions (Figs. 606, 607) develop from small transparent vesicles, particularly on the sides of the tongue and the angles

Fig. 606. Chronic recurrent aphthae: blistering stage.

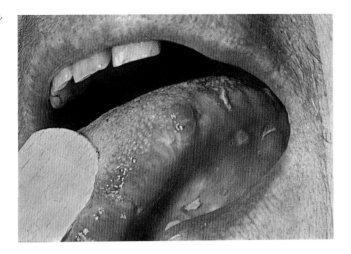

Fig. 607. Chronic recurrent aphthae.

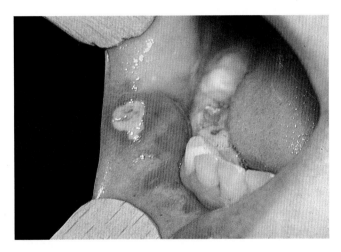

Fig. 608. Periadenitis mucosae necrotica recurrens (Sutton's ulcer).

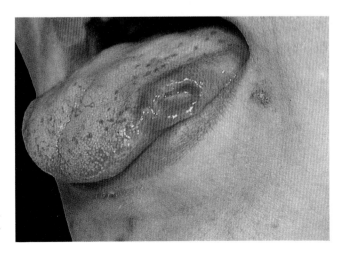

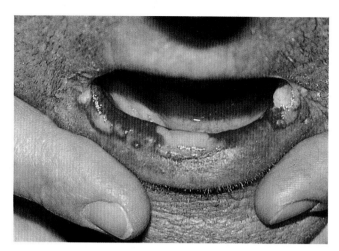

Fig. 609. Labial erosions in methotrexate treatment.

of the mouth. The erosions are typically surrounded by a highly inflammatory, red margin. In contrast to stomatitis aphthosa only a few aphthae appear, and almost never affect the gingiva. Furthermore, recurrent lesions are exceptional in stomatitis aphthosa. In questionable cases evidence of the herpes virus or an increased antibody titer is decisive. Occasionally, early Behçet's syndrome (see also Section A6) must be ruled out.[2, 5]

Patients with chronic recurrent aphthae may have one or, infrequently, a few deep mucosal ulcerations with craterlike margins in an interval free of aphthae, or during an eruption of aphthae (Fig. 608). Such *periadenitis mucosae necrotica recurrens* develops from a submucosal nodule, which ulcerates superficially. After the elimination of a central necrotic plug of tissue, an ulceration as large as a bean with a hard elevated border remains for several weeks. Sensitivity to pain varies greatly, and some patients do not request medical treatment. Regional lymph nodes, however, are very often enlarged and tender to pressure. In the differential diagnosis a malignant tumor will almost always have to be excluded by a biopsy. Stomatitis ulceromembranacea, on the other hand, is frequently accompanied by general signs and is almost always very

painful. In contrast to periadenitis mucosae necrotica recurrens, it responds well and promptly to treatment with antibiotics and possesses a typical bacterial flora.[1, 3, 4]

2. So-called **Bednar's aphthae** are not aphthae but are usually mechanically caused erosions (as for example by cleansing the oral cavity of a child by the mother) with subsequent bacterial superinfection. In older people, however, "solitary aphthae" should not be too long observed "clinically" but should be quickly examined histologically to rule out squamous cell *carcinoma*. Aphthous ulcerations of the tonsillar region or at the angles of the mouth require a hematologic examination to eliminate *agranulocytosis* or ulcerous, acute myeloblastic or monocytic leukemias.

3. Stomatitis caused by **drugs** may also be characterized by sharply ragged aphthous ulcerations with hyperemic borders and a tendency to occur in folds. This is at present well illustrated by methotrexate (Fig. 609) and fluorouracil, whereas stomatitides caused by gold or actinomycin C therapy produce large areas of ulcers from the beginning and hardly ever assume an aphthous appearance.

4. Flat, sharply limited mucosal erosions occur also in the course of **lichen planus** (pemphigoides). They are postbullous lesions which lack the typical aspect and hyperemic surroundings of genuine apthae. Further details can be found in Chapter 25, B3 and Chapter 34, B.5. The diagnosis is corroborated by other cutaneous and mucosal changes characteristic of lichen planus. If those are missing, which is possible in rare instances, the diagnosis can be secured by biopsy.[6,7]

5. With regard to **oral submucosal fibrosis**, see Chapter 34, A12. Here it should only be mentioned that in the beginning after rupture of the vesicles, which are about rice-corn size, flat and very tender ulcerations which resemble aphthae develop.

(1) CERNÉA, P., B. DUPERRAT, C. CRÉPI, R. KUFFER, J.-M. MASCARA et M. BAUMONT: La périadénite de Sutton (Periadenitis mucosa necrotica recurrens). Rev. Stomat. (Paris) *67:* 271–286 (1966).

(2) HERRMANN, D.: Zur Morphogenese der chronisch-rezidivierenden Aphthen. Dtsch. zahnärztl. Z. *25:* 993–999 (1970).

(3) HURT, W. C.: Periadenitis mucosa necrotica recurrens. Oral Surg. *13:* 750–755 (1960).

(4) MATHIS, H., und D. HERRMANN: Zur Periadenitis mucosae necrotica recurrens (Sutton). Dtsch. zahnärztl. Z. *25:* 1154–1163 (1970).

(5) NASEMANN, TH.: Virusinfektion der Mundschleimhaut und aphthöse Erkrankungen mit noch unbekannter Ätiologie. Münch. med. Wschr. *110:* 2559–2566 (1968).

(6) SHKLAR, G.: Lichen planus as an oral ulcerative disease. Oral Surg. *33:*376–388 (1972).

(7) UNDEUTSCH, W., H. FISCHER und R. MÜLLER: Rezidivierender pemphigoider und erosiver Lichen ruber planus der Mundschleimhaut mit sklerosierender Makroglossie. Derm. Mschr. *156:* 212–218 (1970).

36. Hemorrhagic Phenomena

Nosologically, *hemorrhagic diatheses* are divided into isolated or combined blood dyscrasias due to disturbances of the *humoral clotting mechanism, blood platelets, and vessels.* In the clinical differential diagnosis visible phenomena act as guideposts. Large, irregular hemorrhages, i.e., *suffusions and suggillations* extending into the outer integument as well as into the inner organs, support a diagnosis of clotting disturbances or coagulopathies. In contrast, punctiform bleedings *(petechiae)* suggest *thrombocytopathia* or *vascular hemorrhagic-diathesis. Thrombocytopathias,* however, may present large areas of bleeding and *hemorrhages from the mucous membranes* in addition to petechial exanthems. The manifestations of such hemorrhages, even after blunt injuries, are as characteristic of thrombocytopathia as bleedings *at the site of trauma* (tooth extraction, puncture from a lancet) are of *coagulopathies.* In spite of these clinical guidelines, special laboratory tests are always reguired to diagnose coagulopathies and thrombocytopathies.[59]

Extensive, massive *hematomalike hemorrhages* occurring at isolated and unusual sites should suggest trauma. An example is the so-called *"penis fracture"* (Fig. 610) or "penis rupture," which generally occurs as a traumatic tear in the corpus cavernosum.[60] However, hemorrhage on the palms or backs of the hands and on the heels, already mentioned as pseudochromohidrosis,[12] may suggest *"hemihidrosis"* in neurotic stigmatized persons.[27,55] In distinctly malnourished children one must consider the possibility that hemorrhages into the skin may be a

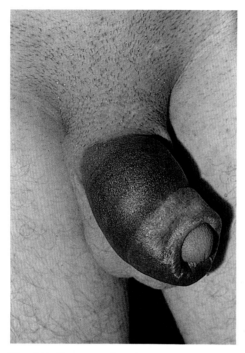

Fig. 610. Fracture of penis.

manifestation of the "battered child" syndrome (Fig. 611).

Another cause of circumscribed and initially puzzling lesions showing bleeding is ectopia or heterotopia of the uterine mucous membrane, i.e., *endometriosis*,

with rice-corn or coin-sized lesions. Their surface is either completely smooth or slightly nodose. They are dark brown-red or dark blue and occur primarily on the umbilicus, the external genitals, or in scarred tissue. Discomfort or pain in these lesions in connection with the menstrual cycle is characteristic.[47, 56] Histologically, the glandular structures and elements of stroma correspond to endometrial tissue. In the differential diagnosis of the rather rare lesions on the extremities, nodose, deeply subcutaneous lesions such as neurofibromas, lymphangiomas, or gummas have to be considered. Solitary umbilical or genital endometriosis with its blue-black color may suggest a melanoma or an ulcerated hemangioma, or, if it has a harder consistency, a sarcoma or epithelioma or, above all, a metastasizing per contiguitatem ascending visceral carcinoma.[28] Other possibilities in the umbilical area are cystic formations originating from the yolk sac or urachus.[43]

On the other hand, more or less extensive macular suffusions, which are not only superficial but also subcutaneously localized and are always found at the same location, are typical of *hemophilia*. It occurs almost exclusively in men, and is characterized by bleeding that apparently stops for a certain time but

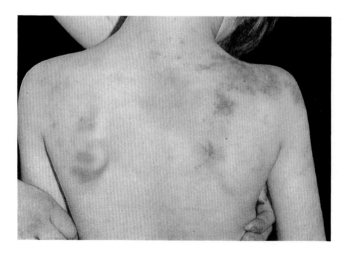

Fig. 611. Hematoma after maltreatment—so-called "battered child" syndrome.

subsequently persists (after consumption of the locally released tissue thrombokinase). In addition to the already mentioned skeletal hemorrhages, extremely painful "pressing" *hemarthroses*, which may sometimes increase the size of the joints in a monstrous way or even perforate them, is also characteristic of hemophilia. The recurrent hemorrhages into the joints may result in an irreversible arthronosis ("arthritis-arthrosis hemophilica"). Furthermore, large visceral blood hematomas, if located in the psoas muscle, may be confused with surgical disorders of the abdominal cavity, since they frequently are accompanied by pronounced generalized signs (increases in temperature, ESR, leukocytes, and alpha$_2$-globulins). In female carriers uterine hemorrhage during pregnancy may be harmful. Aside from pregnancy, prolonged and increased uterine bleedings may occur in carriers of hemophilia B. In principle, the main coagulopathies distinguishable in clotting physiology (deficiency of Factor VIII: hemophilia A; deficiency of Factor IX: hemophilia B, "Christmas disease"; deficiency of Factor X: hemophilia C) cause the same clinical signs.[39]

In addition, in the differential diagnosis dominantly inherited *parahemophilia** due to deficiency of Factor V as well as *inhibitory body hemophilia* must be considered. In the latter – in hemophiliacs – there is apparently a circulating inhibitory body against the missing clotting factor that continues to lower or neutralize the clotting factor given therapeutically. Besides this so-called inhibitory body hemophilia, it has been observed in dermatitis herpetiformis and bullous pemphigoid, among others,[15] that inhibitory bodies of the second clotting phase may become manifest in connection with

---

* In the United States this condition is considered to be recessively inherited. (Tr.)

Schönlein's purpura or even *fulminant purpura*. In *purpura fulminans*, which is especially fulminant in children after infection with scarlet faver, there is present, almost symmetrically and usually beginning on the lower extremities, a deficiency of Factor V with an excess of antithrombin; this manifests itself, sometimes in combination with hematuria and melena, in cufflike cutaneous bleedings with central blister formation and demarcation.[13] In contrast to *thrombotic-thrombocytopenic purpura*,[42] the lack of hemolysis or considerable neurologic signs is important,[34] whereas in *acute toxic epidermolysis*, Lyell's syndrome, vesicle formation does not occur in areas of blood absorption by the skin, in contrast to fulminant purpura. Acute, extensive bleeding skin is characteristic of the *Waterhouse-Friderichsen syndrome*. Such bleeding occurs mostly after meningococcic or pneumococcic infections or more rarely after staphylococcic sepsis, and is caused by synchronous or metachronous hemorrhages into the cortex of the adrenal gland. Such peracute and vitally significant hemorrhagic suffusions lead to the question of pathogenesis and whether the *Sanarelli-Shwartzman phenomenon* is also possible in humans. As in animal experiments, the effects of pregnancy in humans may be influential as preparatory factors. In any case, in a Sanarelli-Shwartzman phenomenon in man, again as in animal models, only hemorrhages and necroses based on a neutrophil inflammation should be present. In contrast, in the Waterhouse-Friderichsen syndrome, morbilliform, urticarial, papular, or nodose elements occur, although they are only transient. In the septicemic stages on the trunk and extremities, hemorrhagic phenomena predominate; on the extremities there may also be gangrenous changes.

In contrast to the Waterhouse-Friderichsen syndrome, *meningococcic sepsis*, even in serious cases (Fig. 612), lacks the

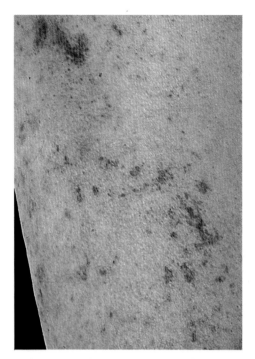

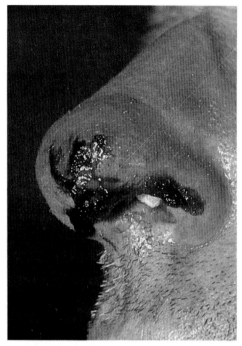

Fig. 612. Bleeding into the skin in meningococcic sepsis.

Fig. 613. Mucosal bleeding caused by overdose of anticoagulants.

phenomena of acute, disseminated intravascular clotting with subsequent consumption coagulopathy; in general, we
are dealing here only with a more or less
discrete petechial exanthem.[35]

Extensive macular skin bleeding, however, is most frequently observed during
therapy with coagulants (the coumarin and
indandione group). Such therapy does
not produce bleeding from membranes,
but between the third and fifth days, i.e.,
still before diminution of the Quick values
(prothrombin time), blue-red areas appear
on the breasts, loins, and thighs. These
areas change into hemorrhagic black
blisters and re-epithelialize only after
several weeks (Fig. 613). For the diagnostic differentiation of a possible overdose
of these coagulants it is important to note
that at the onset of such coumarin
necroses the prothrombin time and the
number of thrombocytes are usually

normal. If, however, the coumarin necroses are located very distally, for
example, on the toes, differentiation from
an acute closure, phlebothrombosis, or
endangiitis obliterans may be difficult at
first.[25]

Extensive confluent areas of cutaneous
bleeding may be caused by a so-called
consumption coagulopathy – that is, the
intravascular utilization in excessive
blood clotting of coagulation Factors II,
V, and VIII and thrombocytes. Changes
of the lungs and kidneys due to the
absence of fibrin are associated. Such
consumption coagulopathies are found in
leukemia and snake bites and in the
Kasabach-Merritt syndrome discussed
earlier with the angiomas, but above all
as a defibrination syndrome with reactive
fibrinolysis in carcinomas, for example of
the prostate, or after abortion involving
premature separation of the placenta.[46]

Vascular hemophilia (also known as angio-hemophilia or constitutional thrombo-pathy) is an autosomal dominant hemorrhagic diathesis. It has a moderately severe tendency toward bleeding from the nose and gums (as after dental surgery) and toward suffusions. To a lesser extent there is a tendency toward hemarthrosis and also to hypermenorrhea and poly-menorrhea.

Hemorrhagic manifestations during the spring and fall are characteristic; vascular hemophilia favors one sex and diminishes in expressivity in later life. This pseudo-hemophilia shows a lack of Factor VIII or IX and a prolonged bleeding time, in contrast to hemophilia which has a normal bleeding time and prolonged blood coagulation. The vascular component of this angiohemophilia is also shown by the additional presence of ecchymoses.

In addition to the petechiae and ecchymoses of the angiohemophilias, *idiopathic thrombocytopenic purpura* (Werlhof's disease) shows suffusions and above all bleedings from the mucous membranes. Temporarily these bleedings may occasionally be the only manifestation of the disease (as with, for instance, exceedingly profuse and long-lasting menses) or (in contrast to Henoch's purpura) there may be painless gastrointestinal bleedings

(Fig. 614). This thrombocytopenic purpura may be idiopathic or it may occur as a manifestation of another disease; two-thirds of the cases occur before the twentieth year of life, and this hemorrhagic diathesis distinctly favors the female sex. The clinical impression should be supported by establishing a prolonged bleeding time, thrombocytopenia (without definite anemia or leukocytopenia), shortening of the life span of thrombocytes, an increase of immature megakaryocytes in the bone marrow, and eventually an immunogenic basis. In addition to a positive direct Coombs' test, a prolonged recalcification time, pathologic clot retraction, and a positive Rumpel-Leede test will further support the diagnosis. Although in childhood acute thrombocytopenic purpura generally follows infectious diseases (for instance, influenza), in adults drugs play the most important role.

A few hours after medication all the signs of Werlhof's purpura develop in full severity; however, after a preceding exanthematic disease it may take three to seven days before the signs appear.[16] *Thrombocytopenias* and all their manifestations may also appear in some dermatologic diseases, for instance, in connection with *Kasabach-Merritt's giant hemangioma* of the skin,[19] as a manifestation of the

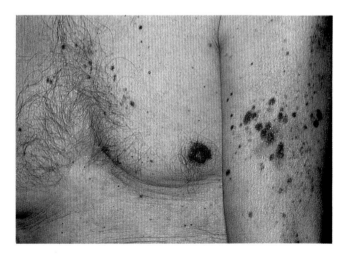

Fig. 614. Werlhof's disease.

Wiskott-Aldrich syndrome with seborrheic and later more lichenified cutaneous changes and a deficiency of IgM,[61] and finally as an apoplectic or pseudomeningitic manifestation that masks the start of systemic lupus erythematosus. Petechial or superficial hemorrhagic areas in the course of Werlhof's disease that are mixed with different pre-existing cutaneous diseases, as in areas of chronic lupus erythematosus, are observed much more rarely. With regard to the cutaneous hemorrhagic signs of thrombocytopenic purpura, the principal triple signs should be emphasized again (punctiform, superficial, and mucosal bleeding areas); it should be added that petechiae predominate on the trunk and proximal extremities, whereas suggillations favor the face and the volar aspects of the hands and feet, if they are involved at all. The petechiae of Werlhof's disease are round, dusky bluish-red efflorescences of pinhead to lentil size which cannot be made to blanch completely by diascopy. The lesions of this disease are primary petechiae and therefore, they do not show the focal bleeding points within elevated erythematous lesions either in retrogression or under diascopy as in Schönlein's purpura. Another contrast with the progressive pigmented purpuras is the fact that the dusky bluish-red petechiae of Werlhof's disease change to a yellowish-green color according to their character as microhematomas, whereas the *pigmented purpuras*[22] have a characteristic rusty brown color owing to the deposition of hemosiderin. The lesions of thrombocytopenic purpura have a certain dependency on the blood vessels in spite of the essential nature of this disease as a platelet deficiency. This relationship is evident by changes in blood pressure,[21] an intrathoracic increase of pressure at defecation, the Rumpel-Leede test (among others) and finally by a certain orthostatic predilection. In contrast to hemophilia, Werlhof's disease lacks petechial exanthems and only rarely shows intra-articular bleeding. Scurvy is characterized by subcutaneous bleeding (in children this may also be subperiosteal), gingival bleeding, and a positive Rumpel-Leede test, and in addition there is the typical chessboardlike arrangement of punctiform hemorrhages, which always develop on the base of a prescorbutic follicular keratosis. All these factors permit an immediate clinical differentiation from Werlhof's disease, so that it is not necessary either to perform thrombocytic studies or to determine coagulation factors. Ecchymoses, sometimes combined with disturbances of coagulation, are also seen with *liver diseases* of different origins or with pancreaticohepatic syndromes. Moreover, massive hemorrhages emanating from all body orifices should arouse suspicion first of *paramyeloblastic leukemia* or *panmyelophthisis* rather than of thrombocytopenia. Hemorrhagic myelophthises are known to occur in several diseases caused by malignant growths (such as carcinomatoses) or as an effect of radiation. *Symptomatic thrombocytopenias* have been seen with *megaloblastic anemias, thrombocythemias* ("thrombocythemia hemorrhagica"),[5] and occasionally also with some *endocrine disorders*, for instance, Graves' disease and Cushing's disease. However, if in contrast to the usual signs of Werlhof's disease, coagulopathy or thrombocytopenia are absent and if only mild trauma, such as pinching, results in formation of hematomas, subcutaneous bleeding, or hemoptysis, one must consider the *Goodpasture syndrome*.[4] Additional signs of this syndrome are hypochromic anemia, the presence of erythrocytes and albumen in the urine, and signs of glomerulonephritis combined with a highly febrile hemorrhagic pneumonia. All these signs occur in young males. In contrast to the Goodpasture syndrome, classic periarteritis nodosa shows pulmonary infiltration only in a few cases. Additional diagnostic help can be obtained from biopsies taken from the nasal mucous membrane and, more importantly, from the kidneys. [4, 40, 63]

Essential pulmonary hemosiderosis (also known as the Ceelen-Gellerstedt syndrome), which has an increased incidence in families and begins even in early infancy, lacks cutaneous and renal changes. However, if renal signs (microhematuria), melena or hematemesis, and mucocutaneous changes take place (as also occurs in thrombocytopenic purpura), one should examine for the presence of not only hemolytic anemia and transitory cerebral disorders but also *thrombotic-thrombocytopenic purpura*. This exceedingly rare disease, which is accompanied by high fever and swelling of the liver and spleen, is supposed to be a collagenosis. Lupus erythematosus among other diseases may show immunocytothrombocytopenic and immunohemolytic anemias (the so-called Evans syndrome).

Thrombasthenia, caused by a congenital autosomal recessive lack of glyceraldehyde dehydrogenase, begins in early infancy with changes resembling those in Werlhof's disease; the number of blood platelets is normal but agglutination is disturbed and clot retraction is absent.

Hereditary familial purpura simplex occurs in families as a simple benign type of purpura; apparently it is only the expression of an isolated weakness of the vascular walls (decreased capillary resistance, prolonged bleeding time, positive Rumpel-Leede test). This hereditary purpura affects women in the premenstruum; however, in the periclimacterium the tendency toward hemorrhaging will recede. Ptosis of the eyelids has been observed as an associated sign. The frequently autosomal dominant congenital *Ehlers-Danlos syndrome* (cutis hyperelastica) may also show vascular purpura as an important additional phenomenon. Bursting of a blood vessel (rhexis hemorrhage) can be explained as a genetic impairment of the orderly structure of the

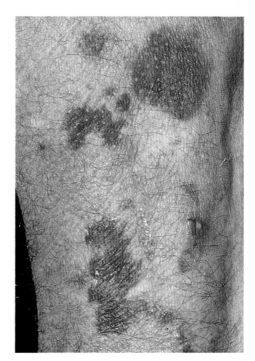

Fig. 615. Senile purpura.

collagen and a weakness of the interlacing of less functionally adequate connective tissue bundles.

In addition to such ecchymoses or petechiae, one observes "hematomas" in the Ehlers-Danlos syndrome, although artificially produced cutaneous wounds bleed very little. Such hematomas in these patients may suggest hemophilia and lead to the appropriate examinations; eventually these hematomas develop into pseudotumors through organization and calcification. Hemorrhages of the gums after brushing the teeth or prolonged postpartum hemorrhages have also been observed.

Senile purpura (Fig. 615) shows a rather characteristic appearance and is today frequently seen in younger people as a phenocopy after cortisone medication; this type of purpura is probably a vascular phenomenon similar to the hemorrhages in Ehlers-Danlos syndrome. Senile purpura and *solar purpura*[7] belong

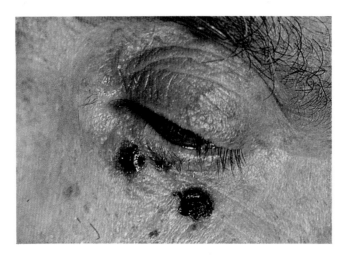

Fig. 616. Hemorrhagic necrosis in Weil's disease.

to closely allied groups; both show cutaneous colloid degeneration and bizarre areas of suggillation with ragged borders on the upper extremities but hardly ever on the face and the lower extremities. Their significance as a sign of old age is

Fig. 617. Microemboli on the fingertips in endocarditis lenta.

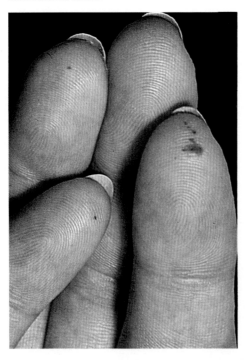

emphasized by the mostly simultaneous presence of senile elastosis, for instance, spontaneous stellate pseudoscars.[11] The solitary lesions of senile purpura cannot be provoked by intense pinching or hitting with a percussion hammer, still less by intradermal injection of bacterial filtrates; however, intradermal injection of heparin causes bleeding.[29] Our own examinations point to a hepatogenic partial factor for the pathogenesis of senile purpura, and therefore this type of purpura in older persons may be a clue to liver damage.[32] Facial lesions resembling senile purpura – that is, larger ecchymoses with ragged borders – will be seen more frequently in dysproteinemic purpura,[18] e.g., cryomacroglobulinemic purpura, and also in infectious diseases, e.g., Oroya fever of the leptospiroses, especially Weil's disease (Fig. 616). On about the fourth or fifth day of the disease such hemorrhages appear in combination with pain in the calves, febrile albuminuria, and jaundice; however, more often there will be urticarial, morbilliform, or similar exanthems. Other infectious diseases such as exanthematic typhus or recurrent fever produce exanthems that are more petechial than ecchymotic. However, ecchymoses or the smaller petechiae, if located mostly on the fingertips or subungually with round blueberry-black hemorrhages, signify the presence of smaller emboli, for instance, subacute bacterial endocarditis (Janeway's spots) (Fig. 617). The differential diagnosis should consider subungual lesions such as a painful glomus tumor; if painless, a subungual melanoma; and if multiple, Osler's nodules also. *Splinter hemorrhages* of the *nailplate*, i.e., dark violet extravasations of 1 to 3 mm in length, are seen with acute trichinosis or with drugs acting as peripheral vasodilators (griseofulvin); however, these splinter hemorrhages do not signify a definite skin disease.[49]

Paroxysmal finger hematoma is a transient, spastic disturbance of the blood supply, probably resulting from a local vascular change. An ecchymosis develops after acute stinging pain.[26] However, if grouped, papular telangiectatic changes without such pain phenomena occur on

the *palms*, isolated capillaritis[41] or *thrombophlebitis* of this region has to be considered. Blue-blackish dots on the heel ("talon noir"), especially in young girls, resemble tattoos or even melanomatous satellites but represent so-called *plantar pseudohidrosis*, which is at least partly a calcaneal petechia or intracorneal hematoma.[6, 12] The spotted eruptive telangiectases at the very onset of progressive scleroderma, which occur on the distal parts of the fingers among other sites, remain light red for the duration. In other dermatoses, for instance, *Darier's disease*, hemorrhagic lesions on the forearms and calves are usually caused secondarily by trauma.[24]

In the pronounced exudative-inflammatory vascular damage of the *leukocytoclastic-hemorrhagic microbid* type, clinically polymorphous (that is, only facultatively or consecutively purpuric)

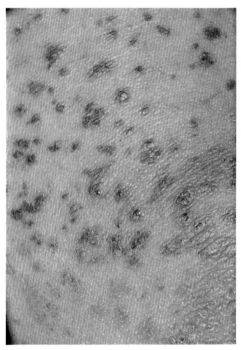

Fig. 618. Schönlein's purpura: elevated erythemas with focal petechiae.

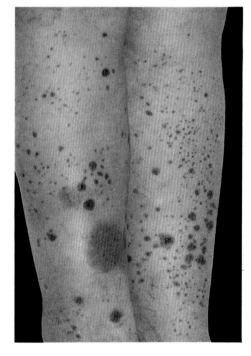

Fig. 619. Schönlein's purpura: older exanthem with vesiculation and necrosis.

phenomena occur; these usually have a purely serous and not hemorrhagic course here and also extracutaneously in other organs such as the muscles and even more in the joints (foot and knee joints). Usually in direct association with infectious-hyperergic causes (sore throat, sinusitis, bronchiectases) or drug-allergic influences, attacks of recurrent lesions favoring the extensor surfaces of the extremities, the flanks, and the gluteal region occur. They may become confluent – especially on the trunk – and form an eruption which in combination with weak filtration pressure resembles cutis marmorata. The individual lesion is sometimes a light red, at other times a more bluish-red erythema, which is distinctly exudative and consequently quite often urticarial and elevated. In the subsequent course it may show a central vesicular change or may be surrounded by a vasoconstrictive halo. Only in the region of such formations – and hardly ever in fresh lesions – will punctiform hemorrhaging occur. These bleeding spots are focal and are not petechiae in themselves; they are often recognized only after they blanch out under diascopy (Figs. 618, 619). In contrast to the long visible and rust-brown deposits of hemosiderin in progressive pigmented purpura, in Schönlein's purpura there are only a few transient, pale-yellow spots of hemosiderin, which because of their annular configuration may be mistaken for "false" purpura Majocchi. Moreover, the polymorphism of Schönlein's syndrome makes it obvious that in the prepurpuric stage, especially if the extensor surfaces of the upper extremities are favored – generally, Schönlein's purpura as *purpura orthostatica* favors the lower half of the body – erythema multiforme should be considered. But even after the occurrence of focal point bleedings in Schönlein's syndrome the cockadelike character is preserved, or it may happen that ecchymoses may group in cockade form on the forearms

and on the face ("early infantile, post-infectious cockade purpura").[37] Rather sparse attacks of Schönlein's purpura may also be mistaken for insect stings or bites, whereas prepurpuric, urticarial eruptions of Schönlein's purpura, perhaps in the course of a sore throat and supported by an appropriate history, are mistaken for urticaria caused by penicillin. Erythema annulare rheumaticum is an evanescent, discrete, macular erythema, which for practical purposes occurs only in the epigastric area. Erythema annulare centrifugum, however, shows hemorrhagic features extremely seldom. Besides, it has continuous, tortuous bands of erythema, which completely lack as minor lesions the approximately penny-sized erythemas with focal petechiae that occur in Schönlein's syndrome. If punctiform hemorrhages do occur in erythema annulare centrifugum, they are associated with telangiectases.[31] In Schönlein's purpura the Rumpel-Leede test may be either positive or negative, and conspicuous or regular changes of other clotting data are lacking. Not only febrile polyarthritic signs but also abdominal colics (with bloody diarrhea) are supplementary signs that are just as important as *renal phenomena*, especially in adolescents. These phenomena range from mere hematuria ("renal purpura") or hemorrhagic cystitis to signs of diffuse glomerulonephritis, which is the most frequently associated sign, leading in a few cases to uremic states. In contrast, Werlhof's disease does not show any comprehensive renal involvement. The several forms of progressive pigmented purpura or the dysproteinemic forms of purpura likewise lack any essential renal involvement. Familial hematuria suggests Osler's disease first, whereas bleeding from the urinary tract in childhood may be the expression of scurvy, i.e., Möller-Barlow's disease. But another important morphologic point must also be stressed: *Petechiae in thrombocytopenic purpura are always*

Fig. 620. Vasculitis hyperergica.

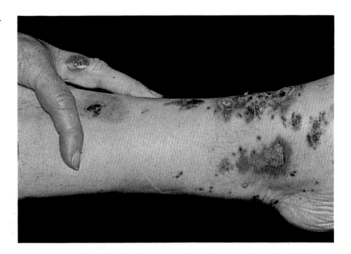

flat, whereas in polymorphic Schönlein's purpura they do not lie on the level of the surrounding skin. At least at the onset of the exanthem, they are distinctly raised urticarially. This behavior is typical not only of Schönlein's purpura but *also of other leukocytoclastic angiitides.*

In these, not only leukocytes and leukoclasia but also the presence of fibrin are important epiphenomena of the vascular changes, characterized by edema, degeneration, and proliferation of the endothelium. These factors form important microscopic differences from

thrombocytopathias and the pigmented purpura group.[51, 52]

Cutaneous eruptions which are evidently related pathogenetically to Schönlein's purpura and which are apparently located at the arterioles and also at the venules and capillaries of the cutis have been designated collectively in recent years as "arteriolitis (vasculitis) allergica cutis" independently of the clinical, hemorrhagic, urticarial, or other "inflammatory" features (Figs. 620, 621).[51, 52, 62]

Similar arteriolitides have been observed in Wegener's granulomatosis

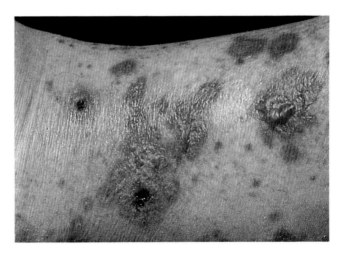

Fig. 621. Vasculitis hyperergica.

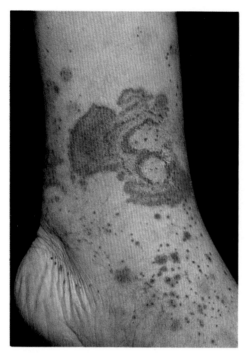

Fig. 622. Purpura in Wegener's granulomatosis.

(Fig. 622). In contrast, *periarteritis nodosa cutis*, which on the skin does not always show the highly characteristic picture of apoplexia cutis but three or four signs of nodular or gangrenous phenomena, represents a syndrome that is serious from the onset. It is a partly septic-febrile syndrome with a sharply increased ESR, leukocytosis and eosinophilia in the blood, urinary findings denoting renal involvement, increased blood pressure, ocular changes, and many others. Either it does not respond at all to the usual drugs or it tends toward spontaneous regression, as does arteriolitis hyperergica, which is situated at a higher level. In these characteristic cutaneous conditions of disease, which are partly designated as *"dermatitis nodularis necrotica"*[8] there are hardly any pathogenetic differences in spite of their various levels of localization. Various precipitating substances in the blood plasma or aggregated gamma globulin, among others, have been found. But these findings are not too "specific" for such "allergic vasculitis." It is clinically more important that *necrotizing vasculitides* especially may herald malignant, lymphoproliferative systemic disease (Hodgkin's disease or lymphosarcoma).[53] The clinical picture of necrotizing vasculitides simulates the vascular changes of endocarditis lenta or ulcerosa, whereas papulonecrotic tuberculids, in spite of their central necrosis, are different owing to their relative monomorphism, their boutlike attacks and rather dense distribution at the distal parts of the extremities and the buttocks, the lack of punctiform bleeding, and the favored location on the osseous protuberances. On the other hand, in cryopathias (cryofibrinogenemia, *cryoglobulinemia*) the favorite location of *purpura cryoglobulinemia* is toward the acra, e.g., around the elbows.[2, 44, 54]

In *cryofibrinogenemia*[48] distinct precipitation starts only in heparinized plasma at 4° C, and in *cryoglobulinemia* it begins only in cooled serum. In both cryopathias the precipitates dissolve again completely when warmed to 37° C.

Electrophoretic examinations and analysis of the sedimentation rate with the ultracentrifuge permit further differentiation from asymptomatic forms, especially in plasmacytoma and macroglobulinemia. Other than *purpura necroticans* or perhaps periarteritis nodosa, functional signs such as Raynaud's phenomenon, cutis marmorata, erythemas, and cold urticaria point to cryoglobulinemia, which, however, might have existed for some time without cutaneous signs. Moreover, one can occasionally elicit purpura or cold urticaria in such patients by applying pieces of ice to the skin, whereas cooling of the conjunctiva with a piece of ice – which may be dangerous with regard to possible sequelae – may result in characteristic but unspecific clumping of erythrocytes ("sludged blood phenomenon"). Purpura necroticans, which may appear on the legs and the scrotum as well as on the acra (ears and hands) and may be associated with the formation of blood blisters on the nose and mouth, leaves brownish spots of hemosiderin when healed. Furthermore, precipitations of protein as deposits in the vascular walls of veins and capillaries or inside aggregates of erythrocytes may be present in the histologic picture of cryoglobulinemia.

Another *viscosity syndrome*, manifesting itself as *hemorrhagic diathesis*, is *macroglobulinemia* (Fig. 623). It presents hemorrhages from the oral and nasal mucous membranes, appearing less often in petechial lesions than in specific plaquelike infiltrates of the skin.[17]

Macroglobulin, which shows up in the serum as a high and weak peak with a migration velocity of the gamma M −, previously beta$_2$M − globulin, has a high molecular weight of about 1 mill. This is also immunobiologically identical with the normal gamma M − globulins and permits a distinction from the proteins in the serum and urine in plasmacytoma. Besides the disturbance of coagulation factors in the plasma as well as the thrombocytes, vascular factors are presumably important for the development of the previously

mentioned hemorrhagic phenomena independent of anatomical findings. If there is any doubt, other indications are the extremely elevated ESR, which should express considerable dysproteinemia, and the so-called Sia reaction (if the serum to be examined is added drop by drop to distilled water, cloudiness caused by precipitation of the macroglobulins will be apparent but will resolve when warmed again, contrary to the findings in other hyperglobulinemias). Determinations of the sedimentation rate with the ultracentrifuge as well as the previously mentioned immunoserologic examinations (immune electrophoresis and others) should be added, especially if the Sia test is positive.

Purpuric phenomena caused by changed circulation and conditioned by viscosity occur in *amyloidoses*. In these, however, proven specific vascular deposits may be etiologically significant. Especially in the systemic forms, *systematized paramyloidosis, skin and muscle amyloidosis,* or *primary amyloidosis,* there are hemorrhagic phenomena that usually appear as petechial bleeding in normal skin or as one of the following manifestations:[9, 14] papular, lichenoid, subcutaneous or sclerodermiform infiltrates, macro-

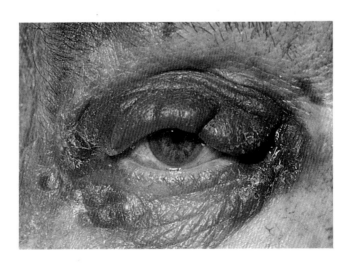

Fig. 623. Waldenström's disease (macroglobulinemia).

glossia, and blister formation following minor trauma. Punctiform bleeding, occurring at the onset or end of the disease, is located mainly on the upper half of the body, especially around the eyes, on the neck, and in the axillary area. Such punctiform bleeding either occurs spontaneously or follows minimal trauma (rubbing of the eyelids, coughing fits, and similar causes).

The tendency toward bleeding in the patient with *plasmacytoma* results from thrombocytopenia (replacement of the bone marrow by plasmacellular proliferation) or a disturbance of the clotting mechanism. These usually collaborate in a complex manner and are responsible for the various clinical forms of disturbed blood pressure, which is also associated with histochemically proven vascular changes. In the same manner, in *undifferentiated reticuloses* the singular macular or papular lesions, which are already red, indicate hemorrhagic components caused by thrombocytopenia and perhaps also increased fibrinolytic activity. Petechiae are also part of the typical picture, interspersed among the papules or in the normal surroundings, especially on the trunk. They are present in several storage reticuloses, usually the disorders with a more acute course, such as *histiocytosis X*, especially *Letterer-Siwe's disease* and *Hand-Schüller-Christian's disease*.[50] However, they are seldom seen in benign, slowly progressive, *eosinophilic granuloma*. But it is this hemorrhagic sign especially that permits clinical differentiation from true Darier's disease of any scaly-crusted papules that sometimes look like lesions of Darier's disease. True Darier's disease usually assumes a hemorrhagic aspect only in the later years of life and only on the palms and soles.[14] In contrast to Letterer-Siwe's disease, seborrheic eczemas are less papularly disseminated. They consist of similarly colored, faded yellowish-brown plaques of erythema. They become interspersed with hemorrhages or

petechiae only in the later years of life, especially in labile hypertonic persons or diabetics.

In general, hemorrhagic phenomena actually manifest themselves conspicuously rarely in the mastocytoses in spite of the clotting changes that are often found and which seem to result from hyperheparinemia. But in cutaneous – visceral *mastocytosis* a relationship to the various urticaria pigmentosa lesions as intrafocal or perifocal petechiae is occasionally found.[3, 10]

Although the cutaneous dysproteinemic types of purpura[18] produce purely petechial exanthems or isolated punctiform hemorrhages, it should be emphasized that Schönlein's purpura, if it follows an eminently chronic course lasting for decades with numerous attacks, will lose the polymorphic character of its eruptions with their facultative purpuric aspect. Schönlein's purpura in such cases will show only pinpoint-sized reddish petechiae which no longer derive mainly or preferably from an urticarial erythematous base. Such chronic cases of the Schönlein syndrome have been known even in the past to present relatively early the final stages of cirrhosis of the liver that were apparently caused by the same syndrome; in addition there were changes of the serum proteins with an increase in the globulins. It is not surprising, therefore, that this course of Schönlein's syndrome showing hypergammaglobulinemia and frequently also hyperproteinemia has been called "purpura hyperglobulinemica."[20] Nevertheless, we prefer to retain the classification of hyperglobulinemic purpura as *"Schönlein's purpura of the Waldenström type,"*[29] although there are no important histologic differences from the usual acute Schönlein's syndrome. This special type must be differentiated from *purpura with cirrhosis of the liver* which usually affects the legs and favors a purely petechial form. The most important differential laboratory test will in both cases furnish a different type of curve of the gamma peak in the electrophoresis diagram.[29] In addition, like some of the other hemorrhagic diatheses, it may be accompanied by hemolytic tendencies; in rare cases, therefore, chronic hyperglobulinemic Schönlein's purpura of the Waldenström type may also show a positive Coombs test or hemolytic anemia.[30, 36]

It is easily understandable that diabetics may frequently have purely *petechial hemorrhages* on the legs, because diabetic vascular changes, especially of the lower extremities, are seen so often. Some time later, in about 5 per cent of cases, such petechial exanthems may be accompanied by peripheral gangrene. In contrast to the usual location on the legs of these closely aligned but finely disseminated lesions of "purpura diabeticorum," the petechiae of systemic fat embolism are sparsely and irregularly distributed on the trunk, for instance, on the shoulders, chest, axillae, and conjunctivae.[58] Such petechiae of systemic fat embolism may occur for example after destruction of the long bones; they are also infrequently a sign of a general hemorrhagic diathesis. *Abortion* induced by the caustic action of *soap*[1] may result in petechial erythrodiapedetic hemorrhages, probably as an expression of a partial consumption coagulopathia similar to purpura after fat embolism. These hemorrhages are frequently accompanied in characteristic fashion by large areas of herpes simplex eruptions (e.g. periorally).

The term *factitious purpura* should be used for recurrent painful ecchymoses induced by trauma; they can be prevented by protective dressings. Similar lesions can even occur in patients sensitized against their own erythrocytes (stroma, hemoglobulin, DNA).[33, 38, 57]

The phenomenon of smaller or larger punctiform hemorrhages has been discussed as a clinical criterion for the analysis of hemorrhagic lesions. The group of conditions included by the term *progressive pigmented purpura* shows as diagnostic signs mostly characteristic reddish-brown, annular deposits of hemosiderin as residua of former petechial hemorrhages. Excluding the *toxic-allergic exanthems of hemorrhagic character* (which occur especially during the summer months and most frequently affect individuals during the sixth and seventh decades [diabetes mellitus, hypertension, sedatives]; these are also more prevalent in women than in men and are found mostly on the legs), the appearance of erythema, very fine petechiae, and washed-out rusty brown pigmentations recurs as a guiding principle for all the special forms of manifestations of this group *(purpura Majocchi, Schamberg's disease, dermatitis lichenoides purpurea et pigmentosa, arciform telangiectatic purpura, eczematidlike purpura, purpura due to adalin,* * *and others)*. On the other hand, as opposed to this triad, capillary ectasias, nodular or eczematoid reactions, and pruritus occur only as epiphenomena with irregular frequency. As a rule, these *pigmented hemorrhagic dermatoses of the lower extremities* may extend up to the middle of the buttocks, or to about the same height as acrodermatitis chronica atrophicans, frostbite, papulonecrotic tuberculids, and similar eruptions. However, unusual extensions of these dermatoses to the arms or upper back do not speak against the diagnosis of a drug reaction; this can be supported by a history of intake of a carbamide derivative, or perhaps also of other sedatives.

Histologically, there are three relevant facts: lymphohistiocytic accumulations of cells, a mild degree of diapedesis of red blood cells, and storage of hemosiderin.[22]

Undeniably it is extremely important to obtain a history of use of sedatives, especially of the adalin group; however, similar hemorrhagic pigmented derma-

---

* A German sedative. (Tr.)

toses that occur in conjunction with a
definite underlying disease – for instance,
disorders of the hepatic porphyrin metabolism ("porphyric purpura") – should
not be overlooked.[23]

The term "ochre-colored dermatitis"
(dermite ocre Favre-Chaix) is applied to
an ochre-yellow to dark brown hyperpigmentation of the lower extremities
with only a few annular but many more
diffuse areas. In contrast to progressive
pigmented purpura, this condition is
hardly ever caused by certain drugs,
labile hypertension, or polycythemia but
rather by chronic venous insufficiency.
Histologically, in contrast to chronic
progressive purpura, this ochre-colored
dermatitis involves atrophy and hyperpigmentation of the básal cell line, and
extravasation of red blood cells not only
into the apices of the papillae but also
into the entire cutis; furthermore, deposits of hemosiderin, perivascular cell
infiltrations, and distinct distention of the
venous plexus of the subcutis are also
seen.[45]

(1) ADAM, W.: Über den morphologischen Nachweis des Seifenabortus. Dtsch. Z. gerichtl. Med. *41:* 416–419 (1952).
(2) ALLEGRA, F.: Zwei Krankheitsfälle mit Kryoglobulinämie. 1. Syndrom des Typus Raynaud, 2. ausschließlich auf die Haut beschränkte Periarteriitis nodosa. Arch. klin. exp. Derm. *217:* 363–376 (1963).
(3) ASBOE-HANSEN, G.: Urticaria pigmentosa haemorrhagica. Acta derm.-venereol. (Stockh.) *30:* 159–162 (1950).
(4) AZEN, E. A., and D. V. CLATANOFF: Prolonged survival in Goodpasture's syndrome. Arch. Intern. Med. *114:* 453–460 (1964).
(5) BAUMGARTNER, W.: Zwei Fälle von Thrombocythaemia haemorrhagica. Helv. med. Acta *23:* 320–324 (1956).
(6) BAZEX, A., A. DUPRÉ et J. FERRERE: La pseudo-chromidrose plantaire, état actuel de la question. Ann. Derm. Syph. (Paris) *94:* 169–186 (1967).
(7) BERLIN, CH.: Purpura solaris. Acta derm.-venereol. (Stockh.) *20:* 77–93 (1939).

(8) BINKLEY, G. W.: Dermatitis nodularis necrotica. Arch. Derm. (Chic.) *75:* 387–393 (1957).
(9) BROWNSTEIN, M. H., and E. B. HELWIG: The cutaneous amyloidoses. Arch. Derm. (Chic.) *102:* 20–28 (1970).
(10) BUCHHOLZ, W.: Ein kasuistischer Beitrag zur hämorrhagischen Mastozytose. Z. Haut- u. Geschl.-Kr. *44:* 113–120 (1969).
(11) COLOMB, D., J.-A. PINCON et J. LARTAUD: Individualisation anatomo-clinique d'une forme méconnue de la peau sénile: les pseudo-cicatrices stellaires spontanées. Ann Derm. Syph. (Paris) *94:* 273–286 (1967).
(12) DUPRÉ, A.: Une "forme majeure" de pseudo-chromidrose plantaire, phlycténulaire et hémorragique – Association à des troubles thrombocytaires – Essai pathogénique. Dermatologica (Basel) *140:* 178–185 (1970).
(13) EGER, H., H. FRISCH, H. HAAS, B. LEDERER und A. PROPST: Purpura fulminans. Med. Welt *21* (N. F.): 2015–2019 (1970).
(14) ENGEL, R.: Purpura bei Paramyloidose. Klin. Wschr. *24/25:* 368–372 (1946/47).
(15) FISCHER, M., K. LECHNER und W. RAITH: Hemmkörperhämophilie bei bullösem Pemphigoid (Lever). Hautarzt *19:* 459–462 (1968).
(16) GEHRMANN, G.: Klinische und immunologische Aspekte des Morbus Werlhof. Dtsch. med. Wschr. *91:* 1069–1074 (1966).
(17) GOTTRON, H. A., G. W. KORTING und W. NIKOLOWSKI: Die makroglobulinämische retikuläre Hyperplasie der Haut. Arch. klin. exp. Derm. *210:* 176–201 (1960).
(18) HAENSCH, R.: Dys- und Paraproteinämien und haemorrhagische Diathese. Hautarzt *10:* 97–105 (1959).
(19) HERZKA, H., K. SCHÄRER und J. P. MÜHLETHALER: Hämangiom mit Thrombocytopenie und Fibrinogenmangel beim Neugeborenen. Schweiz. med. Wschr. *96:* 383–386 (1966).
(20) HOLUBAR, K., K. LECHNER und L. PFLEGER: Zur Pathogenese der Purpura hyperglobulinaemica. Hautarzt *15:* 122–116 (1964).
(21) HOLZMANN, H., und G. W. KORTING: Labiler Hypertonus und Manifestationsrhythmus einer chronisch-thrombocytopenischen Purpura. Arch. klin. exp. Derm. *208:* 502–515 (1959).

(22) ILLIG, L., und K. W. KALKOFF: Zum
Formenkreis der Purpura pigmentosa
progressiva. Hautarzt *21:* 497–505
(1970).

(23) IPPEN, H., G. GOERZ und H. BRÜSTER:
Purpura porphyrica. Arch. klin. exp.
Derm. *223:* 128–156 (1965).

(24) JONES, W. N., TH. E. NIX and W. H.
CLARK: Hemorrhagic Darier's disease.
Arch. Derm. (Chic.) *89:* 523–527 (1964).

(25) JOST, P.: Cumarinnekrosen. Schweiz.
med. Wschr. *99:* 1069–1077 (1969).

(26) JUNG, E. G.: Das paroxysmale Fingerhämatom. Schweiz. med. Wschr. *94:*
458-460 (1964).

(27) KLAUDER, J. V.: Stigmatization. Arch.
Derm. Syph. (Chic.) *37:* 650–659 (1938).

(28) KLIEGEL, H., und K. KRINITZ: Das
Bild der Endometriose an der Haut.
Hautarzt *4:* 445–451 (1953).

(29) KORTING, G. W., und W. ADAM: Purpura Schönleini und Leberzirrhose in
ihrer Abgrenzung von der »Purpura
hyperglobulinaemica«. Derm. Wschr.
131: 121–128 (1955).

(30) KORTING, G. W., und G. BREHM: »Purpura hyperglobulinaemica« mit positi-
vem Coombs-Test. Arch. klin. exp.
Derm. *202:* 449–465 (1956).

(31) KORTING, G. W., und H. EISSNER:
Beitrag zur teleangiektatischen und
purpurischen Erscheinungsform des
Erythema centrifugum anulare (Typus
Gougerot und Patte). Derm. Wschr.
138: 854–863 (1958).

(32) KORTING, G. W., und R. GEBHARDT:
Zur hepatischen Co-Genese der Purpura
senilis. Derm. Mschr. *155:* 124–128
(1969).

(33) KREMER, W. B., C. E. MENGEL,
J. B. NOWLIN and H. NAGAYA: Recurrent ecchymoses and cutaneous hyper-
reactivity to hemoglobin: a form of
autoerythrocyte sensitization. Blood
30: 62–73 (1967).

(34) KREY, W.-D., und F. LEYH: Beitrag
zur Klinik und Pathogenese der thrombotischen thrombopenischen Purpura
(Moschcowitz). Med. Welt *18* (N. F.):
2355–2360 (1967).

(35) KÜNZER, W., F. SCHINDERA, W.
SCHENCK und H. SCHUMACHER: Water-
house-Friderichsen-Syndrom. Abgrenzung, Pathogenese und Therapie mit
Streptokinase. Dtsch. med. Wschr. *97:*
270–273 (1972).

(36) KUHN, E., und R. KOHN: Über Purpura hyperglobulinaemica und erwor-
bene hämolytische Anämie beim glei-
chen Patienten. Schweiz. med. Wschr.
93: 1538–1540 (1963).

(37) LAUGIER, P., N. HUNZIKER, J. REIF-
FERS et M. J. RUDAZ: L'oedème aigu
hémorragique du nourrisson (purpura
en cocarde avec oedème). Dermatologica (Basel) *141:* 113–118 (1970).

(38) LEVIN, R. M., R. CHODOSH and J. D.
SHERMAN: Factitious purpura simula-
ting autoerythrocyte sensitization. Ann.
Int. Med. *70:* 1201–1206 (1969).

(39) MARX, R.: Über Hämophilien. Dtsch.
med. J. *19:* 489–495 (1968).

(40) MISGELD, V.: Das Goodpasture-Syndrom. Z. ärztl. Fortb. *56:* 896–908
(1967).

(41) MOYER, D. G., and S. A. CHERNILA:
Capillaritis of the palms. Arch. Derm.
(Chic.) *99:* 591–592 (1969).

(42) MUELLER-ECKHARDT, C.: Die Diagnose
der idiopathischen thrombozytopeni-
schen Purpura. Dtsch. med. Wschr.
95: 2339–2342 (1970).

(43) NIX, T. E., and C. J. YOUNG: Congenital umbilical anomalies. Arch. Derm.
(Chic.) *90:* 160–165 (1964).

(44) NÖDL, F.: Purpura bei essentieller
Kryoglobulinämie. Arch. klin. exp.
Derm. *210:* 76–85 (1960).

(45) ODEH, F., und M. GOOS: Zur Histopathologie der Dermite Ocre Favre-
Chaix. Z. Haut- u. Geschl.-Kr. *47:*
147–154 (1972).

(46) OHLER, W. G. A., J. FISCHER, W. EN-
DERS und B. KIKILLUS: Hypofibri-
nogenämische hämorrhagische Diathese
bei Prostatakarzinom. Dtsch. med.
Wschr. *91:* 119–124 (1966).

(47) POPOFF, L., R. RAICHEV and V. C.
ANDREEV: Endometriosis of the skin.
Arch. Derm. (Chic.) *85:* 186–189
(1962).

(48) RAITH, W.: Hautnekrosen bei essentieller Kryofibrinogenämie. Z. Haut-
u. Geschl.-Kr. *40:* 409–420 (1966).

(49) REINHART, U.: Über Splitterblutungen
der Nagelplatte und ihre klinische Bedeutung. Schweiz. med. Wschr. *93:*
1229–1232 (1963).

(50) RUCH, D. M.: Cutaneous manifestations of Letterer-Siwe's disease. Arch.
Derm. (Chic.) *75:* 88–95 (1957).

(51) RUITER, M.: Arteriolitis (vasculitis) »allergica« cutis (superficialis). A new dermatological concept. Dermatologica (Basel) *129:* 217–231 (1964).

(52) RUITER, M., und F. H. OSWALD: Weiterer Beitrag zur Kenntnis der Arteriolitis (Vasculitis) »allergica« cutis. Hautarzt *14:* 6–18 (1963).

(53) SAMS, W. M., D. D. HARVILLE and R. K. WINKELMANN: Necrotising vasculitis associated with lethal reticuloendothelial diseases. Brit. J. Derm. *80:* 555–560 (1968).

(54) SCHÜTZ, I.: Purpura necroticans bei Kryoglobulinämie. Z. Haut- u. Geschl.-Kr. *42:* 777–786 (1967).

(55) SCHULTZ, J. H.: Stigmatisierung und Organneurose. Dtsch. med. Wschr. *53:* 1584–1586 (1927).

(56) STECK, W. D., and E. B. HELWIG: Cutaneous endometriosis. J. Amer. Med. Ass. *191:* 167–170 (1965).

(57) STEFANINI, M., and E. T. BAUMGART: Purpura factitia. An analysis of criteria for its differentiation from auto-erythrocyte sensitization purpura. Arch. Derm. (Chic.) *106:* 238–241 (1972).

(58) STEPHENS, J. H., and H. L. FRED: Petechiae associated with systemic fat embolism. Arch. Derm. (Chic.) *86:* 515–517 (1962).

(59) STORCK, H.: Über hämorrhagische Phänomene in der Dermatologie. Dermatologica (Basel) *102:* 197–252 (1951).

(60) THEISEN, H.: Zur Kenntnis der sog. Penis-Fraktur. Z. Haut- u. Geschl.-Kr. *36:* 119–122 (1964).

(61) TYMPNER, K.-D., K. HAGER und P. SCHWEIER: Immunologische Untersuchungen beim Wiskott-Aldrich-Syndrom. Münch. med. Wschr. *110:* 517–521 (1968).

(62) WILKINSON, D. S.: Some clinical manifestations and associations of »allergic« vasculitis. Brit. J. Derm. *77:* 186–192 (1965).

(63) WIRTH, H.: Goodpasture-Syndrom. Münch. med. Wschr. *112:* 189–192 (1970).

37. Angiomas

A. Hemangiomas

Hemangiomas are one of the most frequently encountered human blastomas; oncologically they form a borderline between hyperplasias and hamartomas. Hemangiomas in the narrow sense today comprise only those angioblastomas that are caused by proliferation of capillaries of their arterial or venous components, respectively. The majority of these new formations of blood vessels develop within the skin, usually on the trunk and head.

1. The **cavernous hemangioma** (planotuberous or tuberonodular) in most cases is present at birth or appears within the first few months of life. Appearing first as a red macule or small oval papule, the tumor grows quickly to various sizes, at times as large as hen's eggs. The majority of cavernous hemangiomas do not surpass a diameter of 2 to 4 cm. If they are located in the upper cutis they give the impression of a strawberry or raspberrylike, furrowed, bright red growth resting on a broad base and movable with the skin; the surrounding cutaneous region is otherwise unremarkable (Figs. 624, 625). The surface of these growths is smooth and shows ulceration only after trauma or if the tumors are especially large. Palpation reveals a peculiar rubber spongelike consistency. A large majority of these cavernous hemangiomas regress spontaneously. The first visible sign of beginning involution is grayish-white, branchlike cicatrizing streaks on the surface of the angioma. Hemangiomas located in the deeper cutis present in most cases only a firm elastic bulge; this may make diagnosis difficult. However, because of their content of blood these hemangiomas almost always betray their presence by an indistinct steel-bluish color shining through the skin.

In combination with isolated cutaneous cavernous hemangiomas or even as separate growths, hemangiomas are occasionally found mostly by accident on the inner organs, of which the liver, spleen, and skeleton (vertebrae, top of skull) are the most frequent localizations. About 10 per cent of extracutaneous hemangiomas are found in the striated muscles, the parotid gland, the lungs, and the bronchial system. In rare cases hemorrhages or signs of displacement may lead to clinically relevant findings.[14, 28, 40, 41, 44, 47]

Cavernous hemangiomas of the face or the distal parts of the extremities may lead to hypoplasia of the underlying osseous or mammary tissue. In addition, osseous hemangiomas may result in local fibrous substitution of the affected part of the skeleton or, in exceptional cases, they may be the cause of massive osteolysis. *Gorham's syndrome* is the term given to osteolyses caused by angiomas.[11, 12]

2. In multilocular hemangiomatosis multiple planotuberous cutaneous angiomas are present simultaneously with angiomas interspersed in the internal organs. Like the cutaneous cavernous hemangiomas, this systemic disease appears im-

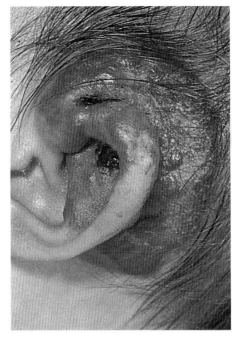

Fig. 624. Cavernous hemangioma with beginning regression.

mediately after birth or within the first few months of life. However, owing to the progressive course of this disease, these children die before the end of the first year of life from hemorrhages or insufficiencies of internal organs (lungs, liver, or intestinal tract). These hemangiomas

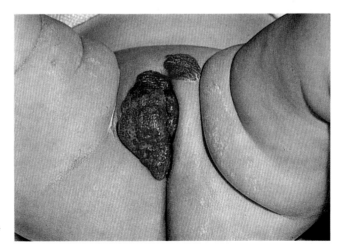

Fig. 625. Cavernous hemangiomas in the vulval area.

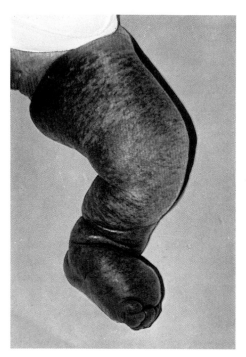

Fig. 626. Giant hemangioma in the Kasa-bach-Merritt syndrome.

differ neither clinically nor histologically from solitary planotuberous angiomas.[1, 10, 37, 42]

3. The **Kasabach-Merritt syndrome** is a combination of giant hemangiomas (Fig. 626) or extensive hemangiomatoses with thrombocytopenia and fibrinogeno-penia. An activation of the fibrinolytic system is present simultaneously, and results in the development of a consump-tion coagulopathia with profuse hemor-rhages. Purpura may develop because of the thrombocytopenia. Kasabach-Merritt syndrome therefore does not appear in-dependently of the form and location of the angioma but depends chiefly on the volume of the angioma.[5, 9, 16]

4. Maffucci's syndrome consists of a com-bination of multiple cutaneous hemangio-mas with an osseous chondromatosis. Here also the hemangiomas are present at birth or shortly thereafter. Besides the hemangiomas, although much more rarely, multiple cutaneous lymphangiomas or a "blue rubber bleb" nevus may be observed. The osseous chondromatosis in most cases attracts attention only at the age when the child learns to walk; however, at an even earlier age the painless hard osseous tumors covered with normal skin can be observed on the fingers and toes. Additional tumors may develop or the already existing ones may enlarge until the end of the growth period. These enchondromas or ecchondromas, located asymmetrically and bilaterally, do not show shortening of the limbs but result in deformities or functional incapacities. Occasionally these chondromas may de-generate into chondrosarcomas. The diag-nosis can be made either clinically or with the aid of radiographs.[2, 3, 39, 45]

5. Ulceromutilating hemangiomatosis is a special type of extensive angioma that endangers the life of infants; the lesions have a cervicofacial localization mainly. The angiosclerosis underlying this heman-giomatosis may also be present on the internal organs.[26]

6. Histologically, cavernous hemangio-mas may also show participation of the eccrine sweat glands. Such **hidroangiomas** (see also Chapter 3, A7) are in most cases an accidental histologic finding because increased sweat secretion may not always be present within the region of the angioma. Clinically, the diagnosis can be suspected only if the angiomatous areas show in-creased sweat secretion.[18]

7. In contrast to multilocular hemangio-matosis, the cutaneous changes in the **blue rubber bleb nevus syndrome** occur much later in childhood or even afterward. Clini-cally, one finds either a few or more than a hundred blue-black angiomas of varying size and with a conspicuously rubbery consistency (Fig. 627). A single heman-

Fig. 627. "Blue rubber bleb nevus" syndrome.

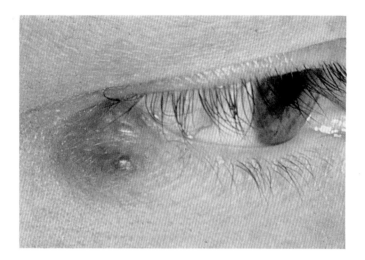

gioma can easily be compressed into a soft mass; after removal of the compression the lesion will quickly refill. The palms and soles often show many angiomas also. An additional important criterion of this disease is the systematization of the angiomas in the gastrointestinal tract. Because they can bleed easily, they may cause life-threatening complications. Multiple glomus tumors may occur in combination with the blue rubber bleb nevus. Histologically, one finds cavernous hemangiomas which have venouslike walls in places. The differential diagnosis must exclude Osler's disease first. The latter disease shows angiomas of much smaller size than those of the blue rubber bleb nevus syndrome, and the trunk almost always remains uninvolved; moreover, the intestine is not involved quite as regularly. Further differences are apparent histologically.[35, 36, 38, 39]

8. Paraproteinemias have been accompanied by multiple eruptive hemangiomas. The histologic examination reveals vascular ectasias and new formations filled with precipitates of albumen. In contrast, pronounced telangiectases are seen more frequently than eruptive hemangiomas in patients with plasmacytoma. Even cutaneous changes similar to telangiectasia

eruptiva perstans have been observed occasionally.[27, 30]

9. Hemorrhagic hereditary telangiectasia or Osler's disease shows character-

Fig. 628. Osler's disease. Additional finding: fibrosed nevus cell nevi on the nose.

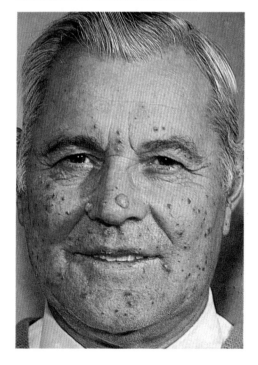

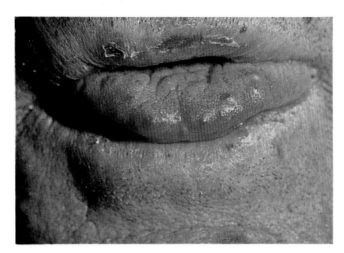

Fig. 629. Osler's disease:
angiomas of the tongue.

istic blue-red, usually completely com-
pressible telangiectases on the skin and
mucous membranes; they may be as large
as pinheads. Bright red, spider-nevilike
telangiectases often develop simultaneously. The lesions favor the mucous membranes of the mouth and nose, the central-
facial region, and the fingers (Figs. 628,
629). The trunk, with the exception of the
middle of the upper chest, almost always
remains free. Clinically, the leading sign is
nosebleeds, but the presence of telangiectases in the stomach, intestines, bladder,
and also within the liver and lung (so-
called arteriovenous pulmonary fistulas)

is also important. The latter manifestation
in some patients may be so conspicuous
that occasionally the cutaneous changes
recede very much into the background.
It must be supposed that patients with
Osler's disease are predestined to disorders
of liver functions; however, there is no
definite increase of cirrhosis of the liver.
Formerly, pathologic-anatomic studies
have emphasized conspicuously dilated
vessels within a diseased region, sometimes occasionally of a thrombotic character and accompanied by changes of the
elastica and collagen; recently emphasis
is laid upon the presence of blocked arte-

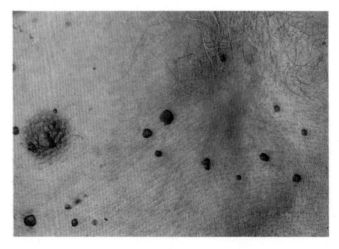

Fig. 630. Senile angiomas.

ries and arteriovenous anastomoses. The fully developed angiomalike Osler-telangiectasia may be based on a conglomeration of latent dysplastic vessels or on other special conditions in the peripheral vascular circulation; all this is caused by quantitatively and qualitatively increased stimuli triggered by certain labile hormonal phases. However, even serial histologic sections may show only "simple" telangiectases.[17, 29, 34]

The apparent combination of Osler's disease with progressive scleroderma should be accepted only with reservations, because this so-called **CRST syndrome** (consisting of calcinosis cutis, Raynaud's sign, sclerodactylia, and telangiectasia) only combines signs that can occur in any stage of typical scleroderma. In the differential diagnosis Osler's disease must be distinguished from multiple senile angiomas, multiple spider nevi occurring in patients with liver disease, and angiokeratoma corporis diffusum (Fabry's disease) (see Table 11).[15, 48]

10. Senile angiomas develop more or less simultaneously, mainly on the trunk and the proximal parts of the extremities (Fig. 630). During the second and third decades mainly and again with another peak during the fourth to sixth decades, the angiomas begin inconspicuously as ruby red, fleabite-like macules. Later on they change into purple-red to dark violet peppercorn-like lesions, and finally develop into soft, protruding, blue-violet, blood-filled, small sacs. Histologically, these lesions are true angioblastomas which are confined in their growth to the upper subpapillary layer. The vicinity of senile angiomas in older persons shows degenerative changes of the elastica and the collagen. In contrast to hemorrhagic hereditary telangiectasia, involvement of the mucosa and hemorrhaging are absent; the latter disease also spares the trunk to a large extent, whereas senile angiomas prefer the location on the trunk and in turn spare the peripheral parts of the extremities. A senile angioma never shows telangiectatic characteristics.[19]

The vermilion part of the lips may have relatively soft, reddish-blue or dusky blue, lentil-sized vascular dilatations, sometimes with a serrated border; they are called **senile angiomas of the vermilion border.** Such angiomas as a rule are present only as single lesions; clinically they resemble a venous node more than a hemangioma (Fig. 631). Such angiomas are limited in their occurrence to persons beyond the fortieth year of life and are supposed to be associated with pulmonary emphysema.[32]

11. The differential diagnosis should consider **spider nevi** (naevi aranei) above all in connection with Osler's disease and

Fig. 631. Angioma of the free vermilion border.

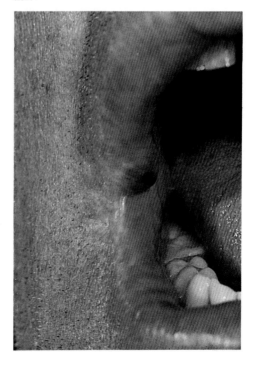

Table 11 Differential Diagnosis: Angiokeratoma Corporis Diffusum (Fabry's Disease) Versus Osler's Disease

	Fabry's Disease	Osler's Disease
Time of onset of first manifestation	As a rule around the 7th–8th year of life, occasionally also later	Usually in the 2nd to 3rd decade, frequently congenital (puberty, pregnancy, or climacterium)
Sex distribution	The male sex is definitely favored	Both sexes are equally affected
Tendency to bleeding	No tendency to bleeding	Cardinal sign: epistaxis, usually even before manifestation of first skin changes; rarely hematuria, melena, or hemoptysis
Paresthesias	Relatively often: tingling and drawing sensations in the arms. Pain from cold	Occasionally, especially subjective Raynaud-like phenomena
Favorite site of skin changes	Centripetal: lower abdomen, umbilicus, buttocks, hands, and extensor surfaces of the large joints	Acral: face, fingers, toes, and genitals
Mucosal involvement	Often lips, not so often buccal mucosa	Almost regularly, nasal mucosa; very often, lips, buccal mucosa, and tongue
Lesions	Point-sized to large pinhead-sized purpuric-red, blue-black angiomas with occasionally a keratotic surface. Usually do not disappear completely on diascopy	Light red micro spider nevi; also blue-red large pinhead-sized, angiomalike lesions which usually disappear completely on diascopy
Cyanosis	–	If arteriovenous pulmonary aneurysms are present
Clubbed fingers	In some cases	If arteriovenous pulmonary aneurysms are present
Edema of feet and and legs	Frequently	–
Sweat production	In some cases hypohidrosis or anhidrosis, but hyperhidrosis has also been observed	Disturbances unknown
Hyperpyrexia	Occasionally, mostly in simultaneous anhidrosis	–
Involvement of inner organs	Often decades after the skin changes: vessels, cardiac muscles, brain, and kidneys	Mucosae of the intestinal and urogenital tracts. Disturbances of liver functions
Hypertension	Almost always in the end stage	–
Heart, EKG	Cardiomegaly, left hypertrophy, abnormal T-wave	No pathologic changes
Lungs	Dyspnea, attacks of asthmatoid bronchitis	So-called arteriovenous pulmonary aneurysms
CNS	Cerebrovascular disturbances, apoplectic insults	–

Table 11 (continuation)

	Fabry's Disease	Osler's Disease
Eyes	Corneal opacities from lipoid deposits, ampullary venectasias in the conjunctiva or retina	No deposits, retinal bleeding
Urinary sediment	Microhematuria, proteinuria, double-refractive substances: "Maltese crosses"	Hematuria
Etiology	Hereditary thesaurismosis: deposit of a sphingosintri-hexosid	"Hereditary vasculopathia," increased development and display of arteriovenous anastomoses and "sluice" arteries
Hereditary	Sex-linked, constant penetrance in the heterozygote male gene carrier and occasional penetrance in the heterozygote female individual	Autosomal, regularly dominant, but occasionally also recessive inheritance
Prognosis	Serious, especially for the male sex; failure of heart or circulation, or uremia	Often undisturbed; anemia from bleeding, death from loss of blood in 5 per cent

senile angiomas. Morphologically these nevi are distinctly characterized by a punctiform vascular ectasia with stellar- or spiderlike extensions (Fig. 632). The lesions occur mainly on the face, V-area of the neck, shoulder blades, and backs of the hands. Spider nevi sometimes show distinct central pulsation and occur more than coincidentally in patients with cirrhosis of the liver or hyperthyroidism or in pregnancy; the purely papular senile angiomas are not associated with the previously mentioned three conditions more often than usual. Isolated spider nevi are also found occasionally in completely healthy persons.

In Osler's disease the angiomalike and somewhat spiderlike vascular changes as a rule precede the clinical manifestations of disturbed liver function, whereas spider nevi may first appear after cirrhosis of the liver.[15, 23, 24]

12. The basic cause of **angiokeratoma corporis diffusum** (Fabry's disease) is a pathological storage of ceramidetrihexos-idase-dihexosidase and -monohexosidase caused by a decrease or absence of the enzyme ceramidetrihexosidase. These deposits of lipoid affect the endothelium and the media of the blood vessels, the perineural sheaths, the cells of the ganglia of the autonomic nervous system, the epithelium of the glomeruli and tubuli, and the cells of the cardiac muscles.

The clinical picture of Fabry's disease is rather polymorphic. Acromegaloid facial features are remarkable. The cutaneous changes consist of purple-red to blackish-blue pinhead-sized macules; in some patients these lesions show a distinctly hyperkeratotic surface (Fig. 634). Their diameter may measure 3 to 4 mm. At times there is considerable clinical similarity between the lesions of Fabry's disease and Osler's disease; therefore, the location of vascular dilatations is of special importance. The angiokeratomas of Fabry's disease are found more or less densely mainly in the region of the lower

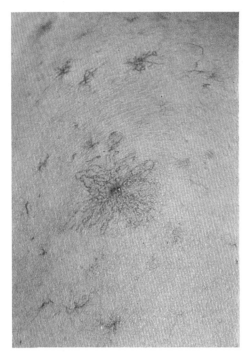

Fig. 632. Spider nevi.

abdomen and buttocks. A leading diagnostic sign is the involvement of the umbilical region (Fig. 635). Similar lesions not covered by keratotic tissue exist on the mucous and transitional membranes. The frequently saclike dilated vessels on the conjunctiva (Fig. 633) are easily

recognizable. For disorders of sweat secretion see Chapter 1, A2 and Chapter 3, B1. Patients with Fabry's disease have a tendency toward crisislike elevations of body temperature due to lack of perspiration, accompanied at times by severe pain in the extremities. Such painful attacks can be triggered by immersion in warm water of more than 38° C; the same is true for water temperatures below 22° C. The central nervous system is involved in about one-third of the cases. Foremost are vascular cerebral signs in younger patients, ranging from fleeting pareses to fully developed unilateral paralyses. Vascular alterations are probably responsible for the frequent complaints of headaches and of pareses of the oculomotor and trigeminal nerves. The kidneys occupy a central place in the course of Fabry's disease. The majority of the patients succumb to uremia, and another portion develops renal hypertension with subsequent cardiac insufficiency or cerebral hemorrhage. Because in most cases males show typical cutaneous changes simultaneously with kidney disorders, it is not difficult to classify such renal disease. However, such a classification is difficult in cases without cutaneous signs, especially in heterozygous female carriers. Here a renal biopsy will help to arrive at the

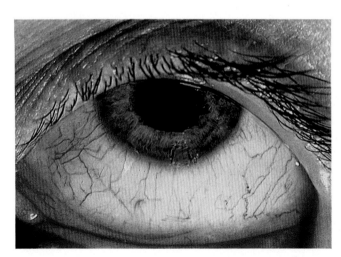

Fig. 633. Angiokeratoma corporis diffusum: ectatically dilated conjunctival vessels.

Fig. 634. Angiokeratoma corporis diffusum: multiple angiomas of the fingertips.

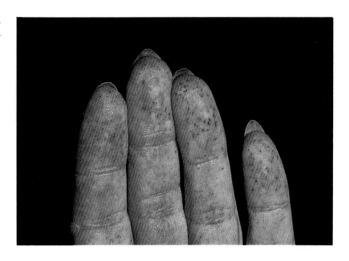

correct diagnosis. A transformation of the glomerular epithelium into fine vacuolar foam cells is characteristic. Many patients in an advanced stage then show clinical, roentgenologic, and electrographic signs of left ventricular hypertrophy. Ocular changes consist of balloonlike and saclike aneurysms of the bulbar conjunctiva, as well as the mandatory corneal opacities arranged in vertexlike yellow-brown lines (cornea verticillata) (Figs. 636, 637). These lines can be found even before the appearance of the first cutaneous and mucous

membrane lesions and are a constant finding also in heterozygous individuals. The third ophthalmologic sign consists of sausagelike venous dilatations in the ocular fundus.

Laboratory examination of the urine will almost always show red and white blood cells and a varying degree of albuminuria. In advanced cases lipoid cylinders

Fig. 636. Angiokeratoma corporis diffusum: cornea verticillata.

Fig. 635. Angiokeratoma corporis diffusum: angiomas of the umbilical pit.

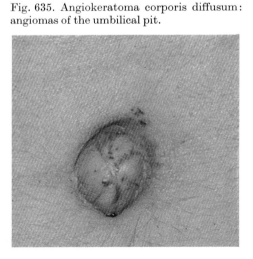

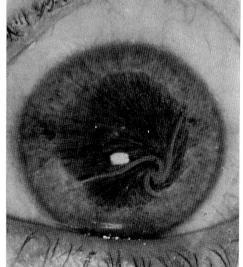

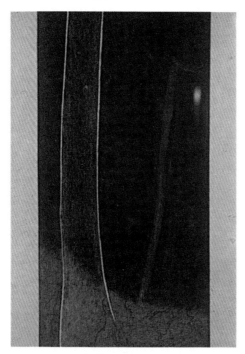

Fig. 637. Angiokeratoma corporis diffusum: cornea verticillata seen by slit lamp.

with typical double refractive Maltese crosses (Fig. 638) and isosthenuria are present.

The diagnosis is not difficult if one is familiar with the clinical facts; in doubtful cases slit-lamp examination of the cornea will quickly help to arrive at the correct diagnosis.[4, 6-8, 13, 21, 22, 31, 33, 43, 46, 49]

13. Caviar tongue is the term given to caviarlike dilatations of blood vessels visible on the undersurface of the tongue in old age (Figs. 639, 640). Macroscopically these lesions resemble the angioma-like lesions observed in Osler's disease, but in this location they must be considered purely venous dilatations.[20, 25]

(1) BABEJ, K.: Multiloculäre Hämangiomatose. Mschr. Kinderheilk. *116:* 107–110 (1968).

(2) BARADNAY, G., J. HOFFMANN und J. OKRÖS: Dyschondroplasie und Hämangiomatose (Maffucci-Syndrom). Zbl. allg. Path. *101:* 296–302 (1960).

(3) BEAN, W. B.: Dyschondroplasia and hemangiomata (Maffucci's syndrome) II. Arch. Intern. Med. *102:* 544–550 (1958).

(4) BRADY, R. O., A. E. GAL, R. M. BRADLEY, E. MARTENSSON, A. L. WARSHAW and L. LASTER: Enzymatic defect in Fabry's disease. Ceramidetrihexosidase deficiency. New Engl. J. Med. *276:* 1163–1167 (1967).

Fig. 638. Angiokeratoma corporis diffusum. (a) Deposits of ceramidetrihexoside in the wall of the vessel (frozen section, polarized light); (b) So-called Maltese crosses in the urine.

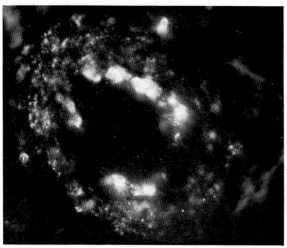
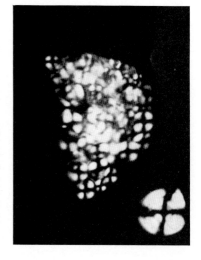

Fig. 639. "Caviar tongue."

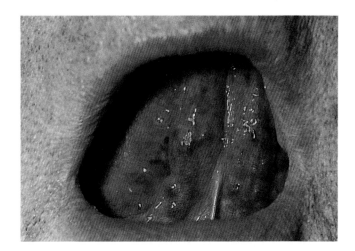

(5) Bureau, Y., H. Barrière, P. Litoux et B. Bureau: L'angiome géant thrombopéniant (syndrome de Kasabach et Merritt). Ann. Derm. Syph. (Paris) *94:* 5–17 (1967).

(6) Denden, A.: Über die diagnostische Bedeutung der Cornea verticillata für die Erkennung des Morbus Fabry-Anderson. Klin. Mbl. Augenheilk. *156:* 49–62 (1970).

(7) Denk, R.: Elektrokardiographische Untersuchungen bei Hautkranken. Arch. Kreisl.-Forsch. *60:* 33–114 (1969).

(8) Denk, R., und G. Sollberg: Skelettmuskelbefunde beim Angiokeratoma corporis diffusum. Hautarzt *17:* 248–252 (1966).

(9) Deutsch, E., M. Fischer und L. Kucsko: Das sogenannte »Kasabach-Merritt-Syndrom« des Erwachsenen. Beitr. path. Anat. *130:* 369–393 (1964).

(10) Fischer, C., und H. Röckl: Ein Fall von systemisierter Hämangiomatose. Hautarzt *12:* 79–82 (1961).

(11) Fost, N. C., and N. B. Esterly: Successful treatment of juvenile hemangiomas with prednisone. J. Pediat. *72:* 351–357 (1968).

(12) Frost, J. F., and R. M. Caplan: Cutaneous hemangiomas and disappearing bones. Arch. Derm. (Chic.) *92:* 501–508 (1965).

(13) Garcin, R., J. Hewitt, S. Godlewski, P. Laudat, H. de Montera et J. Emile: Les aspects neurologiques de l'angiokératose de Fabry. Presse méd. *75:* 435–440 (1967).

(14) Hambach, R.: Knochenhämangiome und -hämangiomatosen. Münch. med. Wschr. *105:* 1268–1272 (1963).

(15) Hauser, W.: Gefäßspinnen – ihre Ursache und Bedeutung, unter besonderer Berücksichtigung der progressiven Sklerodermie. Dtsch. med. Wschr. *93:* 2010–2013 (1968).

Fig. 640. Phlebectasias of the oral mucosa.

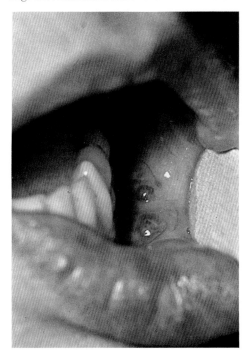

(16) HERZKA, H., K. SCHÄRER und J. P. MÜHLETHALER: Hämangiom mit Thrombocytopenie und Fibrinogenmangel beim Neugeborenen. Schweiz. med. Wschr. *96:* 383–386 (1966).

(17) HUBER, H., und K. HEINRICH: Die Kombination des Morbus Rendu-Osler-Weber mit arteriovenösen Lungenfisteln. Dtsch. med. Wschr. *88:* 1438–1444 (1963).

(18) HYMAN, A. B., H. HARRIS and M. H. BROWNSTEIN: Eccrine angiomatous hamartoma. N. Y. J. Med. *68:* 2803–2806 (1968).

(19) KELLER, R.: Zur Klinik und Histologie der senilen Angiome. Dermatologica (Basel) *114:* 345–359 (1957).

(20) KOCSARD, E., F. OFNER and V. ST. E. D'ABRERA: The histopathology of caviar tongue. Dermatologica (Basel) *140:* 318–322 (1970).

(21) KORTING, G. W., und R. DENK: Über die klinischen Unterschiede zwischen Fabry-Krankheit und Morbus Osler. Med. Welt. *17* (N. F.): 851–855 (1966).

(22) KREMER, G. J., und R. DENK: Angiokeratoma corporis diffusum (Fabry). Lipoidchemische Untersuchungen des Harnsediments. Klin. Wschr. *46:* 24–26 (1968).

(23) MARTINI, G. A.: Über Gefäßveränderungen der Haut bei Leberkranken. Z. klin. Med. *153:* 470–526 (1955).

(24) MARTINI, G. A., und J. STAUBESAND: Zur Morphologie der Gefäßspinnen (»vascular spiders«) in der Haut Leberkranker. Virchows Arch. path. Anat. *324:* 147–164 (1953).

(25) MENDES DA COSTA, S., und G. CREMER: Kaviarähnliche Körner unter der Zunge. Derm. Wschr. *91:* 1206–1209 (1930).

(26) MICHEL, P.-J.: Sur une forme particulière d'angiomes superficiels du nouveau-né à évolution extensive, ulcéro-mutilante et maligne, habituellement mortelle. (Angioscléroplastose de Favre et Fiessinger). Ann Derm. Syph. (Paris) *89:* 152–160 (1962).

(27) MISGELD, V.: Solitäres Plasmocytom der Haut. Ungewöhnliche Manifestation mit perifokaler Mastzellenvermehrung unter dem Bilde einer »Teleangiectasia non maculosa perstans«. Hautarzt *21:* 265–270 (1970).

(28) MÖRL, F. K., und J. DORTENMANN: Hämangiome des Dickdarms. Med. Welt. *19* (N. F.): 2483–2485 (1968).

(29) NÖDL, F.: Zur Histopathogenese der Teleangiectasia hereditaria haemorrhagica Rendu-Osler. Arch. klin. exp. Derm. *204:* 213–235 (1957).

(30) OEHLSCHLAEGEL, G., K. STOLLMANN und F. SCHRÖPL: Ungewöhnliche Hämangiomatose der Haut bei Plasmocytose. Hautarzt *19:* 210–215 (1968).

(31) OPITZ, J. M., F. C. STILES, D. WISE, R. R. RACE, R. SANGER, G. R. VON GEMMINGEN, R. R. KIERLAND, E. G. CROSS and W. P. DE GROOT: The genetics of angiokeratoma corporis diffusum (Fabry's disease) and its linkage relations with the Xg locus. Amer. J. Human Genet. *17:* 325–342 (1965).

(32) PASINI, A.: Über das senile Angiom des freien Lippenrandes. Mh. prakt. Derm. *44:* 275–287 und 342–350 (1907).

(33) PHILIPPART, M., L. SARLIEVE and A. MANACORDA: Urinary glycolipids in Fabry's disease. Their examination in the detection of atypical variants and the pre-symptomatic state. Pediatrics *43:* 201–206 (1969).

(34) PIETSCHMANN, H., und G. KOLARZ: Hereditäre hämorrhagische Teleangiektasie (Morbus Osler). Bericht über 24 Patienten, insbesondere über deren Leberbefunde. Münch. med. Wschr. *111:* 2489–2493 (1969).

(35) RICE, J. S., and D. S. FISCHER: Blue rubber-bleb nevus syndrome. Generalized cavernous hemangiomatosis or venous hamartoma with medulloblastoma of the cerebellum. Arch. Derm. (Chic.) *86:* 503–511 (1962).

(36) RICHTER, G.: »Blue Rubber-Bleb Nevus Syndrom« als Anämieursache. Z. Haut-u. Geschl.-Kr. *39:* 256–261 (1965).

(37) ROSS, W.: Multilokuläre Hämangiomatose im Säuglingsalter mit besonderem Befall der Leber. Acta Hepatosplenol. (Stuttg.) *11:* 207–217 (1964).

(38) DE SABLET, M., et J.-M. MASCARO: Tumeurs glomiques multiples et blue rubber bleb naevus. Ann. Derm. Syph. (Paris) *94:* 35–46 (1967).

(39) SAKURANE, H. F., T. SUGAI and T. SAITO: The association of blue rubber bleb nevus and Maffucci's syndrome. Arch. Derm. (Chic.) *95:* 28–36 (1967).

(40) SCHNYDER, U. W.: Zur Klinik und Histologie der Angiome. Arch. klin. exp. Derm. *204:* 457–471 (1957).

(41) SCHNYDER, U. W.: Hämangiome. Dtsch. med. Wschr. *94:* 1990–1991 (1969).

(42) SOMMACAL, D.: Ein Fall von multipler Hämangiomatose im Säuglingsalter. Helv. paediat. Acta *12:* 666–678 (1957).

(43) SPAETH, G. L., and P. FROST: Fabry's disease. Its ocular manifestations. Arch. Ophthal. (Chic.) *74:* 760–769 (1965).

(44) STEIN, G., K. H. WOEBER und S. SCHÖNBOHM: Zur Klinik kavernöser Hämangiome an Haut und inneren Organen. Arch. klin. exp. Derm. *218:* 177–190 (1964).

(45) SURINGA, D. W. R., and A. B. ACKERMAN: Cutaneous lymphangiomas with dyschondroplasia (Maffucci's syndrome); a unique variant of an unusual syndrome. Arch. Derm. (Chic.) *101:* 472–474 (1970).

(46) SWEELEY, C. C., and B. KLIONSKI: Fabry's disease: classification as a sphingolipidosis and partial characterization of a novel glycolipid. J. Biol. Chem. *238:* 3148–3150 (1963).

(47) WENDER, CH., and J. E. ACKER: Constrictive pericarditis associated with hemangioma of the pericardium. Amer. Heart J. *72:* 255–258 (1968).

(48) WINTERBAUER, R. H.: Multiple telangiectasia, Raynaud's phenomenon, sclerodactyly, and subcutanous calcinosis: a syndrome mimicking hereditary hemorrhagic telangiectasia. Bull. Johns Hopk. Hosp. *114:* 361–383 (1964).

(49) WISE, D., H. J. WALLACE and E. H. JELLINEK: Angiokeratoma corporis diffusum. Quart. J. Med. *31:* 177–206 (1962).

B. Telangiectatic Angiomas

In contrast to cavernous hemangiomas, so-called cutaneous hemangiomas are **telangiectatic nevi,** which are located either medially and symmetrically or unilaterally, most frequently on the head. Telangiectatic nevi are usually present at birth and tend toward occasional nodose transformation only at a late age. They follow a segmentary distribution and rather frequently involve the ocular and oral mucosae. Occasionally they are combined with lymph vessel dilatations. At the onset, cutaneous hemangiomas have a distinctly functional character, which can be recognized by their variable color saturation, for example, from thermic influences, in crying or sleeping, or from the complete blanching that occurs after death. Rare post-traumatic manifestations seem to be possible (see Chapter 18, F2).

Angiophakomatoses are those syndromes of anomalies whose systematized vascular changes affect the skin, eyes, and central nervous system. There are also hyperplasias and, much more rarely, hypoplasias of the soft tissue and bones. According to their respective erythematous characters, the *Sturge-Weber syndrome* is discussed in Chapter 18, F4, the *Klippel-Trenaunay-Weber syndrome* in Chapter 18, L5 and Chapter 10, B15, and *ataxia telangiectatica* in Chapter 18, F3. With regard to *familial telangiectases of the cheeks* and *generalized telangiectasia,* consult also Chapter 18, F3. Multiple telangiectases are also part of the clinical picture of various poikilodermas, whose details are discussed in Chapter 23. For rosacea see Chapter 30, B1.

1. The **Bonnet-Dechaume-Blanc syndrome** is facultatively accompanied by unilateral telangiectases or large hypertrophic angiomas on the face. But more important are the likewise unilateral angioma racemosum of the retina as well as juxtathalamic or juxtamesencephalic arteriovenous aneurysms with related ocular and nervous deficiencies.[2, 5]

2. Angioma serpiginosum has differential diagnostic significance. It represents superficial new vascular formations which favor girls or young women and appear spontaneously without any preceding disorders. It is located on the thighs and buttocks, but the arms and parts of the trunk near the extremities may also be involved. At first only pinhead-sized, shiny red points that blanch under diascopy are recognizable (Fig. 641). If addi-

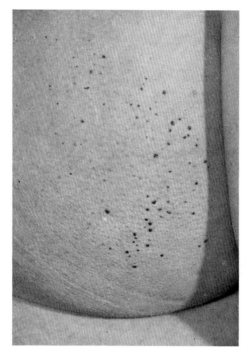

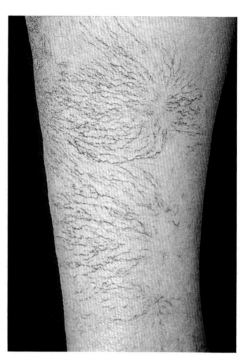

Fig. 641. Angioma serpiginosum.   Fig. 642. Broomstraw-like varicosities.

tional newly formed vessels occur, they may assume arched or serpiginous shapes. The epidermis covering the angiomas remains smooth, and the entire angioma rises neither visibly nor palpably above the surrounding level of the skin. The lesions heal without atrophy. Histologically, subepidermally located vascular dilatations and new-formed vessels are present. Inflammatory infiltrates or vas-

Table 12 Differential Diagnosis: Angioma Serpiginosum–Progressive Pigmented Purpura

	Angioma Serpiginosum	Progressive Pigmented Purpura
History	–	Intake of drugs containing bromides
Sex distribution	90% females	Neither sex is favored
Topographic distribution	Asymmetrical, palms and soles free, extremities	Usually asymmetrical on the legs
Course	Usually progressive; spontaneous regression without remnants possible	Healing often with superficial atrophy; long-persisting pigmentation of hemosiderin
Histology	Dilatation and new formation of vessels in the papillary body, no deposits of hemosiderin and no infiltrate	Telangiectases, extravasates of erythrocytes, deposits of hemosiderin. Inflammatory changes of vascular walls

cular changes are never observed. In contrast to the manifestations of progressive pigmentary purpura, which also occasionally prefers the location on the lower half of the body, the phenomenon of purpura (and therefore of any rust-brown pigmentation) as well as regression with moderate atrophy is missing. Other differential diagnostic criteria are summarized in Table 12.[1, 3, 4, 6]

3. Those vascular dilatations that either originate in the course of venous stasis or are considered to be the initial stage of a constitutional tendency toward varicosities must be differentiated from telangiectatic angiomas. **Broomstraw-like varicosities** are found on the thighs and legs of pregnant, older, and often obese persons. The dark blue-red, 0.5 to 2 mm wide, small cords of varicosities have an irregularly tortuous course. At various distances they dilate to form ampullalike or nodose ectasias. In contrast to essential telangiectases, their circumference is somewhat reduced if they are elevated, but complete blanching is not possible any longer. In the area of the internal malleolus broomstraw-like varicosities occasionally extend into a wide reticulated network that affects the sole of the foot also. Together with small blue-red spots they form the so-called corona phlebectatica. In some patients there are only fanlike circular venous dilatations that are even smaller but can still be fully blanched. These "brushlike figures" may give the first hint of insufficient venae perforantes (Fig. 642).

4. In older patients fine vascular dilatations are frequently observed on the lower thoracic aperture (Fig. 643). This so-called **Sahli's circle of veins** occurs relatively often in healthy men over fifty years of age. However, it may also be an indication of a chronic intrathoracic increase in pressure, for instance, in pulmonary emphysema, and it is then an ex-

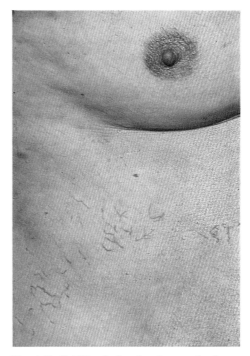

Fig. 643. Sahli's circle of veins on the lower thorax.

pression of an additionally established venous collateral circulation.

(1) BARABASCH, R., und M. BAUR: Angioma serpiginosum. Ein Name für verschiedene dermatologische Krankheitsbilder. Hautarzt *22:* 436–442 (1971).
(2) BONNET, P., J. DECHAUME et E. BLANC: L'anévrysme cirsoïde de la rétine (anévrysme racémeux). Ses relations avec l'anévrysme cirsoïde de la face et avec l'anévrysme cirsoïde du cerveau. J. méd. Lyon *18:* 165–178 (1937).
(3) LAUGIER, P.: L'angiome serpigineux de Hutchinson. Dermatologica (Basel) *135:* 369–374 (1967).
(4) NEUMANN, E.: Some new observations on the genesis of angioma serpiginosum. Acta derm.-venereol. (Stockh.) *51:* 194–198 (1971).
(5) PAILLAS, J. E., J. BONNAL et C. RIGHINI: Angiome encéphalo-rétino-facial (syndrome de Bonnet, Dechaume et Blanc). Rev. neurol. *101:* 698–707 (1959).
(6) STEVENSON, J. R., and C. S. LINCOLN: Angioma serpiginosum. Arch. Derm. (Chic.) *95:* 16–22 (1967).

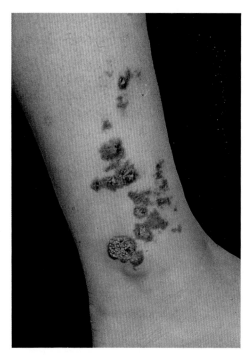

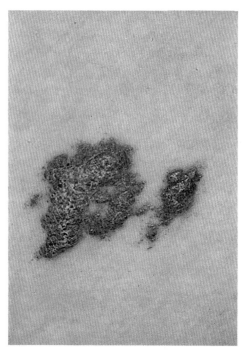

Fig. 644. Angiokeratoma circumscriptum.   Fig. 645. Angiokeratoma circumscriptum.

C. Angiokeratomas

1. The **verrucous hemangioma** is a struc-tural variant of the capillary or cavernous hemangioma. This hemangioma has a wartlike surface as a result of hyperkera-tosis and acanthosis of the overlying epidermis. Like most hemangiomas it is already present at birth or may develop during the first months of life. Verrucous hemangiomas are especially frequent on the lower extremities; they develop slowly

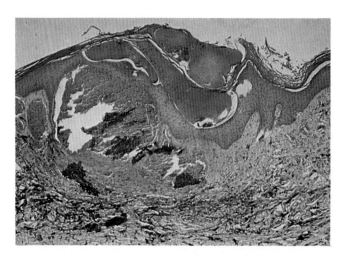

Fig. 646. Angiokeratoma cir-cumscriptum: intraepider-mal blood extravasates, sub-epidermal angioma, massive deposits of hemosiderin in the corium. Berlin blue reac-tion stain, 30 × .

and occasionally more angiomas appear like satellites in their immediate vicinity. Only histologic examination permits a distinction from angiokeratoma circumscriptum because an old angioma is present within a verrucous hemangioma.[6, 10]

2. In contrast to such warty hemangiomas, the angiokeratoma develops from telangiectases. Whereas the verrucous hemangioma extends into the deep cutis and the subcutis, the **circumscribed angiokeratoma** is confined to the papillary body (Figs. 644, 645, 646); even at birth it has already developed to its full extent on the lower extremities, and to a lesser extent on the trunk. Seldom will such an angiokeratoma first appear during childhood or in an adult. In most cases there are several closely aggregated, blue to reddish-black, about pinhead-sized telangiectases that cannot be compressed. However, such papular telangiectases may extend in a segmental arrangement over large cutaneous regions. Nosologically there is a certain similarity with the angiophakomatoses because a nevus flammeus (telangiectatic nevus) may coexist within the same segment; it is also not uncommon to find an association with venous ectasias and osteohypertrophies. The differential diagnosis must include the possibility of a melanoma, especially in lesions on the soles of the feet.[3, 5]

3. Angiokeratoma acroasphycticum of fingers and toes has a certain familial disposition and is found mostly in vagotonic persons who are inclined toward acrocyanosis and frostbite. The first cutaneous changes develop around the time of puberty and favor the female sex. The macules are small and erythematous at first, developing slowly into rice-cornsized, dark blue vascular dilatations with a rough surface. Like Osler's disease and angiokeratoma corporis diffusum, the fingers and toes are the favored locations, but exceptionally the dorsal aspects of the

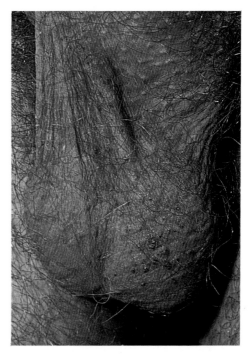

Fig. 647. Angiokeratoma of the scrotum.

hands and feet as well as the elbows and knees may show angiokeratomas of a corresponding type; however, in contrast to the former diseases, angiokeratoma is not a systemic disease.[4, 7]

4. The **angiokeratoma of the scrotum or vulva** does not have an acroasphyctic character. In contrast to circumscribed angiokeratoma and angiokeratoma acroasphycticum of the fingers and toes, the telangiectatic lesions of the scrotum or vulva appear only in older persons. The cause of the vasodilatations may be increased venous pressure (varicocele). Clinically the lesions consist of isolated or multiple, pinhead- to lentil-sized ectasias that are at first light red and later bluishred with a verrucous surface (Fig. 647). In the differential diagnosis angiokeratoma corporis diffusum (see Section A 12) must be excluded.[1, 2, 8, 9]

5. Angiokeratoma corporis diffusum was
discussed in Section A12 of this chapter
because of its similarity to Osler's disease.

(1) Agger, P., and P. E. Osmundsen:
Angiokeratoma of the scrotum (For-
dyce); a case report on response to
surgical treatment of variocele. Acta
derm.-venereol. (Stockh.) *50:* 221–224
(1970).

(2) Blair, C.: Angiokeratoma of the vulva.
Brit. J. Derm. *83:* 409–411 (1970).

(3) Dammert, K.: Angiokeratosis naeviformis – a form of naevus teleangi-
ectaticus lateralis (naevus flammeus).
Dermatologica (Basel) *130:* 17–39 (1965).

(4) Dostrovsky, A., and F. Sagher:
Abortive form or early form of angiokeratoma. Dermatologica (Basel) *96:*
412–417 (1948).

(5) Fischer, H., und H. C. Friederich:
Angiokeratoma corporis circumscriptum
naeviforme mit Venektasien und Osteo-
hypertrophie. Derm. Wschr. *151:* 297–
306 (1965).

(6) Halter, K.: Haemangioma verruco-
sum mit Osteoatrophie. Derm. Z. *75:*
271–279 (1937).

(7) Haye, K. R., and D. J. A. Rebello:
Angiokeratoma of Mibelli. Acta derm.-
venereol. (Stockh.) *41:* 56–60 (1961).

(8) Imperial, R., and E. B. Helwig:
Angiokeratoma of the vulva. Obstet.
and Gynec. *29:* 307–312 (1967).

(9) Imperial, R., and E. B. Helwig:
Angiokeratoma of the scrotum (For-
dyce type). J. Urol. *98:* 379–387 (1967).

(10) Imperial, R., and E. B. Helwig:
Verrucous hemangioma. Arch. Derm.
(Chic.) *96:* 247–253 (1967).

D. Lymphangiomas

1. The most frequent form of lymphangioma is **lymphangioma circumscriptum
cutis.** Like hemangiomas most of them are
either already present at birth or appear
within the first years of life. However, in
contrast to cavernous hemangiomas they
lack a definite tendency toward regression.
Preferred sites are the chest, back, and
back of the neck, and also the proximal
parts of the extremities. However, the
mucous membranes of the mouth and
genitals may also be the sites of such
lymphangiomas. Clinically the lesions
show closely adjacent "vesicles" that may
be as large as pinheads and resemble
frogs' eggs in appearance; lymph is
obtained upon puncture. Some angiomas
contain a milky or hemorrhagically cloudy
fluid that gives a red to reddish-brown
color to the lesion (Fig. 648). After a
long period the surface may become
hyperkeratotic and a more wartlike appearance results. The size of the cutaneous
area affected by lymphangioma circumscriptum cutis varies considerably from 1
to several centimeters. If surgery is con-
templated a determination of the depth is
especially important. This is relatively
easy to discover with the aid of isotope
lymphography.[2, 3]

2. Lymphangioma simplex is found much
more rarely than circumscribed lymphangioma. Its most frequent site is the tongue
and above all the scrotum. The lesions
consist of small, often grouped nodules
that are either flesh colored or grayish-
red; occasionally this color leads to the
mistaken diagnosis of a hemangioma. The
individual angiomas can be expressed.[3]

3. Cavernous lymphangioma appears
simply as a tumorous growth with unchanged overlying skin. The soft mass can
be demarcated relatively well but it may
lead to a considerable enlargement in the
volume of the involved cutaneous areas
(as for instance in macrocheilia, macroglossia, "persistent swelling of the cheeks,"
and similar conditions). Cavernous lymphangioma, unlike lymphangioma simplex,
will not be emptied under pressure. A
definite diagnosis can be established only
by histologic examination or, better still,
by isotope lymphography. A monstrous
congenital variant of lymphangioma cavernosum is the **cystic hygroma.** Here the

Fig. 648. Hematolymphangioma cysticum circumscriptum.

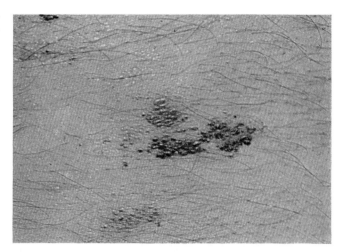

deep extension of the lymphangioma will often reach from the neck region down to the shoulder or to the upper chest area. Similar lymphangiomas may also be seen in the axillae and popliteal spaces.

The skin over the mostly fluctuating lymphangiomas is either immovably attached to the tumor or can be lifted up widely, as in the case of cutis laxa. The amount of fluid may change relatively quickly, so that the intensity of the swelling is variable. Especially in the cervical region manifestations of displacement may cause life-threatening complications that require immediate surgical intervention.[1, 4]

(1) KNORR, G.: Das cystische Lymphangiom des Halses. Virch. Arch. path. Anat. *319:* 347–372 (1951).

(2) PEACHEY, R. D. G., C.-C. LIM and I. W. WHIMSTER: Lymphangioma of skin. A review of 65 cases. Brit. J. Derm. *83:* 519–527 (1970).

(3) PEVNY, I., G. BECKER und G. BONSE: Das Lymphangioma circumscriptum cutis und seine Diagnostik mit Hilfe der Isotopenlymphographie. Hautarzt *18:* 401–408 (1967).

(4) REGENBRECHT, J.: Das Lymphangiom. Münch. med. Wschr. *101:* 2197–2205 (1959).

E. Vascular Neoplasias

1. Kaposi's sarcoma (sarcoma idiopathicum multiplex haemorrhagicum) begins with soft, loose, not-reddened edema of the feet, legs, or hands. The arms and thighs remain unaffected even after a long course of illness. The disorder almost always begins on the skin, and only later do similar tumors appear in the respiratory and gastrointestinal tracts. The disease occurs conspicuously more often in men than in women. In the beginning there are pitting edemas; however, they are soon followed by stable swellings which, in contrast to stasis-edemas, are resistant to diuretic drugs. In addition, the skin of these occasionally almost sclerodermatically indurated edemas darkens until it reaches a dark brown color (Figs. 649,650). For a while macular changes are predominant, and then frequently round and nodose, rarely plaquelike, infiltrates develop. In any case, in Kaposi's disease the nodose groups, like the preceding bilateral edematous phase, also develop symmetrically. They become depressed in the center later and are less frequently transformed into hemorrhagic blisters or ulcers. The nodes and infiltrates, however, continue to develop in depth. The color of the individual nodes varies according to the num-

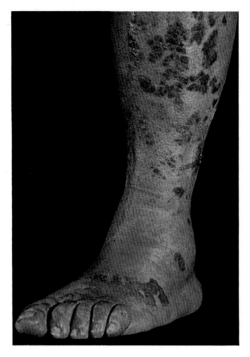

Fig. 649. Kaposi's sarcoma.

The clinical diagnosis of this angioneoplasia is based on the state of general undisturbed health which, except for moderate anemia, lasts for a long time. Other clinical signs are localization on the acra, favoring the lower extremities, and nodose infiltrations found at the sites of the preceding edema. Above all, the bluish-black color of the nodular manifestations seems rather remarkable; also, in complete contrast to other "specific" granulomas or other tumors of the sarcoma group, the nodes may be accompanied by considerable local hyperthermia.

Kaposi's disease is associated more than coincidentally with other malignant tumors or diabetes mellitus, which develops as a subsequent disorder. Histologically, as in hemangioendothelioma, various structures exist next to one another in Kaposi's disease. "Inflammatory" granulomatous processes occur as well as circumscribed spontaneous regressions and neoplastic transformations. The histologic findings are best described as an immature fibrosarcoma with many cells and a poorly differentiated capillary net. In typical cases the picture is completed by excessive deposits of hemosiderin. Aggregations of perifocal round cells convey granulomalike features to this composite picture. In later stages the vascular forma-

ber of blood vessels and hemorrhages inside, but usually bluish-red or bluish-black rather than red or copper-red colors predominate. If residual regressions occur at all they form circumscribed, pigmented, and atrophic areas.

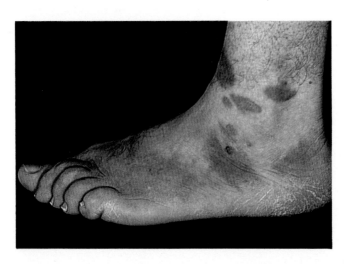

Fig. 650. Kaposi's sarcoma.

tions, which have either thin or thick walls, regress, and proliferations of fibroblasts take over. They are finally replaced by fibrous connective tissue with a few cells. Electron-microscopically, Kaposi's carcinoma is an angiomatosis, which is composed of immature and pluripotent vascular cells, and both endothelial and perithelial elements. The latter change to immature phagocytic fibroblasts. In some instances the absence of nervous elements in these processes has been stressed.[4, 6, 13, 17]

2. Another angioplastic sarcomatous type of chronic edema is known as the **Stewart-Treves syndrome.** This refers solely to those eruptive angiosarcomatoses that develop practically exclusively in females of a higher age group. They occur unilaterally, again on the basis of a chronic, gradually increasing sclerosing lymphedema, such as may occur subsequent to mastectomy because of a mammary carcinoma. This acrosarcomatosis frequently has a stormy course and sometimes begins with hemorrhagic-macular lesions, which change to fast-growing nodules surrounded by petechiae and telangiectases.

A single nodule may be as large as a hazelnut or plum. Several may become confluent, forming nodose groups of tumors. Some rather flat tumorous infiltrates occasionally fluctuate or have a spongy-cystic consistency. The period of latency following removal of the breast is about eight to ten years, and the sarcomatosis itself takes about one and a half years on the average to develop. The Stewart-Treves syndrome differs from sarcoma idiopathicum multiplex haemorrhagicum in its location, which is determined by the site of the chronic lymph stasis, its more frequent occurrence in females, and its biologic character. Kaposi's disease, in spite of the late development of manifestations in the inner organs, behaves like a multiple autochthonous sarcomatous systemic disease, whereas the Stewart-Treves syndrome represents a genuine metastasizing angioplastic sarcoma. Macroscopically, the Stewart-Treves syndrome differs from metastases of a mammary carcinoma by its darker color, hemorrhagic inhibition, and soft spongy consistency. The differentiation of the Stewart-Treves syndrome from nodular changes of reticuloses, reticulogranulomatoses, and hemoblastoses is also easy (history: no limitation to one extremity, among other signs); it can also be easily confirmed histologically.[3, 7, 24]

3. In **proliferating systematized angioendotheliomatosis** the clinical manifestations are equivocal. In some cases mildly itching eruptions occur in conjunction with chills and fever. The rash consists of blue- to brownish-red, poorly demarcated spots or nodose infiltrates of fingernail to palm size. Some areas simulate tuberoserpiginous syphilis, but cutaneous changes resembling those of mycosis fungoides, leukosis, or panniculitis non suppurativa have also been observed. The mucous membranes are not involved and palpable lymph nodes are absent. However, the heart, brain, thyroid and other internal organs may be affected. In contrast to the only slightly characteristic picture, the histologic findings are rather typical. The dilated conglomerate capillaries are densely packed with mononuclear cells. These cellular elements, which apparently originate in the endothelium, do not penetrate the vascular walls. In addition, there are solitary hyalinized thromboses in the affected capillaries, whereas perivascularly only minor and uncharacteristic cell masses are present. A diagnosis and, especially, a differentiation from Kaposi's disease are therefore possible only histologically.[2, 5, 12, 19]

4. Rapidly developing, eruptive angiomas are usually classified as granulating tumors, which are filled with blood and are infectious. They are more aptly called benign telangiectatic granulomas. They occur in adults and their origin and growth are caused by trauma and secondary infection. In appearance the lesions are meaty-red, and usually rest on a small base. They bleed easily, and after reaching a certain size they remain stationary and show no tendency to regress. In typical cases the base of such a tumor is surrounded by a margin of epithelium in folds (Fig. 651). If the tumor already has already been present for some time, its surface may have a brown discoloration of varying intensity caused by deposits of hemosiderin. This discoloration and the tumor's vulnerability may lead to confusion with a malignant melanoma. Furthermore, the corymbiform spreading of small satellites around a larger telangiectatic granuloma may arouse suspicion of a malignant tumor. In exceptional cases several such benign telangiectatic granulomas also occur disseminated over wide

Fig. 651. Benign pedunculated granuloma.

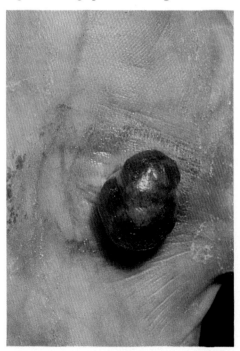

areas of the skin. Their recognition is facilitated by the history of a trauma (such as invasion of foreign bodies at an explosion). Histologically, in contrast to pure angiomas, angiomatous and granulomatous features occur next to each other.[8, 10, 12]

5. Clinically, a hemoangioendothelioma may be very similar to a benign telangiectatic granuloma. Besides the skin, the chief locations are the thyroid gland and liver, and occasionally the gastrointestinal tract. In the beginning there is, on the upper parts of the face or on the scalp, a dark, sometimes slightly fluctuating, nodose tumor, which is occasionally laced with hemorrhages or has a macular base. It tends to show an ulcerative rupture relatively late. If it is situated near the eyes, its clinical manifestations resemble those of chronic lymphadenosis or hemorrhagic tumorlike macroglobulinemia. For the most part, it spreads continuously locally and reaches a greater depth than is apparent. Occasionally, distant metastases to unusual places (spleen, heart, and intestines) may occur. On the other hand, such spongelike hemangioendotheliomas may, even if observed for a long time, remain constant with no recurrence or metastases. Oncologically, a hemangioendothelioma represents a mixed form, which consists of capillary proliferation, especially of the endothelium, and of reticular mesenchymal structures with telangiectatic features. The mesenchymal structures are chiefly responsible for the proliferation potency of the tumor. "Mature" or "immature" parts, or whether cavernomalike, carcinomalike, or sarcomalike formations predominate, are distinguished in this polymorphous tumor.[20, 23]

Compared to these rather dark hemangioendotheliomas, the vascular tumor called a gemmangioma is macroscopically a light, soft fibroma. It is much more benign than the hemangioendothelioma. Histologically, the gemmangioma – in the

Fig. 652. Hemangiopericytoma: capillary lumina surrounded by proliferating pericytes. Hematoxylin and eosin, 160×.

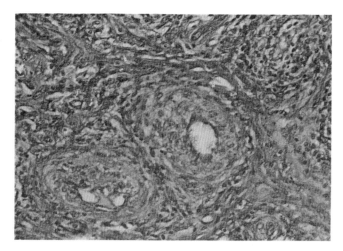

absence of large vessels – shows a capillary net embedded in abundant ground substance, which clearly predominates. In the histologic differential diagnosis, capillary proliferations in common granulation tissue will have to be considered.[14, 18]

6. Angioplastic reticulosarcomas occur especially often on the scalps of older people. They consist of rapidly growing, slightly elevated, infiltrated patches developing from small nodules; in the final stage these lesions may occupy large portions of the scalp and face. The infiltrations show inflammatory redness and advance peripherally with tonguelike extensions. In numerous places there are small cystic protrusions which continuously discharge lymphatic fluid. Solitary or multiple ulcerations also exist to a varying extent. Even wide excisions do not prevent local recurrences. Metastasis into inner organs is a definite possibility. The histologic picture corresponds to that of the Stewart-Treves angiosarcoma.[16, 22]

7. The hemangiopericytoma shows blastomatous development in the perithelial or pericapillary space, which means it takes place outside of the vascular basal membrane and is demonstrable by silver impregnation. Such a tumor may macroscopically resemble a leiomyoma. The circumscribed nodular formations reach a size of 0.5 to 2.0 cm, and occasionally even larger. About half of the pericytomas are embedded in the depth of the cutis or subcutis, as well as in the muscles of the extremities. The hemangiopericytoma is a tumor with a tendency toward considerable variation; it develops before the fourth decade of life, without favoring either sex, and after removal it may recur frequently with a possibility of malignant degeneration. Histologically (Fig. 652), hemangiopericytomas represent angioplastic sarcomas; apparently the prognosis of the cutaneous types of these pericytomas is worse than those with a visceral location. Also, multiple cutaneous hemangiopericytomas have been observed. Since pericytomas may occasionally be painful, the differential diagnosis must consider glomus tumors; these two tumors have many similarities.[1, 9, 11, 15]

(1) BIANCHI, O., J. ABULAFIA et L. MIRANDE: Hémangiopéricytome cutané (Stout et Murray). Ann. Derm. Syph. (Paris) *95:* 269–284 (1968).

(2) BRAVERMAN, I. M., and A. B. LERNER: Diffuse malignant proliferation of vascular endothelium. Arch. Derm. (Chic.) *84:* 72–80 (1961).

(3) BRUNNER, U.: Über das angioplastische Sarkom bei chronischem Lymphödem (Stewart-Treves-Syndrom). Schweiz. med. Wschr. *93:* 949–957 (1963).

(4) DEGOS, R., R. TOURAINE, J. CIVATTE, S. BELAICH et D. FRANCK: Maladie de Kaposi. Ann. Derm. Syph. (Paris) *91:* 113–126 (1964).

(5) FIEVEZ, M., C. FIEVEZ and J. HUSTIN: Proliferating systematized angioendotheliomatosis. Arch. Derm. (Chic.) *104:* 320–324 (1971).

(6) HASHIMOTO, K., and W. F. LEVER: Kaposi's sarcoma. J. Invest. Derm. *43:* 539–549 (1964).

(7) HERY, B., R. MASSE et J.-M. LE FUR: Le syndrome de Stewart Treves. Un nouveau cas rapporté. Revue de la littérature. Bull. Cancer *59:* 269–298 (1972).

(8) JUHLIN, L., S.-O. HJERTQUIST, J. PONTÉN and J. WALLIN: Disseminated granuloma pyogenicum. Acta derm.-venereol. (Stockh.) *50:* 134–136 (1970).

(9) KAUFFMAN, S. L., and A. P. STOUT: Hemangiopericytoma in children. Cancer *13:* 695–710 (1960).

(10) MADŽAROV, I.: Zur Entwicklung und Behandlung des multiplen Granuloma teleangiectaticum. Derm. Mschr. *156:* 108–114 (1970).

(11) METZ, J., und R. BARABASCH: Das Hämangiopericytom. Z. Haut- u. Geschl.-Kr. *46:* 95–98 (1971).

(12) MIDANA, A., et F. ORMEA: A propos d'un cas d'»angioendotheliomatosis proliferans systematisata« (de Tappeiner et Pfleger). Ann. Derm. Syph. (Paris) *92:* 129–138 (1965).

(13) MOTTAZ, J. H., and A. S. ZELICKSON: Electron microscope observations of Kaposi's sarcoma. Acta derm.-venereol. (Stockh.) *46:* 195–200 (1966).

(14) ORSÓS, F.: Gefäßsproßgeschwulst (Gemmangioma). Beitr. path. Anat. *93:* 121–139 (1934).

(15) RAAB, W.: Multiple Haemangiopericytome mit maligner Entartung. Z. Haut- u. Geschl.-Kr. *33:* 243–252 (1962).

(16) REED, R. J., F. E. PALOMEQUE, M. A. HAIRSTON and E. Z. KREMENTZ: Lymphangiosarcomas of the scalp. Arch. Derm. (Chic.) *94:* 396–402 (1966).

(17) RONCHESE, F., and A. B. KERN: Lymphangioma-like tumors in Kaposi's sarcoma. Arch. Derm. (Chic.) *75:* 418–427 (1957).

(18) SCHNEIDER, W., und W. UNDEUTSCH: Seltene Blutgefäßgeschwülste der Haut. Klinik, pathologische Anatomie und Histologie sowie Systematik. Hautarzt *18:* 437–445 (1967).

(19) TAPPEINER, J., und L. PFLEGER: Angioendotheliomatosis proliferans systemisata. Hautarzt *14:* 67–70 (1963).

(20) UNDEUTSCH, W.: Das Hämangioendotheliom der Haut. Arch. klin. exp. Derm. *225:* 181–193 (1966).

(21) WARNER, J., and E. WILSON-JONES: Pyogenic granuloma recurring with multiple satellites. Brit. J. Derm. *80:* 218–227 (1968).

(22) WEIDNER, F., und O. BRAUN-FALCO: Über das angioplastische Reticulosarkom der Kopfhaut bei älteren Menschen. Hautarzt *21:* 60–66 (1970).

(23) WILSON-JONES, E.: Malignant angioendothelioma of the skin. Brit. J. Derm. *76:* 21–39 (1964).

(24) WOLFF, K.: Das Stewart-Treves-Syndrom. Arch. klin. exp. Derm. *216:* 468–496 (1963).

38. Tumors

In the following discussion a growing cutaneous mass will be called a tumor. Therefore, increased growths that do not correspond to the anatomic-pathologic concept of a blastoma will be included. On the other hand, genuine blastomas have been discussed already in other chapters for clinical differential diagnostic reasons. Reference is made here to Chapter 8, juxta-articular nodes; Chapter 10, recurrent and persistent swellings; Chapter 33, ulcers; and Chapter 37, angiomas. A thorough discussion of well-differentiated rare tumors, however, will not be undertaken because their diagnosis is only possible by histologic examination. Accordingly, we shall try to describe a differential diagnosis of several types of tumors on the basis of obvious clinical manifestations.

A. Painful Tumors

As far as the question of painful cutaneous growths is concerned, it is remarkable that most cutaneous tumors lack pain as a meaningful warning sign. In addition, the large majority of the different neurogenic tumors (for instance, the multiple ganglioneuromas, the genuine fibrillary neuromas, and others), are not accompanied by pain.

1. The **glomus tumor** (glomangioma) is a classic painful cutaneous tumor; its guiding clinical sign is pain. Only in the very beginning of the development of this tumor or in instances of the much rarer multiple glomus tumors will painful phenomena be absent. The typical isolated glomus tumor appears as a rounded, sometimes spherical, protruding, red or bluish node with a smooth surface (Fig. 653). The size of a single tumor varies from a few millimeters to 1 or, at the most, 2 centimeters. The favorite site is the matrix of the fingernails or toenails, a location seen somewhat more frequently in women than in men, although the tumor itself does not favor either sex. In the immediate vicinity of a glomus tumor the bones may show pressure defects, and calcification can take place around the lesion. Pain may be elicited by the sensation of cold or touch; less often it is caused by heat or occurs spontaneously. Frequently the entire affected extremity or only the periphery of the tumor shows hyperhidrosis. At times the slightest touch, a minimal movement of the overlying skin or a barely perceptible change of temperature may trigger the typical lancinating attack of pain, which radiates far into the surrounding tissue. Because repeated trigger effects slowly increase the amount of pain, the patient lives in constant fear of possible new attacks of pain; this situation is similar to that in trigeminal neuralgia in which the patient continuously dreads the return of his pain. Especially painful are the tumors located in the subungual tissue. In exceptional cases heavy pressure on a tumor already

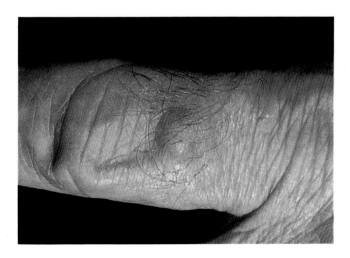

Fig. 653. Glomus tumor.

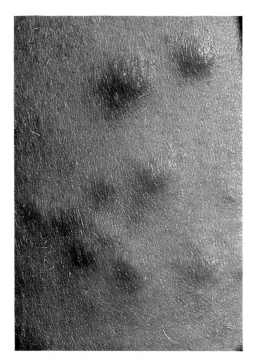

Fig. 654. Multiple leiomyomas with distinctly recognizable groups of arrectores.

ules showing a bluish tint deep in the cutis, sometimes even becoming painful by pressure, are observed. However, considering the quite different polymorphous signs of glomus tumors and neurofibromatosis, it should not be difficult to differentiate between the two diseases; probably both diseases are inherited in autosomal dominant fashion.

Histologically, multiple glomus tumors show fewer epithelioid cells as compared with the solitary type; therefore, they are more similar at first to cavernous hemangiomas.

2. Leiomyomas also involve attacks of a painful character. Often these tumors occur in disseminated form within a small cutaneous area, and they may also be seen in segmental distribution. The individual lesions are about hazelnut-sized, protruding semispherical, brownish-red nodes. Although they are rather easily moved on their undersurface, they are firmly attached to the epidermis in most instances (Fig. 654). These painful multiple leiomyomas of the skin develop histologically from the arrectores pilorum muscles (Fig. 655a, b). Their characteristic pain can be triggered by pressure from the side or in general by displacement from their base, as well as by cold or by drugs having a contracting effect (caffein, Coca-Cola, and others). The painful attacks may be associated with other vegetative stimuli, for instance, segmentary hyperhidrosis. Moreover, even after removal of these tumors segmentary hyperesthesia may remain. The pain of multiple leiomyomas is so typical that other cutaneous tumors resembling these growths (for instance, fibromas, keloids, some nevi) can be excluded simply by their absence of pain.[3, 7, 12]

causing pain may bring about interruption of the complaints, probably due to vascular evacuation. In any case, there is no connection between the size of the glomus tumor and the intensity of the pain; accordingly, extremely painful attacks in some patients may be caused by very small hemangiomalike tumors.[14, 16]

Multiple glomus tumors may be generalized over the entire cutaneous surface or disseminated within a circumscribed region. A simultaneous subungual localization is not seen as a rule. As mentioned before, painful sensations are lacking in multiple glomus tumors. The pea- to bean-sized tumors are covered by normal skin. Sometimes the lesions shine through the epidermis with a bluish tint, leading to a mistaken diagnosis of diffuse phlebectasia or deep subcutaneous multiple cavernous hemangiomas. Similarly, in generalized neurofibromatosis, neurofibromatous nod-

3. The **eccrine spiradenoma** is another cutaneous tumor characterized by pain. Its favorite locations are the face, trunk, and occasionally the extremities. The skin overlying the growth is either unchanged or has a reddish-blue or brownish-yellow hue (Fig. 656). The spiradenoma appears almost always as a solitary tumor measuring on the average 1 cm in diameter. Growing slowly, a moderately firm, protruding semispherical node will develop; it is firmly attached to the overlying skin but remains freely movable on its undersurface. A definite distinction from the glomus tumor can be made only by histologic examination. Preliminary examination of a histologic section with a magnifying glass at first suggests a solid basal cell epithelioma; however, regular microscopy shows that the parenchyma of the tumor is composed of two types of cells of different sizes. The larger cells form alveolar or tubular structures; each cell has a basophilic nucleus with fine chromatin granules and a distinct nuclear membrane. The smaller cells have small hyperchromatic nuclei. These groups of cells are separated by an underdeveloped thin membrane (Fig. 657a, b). The vicinity of the tumor fails to show any reaction.[9, 11, 13]

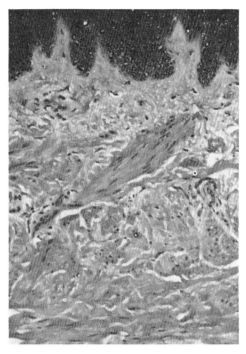

Fig. 655a. Leiomyomas: increased muscular tissue in the corium. Hematoxylin and eosin, 63×.

4. Chondrodermatitis nodularis chronica helicis involves an occasionally extremely painful "tumor"; the slightest touch, for instance, with the pillow case, causes so much pain that the patients cannot sleep on the side of the affected ear. The helix of the ear shows a lentil- to cherrystone sized flat nodule frequently covered with a central crust (Fig. 658). Histologically,

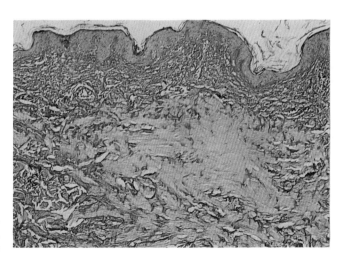

Fig. 655b. Leiomyoma: increased muscular tissue in the corium. Van Gieson, 25×.

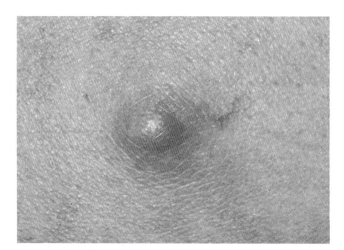

Fig. 656. Eccrine spiradenoma.

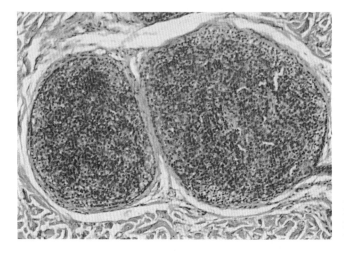

Fig. 657a. Eccrine spiradenoma: encapsulated solid tumors in the corium. Hema-
toxylin and eosin, 63×.

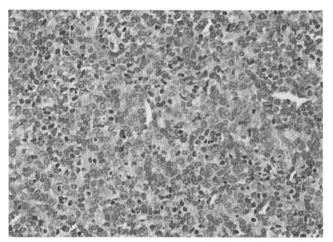

Fig. 657b. Eccrine spiradenoma: Part of 657a. Two
types of cells are recognizable: large, weakly stained
cells with chromatin-poor
nuclei and small, undifferentiated cells with nuclei showing dense chromatin. Hematoxylin and eosin, 100×.

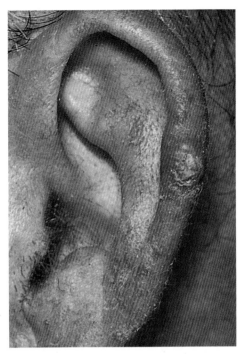

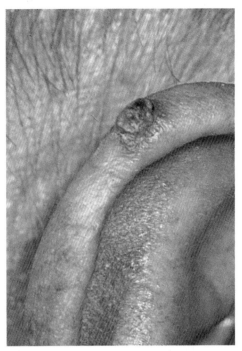

Fig. 658. Chondrodermatitis nodularis chronica helicis.

Fig. 659. Bowen's disease appearing as a painful auricular nodule.

the lesion is composed of histiocytic granulation tissue with angiomatous or endotheliomatous features. The changes of the cartilage may vary widely; definite regressions of the cartilage may occur without a corresponding development of a painful auricular node. The differential diagnosis must include squamous cell cancer, *Bowen's disease* (Fig. 659), and *senile keratosis*. Pain or lack of pain are not decisive criteria. Even with the typical location on the upper ridge of the helix, histologic proof is still required. A *gouty* auricular *tophus* is found most frequently between the free border of the helix and the antihelix; such uric acid tophi, however, develop only after systemic gout has been present for some time. The color of such tophi is a faint milky yellow and, most important, they lack the central crust of the painful tumor of chondrodermatitis nodularis (Fig. 660). However,

the gouty nodule discharges creamy or crumbly material composed of sodium urate crystals (they can be identified by the murexid test); the lesion then forms a stellate or radial scar. Nodular formations of the auricle located on locations other than the helix may be a partial manifestation of *granuloma annulare* (Fig. 661), *sarcoid, xanthomatosis,* or *calcinosis.* In addition, painless, multiple auricular nodules may have a rheumatic basis or may be the result of a marked actinic elastosis known as *"elastotic nodules of the antihelix."* [2, 8,18]

5. Even physiologically the subcutaneous fatty tissue has a lower threshold of pain due to pressure than other tissues. Marked adiposity, when there is either a generalized or proportionate increase of fatty tissue, may be accompanied by moderate sensitivity to pain caused by

Table 13 Differential Diagnosis of Painful Cutaneous Tumors

	Leiomyoma	Isolated Glomus Tumor	Systemized Glomus Tumors	Eccrine Spiradenoma	Lipomatosis Dolorosa
Localization	Trunk and extensor surface of proximal extremities	Males: arms and legs equally affected; rarely subungual. Females: arms favored; preponderantly subungual	Entire integument or segmentary distribution	Mainly face and trunk; absent on palms and soles and in areas of apocrine sweat glands	Trunk; often symmetrical on extremities
Color of skin	Pinkish-red to dark brown	Dark red to bluish-red; subungually: blue	Usually unchanged	Unchanged or bluish	Unchanged or bluish due to venectasias
Number of tumors	(a) Solitary (b) Multiple (hereditary)	Solitary	Multiple	Solitary	Multiple
Size of tumor	Diameter up to 1.5 cm	Diameter of a few mm to 2 cm	Diameter up to several cm possible	Diameter usually about 1 cm, but giant tumors (5 cm) reported	Pea- to orange-sized
Location in the skin	Corium	Corium or subcutis	Corium or subcutis	Corium, rarely extending to subcutis	Subcutis
Sensitivity	In the beginning painless; later violent paroxysms when pressed from the side	Very pronounced; spontaneous or under the influence of cold or from pressure	Usually without pain	Very pronounced	Spontaneous or on pressure
Sex distribution	Males: females – 2:1	Males: females – 1:1	Males slightly more affected than females	Males slightly more affected than females	Males: females – 1:4

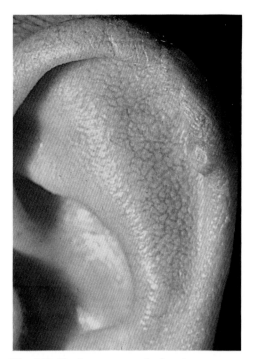

Fig. 660. Tophus composed of urates.

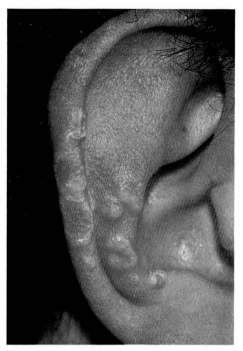

Fig. 661. Granuloma annulare of the auricle.

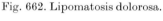

Fig. 662. Lipomatosis dolorosa.

pressure. Such "adiposis dolorosa" must be strictly separated from **lipomatosis dolorosa,** which has almost symmetrical but not equally large, nodular or bulging increases of fatty tissue (Fig. 662). Women suffer from this lipomatosis much more frequently than men, in a proportion of about 4 to 1. Most of the patients are between 30 and 50 years old. Most of the lesions are located on the extremities (arms) and trunk, while the head, hands, and feet almost always remain uninvolved. The number and size of the lipomas are extremely variable. The skin over the individual lesions is movable and can be easily lifted up. Only when a lipoma grows rapidly will the skin remain rather taut but elastic over the tumor. In contrast to indolent lipomas, the tumors of lipomatosis dolorosa grow by repeated attacks accompanied by pain. The painfulness of these lipomas is the main sign during the entire course of the disease;

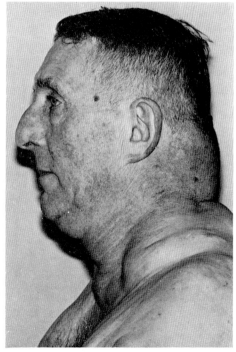

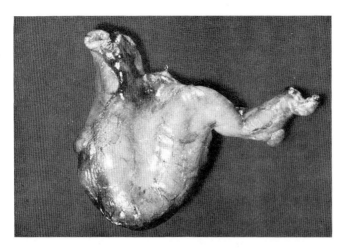

Fig. 663a. Specimen of a painful, neuroma plexiforme obtained at operation.

it may be either spontaneous pain or pain caused by pressure that is far more severe than normal. Prodromal pain and paresthesias may precede the development of lipomas by months. The spontaneous pain is described as either griping, dull, or burning and frequently is mistaken for "rheumatic" pain. Lipomatosis dolorosa has been ascribed to either constitutional factors or a disturbance of the synthesis of fatty acids. In the differential diagnosis only multiple neurinomas or generalized neurofibromatosis must be considered. The latter can be recognized by its areas of pigmentation or, should these be absent, by the histologic findings. [4, 5, 6]

The **lipomatous syndrome of the sacral bone** (subcutaneous fatty nodes in the sacroiliac area, lipomatose nodulaire circonscrite) consists of approximately cherry-sized protrusions in the sacroiliac area that are painful when pressed. This is a special localization of lipomatosis dolorosa and does not represent a special entity. Superficial examination may easily lead to a mistaken diagnosis of painful conditions of the vertebral column. [10, 15, 17]

6. Multiple neurinomas (Fig. 663a, b) and **generalized neurofibromatosis,** as mentioned before, should be considered in exceptional cases of painful tumors. Although generalized neurofibromatosis

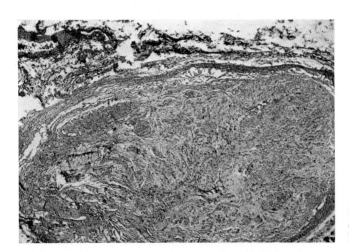

Fig. 663b. Excessive increase of thick nervous fibers. Hematoxylin and eosin.

does not present any diagnostic difficulty as a rule, neurinomas, even when they occur along the distribution of a nerve, can be definitely diagnosed only by histologic examination.

7. Myogeloses are pea-sized, not especially elastic, pressure-sensitive nodules. Because of their muscular origin, they are located deeper than lipomas; although the skin above the nodules is freely movable, at a lower level they are immovably fixed. Frequently they can be palpated on the anterior thorax within the intercostal muscles and the trapezius muscle. The nodules in the intercostal region may be mistaken for cardialgia. However, a patient will describe cardialgia as a widely painful sensation with the flat of the hand applied; myogelosis, on the other hand, will be described as a pointlike sensation with the touch of the fingertip.

8. Tietze's syndrome is caused by a painful swelling of the costal cartilages; it is discussed in Section G 13 of this chapter.

(1) BERGER, H., und M. HUNDEIKER: Multiple Glomustumoren als Phakomatose. Derm. Wschr. *153:* 673–678 (1967).

(2) CARTER,.V. H., V. S. CONSTANTINE and W. L. POOLE: Elastotic nodules of the antihelix. Arch. Derm. (Chic.) *100:* 282–285 (1969).

(3) FISHER, W. C., and E. B. HELWIG: Leiomyomas of the skin. Arch. Derm. (Chic.) *88:* 510–520 (1963).

(4) FRITZSCH, W.: Ein Beitrag zur Lipomatosis dolorosa. Arch. Geschwulstforsch. *3:* 204–212 (1951).

(5) GÜNTHER, H.: Die Lipomatose und ihre klinischen Formen. Arbeiten aus der medizinischen Klinik zu Leipzig, H. *5:* (1920).

(6) GÜNTHER, H.: Die Beziehung des Geschlechts zur Geschwulstbildung. Z. Krebsforsch. *29:* 91–111 (1929).

(7) HALTER, K., und M. HORNEMANN: Zur Genese der Schmerzempfindung in Dermatoleiomyomen. Z. Haut- u. Geschl.-Kr. *12:* 243–251 (1952).

(8) HERZBERG, J.-J.: Zur Histogenese der Chondrodermatitis nodularis helicis Winkler. Hautarzt *9:* 495–500 (1958).

(9) KERSTING, D. W., and E. B. HELWIG: Eccrine spiradenoma. Arch. Derm. (Chic.) *73:* 199–227 (1956).

(10) KORTING, G. W.: Lipomatöses Kreuzbeinsyndrom. Derm. Wschr. *137:* 394 bis 395 (1958).

(11) MUNGER, B. L., B. M. BERGHORN and E. B. HELWIG: A light- and electronmicroscopic study of a case of multiple eccrine spiradenoma. J. Invest. Derm. *38:* 289–297 (1962).

(12) NÖDL, F.: Multiple Leiomyome der Haut, ein neurocutanes Syndrom. Hautarzt *4:* 365–371 (1953).

(13) NÖDL, F.: Zur Histogenese der ekkrinen Spiradenome. Arch. klin. exp. Derm. *221:* 323–335 (1965).

(14) RODERMUND, O.-E., G. KLINGMÜLLER und Y. ISHIBASHI: Über Glomustumoren. Kasuistik und elektronenmikroskopische Befunde. Z. Haut- u. Geschl.-Kr. *44:* 1005–1014 (1969).

(15) SCHMIDT-VOIGT, J.: Das lipomatöse Kreuzbeinsyndrom. Med. Welt *1953:* 772–775.

(16) SCHNEIDER, W., und E. EISENLOHR: Über Glomustumoren. Derm. Wschr. *121:* 225–234 (1960).

(17) SUTRO, C. J.: Subcutaneous fatty nodes in sacroiliac area. Amer. J. Med. Sci. *190:* 833–837 (1935).

(18) WINKLER, M.: Knötchenförmige Erkrankung am Helix (Chondrodermatitis nodularis chronica helicis). Arch. Derm. Syph. (Wien, Leipzig) *121:* 278–285 (1916).

B. Tumors Containing Pigment

Pigmented tumors are of special interest in differential diagnosis, since the melanoma, for which only' early recognition and operative treatment offer chances for a cure, is one of them. Besides those

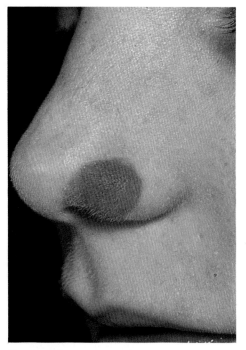

Fig. 664. Nevus cell nevus.

tionary dynamics. This is illustrated by the fact that the average number of nevus cell nevi found in persons in the third decade is 20; only about three nevus cell nevi are still present after the sixth decade, and a 90-year-old person is practically free from pigmented nevus cell nevi. This statement, however, exempts the pigment-free, persistent forms, which develop by fibrosis or impregnation with fatty tissue. The sudden appearance of new nevus cell nevi or a distinct new growth of such nevi already present is observed before puberty and above all during pregnancy, and at such times a melanoma should be ruled out. Histologically, nevus cell formations are divided into:

1. nevus cell nevi occurring in the epidermis at the border of the corium (border nevi, junction nevi).
2. nevus cell nevi occurring in the corium (dermal nevi).
3. nevus cell nevi occurring in the epidermis and in the corium (compound nevi).

Junction nevi occur primarily in childhood, compound nevi until the time of puberty, and dermal nevus cell nevi almost always in adults only. On the palms, soles, and genitals, nevus cell nevi

there are other tumors that only exceptionally or as special forms of otherwise pigment-free tumors contain increased melanin or hemosiderin.

1. The **nevus cell nevus** is characterized by astounding evolutionary and involu-

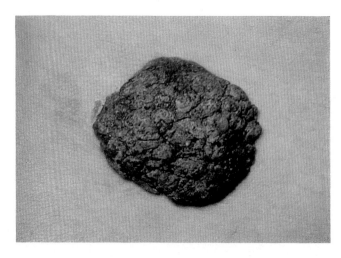

Fig. 665. Hyperkeratotic nevus cell nevus.

tumors that always contain pigment, remain at the stage of junction nevi for the rest of the person's life. In principle, however, because the varieties differ according to micromorphologic points of view, they represent various developmental phases of the single nevus cell nevus.

Nevus cell nevi are light to dark brown, sometimes almost black tumors, which are a few millimeters to a few centimeters in size, and are slightly plaquelike or semispherical and elevated. The brown color is generally homogeneous, but occasionally darker areas may be interspersed. Small nevi, especially junction nevi, have a smooth hairless surface. Later, especially in dermal nevi, they are nodular or papillomatous and often covered with particularly strong body hairs (Figs. 664, 665). Fibrosed and completely pigment-free nevus cell nevi of old people are recognizable macroscopically, usually by this increased hairiness.[21, 56, 57, 60]

Nevus cell nevi on the oral mucosa (see also Chapter 24, F3) are usually slightly elevated, have a smooth surface, and favor the palate. Their content of pigment is variable. The differential diagnosis must include, among other conditions, fibromas, neuromas, papillomas, and lipomas, and, if located near a body opening, (glassy) salivary granulomas should also be considered.[1, 58]

A **balloon cell nevus** is a special form of nevus cell nevus, which can be diagnosed only histologically. It is conceivable that a visibly lightening protrusion of a nevus cell nevus or a light yellowish halo can be explained by a balloon cell transformation. Such a change, however, requires the elimination of a melanoma. The histologic substrate of a balloon cell nevus is absolutely characteristic. The nevus cells are dilated like a honeycomb and are water-clear. The typical nevus cell structures, which are also present nearby, rule out a xanthoma. They are, however, somewhat similar to a so-called myo-

blastomyoma, which is characterized not only by epithelial hyperplasia resembling antlers and a strong rhodiochromia of the stain of the inclusions, but also by a PAS reaction which is often diastase-resistant.[7, 30, 45]

Another special form of the nevus cell nevus is the so-called **Sutton's nevus** (see also Chapter 24, A 10). Clinically, it represents a nevus cell nevus which may reach the size of a lentil and is surrounded by a wide, pigment-free halo (Fig. 369). This loss of pigment starts as a small white ring around a pre-existing nevus cell nevus and extends to a larger area. At the same time regression of the central nevus cell nevus may begin. After an interim stage consisting of an inconspicuous depigmented spot, repigmentation to match the surrounding skin color may ensue. It is not yet clear if this leukoderma represents a nevus depigmentosus, perineval vitiligo, or loss of pigment due to another cause. If, however, the central cell nevus in such a depigmented zone increases in size and protrudes further, a melanoma has to be ruled out, since it may also show perifocal depigmentation. Histologically, in Sutton's nevus there is quite often a massive lymphohistiocytic infiltration of part of the nevus cells. Heavy infiltration may render the nests of the nevus cells atypical.[26, 35]

The majority of nevus cell nevi remain less than 1 cm in diameter. An exception is the large nevus cell nevi that are always already present at birth. They are called **giant pigmented hairy nevi,** and their increased hair growth and especially dark pigmentation (Fig. 98) are conspicuous. The surface is not smooth or somewhat rough as in most nevus cell nevi but is definitely nodular and is interspersed with multiple, coarse, nodular formations, occasionally as large as peas. These giant pigmented hairy nevi at first grow only as fast as the body surface, but they may, like all nevus cell nevi, show increased growth at puberty and in pregnancy; in

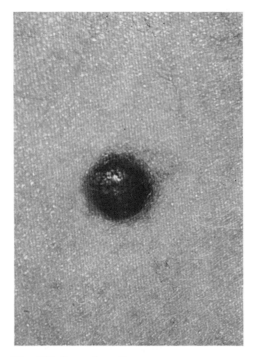

Fig. 666. Juvenile melanoma.

these instances the suddenly appearing intraneval nodules and hyperpigmentations again make a differentiation from a melanoma imperative. The earlier, often repeated statement that no melanoma arises from a giant pigmented nevus has been refuted by observations of patients. Histologically, it is composed mainly of structures of a compound nevus. Schwann's cells are also present, thus creating a certain similarity with neurofibromas. The following paragraph 3 in this section (p. 627) deals with the differential diagnostic criteria of neurocutaneous melanoblastosis.[27, 42, 44, 57]

2. Juvenile melanoma (spindle cell nevus) is a special, clinically distinct form of nevus cell nevus. It appears mostly between the third and eighth years of life, but is occasionally also observed in adults. The term "melanoma" is based less on the macroscopic than the histo-

logic similarity with that tumor. The calottelike protruding juvenile melanoma in general does not surpass a diameter of 0.8 to 1 cm. Its surface is smooth and mostly hairless, and is often covered by telangiectases. The color varies between brick-red and light brown (Fig. 666); only rarely does it assume a dark brown to blackish-brown intensity. Small tumors may be mistaken for lupus nodules because of their lupoid color, but this error may be avoided by testing for fragility with a probe. The face is favored as a site of the lesion, but juvenile melanomas may occur on any area of the body, including the mucous membranes. As a rule, the juvenile melanoma occurs as a single tumor but multiple melanomas are not infrequent (Fig. 667). They occur as aggregated nodules, which may be distributed over a circumscribed surface.

Compared to these multiple juvenile melanomas, nevoxanthoendotheliomas, which are more yellow-brownish in color and more irregularly disseminated, do not create any problem. Multiple leiomyomas cause pain from cold or pressure. Reticulosis with small nodules can be distinguished not only by the histologic picture but also by the absent irregularity of the eruptions and the patient's general well-being.

The histologic analysis (Fig. 668) shows junctional formations of large spindle cell-like cells with round or ragged nuclei and one or two nuclear bodies. The pigmentary content of the cell is not excessive. Diagnostically important are the vascular dilatations and even more, the giant cells that resemble the Touton type. Mitoses may be present, but atypical mitotic figures are absent. Distinct edematization may exist in the subepidermis. In the epidermis irregular acanthosis or pseudoepitheliomatous hyperplasia is present. Evidence of unspecific cholinesterase is sometimes characteristic of juvenile melanoma.[2, 6, 7, 22, 40]

3. If a pigmented giant hairy nevus (on the trunk) is associated with multiple nevus cell nevi, which were already present at birth, **neurocutaneous melanosis** should be considered. This phakomatosis, which favors the female sex, is accompanied by a proliferating melanocytosis of the soft cerebral and spinal meninges along the vessels of the brain; the dura, however, remains unaffected. The melanocytosis in the subarachnoid space causes closing of the arachnoidal lacunae, perineural lymph sheaths, and pacchionian granulations. This results in a massive internal hydrocephalus, and death occurs before the second year of life. Even before the developing hydrocephalus is recognized, cerebral spasms may suggest cerebral melanocytosis. In exceptional cases congenital defects of the bones of the skull are present at the same time; they appear as osseous defects covered by connective tissue of the parietal and frontal bones. These are not worn out by pressure on the calotte of the skull, as this occurs later in internal hydrocephalus.[3, 5, 33, 53]

4. There are two types of **blue nevi** (nevi caerulei), a common type and one that is filled with cells. The common type is much more frequent. It may be present at birth but may also appear for

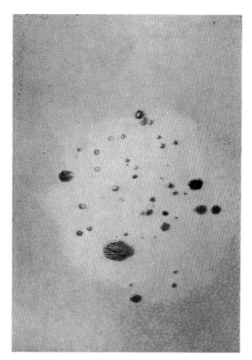

Fig. 667. Multiple juvenile melanomas.

the first time at any other time of life. Favorite locations are the face (forehead) and the extremities (backs of hands and feet). Only very rarely does a blue nevus appear on the mucous membranes. Their light to dark blue color, which is dependent on the depth of the aggregation of

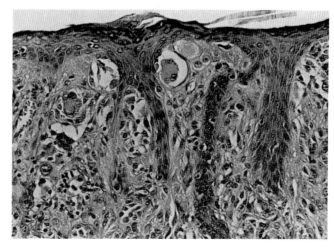

Fig. 668. Juvenile melanoma: distinct junctional activity, nestlike conglomeration of spindle-shaped and oval nevus cells and multiple giant cells with one nucleus or multiple nuclei. Hematoxylin and eosin.

melanocytes in the corium, and the relatively coarse consistency of the tumors are characteristic. The single blue nevus is rarely larger than 0.5 to 0.8 cm in diameter. Larger tumors usually belong to the cell-rich type. For the diagnosis it is important to know that the common type often has a punctiform light area or, more rarely, several whitish spots as a sign that hair follicles have been spared. The surface always remains smooth and does not show increased hair growth (Fig. 669). Occasionally, a nevus caeruleus and a nevus cell nevus, isolated as well as multiple and disseminated, may occur next to each other, and usually there are no transitional zones present. In the differential diagnosis glomus tumors, hemangiomas, pigmented basal cell epitheliomas or histiocytomas, which store hemosiderin, and, last but not least, melanomas have to be considered. In general, a histologic examination will determine the diagnosis immediately.

Fig. 669. Nevus caeruleus.

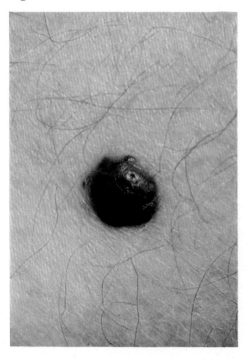

Histologically, the common nevus caeruleus shows fascicular melanocytes and abundant melanogranules in the middle corium. In addition, there are fibrocytes and melanophages and a great dispersion of collagenous fibers in these cell complexes. Occasionally, in the same tumorous tissue typical nevus cells are present as well as the melanocytes. In such a case we are dealing with a combined nevus. The cell-rich nevus caeruleus also contains, besides the spindle-shaped melanocytes, aggregations of light cells which are rich in cytoplasm and have small nuclei. Neural cells may also be part of the proliferation. Under no circumstances is one justified in making a diagnosis of melanosarcoma from areas of sarcomalike structures.

The course of the nevi caerulei is benign with rare exceptions. Malignant transformations occur only in the cell-rich type. Compared with the behavior of melanomas, the cell-rich type changes only after a long time and shows an uneven ulceration of the surface. Metastases may occur only to the regional lymph nodes, but in other patients the course is lethal because of general metastases. Histologically, the cells of the nevus caeruleus which has undergone malignant degeneration are characterized by swelling, vacuolization, and loss of the spindle shape. At the same time, pronounced polymorphism of cells and nuclei and hyperchromia of the nucleus are present. The term "melanosarcoma" should be applied, if at all, only to these malignantly degenerated nevi caerulei.[14, 18, 24, 25, 38, 47, 54]

5. Only exceptionally will a histiocytoma store so much hemosiderin that it appears as a brown pigmented tumor (Fig. 670). These **hemosiderotic histiocytomas** either are raised hemispherically above the surrounding area or are embedded within the skin; they can therefore only be recognized as hard tumors by lifting up a skin fold or by palpation.

Fig. 670. Histiocytoma
storing hemosiderin.

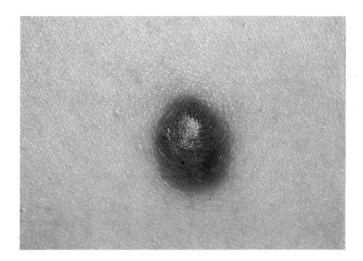

Their surface remains smooth and shows a decrease rather than an increase of hair. Furthermore, they are typically firmly adherent to the overlying skin but remain freely movable against the deeper layers. As a result, a histiocytoma may penetrate in plaquelike fashion into the telescoped skin. Like melanomas, histiocytomas may occasionally be pruritic or may develop concurrently with increased pruritus. At the site of formation an insignificant folliculitis or a minor injury (such as a prick with a thorn or similar trauma) may have preceded the histiocytoma's development. Therefore, most histiocytomas favor the distal parts of the extremities. Sometimes the lesions resemble melanomas, for occasionally the latter may be quite firm; however, there will be no diagnostic difficulty if the patient can state that the tumor has remained unchanged for decades.

Histologically, histiocytomas show more or less densely packed histiocytes and whorls of fibroblasts; the latter decrease with the increasing formation of collagen. The upper portions of the infiltrate occasionally reveal giant cells (chiefly of the Touton type), as well as foamy cells in dissolution. Frequently, histiocytomas may be covered by an atypical hyperplasia of the epithelium, chiefly as broadly tipped, somewhat bizarre acanthosis. The histiocytes of the hemosiderotic histiocytoma have a dense accumulation of brown granules; histochemically they produce a positive iron reaction.[51, 61]

Fig. 671. Basaloma, partly pigmented. Next to it are several senile warts.

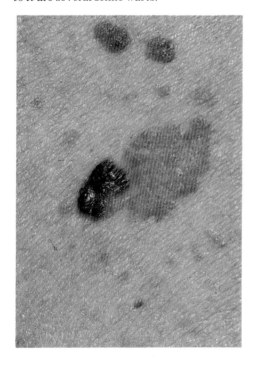

6. The **pigmented basal cell epithelioma** (basaloma) may also require differentiation from melanoma (Figs. 671, 685); the first shows intensive aggregations of pigment either as very small black nodules at the border of the tumor or throughout the entire lesion. As a whole the tumor will be either brown or blackish-blue; however, it will be interspersed with a few lighter yellow-brown nodules. Pigmented basal cell epitheliomas are found more often on the trunk than on the face; they grow slowly and, especially on the trunk, hardly ever result in marked destruction. The diagnosis of pigmented basal cell tumors can be made more readily if at least some of the edge shows a wall-like border similar to a thin string of pearls. Histologically, these pigmented tumors have an intensive accumulation of melanin within the usual structure of a basal cell epithelioma.[62]

The lesions of the **basal cell nevus syndrome** (Fig. 687) also contain a conspicuous amount of pigment (see also Section C3 in this chapter). This is especially true of the disseminated small nodular tumors of the extremities.

7. Seborrheic keratosis (verruca senilis) is as a rule a round to oval tumor resting on a broad base with overhanging edges. The entire lesion may resemble a mushroom (Fig. 672). Cutaneous areas that are subject to tension or lesions that are still at an early stage of development, however, may show a seborrheic wart located almost completely within the level of the surrounding skin. The color of the pigmentation ranges from brownish-yellow to blackish-brown. The surface of a seborrheic wart is finely granular and is covered with a fatty, crumbly hyperkeratosis; it is only in the early stages that it produces the impression of a smooth surface. A large majority of older patients show multiple seborrheic warts, especially on the trunk (anterior and posterior middle portions), and intertriginous areas (Fig. 673) and face. Diagnostic difficulty may arise only with single lesions. One should keep in mind that seborrheic warts appear only after the thirty-fifth to fortieth year of life and that the number of lesions will increase steadily during the subsequent years.

Histologically, seborrheic keratoses show an exophytic sprouting of "basaloid" cells (basal cell papilloma); these are individual cells that correspond neither to basal cell epitheliomatous cells nor to normal basal cells. Because seborrheic

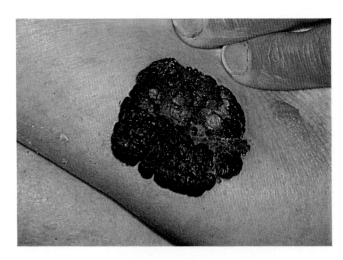

Fig. 672. Senile wart.

warts have distinct differences, they are grouped as keratotic, acanthotic, and adenoid types. The pigment is present as stored melanin within the basaloid cells. Some papillomatous forms simultaneously have many dyskeratoses or keratotic plugs. The number of mitoses is not increased. Normally, parakeratoses and cellular reactions of the stroma are absent; however, they may be present in irritated seborrheic warts. Occasionally whorl-like structures are formed within the hyperplasia of basaloid cells; they consist of keratinocytes and dendritic cells containing large amounts of pigment. Such lesions are called **melanoacanthomas** (Fig. 674). Nevus cells do not belong to the structure of this noninvasive neoplasm.

The question of malignant transformation of seborrheic warts has been discussed frequently; however, in such cases erroneous diagnoses are always based on pseudocancerous or pseudobasal cell epitheliomatous hyperplasias that are seen not infrequently with seborrheic keratoses. In addition, basal cell epitheliomas, sometimes squamous cell cancers, and melanomas may occur in the immediate vicinity of seborrheic warts. As a result of common traumas, "irritated" or "activated" types of seborrheic keratoses may occasionally

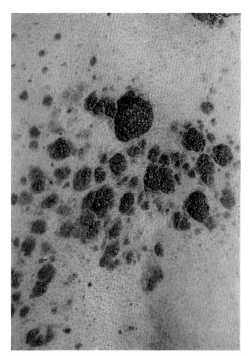

Fig. 673. Multiple senile warts.

assume the features of bowenoid hyperplasia.[4, 10, 13, 50, 55]

The differential diagnosis includes senile keratosis, a circumscribed melanosis, and melanoma. Exceptionally, a **senile keratosis** may show the same brown pigmenta-

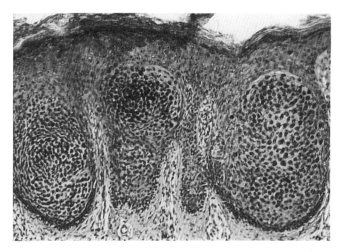

Fig. 674. Melanoacanthoma: increased pigment in epidermally located melanocytes. Hematoxylin and eosin, 63 ×.

tion as a seborrheic wart. However, even palpation will demonstrate a fundamental difference. The seborrheic wart is soft and its surface, consisting of crumbly material, can easily be scratched off. However, a senile keratosis has a hard surface like a nutmeg grater that cannot be scratched off. Also, a senile keratosis will not appear except in chronically light-exposed cutaneous regions. However, a macroscopic differentiation between a senile wart and circumscribed precancerous melanosis (lentigo maligna) may be impossible; a biopsy will have to be performed to be certain of the diagnosis. Certain clues may be available – the extreme rarity of circumscribed precancerous melanosis on the trunk, the variable intensity of pigmentation within a lesion, and the fact that, to a large extent, the surface of circumscribed precancerous melanosis is smooth. The seborrheic wart does not spontaneously regress, whereas in circumscribed precancerous melanosis such a phenomenon is definitely possible. Criteria indicative of the possible presence of a melanoma will be discussed in the section dealing with melanomas. However, if there is the slightest suspicion of a melanoma, a biopsy should not be performed in any case.*

The group of **intraepidermal epitheliomas** also requires differentiation from seborrheic warts. Two varieties of this group are intraepithelial epitheliomas of the Borst type (spinocellular cancer) and those of the Jadassohn type (intraepidermal basal cell epithelioma). Thorough examination of the structural details of tumors of the intraepidermal parts of the hair follicles and of the ducts of eccrine sweat glands has shown the previously little known range of variation of intraepithelial epitheliomas (Fig. 675). The special forms of these intraepidermal tumors will not be discussed in detail; for clinical purposes it is hardly possible to establish definite macroscopic criteria. Clinically, there are similarities with seborrheic warts, superficial basal cell epitheliomas, and Bowen's disease.[9, 29]

The **eccrine poroma**, in brief, shows the following characteristics: it occurs in the epidermal duct portion of the eccrine sweat unit; as a rule it develops slowly on the palms and soles; and it favors men

---

* In the United States, if the size or location of a suspicious lesion is a contraindication to an excisional biopsy, an incisional biopsy is performed. (Tr.)

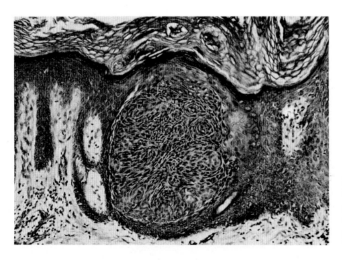

Fig. 675. Intraepidermal epithelioma: in the epidermis are vortices of aggregated epithelial cell elements, which form part of the intercellular bridges.

rather than women around the fortieth to sixtieth years of life. In this location it is frequently mistaken for a fibroma, verruca vulgaris, amelanotic melanoma, or pyogenic granuloma (granuloma telangiectaticum pediculatum benignum). The eccrine poroma has a meaty-red, reddish, or lighter hue, and occasionally a keratotic surface; it is slightly protruding or sessile, and the horny layer around the edge forms a collarette. Histologically, transitional forms to malignant porocarcinomas are seen only seldom.[31, 43, 52]

Inverted follicular keratosis (basosquamous cell acanthoma) consists of a single nodular lesion located in most cases on the upper lip and cheeks and measuring 0.2 to 1.0 cm in diameter. The grayish-brown surface is roughly keratotic and is covered with separate, small, crumbly horny spikes. The edge of such a node may have a wall-like border. The tumor develops from the infundibulum of the hair follicle and simulates invasive growth by penetrating into the epidermis.[17, 46]

The **clear cell acanthoma** is an oval, faintly red or sometimes light brown tumor, 0.5 to 1.0 cm in diameter, with a slightly scaly surface. It is most frequently located on the legs. Histologically, the epidermis shows circumscribed thickening with basal cells that lack melanin but are inconspicuous otherwise. Within a circumscribed area the cells of the epidermis have light, in part visibly empty cytoplasm. These pale keratinocytes abound in glycogen.[16, 19, 20, 59]

Histologically, **sebaceous gland adenoma** (seboadenoma) presents acanthosis, granulosis, hyperkeratosis, and epitheliomatous hyperplasia of the intradermal ductal cells of the so-called free type of sebaceous glands. The separate nodules have a diameter of from 1 to 3 mm, and when examined with a loupe, numerous yellow dots are seen on the surface.

To recapitulate: the macroscopic appearance of the previously mentioned in-

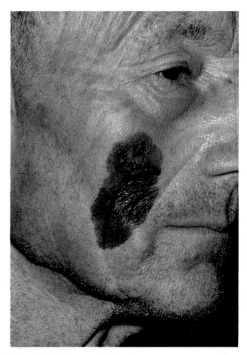

Fig. 676. Circumscribed precancerous melanosis: lentigo maligna.

traepithelial epitheliomas is not characteristic, and only their location may distinguish them from senile warts. A definite diagnosis can be made only histologically.

8. Circumscribed precancerous melanosis (lentigo maligna) is a macular pigmented lesion; only when it develops a nodular protuberance, thereby showing transition into the tumor stage of a melanoma, will it be considered here for differential diagnostic purposes. At first this disease produces a polycyclic macule with slowly enlarging borders and a washed-out light brown color; in the course of years the color becomes a speckled dark brown (Fig. 676). Not infrequently, a marked brownish-black pigmentation is present in combination with circumscribed loss of pigment. Exceptionally, partial spontaneous regressions are observed. The surface is mostly smooth and dry, but occasionally it is also covered with fine scales. Erosions or formations of crusts or bleedings, especially when combined with papillary elevations, must be considered sure signs of transition to a malignant melanoma. Marked inflammatory erythema or infiltration of one part of the lesion or of the immediate vicinity of the entire lesion are equally ominous signs.

Typical locations of circumscribed precancerous melanosis are the upper two-thirds of the face, the backs of the hands, and the extensor aspects of the forearms. However, any other parts of the body, including the mucous membranes adjacent to the skin and the genitals, may be involved. Almost without exception, patients with circumscribed precancerous melanosis are more than 30 years old. An unpigmented form of the disease would resemble Bowen's disease clinically.

Histologically, circumscribed precancerous melanosis does not show nevus cell proliferation but instead an accumulation of typical melanocytes of the dermo-epidermal junction. Simultaneously, proliferation of the rete pegs may occur as in lentigo. Only in the later stages of development will there be formation of ball-like nests composed of atypical melanocytes;

these are indicative of the progression to invasive transformation.[12, 15, 23]

9. The typical **melanoma** is a round or kidney-shaped, or sometimes a clearly polycyclic tumor (Fig. 677). With the exception of an amelanotic melanoma, it has a dark coloring from brown to blue-black. As the pigmentary content of the entire tumor is subject to great variations, light brown or skin-colored areas of the tumor may be adjacent to black parts. If the melanoma is not too dark, there are sometimes fine dark ramifications at the edge. The surface is smooth, glassy, and shiny like frog spawn, and is easily traumatized. Later it may become coarsely papillary or ulcerous. Hyperkeratotic crusts are present only seldom and transform the relatively soft melanoma into a firm tumor. Since a melanoma usually destroys the hair follicles, it is mostly hairless – that is, hairs that were previously present have fallen out. According to the distribution of the melanocytes, a primary melanoma may originate at any site of the body, and even in internal organs. Primary melanomas of the tongue and the oral and genital mucosae (Fig. 678), although rare, must be considered in the differential diagnosis of suspected pigmentary tumors of these

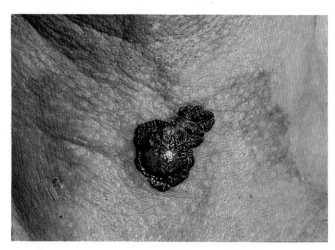

Fig. 677. Melanoma.

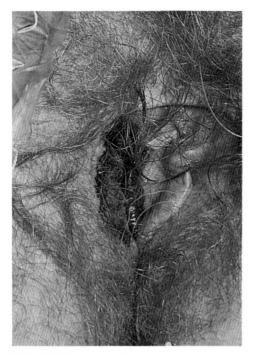

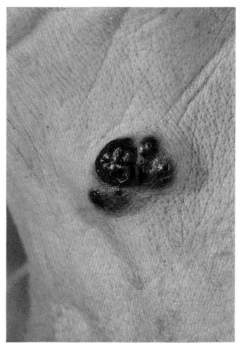

Fig. 678. Melanoma of the vulva.

Fig. 679. Melanomatous metastasis.

regions. In general, the melanoma is characterized by continuous growth and early local, regional, and generalized metastases (Figs. 679, 680). However, even in the presence of extensive, generalized metastases, as long as the vital organs remain unaffected, the course of the dis- ease may last for months or years. Unlike this typical nodular melanoma, the so- called **superficial spreading melanoma** shows adjacent proliferation and regres- sion in the primary tumor. This is rec- ognizable by the disappearance of parts of the tumor and its change to unpigment-

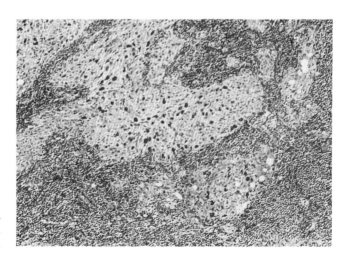

Fig. 680. Melanomatous me- tastasis in a lymph node. Hematoxylin and eosin, 63 ×.

ed, smooth areas that have regressed to the ordinary skin level. In the histologic examination also, this form of melanoma can be differentiated from primary nodular melanoma by its completely intraepidermal growth, yet fluent transitions are possible.

The incidence of the disorder increases rapidly after puberty. Melanomas in children are extremely rare, but they may reach the fetus from a diseased mother via the placenta and are, therefore, already present at birth in exceptional cases. On the other hand, there are also familial instances of the disorder. It should also be kept in mind that multiple primary melanomas may develop in the same patient. In patients with melanomas, multiple and intensely pigmented nevus cell nevi are often present, which makes the recognition of a second melanoma especially difficult.

Although a nevus cell nevus does not represent a melanotic precancerosis, nor does it undergo more frequently than at other sites a transition into a melanoma, it must be considered carefully in the differential diagnosis. A nevus cell nevus may form a suspicious protuberance on a circumscribed area, owing to intrafocal or subfocal abscess formation, the development of epidermal cysts, or a reticulohistiocytic foreign body reaction. Bleeding, another facultative sign of the melanoma, can also be observed in the nevus cell nevus after a trauma if the surface is slightly irritated. Any initially unsuspicious pigmented spot, papule, or node, which either has been present for a long time or has appeared recently, is suspicious of a melanoma if some of the following criteria develop: 1, loss of hair in the area of the preceding lesion or loss of hair of the tumor; 2, sudden change of the surface in the form of scales or crusts; 3, transition of a smooth to an irregularly nodular surface; 4, nodular or glassy frog-egg-like growth or increase in extension within weeks or a few months; 5, hemor-

rhages and ulcerous disintegration without known trauma or following common injuries; 6, intense change of sections of pigmentation to either pigment-free or dark brown to black-brown areas; 7, sudden spotting of pigmentation which had previously been homogeneous; and 8, appearance of basal or marginal erythemas as inflammatory signs or of peritumorous satellites. None of these signs alone is sure evidence of a melanoma, but it should arouse suspicion of a developing melanoma and should lead to immediate confirmation of the diagnosis by ample excision.[11, 28, 34, 39, 42, 48, 49, 57]

Even the histologic picture of the melanoma is extremely variable and may be misdiagnosed, since in places there may be a resemblance to solitary medullary carcinomas, spindle cell sarcomas, or endotheliomas. As in other malignant tumors, a melanoma loses its organoid structure early, although not always in the whole extent of the preceding lesion. Evidence of mitoses is particularly indicative of a melanoma, although absence of mitoses does not rule out the presence of a melanoma. Also, in contrast to other malignant tumors, the so-called stroma reaction may be completely absent. In general, a distinct stroma reaction can be observed only in ulcerated melanomas or in circumscribed precancerous melanosis. The amount of melanin varies not only from melanoma to melanoma but also within a lesion from one area to another. A fine loesslike washing away of melanin is characteristic of a melanoma, as is the transportation of aggregates of isolated melanin cells toward the surface. Other signs of the melanoma are those that occur in other malignant tumors, such as enlargement, distortion, or anaplasia of cells.[11, 41]

The differential diagnosis of the melanoma in certain body sites needs special consideration. Subungual or periungual melanomas may be misdiagnosed for a long time as common felons or paronychias. For the same reason, glomus tumors should be considered. If a dark spot under the nail suggests a subungual hematoma, attention should be paid to the history and whether or not the "spot" moves forward in the course of weeks, which would be typical of a hematoma. Since one should not wait this length of time, the nail can be carefully ground down so that blood coagula can be evacuated. Mycosis caused by Candida may occasionally also show a blackish discoloration of parts of the nailplate, especially if a bacterial mixed infection with *Pseudomonas aeruginosa* is present. On the heel a melanoma may for a while be misdiagnosed as a common hyperkeratosis, clavus, or "mal perforant," especially if peripheral blackish streaks or points are believed to be sequelae of preceding cauterization with silver nitrate. Finally, plantar pseudochromhidrosis may simulate a melanoma with a satellite dissemination. However, in contrast to a melanoma, these changes are predominantly bilateral. On the legs there is a possibility of confusion with angiokeratoma circumscriptum. An angiokeratoma, however, is usually firm and has a keratotic surface (Fig. 681). Under a magnifying glass single thrombosed telangiectases may sometimes be recognized. Like the benign telangiectatic granuloma, the melanoma

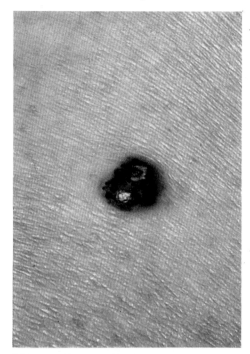

Fig. 681. Circumscribed angiokeratoma.

has a tendency toward erosions and hemorrhages. The deposits of hemosiderin of the pyogenic granuloma may simulate a melanin-containing tumor. However, the basal collarette, pedunculated growth, and the history permit the differentiation. In exceptional cases, cutaneous metas-

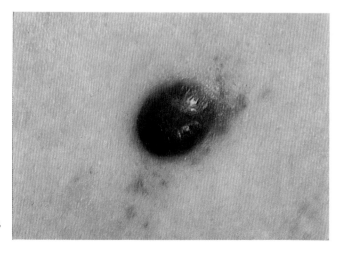

Fig. 682. Hemorrhage into a sebaceous retention cyst.

tases of a primary tumor elsewhere (e.g., a mammary carcinoma) contain so much brown pigment that they may be confused with a melanoma. Hemorrhages into a sebaceous retention cyst may lead to a suddenly enlarging blue-red tumor (Fig. 682), thus creating the suspicion of a melanoma.[32, 36]

(1) ACEVEDO, A., and C. D. LANE: Nonpigmented intradermal nevus of the gingiva. Arch. Path. (Chic.) *85:* 448–449 (1968).

(2) ALLEN, A. C.: Juvenile melanomas of children and adults and melanocarcinomas of children. Arch. Derm. (Chic.) *82:* 325–335 (1960).

(3) BALTZER, J.: Ein Beitrag zu den Melanophakomatosen. Beitr. path. Anat. *137:* 99–119 (1968).

(4) BARON, G., und H. KRESBACH: Zur Histopathologie der Verrucae seborrhoicae und zur Frage ihrer malignen Entartung. Derm. Wschr. *154:* 821–829 (1968).

(5) BATTIN, J., CL. VITAL, J. ALBERTY, J.-P. GUYONNET-DUPERAT, H. LEGER et A. FONTAN: La mélanose neurocutanée. Arch. franç. Péd. *25:* 277–289 (1968).

(6) BOURLOND, A.: Multiple juvenile Melanome. Klinische Beobachtungen mit histologischer und elektronenmikroskopischer Untersuchung. Hautarzt *22:* 144–149 (1971).

(7) BROWNSTEIN, W. E.: Multiple agminated juvenile melanoma. Arch. Derm. (Chic.) *106:* 89–91 (1972).

(8) BRUNCK, H.-J.: Über den kindlichen Blasenzellnaevus. Arch. klin. exp. Derm. *205:* 48–52 (1957).

(9) CABRÉ, J., und H. HOLZMANN: Zur morphologischen Variationsbreite der intraepidermalen Epitheliome der Haut. Derm. Wschr. *150:* 57–75 (1964).

(10) CHRISTELER, A., et J. DELACRÉTAZ: Verrues séborrhéiques et transformation maligne. Dermatologica (Basel) *133:* 33–39 (1966).

(11) CLARK, W. H. JR., L. FROM, E. A. BERNARDINO and M. C. MIHM: The histogenesis and biologic behavior of primary human malignant melanomas of the skin. Cancer Res. *29:* 705–726 (1969).

(12) COSTELLO, M. J., S. B. FISHER and CH. P. DEFEO: Melanotic freckle. Lentigo maligna. Arch. Derm. (Chic.) *80:* 753–766 (1959).

(13) CRAMER, H. J.: Verruca seborrhoica und sog. »Basosquamous Cell Acanthoma«. Arch. klin. exp. Derm. *212:* 49–63 (1960).

(14) CRAMER, H. J.: Über den »Neuro-Nevus blue« (Masson). Hautarzt *17:* 16–21 (1966).

(15) CRAMER, H. J.: Unpigmentierte Melanosis praeblastomatosa. Hautarzt *18:* 203–206 (1967).

(16) DEGOS, R., and J. CIVATTE: Clear-cell-acanthoma. Experience of 8 years. Brit. J. Derm. *83:* 248–254 (1970).

(17) DEGOS, R., J. CIVATTE, J. DELORT et S. BELAICH: »Inverted follicular keratosis.« Ann. Derm. Syph. (Paris) *95:* 23–28 (1968).

(18) DORSEY, C. S., and H. MONTGOMERY: Blue nevus and its distinction from mongolian spot and the nevus of Ota. J. Invest. Derm. *22:* 225–236 (1954).

(19) EBNER, H.: Das Klarzellakanthom (Acanthome á cellules claires). Z. Haut-u. Geschl.-Kr. *43:* 53–58 (1968).

(20) FINE, R. M., and M. E. CHERNOSKY: Clinical recognition of clear-cell acanthoma (Degos'). Arch. Derm. (Chic.) *100:* 559–563 (1969).

(21) FREEMAN, R. G., and J. M. KNOX: Epidermal cysts associated with pigmented nevi. Arch. Derm. (Chic.) *85:* 590–594 (1962).

(22) GARTMANN, H.: Das sog. juvenile Melanom. Münch. med. Wschr. *104:* 587–592; 633–635 (1962).

(23) GARTMANN, H.: Besteht ein histologischer Unterschied zwischen der präblastomatösen Melanose und dem »activated junctional nevus« (Allen)? Ein Beitrag zur Entstehungsweise des Melanoms. Hautarzt *13:* 507–511 (1962).

(24) GARTMANN, H.: Neuronaevus bleu Masson – cellular blue nevus Allen. Arch. klin. exp. Derm. *221:* 109–121 (1965).

(25) GARTMANN, H., und G. LISCHKA: Maligner blauer Naevus (Malignes dermales Melanocytom). Hautarzt *23:* 175–178 (1972).

(26) GOLDMAN, L., R. G. WILSON, R. GLASGOW and R. RICHFIELD: Perilesional leucoderma in metastatic melanoma. Acta derm.-venereol. (Stockh.) *47:* 369–372 (1967).

(27) GOODMAN, R. M., J. CAREN, M. ZIPR-
KOWSKI, B. PADEH, L. ZIPRKOWSKI and
B. E. COHEN: Genetic considerations in
giant pigmented hairy naevus. Brit. J.
Derm. *85:* 150–157 (1971).

(28) HERFERT, O.: Das Melanom der Mundhöhle als maligner Primärtumor. Stoma
(Heidelberg) *1962:* 38–63.

(29) HOLUBAR, K.: Das intraepidermale
Epitheliom (sog. Borst-Jadassohn): Ver-
körpert dieser Begriff eine Entität im
histopathologischen Sinne oder nicht?
Z. Haut- u. Geschl.-Kr. *44:* 391–418
(1969).

(30) HORNSTEIN, O.: Zur Kenntnis des sogenannten Blasenzellnaevus. Arch. klin.
exp. Derm. *226:* 97–110 (1966).

(31) HYMAN, A. B., and M. H. BROWNSTEIN:
Eccrine poroma. An analysis of forty-
five new cases. Dermatologica (Basel)
138: 29–38 (1969).

(32) JUHLIN, L., and B. PONTÉN: Plantar
pseudochromohidrosis simulating malignant melanoma. Acta derm.-venereol.
(Stockh.) *47:* 255–258 (1967).

(33) KETELS-HARKEN, H.: Zur Kasuistik der
neurokutanen Melanoblastose. Zbl. allg.
Path. *104:* 396–403 (1963).

(34) KLEEMANN, W.: Das multiple primäre
maligne Melanoblastom. Z. Haut- u.
Geschl.-Kr. *43:* 677–682 (1968).

(35) KOPF, A. W., S. D. MORRILL and I. SIL-
BERBERG: Broad spectrum of leuko-
derma acquisitum centrifugum. Arch.
Derm. (Chic.) *92:* 14–35 (1965).

(36) KORTING, G. W.: Mammacarcinom-
Metastasen der Kopfhaut mit pigmen-
tierten Dendritenzellen. Arch. klin. exp.
Derm. *214:* 504–512 (1962).

(37) KORTING, G. W.: Ungewöhnlich zentral
protuberierender Sutton-Naevus. Med.
Welt (Stuttg.) *1965:* 2562.

(38) KORTING, G. W.: Über nachbarschaft-
liches Vorkommen von Blauem Naevus
und Pigmentnaevus in isolierter wie
disseminierter Weise. Z. Haut- u.
Geschl.-Kr. *42:* 1–4 (1967).

(39) KORTING, G. W., und G. BREHM:
Multiples primäres und familiäres Melanom. Z. Haut- u. Geschl.-Kr. *44:* 87–90
(1969).

(40) KORTING, G. W., G. BREHM und F.
NÜRNBERGER: Zur klinischen Variationsbreite des sog. juvenilen Melanoms.
Z. Haut- u. Geschl.-Kr. *43:* 233–238
(1968).

(41) KORTING, G. W., H. HOLZMANN und
N. HOEDE: Bemerkungen zur Stroma-
reaktion beim Melanom. Med. Welt *18*
(N.F.): 1786–1794 (1967).

(42) KREYSEL, H. W., F. SCHANDELMAIER,
P. J. UNNA und E. WOTZKA: Malignes
Melanom auf Tierfellnaevus. Z. Haut- u.
Geschl.-Kr. *39:* 66–75 (1965).

(43) KRINITZ, K.: Malignes intraepidermales
ekkrines Porom. Z. Haut- u. Geschl.-Kr.
47: 9–17 (1972).

(44) KRINITZ, K., und K.-D. WOZNIAK:
Malignes Melanom und Tierfell-Naevus.
Derm. Mschr. *158:* 130–139 (1972)

(45) LEWIS, B. L.: Clinical appearance of a
balloon cell nevus. Arch. Derm. (Chic.)
100: 312–313 (1969).

(46) MEHREGAN, A. H.: Inverted follicular
keratosis. Arch. Derm. (Chic.) *89:*
229–235 (1964).

(47) MERKOW, L. P., R. C. BURT, D. W.
HAYESLIP, F. J. NEWTON, M. SLIFKIN
and M. PARDO: A cellular and malignant
blue nevus. Cancer *24:* 888–894 (1969).

(48) MILLER, A. S., and P. A. PULLON:
Metastatic malignant melanoma of the
tongue. Arch. Derm. (Chic.) *103:*
201–205 (1971).

(49) MILLER, T. R., and G. T. PACK: The
familial aspect of malignant melanoma.
Arch. Derm. (Chic.) *86:* 35–39 (1962).

(50) MISHIMA, Y., and H. PINKUS: Benign
mixed tumor of melanocytes and malpighian cells. Arch. Derm. (Chic.) *81:*
539–550 (1960).

(51) NIEMI, K. M.: The benign fibrohistiocytic tumours of the skin. Acta derm.-
venereol. (Stockh.) *50:* Suppl. 63, 1–66,
(1970).

(52) PINKUS, H., and A. H. MEHREGAN: Das
ekkrine Porom und seine klinischen
Varianten. Hautarzt *15:* 561–562 (1964).

(53) REED, W. B., S. W. BECKER, S. W.
BECKER JR. and W. R. NICKEL: Giant
pigmented nevi, melanoma, and lepto-
meningeal melanocytosis. Arch. Derm.
(Chic.) *91:* 100–119 (1965).

(54) RODRIGUEZ, H. A., and L. V. ACKER-
MAN: Cellular blue nevus. Clinicopatho-
logic study of forty-five cases. Cancer
(N.Y.) *21:* 393–405 (1968).

(55) SANCHEZ YUS, E., y P. SIMON HUARTE:
Verruga seborreica y melanoacantoma.
Son ambos tumores una misma cosa?
Actas dermo-sif. (Madr.) *60:* 73–87
(1969).

(56) SAYLAN, T., R. MARKS and E. WILSON-JONES: Fibrous papule of the nose. Brit. J. Derm. *85:* 111–118 (1971).

(57) SCHAUER, A., und A. VOGEL: Die Pigmentgeschwülste. Untersuchungen über das biologische Verhalten. Med. Welt *18* (N.F.): 101–109; 149–159 (1967).

(58) WEATHERS, D. R.: Benign nevi of the oral mucosa. Arch. Derm. (Chic.) *99:* 688–692 (1969).

(59) WELLS, G. C., and E. WILSON-JONES: Degos' acanthoma (acanthome á cellules claires). A report of five cases with particular reference to the histochemistry. Brit. J. Derm. *79:* 249–258 (1967).

(60) WINKELMANN, R. K., and G. ROCHA: The dermal nevus and statistics. An evaluation of 1200 pigmented lesions. Arch. Derm. (Chic.) *86:* 310–315 (1962).

(61) WORINGER, F.: L'histiocytome hémosidérique de Diss. Bull. Soc. franç. Derm. Syph. *60:* 339–341 (1953).

(62) ZELICKSON, A. S.: The pigmented basal cell epithelioma. Arch. Derm. (Chic.) *96:* 524–527 (1967).

C. Predominantly Facial Tumors

Many of the facial tumors to be discussed here also occur on other parts of the body. In a typical case, however, they favor the facial region with some regularity, so that such a manifestation leads to differential diagnostic considerations. Localization on the face is encountered on the one hand in primary malignant tumors (squamous cell and basal cell epitheliomas, sarcomas, and especially reticulum cell sarcomas), on the other hand in metastatic tumors, and finally, in the development of tumors arising from adjacent parts of the body. In addition, some phakomatoses such as Pringle's disease (sebaceous adenoma), cylindroma, and the basal cell nevus syndrome are frequently located on the face.

1. Basal cell epitheliomas occur on the face in about 80 to 90 per cent of cases and on the scalp in only about 2 per cent. After the face, the next most frequent location is the skin of the trunk, with an incidence of about 5 per cent of all basal cell epitheliomas.

Some special types have been mentioned before: the pigmented basal cell epithelioma in the preceding section B6, the ulcerated basal cell epithelioma (rodent ulcer) and the "ulcus terebrans" in Chapter 33, A1, and the sclerosing morphealike basal cell epithelioma in Chapter 16, A6; the multiple basal cell epithelioma of the trunk is discussed in the following section G10.

The basal cell epithelioma is supposedly derived either from the normal epithelial cells or from the so-called primary epithelial germ cell, and an important role in the development of this disorder may also be ascribed to the adjacent connective tissue. The basal cell epithelioma is fundamentally an epithelial tumor attached to the epithelium spreading into the corium. The character of the basal cell epithelioma as a hamartoma is also substantiated by the absence of a tendency to metastases. In extremely rare cases and only with an especially long period of active growth, the basal cell epithelioma may "become wild" – that is, it will change into an aggressive carcinoma. In such a case we are dealing with a basal cell cancer with all the biological attributes of a genuine malignant neoplasm of the epidermis.

As a rule the typical basal cell epithelioma is an isolated tumor favoring the upper half of the face (cheeks, alae nasi, temporal region) (Fig. 683). As opposed to the squamous cell cancer, which occurs especially often on the lower lip, the basal cell epithelioma develops more frequently on the upper lip (Fig. 684). On the scalp it often occurs in the immediate vicinity of a sebaceous nevus or a syringocystadenoma papilliferum (Fig. 685). An isolated basal cell epithelioma grows so slowly that several years may elapse before a distinctly visible tumor has developed. In most cases the tumor is very hard and may be so slightly elevated

Fig. 683. Nodular basaloma.

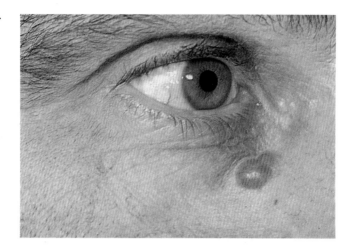

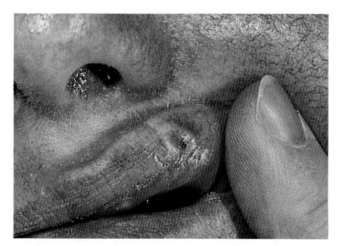

Fig. 684. Nodular basaloma
of the vermilion border.

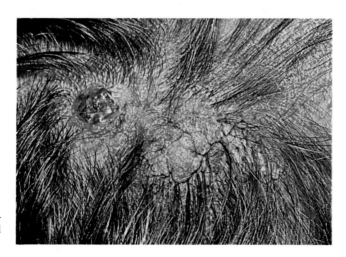

Fig. 685. Pigmented basaloma in a sebaceous gland
nevus.

above the level of the surrounding skin that only upon stretching of the skin will it become more distinctly visible; later it is possible to visualize one or more grayish-red to pearl gray, smooth and faintly shiny nodules. As these nodules form the edge of the tumor, the center has an umbilicated depression; later this center will develop into the characteristic flat epithelial defect that forms the ulcerated basal cell epithelioma (ulcus rodens). As further growth of the tumor as an isolated node occurs, or as the peripheral nodules increase to about pinhead size, slowly growing, long extended telangiectases become visible; they appear initially within the surrounding skin and then cover the tumor. The development of these telangiectases is purely mechanical by extension of the papillary body over the growing nodular tumor in the corium; such telangiectases can be observed over any node enlarging in the corium and have no special significance. Although basal cell epitheliomas can be diagnosed relatively easily, even macroscopically, histologic proof should be secured in order to avoid confusion with such conditions as cutaneous metastases of carcinomas of the inner organs, the different tumors originating from cutaneous appendages, and senile hyper-

plasias of sebaceous glands (see also Section C13). It is especially difficult to distinguish retention cysts of Moll's glands (ciliary glands of the conjunctiva) from small basal cell epitheliomas of the eyelids and the ciliary border. **Syringomas of the lids** frequently grow as large as pinheads in a few weeks. Their semispherical surface either is inconspicuous or has a waxy shine and is covered with individual telangiectases. Lateral transillumination will show a cystic lesion. The lower lids are affected more frequently and often in a conspicuously symmetrical fashion.[12, 13, 20, 21, 23, 25, 40, 42, 74]

2. Pseudorecurrences following contact radiotherapy, not only of basal cell epitheliomas but also of other cutaneous tumors, have been observed; they require careful distinction from further continuous peripheral growth of the original tumor. Such pseudorecurrences begin days or a few weeks after the erosive reaction and are characteristically limited to the edge of the cone. The always circular wall diminishes steeply in the center but gradually toward the edge; its consistency is variable. Seldom will it become as hard as a basal cell epitheliomatous node. The epithelial covering of a pseudorecurrence

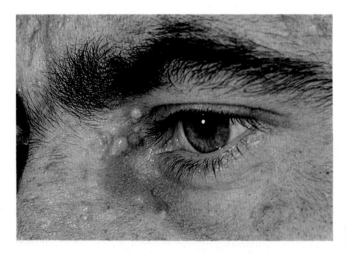

Fig. 686. Basal cell nevus syndrome: multiple small nodular basalomas.

may be affected by the erosive reaction or it may remain unaffected. Telangiectases are absent. Regression takes place after a few weeks with no therapy. Histologically, one observes a papillary epithelial hyperplasia similar to a seborrheic wart or a keratoacanthoma.[17, 49]

3. The **basal cell nevus syndrome** is characterized by the familial occurrence of multiple (up to 100 or more) basal cell epitheliomas in early childhood or adolescence. In contrast to the likewise multiple epitheliomas of the trunk that result from chronic arsenical intoxication, those of the basal cell nevus syndrome occur as nodular, partly pigmented lesions not restricted to the trunk (Figs. 686, 687). The closely adjacent nodes of this syndrome are found primarily on the face (nasolabial folds, forehead, and eyelids), the back of the neck, forearms, and thighs. Obviously, chronically light-exposed areas are not favored sites, in contrast to the locations of "common" basal cell epitheliomas. The rate of growth of these nevoid tumors is especially slow and they may remain stationary in size for years. On the other hand, some of these lesions may suddenly change without apparent cause into an expansive stage of growth with widespread ulceration and destruction. In addition to the characteristic morphologic cutaneous findings, there are a number of associated signs that appear with various degrees of regularity. The pitted lesions of the palms and soles that are occasionally observed are discussed in Chapter 28, D3. The maxilla and the mandible regularly show multiple cysts. These are solely follicular cysts which in exceptional cases may degenerate into fibrosarcomas or ameloblastomas (neuroectodermal tumor). In the skeletal system frequent signs are costal synostoses, absence of some ribs, forked ribs, cervical ribs, occult spina bifida, and congenital kyphoscoliosis. Many patients with the basal cell nevus syndrome are mentally retarded or have psychic anomalies. Organic brain diseases such as hydrocephalus or, very often, calcification of the falx cerebri and the plexus chorioideus have been encountered. Also noteworthy are calcifications of the ovary as well as ovarian fibromas and mesenteric cysts. Some patients with this syndrome have, in addition, a disturbance of the tubular phosphate reabsorption as seen in pseudohyperparathyroidism.

The basal cell nevus syndrome is inherited as an autosomal dominant trait

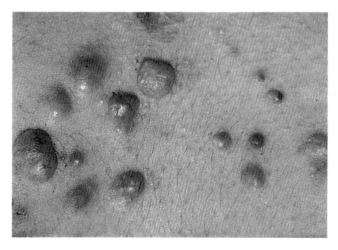

Fig. 687. Basal cell nevus syndrome: multiple nodular basalomas.

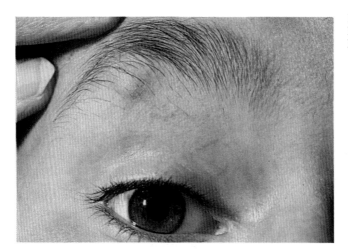

Fig. 688. Calcifying epithelioma in the area of the lateral part of the eyebrows.

with variable expressivity. On the one hand, the cerebral and osseous signs may be present even before the appearance of the basal cell epitheliomas; on the other hand, in abortive cases these signs may be the only pathological findings. Analysis of chromosomes so far has shown only unremarkable karyotypes. The various proven changes of the chromosomes (breaks or recombinations) in fibroblastic and lymphocytic cultures, however, may be considered an expression of an increased disposition toward malignant transformation.[8, 9, 26, 27, 33, 38, 72, 86, 90]

4. A calcified epithelioma (pilomatricoma, Malherbe's calcifying epithelioma) is a tumor located in the deep corium or in the subcutis; macroscopically it can be suspected but not diagnosed with certainty. The tumor is a suborganoid hamartoma deriving from the matrix cells of the intrafollicular portion of the hair follicle; this explains the frequent presence of pilomatricomas on the head (periorbital region – Fig. 688) and their absence on the palms and soles. Other sites of predilection are the extensor aspects of the upper arms and the upper trunk. The tumor is solitary and is seldom larger than a bean; exceptionally, multiple calcifying epitheliomas have been observed. Because

this tumor is discovered only after it has reached a certain size, and even then only accidentally, definite information as to the age of the patient at the beginning of the lesion's development does not exist. In any case it is not infrequently observed even in childhood. The tumor itself is rather hard and after long duration may assume an osseous consistency. It is easily movable on its base, and the epidermis over the tumor is not fixed. In general, the skin overlying the pilomatricoma shows only a suggestion of a yellow or gray hue. A definite diagnosis depends entirely on the characteristic histologic findings. The tumor is encapsulated by connective tissue containing masses of basophilic cells, which slowly lose their basophilic granula and change into shadow cells with increasing eosinophilia. These eosinophilic shadow cells have well-defined cellular borders but only visibly empty centers corresponding in size to the former nuclei of the cells. Calcified granula are also deposited within the shadow cells, with formation of bone (containing bone marrow) in the immediate vicinity of the solid masses of shadow cells. The formation of bone is due to the presence of osteoblasts developing from the stroma of the tumor; these osteoblasts are not derived from the shadow cells. Frequently, hair folliclelike structures and sebaceous glandular cells are observed between the components of the tumor. The differential diagnosis must include lipomas, osteomas, hard fibromas, and dermoid cysts.[53, 62, 68, 93, 94]

5. Extraoral dental fistulas are discussed in Chapter 14, B1. Here it should be emphasized again that during an interval with only mild inflammation such odontogenous fistulas have relatively soft, erythematous nodules; at this time a fistulous duct may not be evident. The skin over the mandibles and the region of the chin are characteristic locations. Unusual sites, such as the infraorbital region and the neck, do not exclude a diagnosis of dental fistula. After a longer period the growth is firmly attached to its base and its center is slightly retracted. Histologic examination will generally show only unspecific granulation tissue, but it may be accompanied by marked pseudoepitheliomatous hyperplasia, simulating a malignant tumor. On the other hand, lymphadenosis benigna cutis (lymphocytoma cutis), facial eosinophilic granuloma, sarcoid, and lupus vulgaris can be excluded in most cases without difficulty. The starting point of extraoral dental fistulas must be looked for in carious, devitalized, or partly infected teeth; with the collaboration of a dentist there should be no special problems.[7, 61]

6. Osteosis cutis multiplex is a rare disorder consisting of multiple primary osteomas of the face. Multiple skin-colored nodules with no preceding lesions favor the forehead, cheeks, and chin and are occasionally observed on the thorax and the extremities. They only rarely exceed a diameter of 5 mm and are conspicuously hard. Because of their deep location, some of the nodules are first detected by palpation. There are no accompanying disturbances of the calcium metabolism. If the osteomas remain very small, they may easily be mistaken for milia. The diagnosis can be confirmed only histologically. Osteomas of the skull differ from osteosis cutis multiplex in that they originate from secondary bones. Multiple primary cutaneous osteomas have been observed in association with multiple exostoses.[18, 22, 73, 85, 96]

Gardner's syndrome is composed of fibromas, sebocystadenomas, and primary osteomas of the skin. The multiple cysts and connective tissue tumors also occur primarily on the head, but the tumors become considerably larger than those of osteosis cutis multiplex. Occasionally, atheromas occur on the trunk. The osteomas do not appear on the skin only as heterotopic bone formations but are also found in the skeletal system, the mandible and skull calotte being affected most frequently. The long bones, ribs and pelvic bones are only occasionally affected by osteomas, but they sometimes exhibit exostoses. In radiographs osteomas appear as smoothly limited osseous shadows of bone density. Another important sign of Gardner's syndrome is intestinal polyposis. The colon is chiefly affected but single, small polyps may be present throughout the entire small intestine. The presence of intestinal polyposis may be significant, since in about 50 per cent of cases malignant degeneration occurs. Inheritance in Gardner's syndrome is autosomal dominant, and attention should be given especially to cases showing only two signs. Of the three main signs: osseous tumors, intestinal polyposis, and cutaneous tumors, the last shows the greatest variation in manifestations.[19, 24, 45, 70]

7. In the differential diagnosis of small nodular tumors in the facial area, the **trichoepithelioma** (Fig. 689) should be mentioned first because of its histologic similarity to the basal cell epithelioma. It occurs as either solitary or multiple tumors on the face, trunk, or extremities.

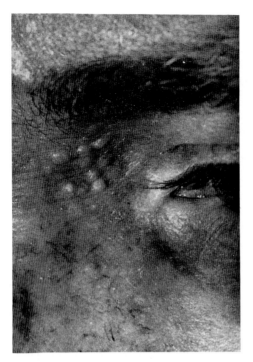

Fig. 689. Trichoepithelioma adenoides cysticum.

The multiple forms often occur in families, simultaneously or alternately in the sibship with cylindromas; for this phenomenon the term Brooke-Spiegler's phako-matosis (Fig. 690) is useful. Favored sites on the face are the nasolabial folds, the eyelids, and the upper lip. Other than in localization and multiplicity, the two varieties of trichoepitheliomas do not vary from each other either macroscopically or microscopically. The tumors are skin-colored and hemispherical and grow no larger than the size of a lentil. The surface is smooth and, except for a few telangiectases, does not show erosions or ulcerations. If epithelial defects develop on top of such a trichoepithelioma, a change into a basal cell epithelioma of the rodent ulcer type is likely. Multiple trichoepitheliomas often appear for the first time peripubertally. A single tumor is limited in its growth, but additional tumors may appear during the patient's life.

Histologically, there are tumors in the corium consisting of epithelial cells as well as several horny cysts. Keratinization in the horny cysts is fully mature and shows no parakeratosis. The surrounding epithelial tissue corresponds to the cellular elements of a basal cell epithelioma. Besides the horny cysts, occasional immature hair follicle structures are also present.[4, 30, 50]

Fig. 690. Pedigree of a family whose members show cylindromas and trichoepitheliomas.

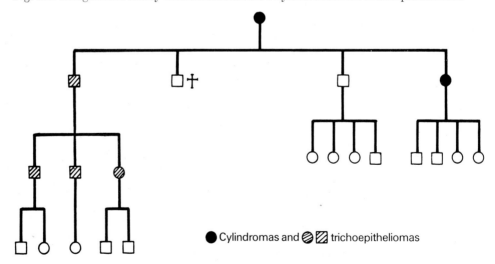

● Cylindromas and ⊘ ▨ trichoepitheliomas

8. Multiple small facial tumors on the root of the nose, nostrils, or eyelids may prove histologically to be **fibrillary neurinomas.** Some patients show macrocheilia simultaneously and therefore the presence of a Melkersson-Rosenthal syndrome is considered first. The cutaneous changes are not always present, but pinhead- to pea-sized firm nodules on the tongue and the vestibulum oris are seen regularly. Cutaneous and mucosal nodules develop chiefly in the first year of life, but subsequent primary manifestations are not unusual. Several irregularly associated signs such as the underdevelopment of the skeletal muscles, genital hypoplasias, centrofacial lentiginosis, or malformations of the foot suggest a complex syndrome of malformations. Histologically, there are clusters of nerve bundles with sheaths of connective tissue and myelinated or demyelinated nerve fibers.[5, 43, 82]

These neurinomas of the lingual, oral, and conjunctival mucous membranes are part of a *mucous membrane neurinoma – carcinoma syndrome.* The neurinomas of the mucous membranes may precede the development of carcinomas of the thyroid gland or adrenal medulla by many years. It is therefore necessary to examine these patients thoroughly for tumors. It should be kept in mind that we are dealing with iodide-inactive thyroid carcinomas.

9. Multiple eruptive milia may also lead to multiple, symptomless facial nodules. In a generalized eruption of milia these elements may also occur on the extremities (extensor and flexor sides) and on the trunk. Familial cases are not unusual. The individual lesion is an isolated, 1 to 5 mm hemispherical nodule, which occasionally has a central comedo (Fig. 691). Otherwise the surface remains unchanged. The whitish-yellow color of these nodules identifies them as milia, but the cyst formation may lie so deep that the skin has a normal color. In contrast to cysts in chloracne and trichoepitheliomas, the milia have rather firm nodules. If the milia are carefully opened with a scalpel, the inner horny mass is easily removed. Histologically, cysts that either originate in the follicle or are isolated in the corium show an epidermislike, stratified structure (stratum spinulosum and stratum granulosum). The content of the cysts consists of horny lamellae with a variable density.[83, 87]

10. In the discussion of the differential diagnosis of basal cell epitheliomas, syrin-

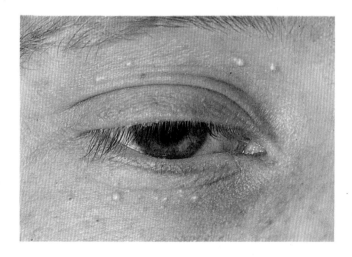

Fig. 691. Multiple milia.

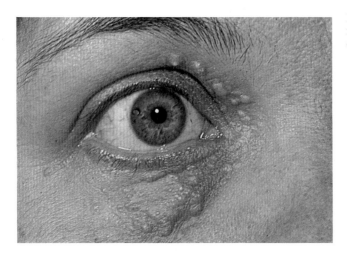

Fig. 692. Multiple syringomas in the area of the inner
canthus.

gomas of the eyelids have already been
considered, so that here only a discussion
of **multiple syringomas** is still necessary.
The histologic findings in the syringomas
at various locations are the same. Multiple
syringomas develop above the orifice of
the sebaceous gland at the point of the
hair follicle where the apocrine glands
originate. Syringomas can occur, therefore, only in those areas in which apocrine
sweat glands are present. Favorite sites
are the lower eyelids, the inner canthus,
the neck, and the ventral upper part of
the thorax. Multiple syringomas are also
present, but only exceptionally, in the

genital area. Occasionally, syringomas
occur in families. The nodules are 1 to
3 mm in size and slightly elevated (Figs.
692, 693). The cystic character is not as
apparent on the trunk as it is on the margin
of the lid. Because the individual soft
nodules may be clumped as in flowerbeds
and may assume a light brown color,
they may be mistaken for plane juvenile
warts. Aside from the characteristic distribution, the diagnosis can be ascertained
only by histologic examination.

11. Small plane juvenile warts hardly
rise above the level of the surrounding

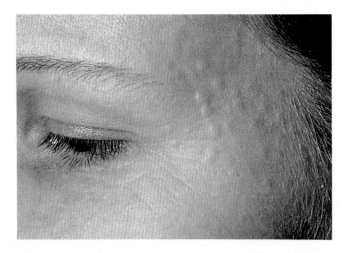

Fig. 693. Multiple syringomas in the temporal area.

skin and frequently have an isomorphic linear distribution. They are a clinical modification of the papovavirus infection in association with a moderate peripheral disturbance of vascularization. It is, therefore, not by chance that the same patients also have common warts simultaneously. Plane juvenile warts are especially typical in children and adolescents. They never occur as solitary lesions, but develop in groups on the forehead, cheeks, chin, or the backs of the hands. Unusually numerous disseminated warts are called verrucae disseminatae or *verrucosis generalisata*. In general, they are pinhead-sized, round or polygonal, flat epidermal lesions; occasionally they are slightly pruritic and have a solid to hard consistency (Fig. 694). They can easily be scratched off, leaving a small, point-sized, psoriasiform bleeding area. The surface of these warts is smooth – only older lesions are slightly verrucous. They are sometimes slightly yellowish, but not so yellow that one would consider them recently erupted xanthomas or syringomas. These, however, are distinctly symmetrical from the beginning. In older persons seborrheic warts on the backs of the hands occasionally suggest plane juvenile warts. Finally, it may be difficult to distinguish between a plane juvenile wart and a common wart whose development is unfinished and which does not yet possess a distinctly papillomatous surface. When located on the face there may be similarities with lichen planus papules because their color in this location is only slightly saturated and thus lighter than on other sites. These warts remain inconspicuous and, because of their smallness, they appear more roundish than polygonal in new eruptions. Also, lichen planus lesions on the face are not pruritic nor do they show Wickham's striae.

12. Eccrine hidrocystomas (eccrine syringocystadenomas) also occur in multiple lesions and in the middle of the face,

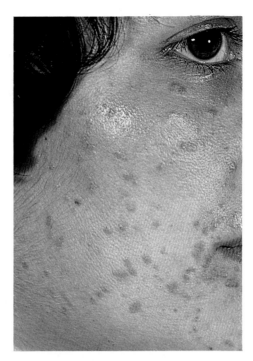

Fig. 694. Plane juvenile warts.

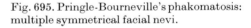

Fig. 695. Pringle-Bourneville's phakomatosis: multiple symmetrical facial nevi.

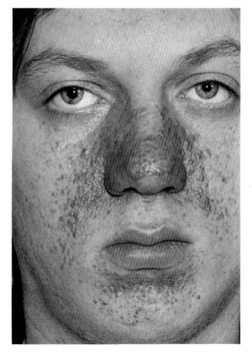

especially on the nose. They swell with heavy perspiration, disappear in cold weather, and are found mainly in individuals with a special tendency to hyperhidrosis. If the semispherical, pinhead-sized lesions are opened, sweat is released. In contrast to syringomas, eccrine syringocystadenomas are cystic dilatations of the eccrine sweat glands.[39]

13. Pringle's tumors (so-called adenoma sebaceum) are also multiple small tumors of the face. In the framework of Pringle-Bourneville's phakomatosis, these facial nevi with their centrofacial location constitute the most important dermatologic sign. The individual nodules usually do not exceed pinhead size and remain skin-colored as a rule (Fig. 695). If, however, telangiectatic vascular dilatations are also present, the tumors assume a reddish appearance. These pinhead- to pea-sized and soft tumors are disseminated most densely in the middle of the face. In the histologic picture no uniform substrate is found. According to the predominant tissue, they may be either connective tissue or vascular tumors; the latter may also contain parts of sebaceous glands.

Other important cutaneous changes of Pringle-Bourneville's phakomatosis are discussed elsewhere: macrulia in Chapter 15, 3, depigmentations in Chapter 24, A5, lumbosacral shagreen skin in Chapter 38, G23, and periungual fibromas in Chapter 38, I12.

The internal organs may be affected in various ways, including cerebral tuberous sclerosis with calcification of the basal ganglia, renal angiomas and angiofibromas, rhabdomyomas of the cardiac muscles, cysts of the skeletal system, and fibroses, cysts, and hamartomas of the lungs. A correct diagnosis of the changes of the internal organs is only possible if the cutaneous findings are known. Pringle-Bourneville's phakomatosis is inherited as an autosomal dominant trait and varies greatly in expressivity. It may be combined with generalized neurofibromatosis (Fig. 696).[16, 37, 63, 65, 88]

14. Older patients often have small, yellow-white papules with a central depression on the forehead and cheeks. These are **circumscribed senile hyperplasias of the sebaceous glands.** They appear mainly as individual or, more rarely, multiple nodules (Figs. 697a, b). The surface remains smooth and the appearance of blood vessels, which are accentuated at the margins, may result in confusion with a beginning basal cell epithelioma. A senile hyperplasia of the sebaceous

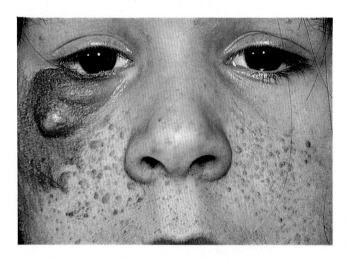

Fig. 696. Pringle-Bourneville's phakomatosis in combination with generalized neurofibromatosis.

Fig. 697a. Senile hyperplasia of the sebaceous glands: multiple lesions on the forehead.

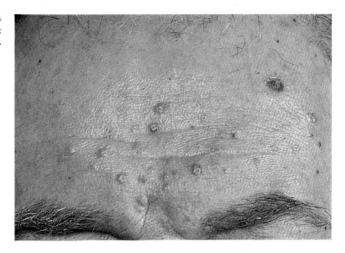

glands always remains, in contrast to a basal cell epithelioma, a soft nodule that does not ulcerate. The patients who are affected belong to the constitutional seborrheic type of individual who rather frequently shows simultaneously a more or less pronounced rhinophyma. Under magnification the entire yellow-white nodule is composed of numerous single stipples, which on the surface correspond to the subepidermally located parts of the sebaceous glands.[1]

15. Among the malignant tumors of the cutaneous appendices we also find the **sebaceous adenocarcinoma** which occurs often in the area of the eyelids, where it originates in the meibomian glands. Other common sites are the face and scalp, but it may originate in other places as well. Clinically it is a poorly defined, yellowish or yellow-reddish protuberant tumor with a verrucous surface. The tumor often ulcerates, and occasionally vermiottelike* particles can be expressed. Growth is inconspicuous at first, but generalized metastases develop relatively rapidly.

* Vermiottes (French for small worms) are so-called cancer pearls. (Tr.)

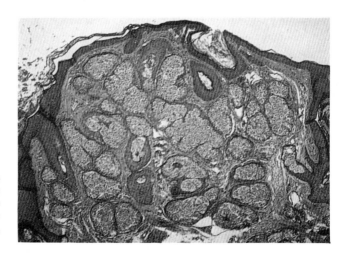

Fig. 697b. Senile hyperplasia of the sebaceous glands: high-lying hyperplasia of the sebaceous glands in the corium. Hematoxylin and eosin, 25×.

Histologically, sebaceous gland carcinomas may contain typical sebaceous gland formations as well as undifferentiated parts of tumors with pathologic mitoses and polymorphous nuclei of cells. In the differential diagnosis, basal cell epitheliomas, squamous cell carcinomas, and keratoacanthomas with sebaceous gland differentiations must be considered.[66, 76, 89]

The **sebaceous gland adenoma** (adenoma seboparum) is as rare as the sebaceous adenocarcinoma. It also favors the face and scalp. These adenomas for the most part occur singly, and consist of soft, well-limited nodes, which do not exceed 1 cm in diameter. A macroscopic diagnosis is not always possible. Histologically, a well-circumscribed tumor is present, containing parts of sebaceous glands as well as rows of basaloid cells. Of special interest is the simultaneous presence of multiple sebaceous gland adenomas and multiple primary carcinomas of the internal organs.[3, 58, 84]

16. Another tumor favoring the face is the **keratoacanthoma,** but other areas that are chronically exposed to light may also be the site of this tumor. On the other hand, single keratoacanthomas of the mucous membranes are extremely rare. Keratoacanthomas do not favor one sex more than the other. They appear with increasing frequency from the fifty-fifth year of life on. With no preliminary signs, the lesion develops rapidly within a few weeks to a hemispherical, bulging tumor on a broad base. In the beginning the surface remains covered by epidermis, which at the most shows a few telangiectases. After it has reached the maximum size, the center of the lesion forms a crater, which is filled with horny masses. Spontaneous regression follows and the horny plug is discharged, so that a basket-shaped ulceration is formed. Healing takes four to six months and leaves a scar. Metastases do not develop. The lesion differs at first from a basal cell epithelioma because it has a different growth rate and no pearly border. Also, a basal cell epithelioma is considerably firmer than a keratoacanthoma. The differential diagnosis from a squamous cell carcinoma is more difficult; however, the latter generally grows considerably more slowly. In addition, a squamous cell carcinoma originates mainly on altered skin, as for example, taut atrophy or senile keratosis. There is also a possibility of metastases and there is no spontaneous healing. In spite of this a histologic distinction between a keratoacanthoma and a squamous cell carcinoma cannot always be made. A mature keratoacanthoma shows a typical epidermal wall surrounding the central horny masses and inverted long-drawn-out lips extending downward. The lateral marginal zones are therefore transformed into sharp edges consisting of epithelium and papillary bodies. At the base of the tumor the infiltrating epithelium extends as far as the sweat gland clusters or the fatty tissue. In the growing epithelium of the tumor there are no conspicuous hyperchromatic cell nuclei or increased or atypical mitoses. The dense surrounding infiltrate, consisting of polymorphous nuclear cells, histiocytes, and lymphocytes, may also contain numerous eosinophilic granulocytes.[31, 35, 36, 46, 75]

Multiple eruptive keratoacanthomas are multiple, partly confluent and extended facial tumors (Fig. 698a, b) that occur almost simultaneously but are rarely observed. In some patients with multiple keratoacanthomas hundreds of single lesions are present as well as mucosal involvement. Keratoacanthomas have a remarkable tendency to form as a response to external irritations (as at injection sites), and they apparently prefer the parts of the skin exposed to light. Like multiple sebaceous gland adenomas, multiple eruptive keratoacanthomas are often associated with malignant disorders such as leukemias, carcinomas, or sideroachrestic anemia.[44, 54, 92]

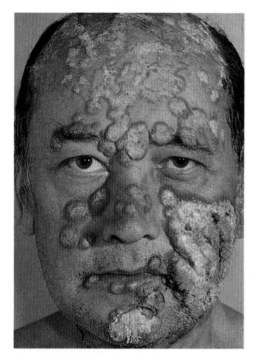

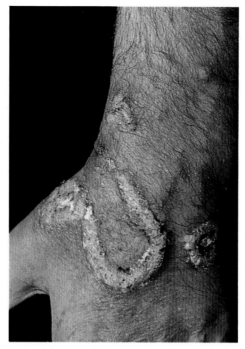

Fig. 698a. Multiple keratoacanthomas in sideroachrestic anemia.

Fig. 698b. Multiple keratoacanthomas in sideroachrestic anemia.

17. Carcinoma spinocellulare, the **keratinizing squamous cell carcinoma of the skin,** likewise occurs mainly in older persons, particularly men. It is found for the most part on the lower lip (Fig. 699), auricles, forehead, backs of the hands, and the extensor surfaces of the forearms, as well as other sites chronically exposed to light. The so-called seaman's skin is in this sense a typical facultative precancerosis. Whereas basal cell epitheliomas and keratoacanthomas always origi-

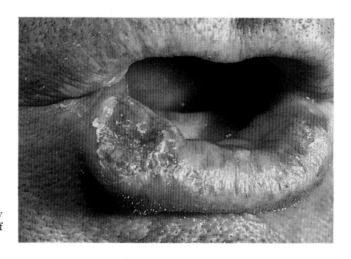

Fig. 699. Ulcerated papillary squamous cell carcinoma of the lower lip.

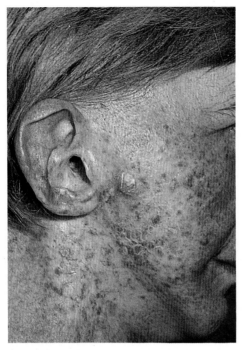

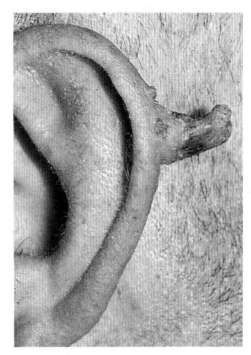

Fig. 700. Squamous cell carcinoma on taut x-ray atrophy.

Fig. 701. Cornu cutaneum.

nate from macroscopically unchanged skin, squamous cell carcinoma usually follows preceding lesions, such as senile keratoses, arsenical keratoses, a taut atrophy (Fig. 700), or a leukoplakia of the mucous membranes. Additional preferred sites of squamous cell carcinomas are the cutaneous areas surrounding the body openings. In this connection the early metastases associated with penile and vulval carcinomas – compared with squamous cell carcinomas at other sites – should be stressed. Carcinomas of the auricle also metastasize early to the regional lymph nodes because of special conditions in the lymph drainage. In the histologic diagnosis it is especially remarkable that occasionally, before typical metastases develop, only tuberculoid or sarcoidlike structures are present in the regional lymph nodes. Keratinizing squamous cell epitheliomas in general grow either exophytically, in a coarsely nodular and wartlike

manner, or endophytically, like an ulcer. It should be emphasized that suddenly appearing vegetations, especially if they occur at the borders of long-existing ulcerations, demand a histologic reexamination. On the lower lip a squamous cell carcinoma usually develops on an atrophic vermilion border, such as that created by the various forms of cheilitis. The development begins with a minimally indurated hyperkeratosis or crust and leads to exophytic or open papillary tumors, which occasionally involve the chin or bottom of the oral cavity, among other sites, with diffuse confluent infiltration. Often such indurated, craterlike ulcerations yield, when pressed, the so-called "vermiottes carcinomateuses," which are grayish-white particles or "cancer pearls." These phenomena, as well as the tendency toward hemorrhages and the unlimited growth, eliminate the possibility of syphilitic or tuberculous primary lesions. It

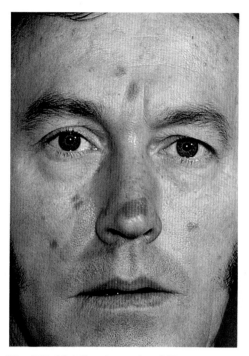

Fig. 702. Multilocular eosinophilic granuloma of the face.

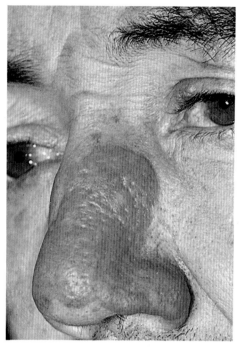

Fig. 703. Orange-peel-like surface of an
eosinophilic granuloma of the face.

should, however, be kept in mind that
granulomatous mycoses (such as blastomycosis or actinomycosis) often show excessive pseudoepitheliomatous hyperplasias.
On the ears the differential diagnosis must
rule out a painful nodule or Bowen's
disease. If multiple squamous cell carcinomas appear at atypical sites, the possibilities include sequelae of chronic arsenical
intoxication or basic hematologic disorders (leukemia, myeloma, or malignant
lymphogranulomatosis). If not only multiple squamous cell carcinomas but also
poikilodermic cutaneous changes and small
spotted pigmentations are present, xeroderma pigmentosum (see also Chapter 24,
E 13) must be ruled out.[6, 14, 55, 71, 79, 95]

18. A cutaneous horn consists of a hyperkeratosis formed like a horn or a cork-
screw and usually found on the ears or
cheeks (Fig. 701). In most cases it is apparently a variant of a senile keratoma

(actinic keratosis). In principle the cutaneous horn represents an etiologically "ambiguous" special form of growth seen with
a number of dermatologic conditions, for
instance, a keratoacanthoma, a squamous
cell cancer, or Bowen's disease. For this
reason histologic control is always necessary.[11]

19. The term **warty dyskeratoma** (isolated dyskeratosis follicularis) describes
hyperkeratotic, warty tumors of the face
and scalp. Macroscopically these lesions
are hardly characteristic – they resemble
perhaps a senile verruca. Histologic findings are a cuplike depression with para-
and orthohyperkeratosis and underlying
irregular acanthosis. Suprabasally one
sees lacunae and cysts filled with dyskeratotic and acantholytic cells.[15, 51, 62, 80]

20. Facial eosinophilic granuloma has a
variety of manifestations. In addition to

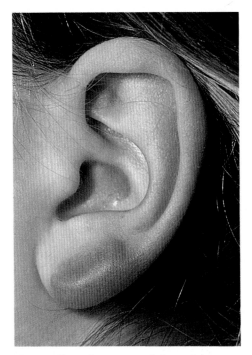

Fig. 704. Lymphocytoma of the earlobe.

flat infiltrates barely elevated above the level of the skin, there are also markedly nodular forms that occur either as solitary lesions or frequently as multiple tumors (Fig. 702). The orange peel-like surface with a brown to brownish-red color is very conspicuous (Fig. 703). Growth proceeds very slowly without formation of ulcera-

tions. In the differential diagnosis one must first exclude hypertrophic chronic discoid lupus erythematosus; this can be done even without a histologic examination because hyperkeratoses, atrophies, and hyperesthesias are lacking. In addition, lymphadenosis benigna cutis and sarcoid have to be eliminated. The histologic findings consist of reticulogranulomatous proliferation with predominantly eosinophilic granulocytes below a free subepidermal zone of connective tissue.[52, 57, 69]

21. Lymphadenosis benigna cutis (lymphocytoma cutis), like eosinophilic granuloma, consists of plaquelike or tumorous infiltrates. Typical sites are the face, especially the earlobes (Fig. 704), breasts, vulva, and scrotal skin. Basically, lymphadenosis benigna cutis may involve any cutaneous location, including the conjunctivae and the oral mucous membranes. The disease is caused by an infectious agent which so far has not been identified. Noteworthy is the simultaneous occurrence of acrodermatitis chronica atrophicans, migrant erythema, and lymphadenosis benigna cutis. All three diseases can be inoculated by a tick bite. Typical lymphadenosis benigna cutis shows an unsharply circumscribed tu-

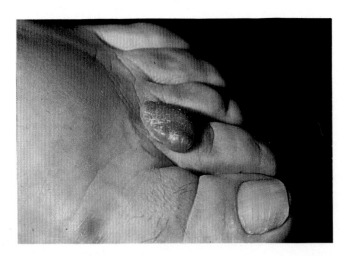

Fig. 705. Atypically located pseudosarcomatous fibroxanthoma.

morous infiltration, the color of which fluctuates between bluish-red and reddish-brown. The surface of the infiltrate occasionally shows mild scaling but otherwise is devoid of secondary changes. Exceptionally, loss of hair may occur within the region of the infiltrate. As a rule spontaneous regression takes place after a few months. There are clinical variants in addition to the typical appearance; however, usually they can be diagnosed only by histologic examination. Such variants include disseminated follicular, small nodular, plaquelike, elevated, and flat forms lying below the level of the skin. The differential diagnosis should include sarcoid, lupus vulgaris (positive probe test), chronic discoid lupus erythematosus (hyperesthesia, follicular keratoses), "lymphocytic infiltration," and a facial eosinophilic granuloma (orange-peel skin). Patients with lymphadenosis benigna cutis show no gross changes in the hemogram, but the differential blood picture and the bone marrow smear reveal lymphocytosis. On the other hand, since specific leukemic cutaneous infiltrates cannot be clinically separated from lymphadenosis benigna cutis, it is important to exclude leukemia in every case. Such definite distinctions can occasionally be made only by histologic examination. Microscopically, lymphadenosis benigna cutis shows mature lymphadenoid cells; in a typical case it has a striking similarity to the structure of a lymph node. The individual cellular nodules are not always well demarcated, and occasionally they penetrate into the surrounding tissue. Besides lymphocytes, plasma cells and reticulum cells appear in varying amounts. Sometimes even pronounced eosinophilia is observed. Nuclear debris is seen rather regularly, either isolated or phagocytized within macrophages. The cellular infiltrate sometimes assumes a definite granulomatous character, as it is interspersed by many blood vessels and capillaries.[2, 60, 64, 68, 78]

22. Pyogenic granuloma is discussed in Chapter 37, E4.

23. Hemangioendothelioma is discussed in Chapter 37, E5.

24. Atypical fibroxanthoma of the skin (pseudosarcomatous fibroxanthoma) is an especially fast-growing tumor similar to keratoacanthoma and pyogenic granuloma. The tumor favors the chronically light-exposed areas of the face (back of the neck, forehead, ears) but occasionally may even appear on the extremities; it occupies an intracutaneous position and reaches a size of 1 to 2 cm in diameter. In rare cases pedunculated tumors have been observed (Fig. 705). In the beginning the skin covering the hard tumor remains unchanged, but during the subsequent course of the disease it has a tendency to develop easily bleeding, shallow ulcerations. The rapid development of the tumor at first suggests a sarcoma, an amelanotic melanoma, or a pyogenic granuloma; all these possibilities in any case must be ruled out. The absence of any tendency toward recurrences or metastasis reflects the benign character of this pseudosarcomatous fibroxanthoma. The histologic examination reveals an ill-defined tumorous tissue without tendency to infiltrative growth; the tissue consists of layers of densely packed polymorphous fibroblasts and histiocytes. Mitoses are present in increased amounts, some in atypical forms. A conspicuous finding is the presence of diffusely distributed multiform giant cells with one or more nuclei. These giant cells often show dendriticlike extensions and vacuolated clearings with positive fat stains.

25. Rhinoscleroma results in a tumor-like distention of the entire nose. The infection with *Klebsiella rhinoscleromatis* leads in the beginning to an ozenalike rhinitis, which is then followed by involvement of the entire respiratory tract. Soon the whitish-yellow infiltration of the septum and conchae nasi results in a conspicuous, unusually hard induration. Finally, a bulging or tuberous distention of the nose follows. The upper lip is so deeply involved that it becomes attached to the dental alveoli. Generally the affected skin or mucous membrane remains smooth with perhaps a faint vascular design; otherwise the area has the aspect of a keloid. Moist rhagades are seldom seen. Later, nodes form on the posterior palate, the pharynx, or the region of the glottis; cicatrization slowly takes place and results in considerable impairment of motility and function. The diagnosis of rhinoscleroma can be firmly established by finding the bacteria in the nasal secretion or by performing a complement fixation test; clinically, the diagnosis can be determined by noting the extraordinary hardness, bilateral development, and slow progression.

Histologically, rhinoscleroma shows an extremely dense accumulation of plasma cells and two other special elements: Russell bodies and Mikulicz cells. The latter are large round cells with a pale netlike plasma and an off-center nucleus; with Giemsa stain they frequently show numerous gram-negative and PAS-positive bacteria. Russell bodies are composed of hyalinized fractured pieces of plasma cells with a variable number of mucoproteins and glycoproteins. However, Russell bodies have no pathognomonic significance (they are seen also in mycosis fungoides, among others). The histologic analysis of the substrate may suggest certain similarities with leishmaniasis, histoplasmosis, or lymphogranuloma inguinale venereum.

In the differential diagnostic considerations, one must keep in mind an exophytic malignancy, tertiary syphilis, leprosy, and, in exceptional cases, even lupus vulgaris.[10, 47, 77, 81]

(1) AUDRY, CH.: De l'adénome sébacé circonscrit. Ann. Derm. Syph. (Paris) 4: 563–571 (1903).

(2) BÄFVERSTEDT, B: Unusual forms of lymphadenosis benigna cutis (LABC). Acta Derm.-Venereol. (Stockh.) 42: 3–10 (1962).

(3) BAKKER, P. M., and S. S. TJON A JOE: Multiple sebaceous gland tumours, with multiple tumours of internal organs. Dermatologica (Basel) 142: 50–57 (1971).

(4) BANDMANN, H.-J., und K. BOSSE: Bericht über hochdifferenzierte Trichoepitheliome bei einem Kind. Hautarzt 19: 394–397 (1968).

(5) BAZEX, A., et A. DUPRÉ: Neuromes myéliniques muqueux á localisation centrofaciale et laryngée. Ann. Derm. Syph. (Paris) 85: 613–641 (1958).

(6) BERG, J. W.: The incidence of multiple primary cancers. I. Development of further cancers in patients with lymphomas, leukemias, and myeloma. J. Nat. Cancer Inst. 38: 741–752 (1967).

(7) CHRISTEN. A. G.: Persistent cutaneous fistulas of dental origin in children: report of two cases. J. Pediatr. 79: 51–54 (1971).

(8) CLENDENNING, W. E., J. B. BLOCK and I. G. RADDE: Basal cell nevus syndrome. Arch. Derm. (Chic.) 90: 38–53 (1964).

(9) CLENDENNING, W. E., J. R. HERDT and J. B. BLOCK: Ovarian fibromas and mesenteric cysts: their association with hereditary basal cell cancer of the skin. Amer. J. Obstet. Gynec. 87: 1008–1012 (1963).

(10) CONVIT, J., F. KERDEL-VEGAS and B. GORDON: Rhinoscleroma. Arch. Derm. (Chic.) 84: 55–62 (1961).

(11) CRAMER, H. J., und G. KAHLERT: Das Cornu cutaneum. Selbständiges Krankheitsbild oder klinisches Symptom? Derm. Wschr. 150: 521–531 (1964).

(12) CRANMER, L., I. M. REINGOLD and J. W. WILSON: Basal cell carcinoma of skin metastatic to bone. Arch. Derm. (Chic.) 102: 337–339 (1970).

(13) DAICKER, B.: Das Lidsyringom. Studien über seinen geweblichen Bau und seine Histogenese. Dermatologica (Basel) 128: 417–463 (1964).

(14) DEGOS, R., J. CIVATTE, S. BÉLAICH et G. TSOITIS: Épithélioma spino-cellulaire avec adénopathie tuberculoïde, puis néoplasique. Ann. Derm. Syph. (Paris) 98: 21–32 (1971).

(15) DELACRÉTAZ, J.: Dyskératomes verruqueux et kératoses séniles dyskératosiques. Dermatologica (Basel) *127:* 23–32 (1963).

(16) DENK, R.: Elektrokardiographische Untersuchungen bei Hautkranken. Arch. Kreisl.-Forsch. *60:* 33–114 (1969).

(17) DÖLCHER, W., und H. WEYHBRECHT: Ein Beitrag zur Frage der sogenannten »Pseudorezidive« nach Chaoulscher Nahbestrahlung mit besonderer Berücksichtigung des Gewebsbildes. Derm. Wschr. *125:* 153–158 (1952).

(18) DONALDSON, E. M., and R. SUMMERLY: Primary osteoma cutis and diaphyseal aclasis. Arch. Derm. (Chic.) *85:* 261–265 (1962).

(19) DUNCAN, B. R., V. A. DOHNER and J. H. PRIEST: The Gardner syndrome: need for early diagnosis. J. Pediatr. *72:* 497–505 (1968).

(20) EHLERS, G.: Zur Klinik der Basalzellepitheliome unter Berücksichtigung statistischer Untersuchungen. Z. Haut- u. Geschl.-Kr. *41:* 226–238 (1966).

(21) EPSTEIN, E., N. N. EPSTEIN, K. BRAGG and G. LINDEN: Metastases from squamous cell carcinomas of the skin. Arch. Derm. (Chic.) *97:* 245–251 (1968).

(22) EVERETT, F. G., and C. H. FIXOTT: Multiple miliary subdermal osteoma. Oral Surg. *24:* 670–673 (1967).

(23) FRIEDERICH, H.C., und G. LÜDERS: Basaliomartige hämatogene Fernmetastase der Nasenspitze als Frühzeichen allgemeiner Metastasierung bei Mammacarcinom. Z. Haut- u. Geschl.-Kr. *43:* 1–8 (1968).

(24) GARDNER, E. J.: Follow-up study of a family group exhibiting dominant inheritance for a syndrome including intestinal polyps, osteomas, fibromas and epidermal cysts. Amer. J. Hum. Genet. *14:* 376–390 (1962).

(25) GEISENHAINER, U.: Basaliome im Lippenbereich. Hautarzt *21:* 167–170 (1970).

(26) GERBER, N. J.: Zur Pathologie und Genetik des Basalzell-Naevus-Syndroms. Humangenetik *1:* 354–373 (1965).

(27) GORLIN, R. J., R. A. VICKERS, E. KELLEN and J. J. WILLIAMSON: Multiple basal cell nevi syndrome: An analysis of a syndrome consisting of multiple nevoid basal cell carcinoma, jaw cysts, skeletal anomalies, medulloblastoma, and hyporesponsiveness to parathormone. Cancer (Philad.) *18:* 89–104 (1965).

(28) GORLIN, R. J., H. O. SEDANO, R. A. VICKERS and J. ČERVENKA: Multiple mucosal neuromas, phaeochromocytoma and medullary carcinoma of the thyroid; a syndrome. Cancer *22:* 293–299 (1968).

(29) GRAY, H. R., and E. B. HELWIG: Epithelioma adenoides cysticum and solitary trichoepithelioma. Arch. Derm. (Chic.) *87:* 102–114 (1963).

(30) GROTERJAHN, A.: Die Talgdrüsengeschwülste mit besonderer Berücksichtigung des Talgdrüsenadenoms. Hautarzt *1:* 319–321 (1950).

(31) GRÜDER, B., und M. HUNDEIKER: Keratoakanthom und Karzinom. Derm. Mschr. *159:* 122–133 (1973).

(32) HAENSCH, R., G. ARETZ und O. P. HORNSTEIN: Zur Histotopie und Histogenese der multiplen Syringome. Arch. Derm. Forsch. *240:* 245–258 (1971).

(33) HAPPLE, R., G. MEHRLE, L. Z. SANDER und H. HÖHN: Basalzellnävus-Syndrom mit Retinopathia pigmentosa, rezidivierenden Glaskörperblutungen und Chromosomenveränderungen. Arch. Derm. Forsch. *241:* 96–114 (1971).

(34) HASHIMOTO, K., B. G. GROSS and W. F. LEVER: Syringoma. Histochemical and electron microscopic studies. J. Invest. Derm. *46:* 150–166 (1966).

(35) HAUSAMEN, J.-E., und N. HOEDE: Diagnostische und therapeutische Probleme beim Keratoakanthom der Mundhöhle. Zahnärztl. Welt *81:* 70–73 (1972).

(36) HELSHAM, R. W., and G. BUCHANAN: Keratoacanthoma of the oral cavity. Oral Surg. *13:* 844–849 (1960).

(37) HEMMATI, A., und K. G. THIELE: Die angiographischen Nierenveränderungen beim Bourneville-Pringle-Syndrom. Dtsch. med. Wschr. *95:* 1885–1886 (1970).

(38) HERMANS, E. H., J. C. M. GROSFELD and J. A. J. SPAAS: The fifth phacomatosis. Dermatologica (Basel) *130:* 446 bis 476 (1965).

(39) HERZBERG, J. J.: Ekkrines Syringocystadenom. Arch. klin. exp. Derm. *214:* 600–621 (1962).

(40) HOEDE, N., und R. GEBHARDT: Ungewöhnliche Metastasierung eines Bronchialkarzinoms. Med. Welt *21* (N.F.): 369–372 (1970).

(41) HOEDE, N., und G. W. KORTING: Pseudosarkomatöses Xanthofibrom. Arch. klin. exp. Derm. *232:* 119–126 (1968).

(42) HUNDEIKER, M., und H. BERGER: Zur Morphogenese der Basaliome. Arch. klin. exp. Derm. *231:* 161–169 (1968).

(43) JACOBI, H., und H. E. KLEINE-NATROP: Beitrag zum »Syndrom der angeborenen fibrillären Neurome«. Derm. Mschr. *156:* 644–652 (1970).

(44) JOLLY, H. W., and C. L. CARPENTER: Multiple keratoacanthomata. Arch. Derm. (Chic.) *93:* 348–353 (1966).

(45) KÄRCHER, K. H.: Die Röntgen-Symptomatologie des Gardner-Syndroms. Fortschr. Röntgenstr. *107:* 90–95 (1967).

(46) KALKOFF, K. W.: Das Keratoakanthom (Molluscum pseudocarcinomatosum) im Rahmen des Krebsproblems. Strahlentherapie *112:* 163–187 (1960).

(47) KELLETER, R., und H. FELDMANN: Rhinosklerom mit tracheobronchialer Ausbreitung. Dtsch. med. Wschr. *98:* 499–503 (1973).

(48) KEMPSON, R. L., and M. H. McGAVRAN: Atypical fibroxanthomas of the skin. Cancer *17:* 1463–1471 (1964).

(49) KNIERER, W.: Pseudorezidive nach Röntgennahbestrahlung von Hautkarzinomen. Derm. Wschr. *119:* 272–274 (1947).

(50) KNOTH, W., and G. EHLERS: Über das Epithelioma adenoides cysticum als Phakomatose Brooke-Spiegler. Hautarzt *11:* 535–545 (1960).

(51) KORTING, G. W.: Dyskeratoma lymphadenoides. Derm. Wschr. *146:* 534 bis 543 (1962).

(52) KORTING, G. W.: Granuloma eosinophilicum faciale. Med. Welt *17* (N.F.): 397–398 (1966).

(53) KORTING, G. W., und K.-H. HASSENPFLUG: Zur Histogenese des Epithelioma Malherbe und von seinen topischen Bebeziehungen zum Keratoakanthom. Arch. klin. exp. Derm. *222:* 11–22 (1965).

(54) KORTING, G. W., und H. LACHNER: Multiple eruptive Keratoakanthome bei sideroachrestischer Anämie. Med. Welt *21* (N.F): 63–65 (1970).

(55) KREBS, A., und K. SCHWARZ: Rapide Entwicklung von Hautkarzinomen bei chronisch-lymphatischer Leukämie mit immunbiologischen Störungen. Dermatologica (Basel) *127:* 52–61 (1963).

(56) KROE, D. J., and J. A. PITCOCK: Atypical fibroxanthoma of the skin. Report of 10 cases. Amer. J. Clin. Path. *51:* 487–492 (1969).

(57) LANGHOF, H., und E. GÜNTHER: Beitrag zur Behandlung des Granuloma eosionophilicum faciale. Derm. Wschr. *151:* 207–212 (1965).

(58) LEVER, W. F.: Sebaceous adenoma. Review of the literature and report of a case. Arch. Derm. Syph. (Chic.) *57:* 102–111 (1948).

(59) LEVER, W. F., und K. HASHIMOTO: Die Histogenese einiger Hautanhangstumoren im Lichte histochemischer und elektronenmikroskopischer Befunde. Hautarzt *17:* 161–173 (1966).

(60) MACH, K.: Die gutartigen Lymphoplasien der Haut. Zur Nosologie und Klassifizierung der sogenannten Lymphocytome. Arch. klin. exp. Derm. *222:* 325–349 (1965).

(61) MACOMBER, W. B., M. K. WANG and E. GOTTLIEB: Cutaneous lesions of dental origin simulating skin cancer. G.P. (Kansas City, Mo.) *14:* 81–85 (1956).

(62) METZ, J., und F. SCHRÖPL: Zur Nosologie des Dyskeratoma segregans (»Warty dyskeratoma«). Arch. klin. exp. Derm. *238:* 21–37 (1970).

(63) MILLEDGE, R. D., B. E. GERALD and W. J. CARTER: Pulmonary manifestation of tuberous sclerosis: Case report. Amer. J. Roentgenol. *98:* 734–738 (1966).

(64) MULZER, P., und E. KEINING: Über miliare Lymphozytome der Haut. Derm. Wschr. *88:* 293–301 (1929).

(65) NICKEL, W. R., and W. B. REED: Tuberous sclerosis. Special reference to the microscopic alterations in the cutaneous hamartomas. Arch. Derm. (Chic.) *85:* 209–224 (1962).

(66) NIKOLOWSKI, W.: Beitrag zur Klinik und Histologie der Talgdrüsen-Naevi und -Carcinome und deren Beziehungen zum sog. Basalzellen-Carcinom. Arch. Derm. Syph. (Berl.) *193:* 340–362 (1951).

(67) OEHLSCHLAEGEL, G.: Das Epithelioma calcificans (Malherbe) unter besonderer Berücksichtigung seiner Histogenese. Z. Haut- u. Geschl.-Kr. *48:* 133–145 (1973).

(68) PASCHOUD, J.-M.: Die Lymphadenosis benigna cutis als übertragbare Infektionskrankheit. Neue Gesichtspunkte über Verlauf, Histologie und Therapie. Hautarzt *8:* 197–211 (1957).

(69) PEDACE, F. J., and H. O. PERRY: Granuloma faciale. A clinical and histopathologic review. Arch. Derm. (Chic.) *94:* 387–395 (1966).

(70) PIFFARETTI, P. G., et G. FOROGLOU: Syndrome de Gardner. Schweiz. med. Wschr. *95:* 1096–1101 (1965).

(71) Pinkus, H.: Differenzierung bösartiger und relativ gutartiger Spinaliome und Melanome. Med. Klinik *62:* 1160–1162 (1967).

(72) Reed, J. C.: Nevoid basal cell carcinoma syndrome with associated fibrosarcoma of the maxilla. Arch. Derm. (Chic.) *97:* 304–306 (1968).

(73) Reichenberger, M., und J. Löhnert: Osteosis cutis multiplex. Hautarzt *22:* 73–77 (1971).

(74) Rodermund, O.-E., und E. H. Cramer: Zur Frage der Metastasierung von Basaliomen. Z. Haut- u. Geschl.-Kr. *43:* 455–464 (1968).

(75) Rook, A., and R. H. Champion: Keratoacanthoma. Nat. Cancer Inst. Monogr. *10:* 257–273 (1963).

(76) Santini, R., ed G. de Panfilis: Adenocarcinoma sebaceo metastitizzante. Rilievi clinici ed istopatologici. Minerva derm. *44:* 279–284 (1969).

(77) Schönfeld, K.: Beitrag zur Behandlung des Rhinoskleroms. Derm. Wschr. *135:* 613–617 (1957).

(78) Self, S. J., V. H. Carter and R. O. Noojin: Disseminated lymphocytoma cutis. Case reports of miliarial and nodular types. Arch. Derm (Chic.) *100:* 459–464 (1969).

(79) Swanbeck, G.: Aetiological factors in squamous cell skin cancer. Brit. J. Derm. *85:* 394–396 (1971).

(80) Tanay, A., and A. H. Mehregan: Warty dyskeratoma. Dermatologica (Basel) *138:* 155–164 (1969).

(81) Tappeiner, J., L. Pfleger und K. Wolff: Das Vorkommen und histochemische Verhalten von Russelschen Körperchen bei plasmacellulären Hautinfiltraten. Arch. klin. exp. Derm. *222:* 71–90 (1965).

(82) Thies, W.: Multiple echte fibrilläre Neurome (Rankenneurome) der Haut und Schleimhaut. Arch. klin. exp. Derm. *218:* 561–573 (1964) .

(83) Thies, W., und E. Schwarz: Multiple eruptive Milien – ein organoides Follikelhamartom. Arch. klin. exp. Derm. *214:* 21–34 (1961).

(84) Torre, D.: Multiple sebaceous tumors. Arch. Derm. (Chic.) *98:* 549–551 (1968).

(85) Tritsch, H.: Osteome der Haut. Arch. klin. exp. Derm. *221:* 336–347 (1965).

(86) Ullman, S., J. Sondergaard and T. Kobayasi: Ultrastructure of palmar and plantar pits in basal cell nevus syndrome. Acta derm.-venereol. (Stockh.) *52:* 329–336 (1972).

(87) Undeutsch, W.: Beitrag zur Kasuistik der multiplen Follikeldysplasien (Hamartien des primären Epithelkeimes). Hautarzt *22:* 57–63 (1971).

(88) Urbach, E., und A. Wiedmann: Morbus Pringle und Morbus Recklinghausen. Ihre Beziehungen zueinander. Arch. Derm. Syph. (Berl.) *158:* 334–343 (1929).

(89) Urban, F. H., and R. K. Winkelmann: Sebaceous malignancy. Arch. Derm. (Chic.) *84:* 63–72 (1961).

(90) Veltman, G., und S. Adari: Die fünfte Phakomatose. Z. Haut- u. Geschl.-Kr. *46:* 221–240 (1971).

(91) Walker, D. M.: Oral mucosal neuroma-medullary thyroid carcinoma syndrome. Brit. J. Derm. *88:* 599–603 (1973).

(92) Weber, G., H. Stetter, G. Pliess und H. Stickl: Assoziiertes Vorkommen von eruptiven Keratoacanthomen, Tubencarcinom und Paramyeloblastenleukämie. Arch. klin. exp. Derm. *238:* 107–119 (1970).

(93) Wiedersberg, H.: Das Epithelioma calcificans Malherbe. Derm. Mschr. *157:* 867–883 (1971).

(94) Wong, W. K., R. Somburanasin and M. G. Wood: Eruptive, multicentric pilomatricoma (calcifying epithelioma). Arch. Derm. (Chic.) *106:* 76–78 (1972).

(95) Wuketich, S.: Lippencarcinom mit ungewöhnlicher Metastasierung in der Herz- und Skelettmuskulatur. Frankfurt. Z. Path. *76:* 87–94 (1966).

(96) Zabel, R.: Osteosis cutis multiplex faciei. Derm. Mschr. *156:* 798–801 (1970).

(97) Zalla, J. A., and H. O. Perry: An unusual case of syringoma. Arch. Derm. (Chic.) *103:* 215–217 (1971).

D. Leonine Face

Leonine face is the name given to an especially wide and swollen face. The finer facial lines are obliterated, and the furrows of the forehead are thickened and deepened by the formation of raised bulges. Massive infiltrates permeate the eyebrows, the cheeks are pendulous, the nose is thickened and widened, and the lips are bulging, swollen, and shaped like

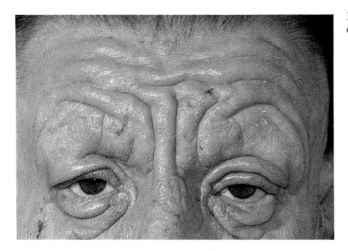

Fig. 706. Leonine face in chronic lymphadenosis.

an elephant's trunk. The thickened epidermis causes the auricles to protrude. Leonine face can be caused by a number of different diseases.

1. Among the chronic leukoses **chronic lymphadenosis** must be considered first. This is mainly a disease of older persons, and sometimes in the beginning it may be masked by other diseases of advancing years. Indefinite cutaneous changes (prurigo, eczematous conditions, generalized herpes zoster, and similar affections) cannot be ascribed to an underlying malignant disease without a correspond-

ing leukemic hemogram. Specific lymphatic-leukemic cutaneous infiltrates frequently affect both sides of the body, favoring the extremities; however, the trunk may show multiple, variably large infiltrates in a certain follicular pattern (Fig. 707) (see also Chapter 22, C2). Plaquelike, flat, and either cordlike or nodular facial tumors may be located on the earlobes, cheeks, eyebrows, nose, or lips, giving the face an acromegaloid appearance (Fig. 706). These tumors are soft and doughlike, resembling lupus vulgaris tumidus; however, infiltrates of cartilagelike consistency have been ob-

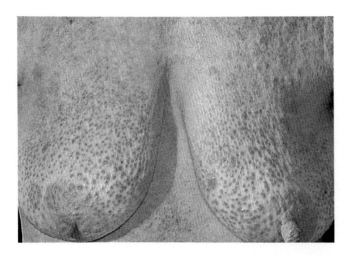

Fig. 707. Chronic lymphadenosis with specific small nodular cutaneous infiltrates.

served. The epidermis of these nonulcerat-
ing tumors is thin and so transparent that
blood vessels can be visualized. The color
is bluish-red, or sometimes more brownish-
red; in the first instance, especially when
seen on the earlobes, a diagnosis of
sarcoid or lymphocytoma should be
considered. In the case of leukemic infiltrates, the blanching produced by
diascopic examination reveals macular
areas of yellowish-brown color similar to
those observed in lupus vulgaris, rather
than the stippled areas typical of sarcoid.

A definite diagnosis can be made only
by considering the entire clinical picture,
such as enlargement of the lymph nodes,
splenomegaly, and the hematologic signs.
No other form of leukemia shows such
marked changes of the serum proteins
(absence of gamma globulins, lack of
antibodies, facultative paraproteins).

Histologically, the cutaneous tumors of
lymphatic leukemia show dense, monotonous proliferation of lymphocytes and
disappearance of the collagenous and
elastic connective tissue. Another important sign is the fact that in chronic
lymphadenosis the epidermis is separated
from the infiltrates of the corium by a
zone of papillary bodies in which cells
are practically absent.[1, 3]

2. Patients with **Sézary's syndrome** are
characterized by a leonine face even more
often than those suffering from chronic
lymphadenosis (Fig. 708). As the dermatologic and clinical findings are almost
identical with those of chronic lymphadenosis, the diagnosis can be verified
only by finding the so-called Sézary cells
(see also Chapter 22, C5).

3. Chronic myeloid leukemia (chronic
myelosis) usually shows, even at the time
the diagnosis is established, a high leukocyte count with a corresponding shift
to the left toward the myeloblasts.
Histochemically, this type of leukemia
shows a lack of alkaline phosphatase in

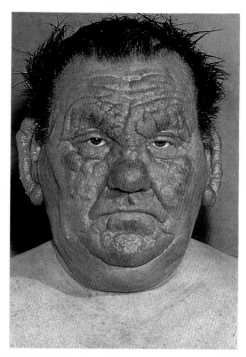

Fig. 708. Leonine face in the Sézary syndrome.

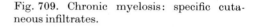

Fig. 709. Chronic myelosis: specific cutaneous infiltrates.

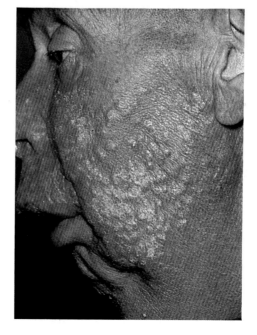

Table 14 Cytochemistry of Hemoblastoses (According to A. HELLER, 1971)

	AlP Blood Smear	AcP	Naphthol As-acet. Esterase	Sof	LAP	Chloracetate Esterase	Alpha-naphthylacet. Esterase	ATP	Beta-glucuronidase	PAS
Chronic myelogenous leukemia	0	(+)	+ normal	+ normal	+ normal	++ normal	+ normal	++ normal	+ normal	++ diffuse
Attack of blastosis	+/++	(+)	(+)	(+)	0	(+)	(+)	0	0	0
Acute myelogenous leukemia	0/+	(+)	(+)	(+)	0	(+)	(+)	0	0	0
Promyelocytic leukemia	0/+	+	+/++	+/++	0	+++	+	(+)	0	0
Monocytic leukemia	0/+	+	+/++	0	+++	(+)	(+)	0	0	0
Acute lymphoblastic leukemia	0/+	0	0	0	0	0	0	0	+	++ coarsely clumped
Erythroleukemia	0/+	0	(+)	(+)	(+)	0	+++	+++	0	++ diffuse coarsely clumped

AlP = alkaline phosphatase, AcP = acid phosphatase, Sof = sodium fluoride, LAP = leukinaminopeptidase, ATP = adenosine-5-triphosphate. The darkly printed boxes are the so-called essential enzymes of the various hemoblastoses.

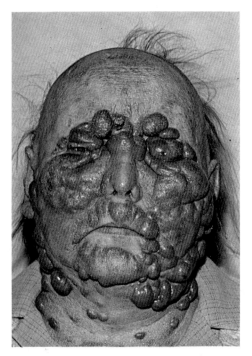

Fig. 710. Mycosis fungoides, tumor stage.

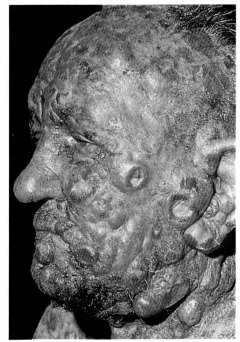

Fig. 711. Leonine face in diffuse reticulum sarcomatosis.

the mature neutrophilic granulocytes (Table 14). Finally, the Philadelphia chromosome, which shows a reduction in size of the twenty-first chromosome, is typical of chromosomal aberrations in myeloid leukemia. Although the acute leukemias show a higher degree of anemia and thrombocytopenia with hemorrhagic diathesis, chronic myeloid leukemia is characterized by general signs of weakness (increased perspiration, cardiac complaints, abdominal pressure due to a splenic tumor, and similar complaints); the usual dermatologic signs are pyodermas, as well as urticarial or pruriginous eruptions. Specific myeloid cutaneous lesions have a brown-red or reddish color similar to that seen in chronic lymphadenosis, however, grouped formations of nodes are almost always observed (Fig. 709). These nodes favor the trunk and the extremities and occur in isolation on the head rather seldom. The cutaneous tumors of myeloid

leukemia, in contrast to those of chronic lymphadenosis, often rupture to form ulcerations. A fully developed leonine face occurs only exceptionally in chronic myeloid leukemia, but specific infiltrations causing enlargement of the nose and trunklike swellings of the upper lip are seen occasionally. Histologic examination shows an infiltrate consisting of myeloid cells in various degrees of maturity. There is a cell-free subepidermal zone of the corium similar to that observed in chronic lymphadenosis.[2, 3-6]

4. In unusual cases **mycosis fungoides** may also show marked infiltrations of the face that results in a leonine face (Fig. 710). However, these lesions are not the plaque-like, diffuse, bulging formations of chronic myeloid leukemia but conglomerations of the closely adjacent nodes of mycosis fungoides. The diagnosis depends on other

cutaneous findings of mycosis fungoides and on the histologic substrate.

5. Lepromatous leprosy often causes a leonine face because lepromas occur on the eyebrows, nose, and earlobes. Above all, a bulging nose with its subsequent mutilations and a chronic hemorrhagic rhinitis point to the existence of leprosy. In addition, the tendency of lepromatous infiltrates to ulcerate – for instance, on the earlobes – may offer another clinical difference from chronic lymphadenosis. However, the diagnosis depends entirely on the presence of the Hansen bacilli.

The term "facies leprosa" in lepromatous leprosy is applied to inflammations of the nasal cavity, atrophy of the anterior nasal spine, and also a distally beginning atrophy of the alveolar process of the maxilla.

(1) FAYOLLE, J., P. COEUR, P.-A. BRYON, O. GENTILHOMME, G. MOULIN et P. MOREL: Les manifestations cutanées des leucémies lymphoïdes chroniques (LLC). À propos de 44 cas d'une statistique personnelle de 430 LLC. Ann. Derm. Syph. (Paris) *100:* 5–24 (1973).

(2) HELLER, A.: Zytochemische Diagnostik der akuten Leukosen. Med. Welt *22* (N.F.): 213–215 (1971).

(3) KEINING, E.: Besondere Vorkommnisse bei leukämischen Erkrankungen der Haut. Arch. Derm. Syph. (Berl.) *189:* 303–310 (1949).

(4) KORINTHENBERG, I.: Chronische Myelose der Haut mit bisher ausschließlicher Krankheitsmanifestation im Gesichtsbereich. Z. Haut- u. Geschl.-Kr. *33:* 372–379 (1962).

(5) PARADE, G. W., und H. VOEGT: Zur Frage der Hautleukämie. Dtsch. Arch. klin. Med. *185:* 265–270 (1939).

(6) PAUL, J. T., and L. R. LIMARZI: Specific cutaneous lesions in chronic myeloid leukemia. Arch. Derm. Syph. (Chic.) *45:* 897–905 (1942).

E. Tumors Favoring the Scalp

In this section only a rough list of certain tumors in this location can be given, based on general clinical experience. It is possible that these tumors are also present in other skin areas.

1. The scalp is the typical site of single or multiple **atheromas** (trichilemmal cysts). In older patients especially the tumors are almost always multiple. As mentioned before, trichilemmal cysts are also a manifestation of Gardner's syndrome. The hemispherical, tensely elastic, cystic new formations are pea-sized to egg-sized and lie in the deep corium or subcutis. The covering skin remains unchanged at first but becomes smooth, shiny, and atrophic as the size of the tumor increases. Because of the pressure atrophy of the hair roots, the surface of the tumor becomes hairless. The thick-walled trichilemmal cysts have no connection with the epidermis or the hair root, so that in contrast to genuine retention cysts they become infected and purulent only occasionally. Histologically, the wall of the cyst consists of multilayered epithelium over a basal membrane. The individual cells disappear without distinct keratohyaline formation but with "blisterous" swelling of the cytoplasm into the central mass of keratin.[27]

The atheromalike follicular and **sebaceous gland retention cysts** develop from a keratotic blockage of the excretory duct. They are easily infected and subsequently discharge their ill-smelling content over the perforation site. Because of their origin from sebaceous glands they are encountered less frequently on the scalp than on the skin of the face and back, which is rich in sebaceous cysts.

Histologic examination of the wall of the cyst will show the remnants of alveoli of the sebaceous glands or hair sheaths. Since the wall of the cyst is often very thin, the cyst's contents may discharge

Fig. 712. Multiple cylindromas on the scalp.

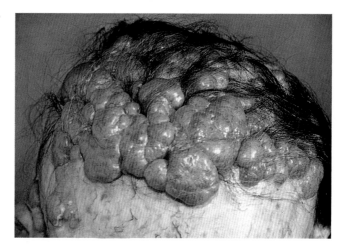

into the surrounding tissue, leading to various inflammatory reactions.

Clinically, however, a distinction between cysts of the atheroma type and retention cysts is not always possible without further study.[11]

Histologically, tumors of the scalp that have been clinically diagnosed as atheromas may show unusual tendencies toward proliferation. This may lead to a consideration of malignant degeneration. The growth impulses, however, generally originate from wall particles of ruptured atheromas and are considered to be benign growths ("**pilar tumor of the scalp**" or proliferating trichilemmal cysts), since atypical mitoses and invasive penetration of single cells or conglomerates of cells are lacking. The presence of giant cells and shadow cells should likewise be considered a residuum of a ruptured atheroma.[19, 33]

2. Cutaneous cylindromas (Spiegler's tumors) may be isolated or multiple or may occur in combination with the trichoepitheliomas mentioned in Section C7. Although the scalp is a distinctly favorite site (Fig. 712), other skin areas are also affected (Figs. 713, 714). Some

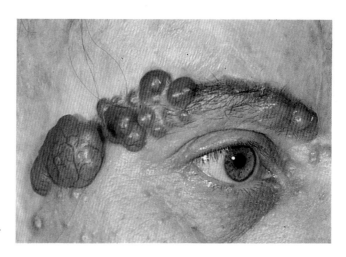

Fig. 713. Multiple cylindromas along the eyebrow.

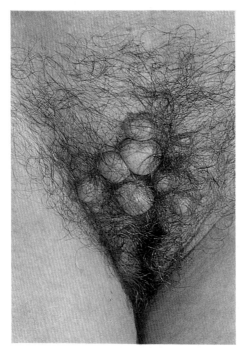

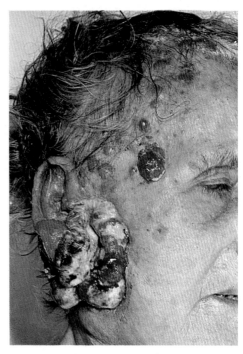

Fig. 714. Multiple cylindromas in the pubic area.

Fig. 715. Maligantly degenerated cylindroma.

patients may have a hundred or more tumors distributed over the entire body. The disorder is conspicuously familial and women show it twice as often as men. The age of manifestation is during the third or fourth decade of life, but occasionally the first tumors may appear in childhood. It seems to be inherited as an autosomal dominant trait with variable penetrance. Individual cylindromas grow very slowly and reach various sizes but seldom attain a diameter of more than 4 to 6 cm. At first the skin- to reddish-colored tumors are raised above the surrounding skin as calottes; with additional growth they later assume semispherical forms.

The surface is smooth, tense, and, because of destruction of the hair follicles, hairless. As in a nodular basaloma, long-extended telangiectases are present. The individual tumors do not remain in isolated formations as cysts on the scalp but form dense, closely grown-together aggregates of tumors. Larger cylindromas may soften in the center and form ulcers. In these cases malignant degeneration to a carcinoma (Fig. 715) with subsequent metastases to regional lymph nodes and inner organs must be considered in spite of the usually benign character of these lesions.

Histogenetically, the cylindromas start from the ducts of the (apocrine ?) sweat glands. The nodular tumors, which consist of single lobules, are separated from each other by a homogeneously hyaline sheath. This hyaline material is also found in the parenchyma of the tumor and gives the impression in part of a cross-section of a cylinder. The tumor parenchyma itself is composed of (1) palisade-shaped peripheral cells with small, darkly stained nuclei, and (2) conglomerations of cells with large pale nuclei located at some distance from the edge.[8, 20]

3. The **mixed tumor of the skin** occurs predominantly on the scalp, neck, and parotid gland, but other locations are also known. It may appear at any age. Clinically, it is a firm, intradermal or subcutaneous, very slow-growing tumor, which remains movable on its base. Usually, a single tumor, which is not larger than 2 to 3 cm in diameter, is present. The overlying skin may be slightly reddened and covered by telangiectases. A macroscopic diagnosis is impossible. Histologically, a differentiation between eccrine and apocrine types is made according to the tissue of origin. Both types consist of tubular lumina, which contain eccrine or apocrine cells. The surrounding stroma contains many cells and forms a rich mucinous ground substance. At certain places it seems dense and is interspersed with isolated cells that lie in lacunae, so that it assumes the appearance of a cartilagelike tissue.[15, 16, 21, 23]

4. Osteomas of the scalp are either single or sparse, very hard tumors. They seldom exceed a diameter of 0.5 to 1.0 cm, but the close proximity of individual nodes simulates a single, large, nodular tumor. Since the surface remains unchanged, the macroscopic diagnosis may be suggested by the unusually hard sensation on palpation. Osteomas are not attached to the calotte of the skull, but remain freely movable on the base. For the histologic findings see Chapter C6.[6, 9, 32]

5. So-called **encephalocraniocutaneous lipomatosis** causes epileptiform attacks, mental retardation, and spastic paralysis of the extremities. Cutaneous lipomatosis shows unusually severe thickening of the scalp, the temporofrontal region, and the neck. The cutaneous involvement of lipomatosis is not always limited to the skull but may also be present on the trunk. It is, however, important that the lipomatous changes extend also to the meninges, the CNS, the heart, and other internal organs, becoming the cause of the manifold signs and symptoms of this disease.[4, 12]

6. Associated with multiple, pea-sized, firm tumors on the back may be similar tumors on the face, and above all, on the scalp. As the growth of the tumor progresses, these **hamartomas of the hair follicles** lead to complete loss of hair. This is discussed in Chapter 11, A22.

7. Syringocystadenoma papilliferum is a hamartoma that develops after puberty. It is often associated with a nevus sebaceus or a basaloma. It occurs most frequently on the scalp, but also in other locations such as the face, neck, armpits, groins, and genital region. It shows irregular streaks or areas of aggregated papules, whose size varies between 1 and 5 cm; some papules have a central depression, and under a magnifying glass tiny cysts can be detected. Occasionally, however, there is only a verrucous surface. Histologically, the tumor, which originates from the duct of an eccrine or apocrine sweat gland, shows acanthotic papillomatosis extending downward like a goblet. The papillae are covered by two layers of epithelium. The basal cells of the epithelium have a cubic form and darkly stained nuclei, whereas those toward the lumen are cylindrical with light, palely tinged nuclei. The stroma of the tumor is often interspersed with distinctly plasmacellular infiltration.[13, 17, 25]

8. Eccrine sweat gland carcinomas (hidradenocarcinomas) may occur in principle in any location, but in large series a conspicuous incidence on the scalp becomes evident. There is no characteristic clinical picture. In general, these carcinomas are pearl-colored, often ulcerated and crusted or verrucous nodes, which show sweat secretion on the surface

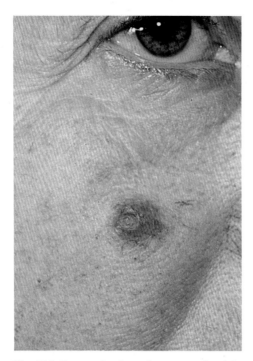

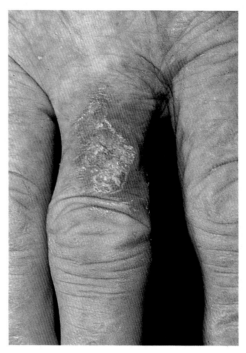

Fig. 716. Sweat gland carcinoma on the right cheek.

Fig. 717. Sweat gland carcinoma of the right ring finger.

(Figs. 716, 717). Because the growth of the tumor progresses slowly, a malignant tumor is not usually considered. In the region of the hand especially, confusion with a common wart is possible, and unsatisfactory treatment results. There is a strong tendency to local recurrence. Beyond that, extensive metastasizing into internal organs is possible. Histopathologically, there are regular adenomatous structures of an anaplastic character with distorted cells and vacuolization, among other features. The large tumor cells are usually rich in glycogen (Figs. 718a, b). [3, 7, 10, 31]

9. Another tumor originating from the excretory duct of the eccrine sweat glands is the **clear cell hidradenoma** (clear cell myoepithelioma). It occurs in most cases in adults as a solitary lesion on the face, scalp, and chest. The unspecific tumors, which may measure up to 3 cm, become attached to the epidermis but are easily movable against the subcutis. If they ulcerate in the center, there may be a certain similarity to a rodent ulcer. The clear cell hidradenoma has been described as partly solid and partly cystic and also pedunculated. Histologically, in the corium of tumors connected with the epidermis there are epithelioid cells arranged in lobules. Also there are small, elongated, and darkly stained cells at the margins of ductlike cavities, and most important, hydropic clear cells, which look like plant cells and have a sharply circumscribed cytoplasmic membrane.

Malignant transformation with metastases is possible, but rare. The local destructiveness of these tumors is remarkable. In the malignant clear cell hidradenoma, groups of cells may resemble a hypernephrotic blastoma because of their light plasma and may suggest that such a cutaneous tumor is a metastasis. [14, 18, 30, 33]

10. Angiolymphoid hyperplasia with eosinophilia occurs in adults on the scalp and the ears as single or multiple tumors that measure from 2 to 40 mm. The surface of the tumors is nodular and devoid of hair but free of secondary changes. Some of the tumors are located relatively high within the corium, and others may extend downward to the subcutaneous fatty tissue, where they cannot be moved. Clinically, angiolymphoid hyperplasia with eosinophilia is frequently mistaken for atheroma, retention cyst of a sebaceous gland, cylindroma, or hemangioma. It differs from pyogenic granuloma in the presence of a complete covering of epithelium, the absence of a basal epithelial scaly border, and the lack of a tendency to bleed. Histologically, this hyperplasia has a vascular portion with thick-walled vessels of normal structure and, in addition, numerous short vascular sprouts, many still without lumen and composed of only slightly differentiated cellular elements. The cellular part of the tumor, with lymphocytes, histiocytes, many eosinophils, and a few mast cells, varies considerably. The "inflammatory" cellular infiltrate can be so dense that the equally present vascular proliferations are completely hidden. Another peculiarity is the formation of structures resembling follicular lymph nodes; these are frequently found only in the deeper subcutaneous parts of the tumor.[22, 34, 36]

11. Trichophytia profunda (kerion celsi) of the scalp may occasionally show reddish-blue nodular infiltrates with peripheral crusts that may grow as large as apples (Fig. 118). When pressed, a honeycomblike, pustular secretion exudes through numerous openings. The presence of areas of superficial trichophytosis on

Fig. 718a. Sweat gland carcinoma: histologic survey. Hematoxylin and eosin, 63 ×.

Fig. 718b. Detailed section with tubular rows of multiple carcinomatous cells. Hematoxylin and eosin, 100 ×.

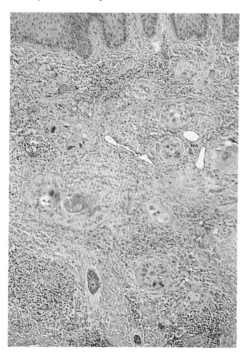

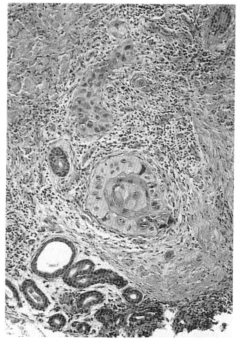

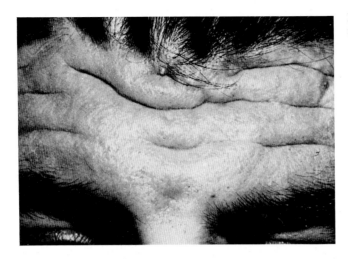

Fig. 719. Cutis gyrata of the forehead.

other parts of the body supports a diagnosis of the fungus infection. Inoculation of a culture plate with easily plugged hairs will verify the diagnosis. Similar types of kerion celsi are also found in the bearded region of the face as nodular soft tumor formations (sycosis parasitaria).

12. Cutis verticis gyrata is discussed in this chapter because at times it may have a tumorlike appearance; cutaneous folds are arranged in juxtaposition, and when deep, a picture resembling cerebral gyri results through coalescence. The main localization is the scalp (Fig. 720), but similar changes are present on the forehead and back of the neck (Fig. 719). The number, length, and thickness of each cutaneous fold vary considerably. However, cutis verticis gyrata is only a sign of several underlying diseases. Histologically, all cases of a "genuine" cutis verticis gyrata simply show gross furrowing of an otherwise normally structured skin.[25]

If the cutaneous folds are already present at birth or become manifest in early childhood, they are usually known as a cerebriform nevus originating from various tissues. As opposed to the genuine cutis verticis gyrata, such nevi are distinctly

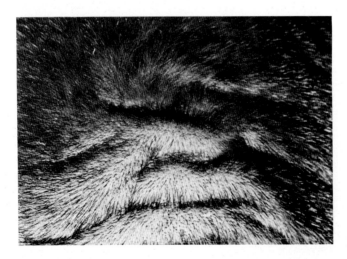

Fig.720. Cutis verticis gyrata.

raised above the surrounding skin and are relatively sharply separated from it. There is no special sex preference, and associated signs are absent. Sometimes the abnormal formation of folded skin may extend over the entire body surface owing to an underlying lipomatous nevus ("the Michelin tire baby").[29]

In exceptional cases "genuine" cutis verticis gyrata may even be present at birth. Such patients should be examined for associated signs such as *acanthosis nigricans* and malformations of the bones and teeth (see also Chapter 24, D20).[5]

In addition, cutis verticis gyrata is not infrequently seen in combination with primary pachydermoperiostosis. This disease affects males almost exclusively. The cutaneous changes become evident after puberty (see also Chapter 7, M2). Sometimes acromegaly is accompanied by cutis verticis gyrata.[37]

The combination of *acromegaly, corneal leukoma,* and *cutis verticis gyrata* is a special syndrome. This syndrome is inherited in autosomal dominant fashion with no preference for either sex. The earliest corneal changes occur even before the tenth year of life, at first unilaterally, but later both eyes are affected. The progress of the disease lasts a few years, and will result slowly in blindness. Acromegalic growth also starts in childhood, whereas cutis verticis gyrata develops at about the fortieth year of life. Radiologic and endocrine examinations fail to show evidence of a tumor of the hypophysis. However, the most striking change visible in radiographic examination of the skeleton is thickening of the frontal bone and of the osseous part of the lateral section of the orbital wall.[28]

In the previously mentioned diseases no connection with defects of the CNS is evident. A special syndrome results from the combination of cutis verticis gyrata with congenital mental retardation. This syndrome affects males almost exclusively; their mental development remains at the stage of earliest childhood, and only rarely will permit occupational activity. In addition to mental retardation these patients suffer from epileptic attacks and spastic paralyses. Furthermore, ocular diseases (strabismus, cataract, nystagmus, blindness) occur more than coincidentally. In this syndrome the cutaneous furrows on the head probably appear only after puberty. Inheritance has not been proven but in quite a percentage there is consanguinity of the parents.[1, 2]

(1) ÅKESSON, H. O.: Cutis verticis gyrata and mental deficiency in Sweden. I. Epidemiologic and clinical aspects. Acta med. scand. *175:* 115–127 (1964).

(2) ÅKESSON, H. O.: Cutis verticis gyrata and mental deficiency in Sweden. II. Genetic aspects. Acta med. scand. *177:* 459–464 (1965).

(3) BAES, H., and D. SUURMOND: Apocrine sweat gland carcinoma. Report of a case. Brit. J. Derm. *83:* 483–486 (1970).

(4) BANNAYAN, G. A.: Lipomatosis, angiomatosis, and macrencephalia. A previously undescribed congenital syndrome. Arch. Path. *92:* 1–5 (1971).

(5) BEARE, J. M., J. A. DODGE and N. C. NEVIN: Cutis gyratum, acanthosis nigricans and other congenital anomalies. A new syndrome. Brit. J. Derm. *81:* 241–247 (1969).

(6) COMBES, F. C., and R. VANINA: Osteosis cutis. Arch. Derm. Syph. (Chic.) *69:* 613–615 (1954).

(7) DAMSGAARD-SORENSEN, P., and A. SOEBORG OHLSEN: Multiple metastasizing sweat gland carcinomas. Acta derm.-venereol. (Stockh.) *49:* 314–318 (1969).

(8) FEYRTER, F., H. GOTTRON und W. NIKOLOWSKI: Über das Cylindrom der Haut. Arch. klin. exp. Derm. *214:* 54–104 (1961).

(9) FRANKE, H.: Beitrag zum Krankheitsbild der Osteosis cutis circumscripta. Hautarzt *7:* 270–272 (1956).

(10) FRESEN, O.: Über das Carcinom der Hautdrüsen am Beispiel eines Schweißdrüsenkrebses der Hohlhand. Hautarzt *11:* 15–23 (1960).

(11) GROSS, ST.: Sebaceous cysts. Correlation of clinical and pathological diagnoses in threehundred cases. J. Amer. Med. Ass. *152:* 813–814 (1953).

(12) HABERLAND, C., and M. PEROU: Encephalocraniocutaneous lipomatosis. A new example of ectomesodermal dysgenesis. Arch. Neurol. (Chic.) *22:* 144–155 (1970).

(13) HASHIMOTO, K.: Syringocystadenoma papilliferum. An electron microscopic study. Arch. Derm. Forsch. *245:* 353–369 (1972).

(14) HASHIMOTO, K., R. J. DIBELLA and W. F. LEVER: Clear cell hidradenoma. Arch. Derm. (Chic.) *96:* 18–38 (1967).

(15) HEADINGTON, J. T.: Mixed tumors of skin: eccrine and apocrine types. Arch. Derm. (Chic.) *84:* 989–996 (1961).

(16) HIRSCH, P., and E. B. HELWIG: Chondroid syringoma. Mixed tumor of skin, salivary gland type. Arch. Derm. (Chic.) *84:* 835–847 (1961).

(17) JANCAR, J.: Naevus syringocystadenomatosus papilliferus with skull and brain lesions, hemiparesis, epilepsy and mental retardation. Brit. J. Derm. *82:* 402–405 (1970).

(18) KERSTING, D. W.: Clear cell hidradenoma and hidradenocarcinoma. Arch. Derm. (Chic.) *87:* 323–333 (1963).

(19) KORTING, G. W., und N. HOEDE: Zum sogenannten »Pilar tumor of the scalp«. Arch. klin. exp. Derm. *234:* 409–419 (1969).

(20) KORTING, G. W., N. HOEDE und R. GEBHARDT: Kurzer Bericht über einen maligne entarteten Spiegler-Tumor. Derm. Mschr. *156:* 141–147 (1970).

(21) KRESBACH, H.: Ein Beitrag zum sogenannten Mischtumor der Haut. Arch. klin. exp. Derm. *221:* 59–74 (1964).

(22) MEHREGAN, A. H., and L. SHAPIRO: Angiolymphoid hyperplasia with eosinophilia. Arch. Derm. (Chic.) *103:* 50–57 (1971).

(23) MENDOZA, S., and E. B. HELWIG: Mucinous (Adenocystic) carcinoma of the skin. Arch. Derm. (Chic.) *103:* 68–78 (1971).

(24) MERENLENDER, I. J.: Atypical cutis gyrata. Arch. Derm. (Chic.) *77:* 669–675 (1958).

(25) NÖDL, F.: Beitrag zum Naevus syringocystadenomatosus papilliferus. Arch. Derm. Syph. (Berl.) *178:* 697–713 (1939).

(26) OTA, M.: Cutis gyrata der Stirnhaut, besonders ihr histologischer Befund. Derm. Wschr. *92:* 345–349 (1931).

(27) PINKUS, H.: »Sebaceous cysts« are trichilemmal cysts. Arch. Derm. (Chic.) *99:* 544–555 (1969).

(28) ROSENTHAL, J. W., and H. W. KLOEPFER: An acromegaloid, cutis verticis gyrata, corneal leukoma syndrome. Arch. Ophthal. (Chic.) *68:* 722–726 (1962).

(29) ROSS, C. M.: Generalized folded skin with an underlying lipomatous nevus. »The Michelin tire baby«. Arch. Derm. (Chic.) *100:* 320–323 (1969).

(30) SANTLER, R., und CHR. EBERHARTINGER: Malignes Klarzellen-Myoepitheliom. Dermatologica (Basel) *130:* 340–347 (1965).

(31) TELOH, H. A., R. B. BALKIN and J. P. GRIER: Metastasizing sweat-gland carcinoma. Arch. Derm. (Chic.) *76:* 80–86 (1957).

(32) TRITSCH, H.: Osteome der Kopfhaut. Arch. klin. exp. Derm. *221:* 336–347 (1965).

(33) UNDEUTSCH, W., und H. BRAUNER: Das Klarzellenhidradenom der Haut. Derm. Wschr. *151:* 649–656 (1965).

(34) WELLS, G. C., and I. W. WHIMSTER: Subcutaneous angiolymphoid hyperplasia with eosinophilia. Brit. J. Derm. *81:* 1–15 (1969).

(35) WILSON-JONES, E.: Proliferating epidermoid cysts. Arch. Derm. (Chic.) *94:* 11–19 (1966).

(36) WILSON-JONES, E., and ST. S. BLEEHEN: Inflammatory angiomatous nodules with abnormal blood vessels occurring about the ears and scalp (pseudo or atypical pyogenic granuloma). Brit. J. Derm. *81:* 804–816 (1969).

(37) ZEISLER, E. P., and L. M. WIEDER: Cutis verticis gyrata and acromegaly. Arch. Derm. Syph. (Chic.) *42:* 1092–1104 (1940).

F. Tumors of Tongue and Oral Mucosa

Carcinomas of the oral cavity and the tongue look like either circumscribed leukoplakias (see also Chapter 34, 4), verrucoid nodes, or granulomatous ulcerations. A decision between the benign or malignant

Fig. 721. Papilloma at the angle of the mouth.

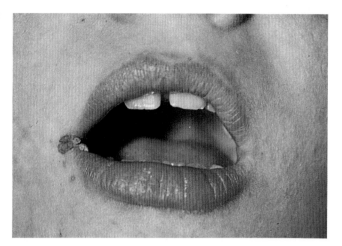

character of verrucous-tumorous vegetations on the labial or oral mucous membrane may be macroscopically and histologically difficult because of the great similarity with carcinomas.

1. On the labial mucous membrane a **squamous cell carcinoma** often originates from an abrasive cheilitis or a leukoplakia. But not every patient has a preceding lesion. At first there is only a small ulceration, which conspicuously lacks a tendency to epithelialize. It develops into either a larger, scarcely painful ulcer or, more often, an open papillary, firm, and easily bleeding tumor (Fig. 699). If the surface of the tumor is definitely verrucous, the possibility of an unusually localized common wart (Fig. 721) must be kept in mind in the differential diagnosis. The diagnosis of a squamous cell cancer should be confirmed in every case by the histologic findings; then a differentiation from a keratoacanthoma, Bowen's disease, and chronic vegetating pemphigus can follow.

The squamous cell carcinoma of the tongue (Fig. 722) or tonsils likewise represents an ulceration or a firm tumor. On the tongue the carcinoma often develops from a profound interstitial glos-

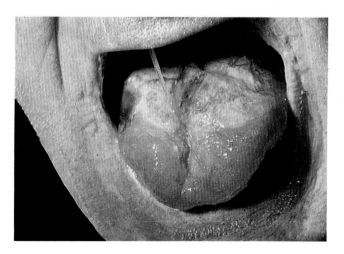

Fig. 722. Carcinoma of the tongue.

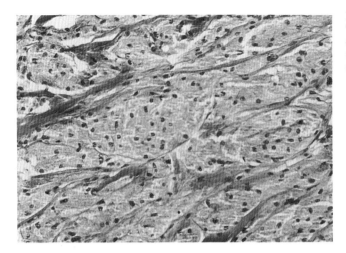

Fig. 723. Myoblastomyoma: Typical large cells with pale, eosinophilically granulated cytoplasm. Hematoxylin and eosin, 157 × .

sitis (Wassermann and Nelson tests). It is initially palpable as a hard infiltrate lying in the tongue. Histologic proof of the macroscopic findings should not be omitted. In squamous cell carcinomas of the mucous membranes, metastases into the regional lymph nodes are more frequent than in other locations.

2. A **myoblastomyoma** (granular cell myoblastoma) is a solitary, pea-sized, and firm tumor, occasionally with a leukoplakic surface, that must be differentiated from a squamous cell carcinoma. This tumor may occur anywhere on the entire cutaneous surface but is frequently observed on the oral mucous membranes and the lingual muscles. In contrast to squamous cell carcinoma, a myoblastomyoma arises without preceding changes and occurs even in children and adolescents. It may in exceptional cases be present at birth. Even if it lasts a long time, the tumor does not exceed a size of 2 cm and does not ulcerate on the surface. The diagnosis can be made only histologically. Closely aggregated oval or polygonal cells, whose cytoplasm is coarsely granulated (Fig. 723), are present. The individual granules are eosinophilic. An accompanying infiltrate or capsule of the tumor is lacking. The tumor, which is basically benign, may become malignant in exceptional cases.[5, 8]

Fig. 724. Glossitis rhomboidea mediana.

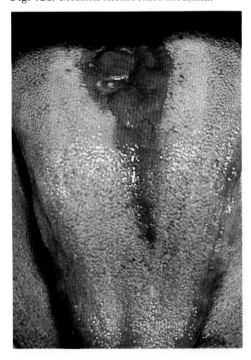

3. Glossitis rhombica mediana is located on the middle third of the dorsum of the tongue. It usually consists of a smooth

Fig. 725. Heterotopic lingual tonsil.

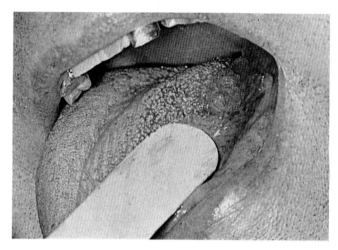

red spot without papillae, and its longitudinal axis lies exactly in the midline of the tongue. Instead of a smooth spot, nodular elevations of varying size (Fig. 724) may be present. Small leukoplakic areas may be present as secondary changes. Glossitis rhombica mediana is usually found by chance. Some patients, however, experience burning of the lingual area if they consume highly seasoned food. Histologically, circumscribed sclerosis of the connective tissue and an unspecific inflammation are present. It is believed that a poorly regressed tuberculum impar constitutes a special locus minoris resistentiae for such inflammatory processes. The fact that glossitis rhombica mediana occurs relatively late in life is evidence of the importance of exogenous factors. Since glossitis rhombica mediana occurs predominantly in older men, suspicion of a carcinoma is often expressed. This can readily be excluded on the basis of the characteristic clinical findings, but in doubtful cases a biopsy should be performed.[1, 11]

4. A heterotopic lingual tonsil is, like the lingual carcinomas, located at the side of the tongue, always on the posterior half. This soft, often glassy looking tumor, which is partly reminiscent of cerebral gyri, is easily recognizable macroscopically (Fig. 725). Such a heterotopic tonsil is always present as a malformation from the time of birth, and causes no difficulty for the patient except acute inflammations such as tonsillary angina.[3]

5. A ranula is a cystic protuberance next to the frenulum linguae. It is a retention cyst of the sublingual glands. The individual cyst may reach the size of a pea (Fig. 726). Some patients experience enlargement of the cyst during a meal.

6. Mucous retention cysts occur mainly at the entrance to the oral cavity. They are hemispherical protuberant tumors measuring up to 1 cm with a smooth surface. The color is that of the surrounding mucous membrane. The tumor results from the rupture of an excretory duct of a mucous gland with an outpouring of mucin into the surrounding mucous membrane. Accordingly, the histologic findings show unspecific granulation tissue filled with or surrounded by mucin. In taking a biopsy it is important to know that the inferior labial artery may protrude tumor-like on the inner labial margin and may imitate a mucous retention cyst. In that case there is the danger that a massive hemorrhage may result.[2, 4, 6].

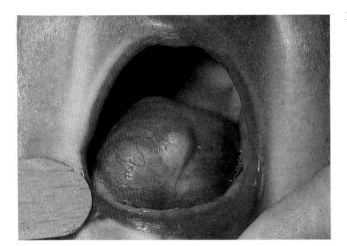

Fig. 726. Ranula.

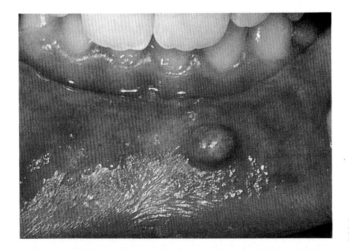

Fig. 727. Mucous cyst granuloma.

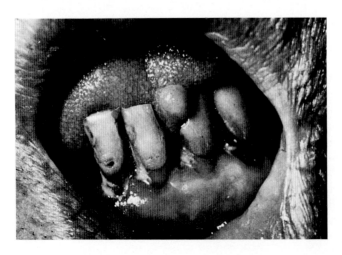

Fig. 728. Lingual proptosis.

Fig. 729. Buccal proptosis.

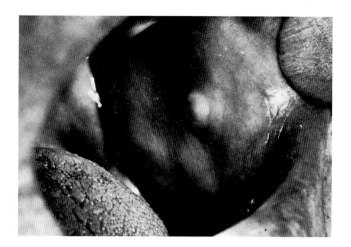

7. In patients who wear dental prostheses, nodose bulging mucous vegetations may develop in the area of the margin of an ill-fitting prosthesis. These **prosthesis fibromas** are for the most part located on the maxilla and the palate. Their base is relatively wide and the surface is covered by smooth mucous membrane. Occasionally, small leukoplakias are located on the bulges. Because of the unphysiological stress on the mucous membrane in the area of the prosthesis, inflammations result, including ruptures of the excretory ducts of the mucous glands. Because of these ruptures, the histologic picture is similar to that of a mucous retention cyst.[7, 10]

8. **Proptosis buccalis** (diapneusis buccalis) results from sucking a piece of mucous membrane into a dental gap. This is a hernialike protuberance of the buccal mucosa or tongue (Figs. 728, 729). If it lasts a long time, this pseudotumor may assume a rough or leukoplakic surface.[9]

9. Characteristic of a **mucosal neurinoma – carcinoma syndrome** are multiple firm nodes at the edge of the tongue or buccal mucosa that may reach a size of 5 mm in diameter (see also paragraph C8).

(1) BREITNER, J.: Glossitis rhombica mediana. Münch. med. Wschr. *92:* 350–351 (1950).
(2) EHLERS, G.: Zur Histogenese der Lippenschleimcysten. Z. Haut- u. Geschl.-Kr. *34:* 77–92 (1963).
(3) HALTER, K.: Über eine atavistische Zungenanomalie (»Tonsilla linguae heterotopica symmetrica«). Arch. Derm. Syph. (Berl.) *194:* 423–427 (1952).
(4) HOWELL, J. B., and R. G. FREEMAN: Prominent inferior labial artery. Arch. Derm. (Chic.) *107:* 386–387 (1973).
(5) MOSCOVIC, E. A., and H. A. AZAR: Multiple granular cell tumors (»myoblastomas«). Case report with electron microscopic observations and review of the literature. Cancer *20:* 2032–2047 (1967).
(6) NIKOLOWSKI, W.: Schleimcysten und sog. Schleimgranulom der Unterlippe. Arch. klin. exp. Derm. *203:* 246–255 (1956).
(7) PIRINGER-KUCHINKA, A.: Über das sogenannte Prothesenfibrom. Öst. Z. Stomat. *64:* 211–219 (1967).
(8) REICH, H.: Der Abrikossofftumor. Hautarzt *9:* 71–77 (1958).
(9) SCHUERMANN, H.: Proptosis buccalis (Diapneusis buccalis). Dtsch. zahnärztl. Z. *14:* 879–882 (1959).
(10) STÖGER, H.: Über sogenannte Prothesenfibrome. Dtsch. zahnärztl. Z. *19:* 401–406 (1964).
(11) WINKLER, J.: Zur Klinik der Glossitis rhombica mediana. Mschr. Ohrenheilk. *97:* 76–81 (1963).

G. Tumors Favoring the Trunk

1. Although **dermatofibrosarcoma protuberans** is located primarily on the trunk, location on the head or extremities is not exceptional. Middle-aged persons are affected most frequently, but even after the tumor has existed for decades, their general health is hardly impaired. After surgical removal of a dermatofibrosarcoma protuberans a high rate of local recurrences has been observed, but metastases into regional lymph nodes or internal organs take place only rarely. If metastases do occur the lungs are usually affected. The initial clinical finding is a hard nodule which slowly develops into a reddish-blue or brownish-yellow hard plaque located in the deeper cutis or subcutis and easily palpated. This plaque later develops into nodular tumors (Fig. 730). Spontaneous ulcerations do not occur. The size of the tumors varies, but as a rule even after a longer duration a diameter of more than 5 cm is hardly ever attained. Multilocular manifestations are rare.

Because dermatofibrosarcoma protuberans closely resembles fibrosarcoma it can be identified more easily clinically than

Fig. 730. Dermatofibrosarcoma protuberans.

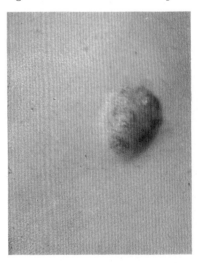

histologically. The stroma of the tumor consists of relatively uniform, spindle-shaped, connective tissue cells arranged in whorls around the blood vessels; atypical cell nuclei and increased mitoses are absent. The tumor cells themselves form fibrillary connective tissue to a varying degree. Giant cells are rare, and histiocytes with phagocytic activity, or those showing storage of lipids and hemosiderin, are almost always absent; these findings make it easier to differentiate the dermatofibrosarcoma from dermatofibromas or sclerosing angiomas. In addition, the cellular dermatofibrosarcoma, which usually shows an atrophic epithelial band, lacks those pseudoepitheliomatous epidermal hyperplasias seen so frequently above collagenized histiocytomas. In contrast, the dermatofibrosarcoma is sometimes abundantly interspersed with blood vessels enlarged into lacunae; these vessels have only one layer of endothelium between the lumen and the surrounding tumor.[16, 36, 56]

2. Multiple hard fibromas of the skin are distributed irregularly, but there is a definite preference for the trunk. As opposed to the frequent occurrence of soft fibromas, the hard variety occurs very seldom. Solitary, rather hard nodes may reach a size of 2 cm. Frequently they protrude hemispherically above the surrounding skin. The epidermis above these nodes remains unaffected. To some extent small tumors lie so deep in the corium that they can only be palpated. Histologically, one finds an intracutaneous fibromalike increase of the connective tissue cells with hyperplasia of the collagenous fibers. Histiocytes, giant cells, and deposits of fibrinoid are absent and with the exception of location, there are almost no clinical differences between a hard fibroma, a dermatofibroma, and a histiocytoma. The differential diagnosis includes above all nodular disseminated connective tissue nevi (see this chapter, Section 23) and a nodular pseudosarcomatous fasciitis (see Section I 17).[21, 22]

3. Generalized neurofibromatosis is characterized as a rule by the simultaneous presence of macular hyperpigmentations ("café-au-lait spots," "axillary freckling"; see Chapter 24, E 7) and multiple cutaneous tumors (Fig. 731). However, each of these manifestations may be present as a single sign and in various degrees of expression. The cutaneous tumors may appear as neurinomas, neurofibromas, and fibromas; they are located along the nerve trunks as painful thickened lesions. In general a certain predominance of localization on the trunk can be observed. The palms and soles remain uninvolved almost without exception. Multiple neurofibromas may even be seen in childhood; during puberty and pregnancy they often increase considerably in number and size. The overlying epidermis is always unchanged because the tumors are located in the cutaneous or subcutaneous tissue. At times the tumors may show a reddish-blue tinge through the skin that may lead to the erroneous diagnosis of angiomas. The size of the tumor varies considerably from pea-size to elephantiasic, lobulated, pendulous tumor masses (Fig. 732). Tumors as large as cherries can be invaginated through a ring in the skin by pressure with the finger, which causes them to snap back like a bell button. In a typical case the diagnosis is not difficult. Similar tumors may appear on the inner organs, giving rise to various clinical signs according to their location. The manifestations of the gastrointestinal tract, the eyes and ears, the skeletal system, and the renal vessels are important. Stenoses of the renal arteries may cause hypertension even in childhood. Many patients suffer from curvature of the spinal column. Sarcomatous degeneration of a neurofibroma is a rare exception; clinically it can be recognized by the rapid growth of solitary tumors into extremely hard and nodular masses

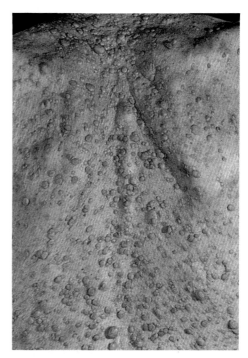

Fig. 731. Generalized neurofibromatosis.

Fig. 732. Lobular elephantiasis in generalized neurofibromatosis.

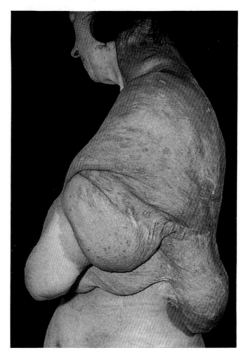

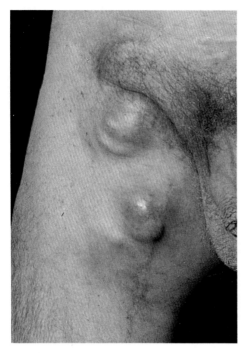

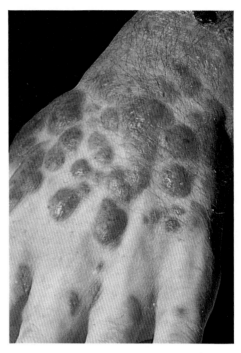

Fig. 733. Sarcomatously degenerated generalized neurofibromatosis.

Fig. 734. Chronic reticulosis.

(Fig. 733). This may result in central
softening and ulceration of the tumor. The
histologic diagnosis of malignancy is made
more difficult because many neurinomas
and neurofibromas show marked cellular
and nuclear polymorphism with giant cells
and, in addition, even infiltrative penetration into the surrounding tissue may be
discerned. Such a sarcoma may at times
contain massive amounts of acid mucopolysaccharides.[9, 13, 18, 31, 37, 38, 46, 57]

4. Formations of multiple nodes of
various sizes on the trunk are also observed in **reticuloses**. They consist of
malignant proliferations of undifferentiated reticular connective tissue; within
the cutaneous region, this tissue is
found around the appendages and the
small vessels. As part of the reticulohistiocytic system it shows special reactivity toward various stimuli. Because the
cellular elements of the reticulohistiocytic
system consist of fixed lymphoid reticulum
cells, histiocytes, and mobile monocytes,
it is easily understandable why in certain
mostly terminal phases monocytes may
appear in the circulating blood, resulting
finally in monocytic leukemia. The clinical
picture of reticuloses is variable and has led
to the establishment of groups of reticuloses (see Table 15). Reticuloses usually
occur between the fifth and seventh decades
of life; the more acute forms are observed
more often in younger than in older persons. In a narrower sense, except for the
multiple nodular infiltrates of the skin,
cutaneous reticulosis at first shows no involvement of the internal organs (lymph
nodes, liver, spleen). A disorder of the
function of the spleen can be discovered
early merely by a scintiscan. In addition,
for a long time there are no changes in the
blood picture. The course of the disease is
variable. Circumscribed, grouped formations of nodes point toward a chronic

course extending over several years (Fig. 734), whereas exanthematic dissemination of infiltrates is frequently indicative of an acute form of the disease which ends in death within a few weeks (Fig. 735). The infiltrates are found predominantly in the deeper parts of the cutis; they are movable against the underlying tissue but not with the upper parts of the skin. The color of the plaquelike as well as the nodular infiltrates varies from a faint to a more saturated brownish- to a bluish-red tone (Fig. 736). Diascopic examination shows a fine brownish-yellow discoloration; sometimes minute petechiae become visible. Ulcerative changes are extremely rare. To a large extent the erythrodermic forms of reticuloses remain confined to the skin; they are discussed in Chapter 22, C4. A third group of reticuloses, which begins primarily as a systemic disease of the reticulohistiocytic system, shows a direct association of the cutaneous infiltrates with

enlargement of the lymph nodes and hepatosplenomegaly. Again, this group may include both acute and chronic courses of reticulosis.

Histologically, reticuloses are usually divided into forms with small cells (lymphoid), medium-sized cells, and large cells. The predominantly monomorphic cellular proliferations of the corium and subcutis start from the appendages or from perivascular tissue. The infiltrate itself may be confined to nodes or it may extend into bands. Frequently a free subepidermal region remains, as in specific leukemic cutaneous infiltrates. Within the region of the infiltrate the bundles of collagenous fibers are split into single fibers with an irregular distribution. There may also be a thick reticular aggregation of fibers. The infiltrates, apart from the erythrodermic forms, tend not to penetrate into the epidermis. Depending on the degree of malignancy, the infiltrates may form a

Fig. 735. Acute malignant reticulosis.

Fig. 736. Plaquelike reticulosis.

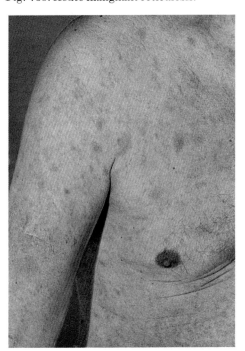

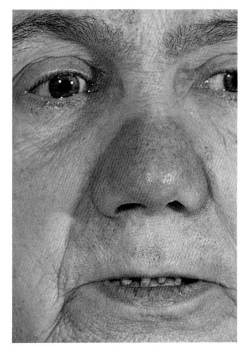

Table 15 Clinical Criteria of the Various Forms of Reticulosis

	Prodromata; Duration	General Condition	Fever	Skin Mucous Membranes
I. Reticuloses of the skin in the narrow sense				
1. Acute or subacute reticulosis, "So-called reticulo-sarcomatosis of the skin," exanthematic form	None; **a few months**	Distinctly impaired	**Septic temperatures**	**Multicentric involvement of skin, plaquelike and nodose lesions, brown to bluish-red, firm, pointed hemorrhages, mucous membranes free**
2. Chronic skin reticulosis, nodose form	**Itching, urticaria, eczemas; several years**	Unimpaired for a long time	Only terminal fever	**Multicentric involvement of skin as in I. l., leonine face, nodes do not ulcerate, mucous membranes free**
3. Erythrodermic cutaneous reticuloses				
(a) Dry, squamous type	**Occasionally itching;** months to years	Burning of skin, attacks of sweating	Terminal	**Scaling erythroderma with uninvolved areas as in exfoliative generalized dermatitis; with pigmentation, mucous membranes occasionally involved**
(b) Edematous oozing type	Occasionally itching; months to years	Burning of skin, attacks of sweating	Terminal	**Erythroderma with edema, erosions on face, genitals and legs, pigmentation, mucous membranes occasionally involved**
II. Polyorganic reticuloses with skin involvement				
1. Leukemic type	**A few months**	**Rapid disintegration, secondary infections**	**Fever** during the whole course	**In 80% gingival swelling** with ulcer formation; in 20% skin involvement: scaling erythemas, papules, plaquelike lesions, hemorrhages
2. Aleukemic type (a) acute (b) chronic	A few months 1–3 years	Poor general condition	With fever Without fever	Often up to pea-sized bluish-red cutaneous nodules

Peripheral Lymph Nodes	Liver, Spleen	Other Inner Organs	Bone Marrow	ESR	White Hemogram	Red Hemogram	Thrombocytes
Often enlarged	0	Sometimes terminal	0	**In most cases unchanged**	In most cases inconspicuous, terminal monocytic leukemia possible	Anemia	Very rarely thrombocytopenia
Affected only after a long time				**In most cases unchanged**	Sub finem leukocytosis (monocytes) up to 30000	Terminal anemia	Terminal thrombocytopenia possible
Enlarged at an early stage	Enlarged after some time		Very rare	At first moderately, later considerably increased	Sometimes eosinophilia; terminal monocytic leukemia possible	Late moderate anemia	0
Enlarged at an early stage	Enlarged after some time		Very rare	At first moderately, later considerably increased	Sometimes eosinophilia; monocytic leukemia possible	Late moderate anemia	0
Enlarged	**Enlarged**		**Interspersed with monocytes and reticulum cells**		**Monocytic leukemia**	Anemia	Thrombocytopenia
Enlarged	**Enlarged**		Uncharacteristic		Uncharacteristic	In advanced cases anemia	Often thrombocytopenia

pseudocapsule by displacing the surrounding collagenous tissue or by destroying the former normal local tissue.[14, 24, 33, 41]

5. Histiocytic medullary reticulosis shows specific nodular infiltrates relatively infrequently. In most cases only unspecific psoriasiform or eczematiform reactions accompany the disease. Histiocytic medullary reticulosis follows an especially foudroyant course with a survival time of only a few weeks; the disease affects patients between the ages of 40 and 60, starting with rapid loss of weight and septic febrile attacks. Enlargement of lymph nodes and hepatosplenomegaly are apparent early in the course of disease. Many patients also develop jaundice. Hematologically, the main features are increasing anemia, leukocytopenia, and thrombocytopenia, which occasionally ends in pancytopenia (aplastic anemia). Purpura almost always is present in the terminal stage. The multiple nodular cutaneous infiltrates may attain a diameter of up to 2 cm and show a brownish-red color. Histologically, this disease is characterized by proliferation of atypical large histiocytes which phagocytize erythrocytes in great numbers. The diagnosis is established either by puncture of the bone marrow or by biopsy of a lymph node or of a specific cutaneous infiltrate.[10, 62]

6. Exceptionally, **reticuloendotheliosis of the infant** occurs congenitally or shortly after birth. This reticulosis may represent a reactive process subject to spontaneous regression after variable periods of time or, on the other hand, it may be a malignant disease which is rapidly lethal. Neither the clinical picture nor the histomorphologic findings permit an early decision, but observation of the clinical course will lead to the correct diagnostic classification. Upon inspection the entire cutaneous surface, especially the trunk, will show hazelnut-sized cutaneous and subcutaneous nodes. The overlying epi-

dermis actually always remains free of secondary lesions such as scaling, crusting, and bleeding. However, the skin may show a color change – depending on the depth of the infiltrate it may be a bluish-red or brownish-red hue. In some infants the infiltrate can only be palpated. The accompanying changes of the inner organs (hepatosplenomegaly, enlargement of lymph nodes) can often be demonstrated only by careful methodical examination. In the early stages cellular changes in the blood smear are almost always lacking, as in the reticuloses of the adult; however, in the terminal stages monocytes will be increased in a peripheral blood smear or in a bone marrow smear. Histologically, one finds a uniform increase of cells with round nuclei in the corium. The areas of cellular proliferation either displace or destroy the regional collagen; a thickened reticular network can be found in its place.[1, 52]

In the differential diagnosis histiocytosis X must be ruled out first. The cutaneous picture easily permits such a differentiation because histiocytosis X almost always forms eczematoid changes, not nodular infiltrates (see also Chapter 21, D4). Such an infiltrate of reticulosis in the genital region may be mistaken at first for a granuloma gluteale infantum (see also Chapter 38, H8).

7. Sympathicogonioma (neuroblastoma sympathicum) is a metastasizing tumor resulting in multiple small nodular growths located on the trunk of infants and children. This hormonally inactive tumor of the adrenal medulla forms metastases primarily in the liver (Pepper type) or in the skeleton (Hutchinson type). Exceptionally, metastasis into the skin alone is observed (Smith type). Even before the appearance of metastases, patients develop irregular attacks of fever, rheumatoid back pain, and a vague anemia. Bony metastases of the skull often result in protrusion of the eyeballs and bilateral

Fig. 737. Circumscribed reticulosis of the skin.

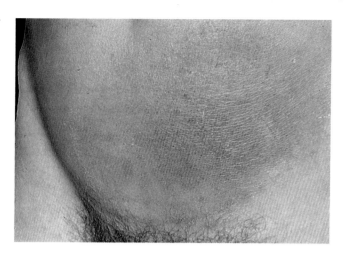

hematoma of the orbits. Cutaneous metastases are attached partly to the epidermis
and partly to the subcutis. The diagnosis
can be established through careful radiologic examination of the adrenals. At
times the sternal marrow may show tumor
cells. As far as the prognosis is concerned,
it is of special importance that permanent
regression of all metastases may occur
spontaneously at any time.[25, 53, 59]

8. Reticulocytosis (reticular hyperplasia)
must be separated from reticulosis as a
reactive hyperplasia capable of spontaneous regression. Reticulocytosis may be
the result of ingestion of drugs (diphenylhydantoin, nitrofurantoin), insect bites
(mites, ticks), or actinic factors (so-called
actinoreticulosis). In many cases the
etiologic factors cannot be ascertained.
The dermatologic findings of reticulocytosis differ from those of reticulosis
only insignificantly in that hemorrhagic
phenomena are practically always absent
(Figs. 737, 738). General signs such as
fever, loss of weight, and asthenia are also
lacking. Although occasionally enlargement of the lymph nodes can be found,
hepatosplenomegaly and changes of the
blood picture are not seen. Often the latter
changes occur in reticuloses only occasionally, so that verification of reticulocytosis

can sometimes be made only in retrospect.
Histologically, reticulocytoses show mainly perivascular infiltrates which have a
more polymorphous composition than
those of the reticuloses; often the infiltrate
contains eosinophilic granulocytes. Near

Fig. 738. Nodular-erosive reticular hyperplasia of the skin.

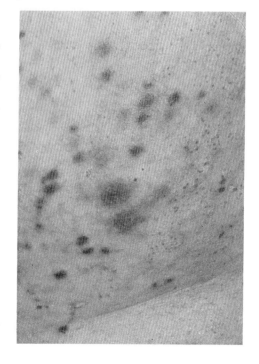

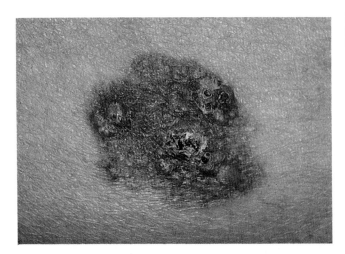

Fig. 739. Basaloma of the trunk (pagetoid type of basaloma).

the deeper tissue the infiltrates have a straight border; however, they penetrate toward and into the epidermis without leaving a free subepidermal zone. This leads to an increase of melanin via a secondary pigmentary incontinence in the border zone of the infiltrate. Unlike reticuloses, in reticulocytosis even the blood vessels take part in the disease process. Their lumina are usually wide and show swelling of the endothelium. The collagenous fibers within the infiltrates are subject to disintegration, however, without showing the reconstructive changes characteristic of the reticuloses. [28, 29, 35]

9. Lipomas should be considered first in the presence of unequally large, subcutaneous, freely movable nodes of the trunk. This type of tumor is discussed in Sections A5 and K1 of this chapter.

10. Multiple basal cell epitheliomas (basalomas) of the trunk are often mistaken for a long time for eczematous or psoriatic lesions. This type of epithelioma consists of very shallow patches which spread outward extremely slowly. The center shows regressive changes with small areas of atrophy, shallow erosions, and scaly crusts (Fig. 739). The typical pearly ridge of the basal cell epithelioma

can be seen in the border area, but frequently only when magnified with a loupe. The pearly ridge itself has a dark black-blue or black-brown pigmentation. Nodules of more than pinhead size and ulcerations are rare and actually are seen only when the affected area is larger than the palm of the hand. In the beginning multiple epitheliomas of the trunk can be separated from areas of Bowen's disease only with difficulty. However, as a rule Bowen's disease shows no signs of regression, and it lacks the pearly and partly pigmented ridge. Paget's disease has to be excluded in the region of the breasts or apocrine sweat glands. Whenever an epithelioma of the trunk does not look quite typical, a biopsy should be taken. Many patients with multiple epitheliomas of the trunk give a history of intake of arsenic; in such a case a further search for other malignancies caused by arsenic (for instance, larynx, bronchial system, liver) should be made. [8, 26, 34]

11. Premalignant fibroepithelioma is another special type of basal cell epithelioma; it favors the lumbosacral, lower abdominal, and inguinal regions. In some patients these fibroepitheliomas are present even on the inner aspects of the thighs. The tumors reach a size of about 1.0 cm in diameter and protrude hemispherically, sometimes on a sessile base. The surface remains unchanged but it can be coarsely nodose or even lobulated. The color of the tumor corresponds to the surrounding skin. Its consistency is rather soft and does not attain the hardness of a nodular basal cell epithelioma. Telangiectases in most cases are absent. Frequently premalignant fibroepitheliomas are present in the immediate vicinity of soft fibromas and senile keratoses. Histologically, this type of basal cell epithelioma shows a conspicuous increase of connective tissue. Bands of epithelial cells composed of only two rows of cells lie between rather vascular connective tissue. The basic epitheliomatous character of this mixed form of epithelial and mesenchymal hyperplasia is emphasized even by the distinctly visible palisadelike, marginal arrangement of the nuclei. The intermediate connective tissue generally shows many fibroblasts, whereas myxoid transformations are seen only rarely.[23, 45, 48]

12. The soft fibroma (fibroma molle) is a tumor that usually occurs as multiple lesions. Preferred sites are regions with soft skin such as the neck, axillae, and inguinal and submammary folds (Fig. 740). Beginning with the fortieth year of life the incidence of fibromas increases perceptibly; adipose individuals often have numerous soft fibromas. Each tumor rests on the skin with a pedicle; its size varies from 2 to 5 mm in diameter. Sometimes such a soft fibroma reaches the size of a hen's egg with the result that the pedicle becomes especially elongated owing to the weight of the tumor. The surface is smooth or finely folded, but squamous or keratotic coverings as well as increased growth of hair are absent; the latter is not part of the clinical picture of a soft fibroma. However, various degrees of a brown pigmentation may be present. The differential diagnosis actually has to consider

only the so-called fibrous nevus cell nevus. These nevi may show a somewhat harder consistency than soft fibromas and have less tendency toward pedicle formation. The presence of several stronger hairs or of well-marked follicular markings favors a fibrous nevus cell nevus. Histologically, soft fibromas consist of normal epidermis that forms a sac around the extended upper layers of corium (collagenous and elastic fibers, blood vessels). The same picture can prevail in the case of a fibrous nevus cell nevus, but careful search will always show the presence of small nests of nevus cells.

13. The **Tietze syndrome** is characterized by painful tumorlike thickening of the ribs. Etiologically, these thickenings are fatigue fractures at the costochondral junction, which, however, cannot always be roentgenologically verified. Initially the disorder causes pain in the area of the cartilages of the first and second ribs when

Fig. 740. Pedunculated fibromas of the axilla

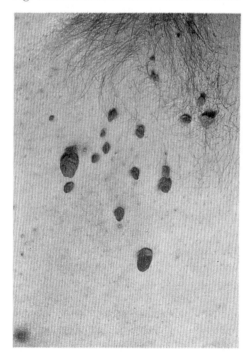

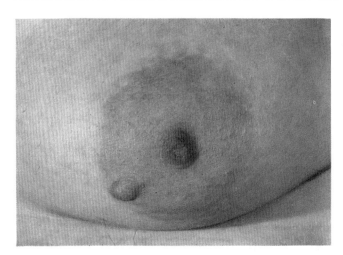

Fig. 741. Myxoma cutis of the areola of the breast.

coughing and moving the arms. Only exceptionally are other ribs involved. Gradually, a firm tumor is formed which is tender on pressure and firmly attached to the cartilage of the rib. The overlying skin can be lifted and shows no inflammatory signs or secondary changes.[50, 60]

14. Among the late stigmas of congenital syphilis, a tumorlike thickening of the medial third of the clavicle **(sign of Higoumenakis)** has been observed relatively frequently. The osseous thickening follows syphilitic ostitis, which appears as a solitary sign at this site of increased demand. Accordingly, in right-handed persons the swelling will occur on the right clavicle and in left-handed persons on the corresponding side. Since this clavicular hyperostosis does not lead to any complaints, it almost always remains unnoticed. In the differential diagnosis the sequelae of a clavicular fracture have to be ruled out.[19, 20]

15. Mammary tumors at first suggest a **mammary cancer.** If mammography does not result in a definite diagnosis, a biopsy is required. Besides a palpable node, sudden pain in the breast, or sudden secretion from the nipple, unilateral flattening or retraction of the nipple, and persistent eczematous changes of the mammary region also suggest a carcinoma. These signs are observed in the mammary carcinomas of both women and men. For the differential diagnosis of *Paget's disease, Bowen's disease of the nipple, primary carcinoma of the nipple, and mamillary adenomatosis,* see Chapter 21, B3. A *myxoma* of the nipple (Fig. 741) may also resemble a malignant tumor. Here also, the diagnosis can be only histologically verified. Further differential diagnostic considerations of a mammary carcinoma from chronic cystic mastopathia and the various forms of mammary fibroadenomas do not belong to the field of the dermatologist. It may be mentioned that diffuse **leiomyomatosis** of the breast may imitate a carcinomatous lymphangiosis, from which it cannot be differentiated mammographically. The diagnosis can be ascertained only by biopsy.[2, 4, 39, 61]

16. Lymphadenosis benigna cutis results in red-brownish or blue-red infiltrates not only at the typical locations on the ear lobe and the scrotum but also in the area of the nipple. They are either multiple small nodules, which affect only part of the areola, or they change the areola into a round, smooth, protuberance in the form of a lozenge (see also Section C21 in this chapter).

17. The so-called **elastic nevus** is a special form of connective tissue nevi which favors the upper thorax. It is either already present at birth or appears in the first years of life, without showing marked tendencies to grow later. The multiple, 2 to 3 millimeter-sized nodules are closely aggregated in a circumscribed area. Their color varies between skin-color and yellow-white. Some of these elastic nevi persist only as a few lentil-sized, flat, elevated tumors. Histologically, the collagenous tissue is increased and the elastic fibers are mostly unaffected.[6, 17, 29]

18. In the umbilical region the only formations that are typical are those which have a biogenetic relationship to this area as embryonic remnants of organs. Thus, congenital umbilical anomalies are of primary dermatologic importance. They are associated with the embryonic allantois, the urachus. Rather frequently there are additional internal anomalies. On the other hand, **congenital umbilical polyps,** as the only remnants of the omphalomesenteric duct, may continue to exist. Such polyps either have a wide base or are pedunculated, and they may therefore simulate a pyogenic granuloma at first. But in contrast to it they have a firmer consistency and a lighter red color. The surrounding area may be affected by an eczema according to the degree of moisture of the polyps. Histopathologically, islands of intestinal mucosa or pancreatic tissue are factors that favor a diagnosis of dysontogenetic umbilical polyps. Dripping urine is in general observed a few days after birth only in children with a totally open urachus. This irritates the surrounding skin, which may lead in turn to the rapid development of acanthomas.

If the urachus remains partially patent, so-called *urachal cysts* may develop; these often become conspicuous when they have reached a special size or have become secondarily infected. Very rare, however, are infraumbilical *mucoepidermoid* tumors of the urachus.[43, 44, 54]

19. Primary cutaneous epitheliomas such as basalomas or squamous cell carcinomas of the umbilical fossa occur very seldom. So-called **secondary umbilical carcinomas,** however, occur more frequently. They originate in primary carcinomas of the abdominal cavity and most probably spread through the lymph vessels of the ligamentum rotundum.

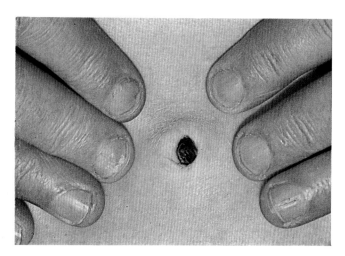

Fig. 742. Horny plug of the umbilical grove.

20. Since dirt in the umbilical fossa apparently adheres well, solid, hard, and dark brown **formations of concrement** (Fig. 742) may develop. They can be removed completely with a pair of pincers without causing any sign of irritation (e.g. erythema) of the bare umbilical skin. Close inspection permits a safe distinction from a melanoma or senile wart in this unusual location.[11]

21. Cutaneous endometriosis is seen most often in the umbilical area and secondly in the inguinal and genital regions. It develops after the menarche but usually is first noticed clinically around the twentieth year of life. According to the skin layer in which they are located, the nodes have a lighter or darker blue color, so that they may be confused with an angioma or metastases from a melanoma. The symptoms – premenstrual feeling of tension or pain – furnish important diagnostic clues. In addition, endometriotic nodules enlarge during menstruation. They usually are attached to the surface and the base and can be moved only slightly. In principle, however, the diagnosis can be made only histologically.[27, 55]

22. In the coccygeal area protuberant nodes denote a **pilonidal sinus** (coccygeal cyst). Since the fistular duct is not apparent in many patients, this condition is often diagnosed as a furuncle. For more details see Chapter 14, B8.

23. Lumbosacral connective tissue nevi are located almost exclusively in the lumbar region. They are signs of Pringle-Bourneville's phakomatosis, and consist of multiple, closely aggregated, distinctly elevated nodules, whose diameter varies from 2 to 10 mm. The color either matches that of the surrounding skin or is somewhat lighter. Histologically, the nodules are formed of increased and hypertrophic collagenous tissue, and in rare cases there

are also changes in the elastic fibers.[6, 7, 42, 58]

24. In **epidermolysis bullosa albopapuloidea** flatly elevated papules also appear in the lumbosacral area beginning in the second decade of life. For details see Chapter 25, A9. In contrast to lumbosacral connective tissue nevi, the individual lesions are slightly smaller and often show a centrally widened follicular opening. Furthermore, their location does not remain strictly limited to the lumbosacral region; they may be distributed in large numbers over the entire trunk. Histologically, although as connective tissue nevi they consist of widened bundles of collagen, they also show disappearance of elastica.[12, 15]

25. In addition to the lumbosacral connective tissue nevus and the nevus elasticus, a third form of the connective tissue nevus exists, the **giant node-disseminated connective tissue nevus,** which is most probably identical with an eruptive collagenoma. The nodes, occurring mainly on the trunk but also on the extremities, are 0.5 to 4 cm large and are scarcely raised at all above the level of the skin. The color of these tumors usually remains unchanged but may occasionally resemble that of a xanthoma. The nodes can be easily moved on their bases but the skin covering the tumors cannot be lifted. Connective tissue nevi manifest themselves even in childhood, but may appear for the first time at an advanced age. They then develop relatively quickly. Familial occurrence is recognized. Histologically, again, only an increase of the collagenous tissue can be found.[5, 17, 32, 49]

26. The **Buschke-Ollendorff syndrome** is a combination of osteopoikilosis with various forms of connective tissue nevi (with the exception of the lumbosacral connective tissue nevi). It is transmitted as an autosomal dominant trait. Cutaneous changes occur even in childhood and may be varied. Some patients show multiple, lentil- to cherrystone-sized firm nodes on the trunk and extremities; these either lie at the level of the skin or protrude hemispherically. Their color varies from skin color to light brown and is similar to that of histiocytomas which store hemosiderin. All connective tissue nevi, however, are different from histiocytomas because of the sole increase of fibers in the presence of explicitly low cells of the tumor tissue. Other patients do not show many individual connective tissue nevi but instead, lesions that are grouped in several places in streaks or distributed segmentally. The individual nevi do not exceed lentil size, have a white-yellowish color, and are closely grouped next to each other, giving the impression of cobblestones. The cutaneous changes may closely resemble those of pseudoxanthoma elasticum. Osteopoikilosis causes no symptoms and is often discovered by chance when radiographs are made for some other purpose. This disorder consists of condensations of about 5 mm in diameter located in the spongiosa. Only exceptionally do osseous cysts coexist. The most frequent sites of osteopoikilosis are the bones of the pelvis

and the extremities. In addition to the cutaneous and osseous changes, which do not cause any symptoms, some patients complain of pain in the joints or extremities, and they may show a pronounced disposition to keloids.[3, 47, 51]

27. In the lumbosacral region a tumor that is already present at birth and varies in size from a pigeon egg to a fist probably contains a **meningocele.** If it has a thin covering, the diagnosis is not difficult. Often, however, the meningocele is completely covered by skin including subcutaneous fatty tissue, so that clinically only a firm elastic tumor in the midline is present. In abortive cases only a **sacral lipoma,** like dorsolumbar hypertrichosis, indicates a spina bifida lying underneath.

28. A **chordoma** is a very rare tumor of the spinal region involving the skin. This is a malignant growth of the ectodermal, embryonic anlage of the chorda. Chordomas are most often located in the sphenooccipital and sacrococcygeal regions. The tumor first begins to grow at an advanced age and leads initially to nonspecific complaints of pain. In progressive stages of the disease neurologic deficits and destruction of the surrounding osseous

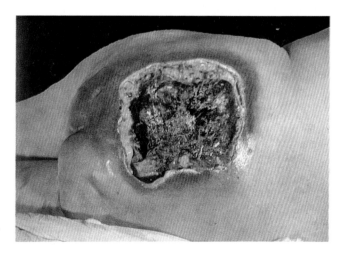

Fig. 743. Ulcerated sacrococcygeal chordoma.

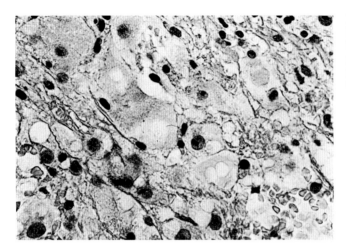

Fig. 744. Chordoma: large balloon cells with ill-defined borders and vacuolized cytoplasm, so-called physaliphorous cells. Hematoxylin and eosin, 680 ×.

tissue ensue, making possible at that time at least a tentative roentgenologic diagnosis. In some patients firm, nodular subcutaneous nodes develop slowly over the sacrum; they later ulcerate (Fig. 743). Histologically, the parenchyma of the tumor consists of rather typical large, light, alveolar cells (Fig. 744).[40]

(1) AMBS, E., P. BIREN und G. KLING-MÜLLER: Über eine angeborene Retikulose. Hautarzt 17: 63–68 (1966).

(2) BECKER, G., und C. W. FASSBENDER: Das Brustdrüsenkarzinom des Mannes. Strahlentherapie 143: 21–26 (1972).

(3) BERLIN, R., B. HEDENSIÖ, B. LILJA and L. LINDER: Osteopoikilosis – a clinical and genetic study. Acta med. scand. (Stockh.) 181: 305–314 (1967).

(4) CORTESE, A. F., and G. N. CORNELL: Carcinoma of male breast. Ann. Surg. 173: 275–280 (1971).

(5) CRAMER, H. J.: Zum Krankheitsbild des sog. »eruptiven Kollagenoms«. Hautarzt 17: 437–440 (1966).

(6) CRAMER, H. J., und G. KAHLERT: Über Bindegewebsnaevi. Hautarzt 19: 251 bis 256 (1968).

(7) DAMMERT, K., and K. M. NIEMI: Naevus elasticus (elastoma juvenile Weidman) and naevus collagenicus lumbosacralis in Pringle's disease. Dermatologica (Basel) 137: 36–45 (1968).

(8) DENK, R., H. HOLZMANN, H.-J. LANGE und D. GREVE: Über Arsenspätschäden bei obduzierten Moselwinzern. Med. Welt 20 (N.F.): 557–567 (1969).

(9) DIEKMANN, L., W. HÜTHER und R. A. PFEIFFER: Ungewöhnliche Erscheinungsformen der Neurofibromatose (von Recklinghausensche Krankheit) im Kindesalter. Z. Kinderheilk. 101: 191 bis 222 (1967).

(10) ENGSTROM, P. F., J. L. AELING and D. W. R. SURINGA: Histiocytic medullary reticulosis with cutaneous lesions. Arch. Derm. (Chic.) 106: 369–371 (1972).

(11) FISHMAN, H. C.: The inspissated umbilical bolus. Arch. Derm. (Chic.) 103: 221–222 (1971).

(12) GASSER, I., und H. WALTHER: Zur Kenntnis der Epidermolysis bullosa et albopapuloidea Pasini. Derm. Wschr. 120: 417–422 (1949).

(13) GEBHARDT, R., und G. W. KORTING: Exzeptionelle Lappen-Elephantiasis. Med. Welt 22 (N.F.): 1692–1693 (1971).

(14) GERTLER, W.: Nosologie und Klinik der kutanen Retikulosen. Derm. Mschr. 155: 621–638 (1969).

(15) GÖTZ, H., und K. MEINICKE: Zur Klinik und Therapie der Epidermolysis bullosa et albo-papuloidea Pasini. Derm. Wschr. 131: 481–487 (1955).

(16) GROETSCHEL, H., und H. J. CRAMER: Multilokulär-symmetrisches Dermatofibrosarkoma protuberans. Derm.Wschr. 153: 574–582 (1967).

(17) HENDERSON, R. R., C. E. WHEELER and D. C. ABELE: Familial cutaneous collagenoma. Arch. Derm. (Chic.) *98:* 23–27 (1968).

(18) HENINGTON, V. M., and A. E. CAROE: Massive fibroma pendulum. Arch. Derm. (Chic.) *80:* 580–583 (1959).

(19) HIGOUMÉNAKIS, G. C.: The »clavicle sign« and its diagnostic value in hereditary syphilis. Urol. Cutan. Rev. (St. Louis) *41:* 799–809 (1937).

(20) HIGOUMÉNAKIS, G. C.: Le signe de la clavicule et sa valeur diagnostique dans la syphilis héréditaire. Ann. Derm. Syph. (Paris) *8:* 939–961 (1937).

(21) HOEDE, N.: Zur Kenntnis der multiplen harten Fibrome der Haut. Z. Haut- u. Geschl.-Kr. *40:* 286–292 (1966).

(22) HOLZMANN, H., K.-H. HASSENPFLUG und B. BEIKIRCH: Zur Frage der Wesensunterschiede von Histiocytom und Dermatofibrom nebst Bemerkungen zu dem bei ihnen zu beobachtenden Verhalten des Follikels. Z. Haut- u. Geschl.-Kr. *40:* 89–95 (1966).

(23) HORNSTEIN, O.: Über die Pinkussche Varietät der Basaliome. Hautarzt *8:* 406–411 (1957).

(24) HORNSTEIN, O.: Bedeutung der Histopathologie für die Diagnostik der Retikulosen. Hautarzt *20:* 210–215 (1969).

(25) HORNSTEIN, O., und G. MÜLKE: Kutan metastasierendes Neuroblastoma sympathicum mit »spontan« regressivem Verlauf. Dermatologica (Basel) *120:* 35–52 (1960).

(26) HUNDEIKER, M., und J. PETRES: Zur Klassifizierung und Differentialdiagnose multipler Basaliome. Derm. Wschr. *154:* 169–176 (1968).

(27) KLIEGEL, H., und K. KRINITZ: Das Bild der Endometriose an der Haut. Hautarzt *4:* 445–451 (1953).

(28) KORTING, G. W., und R. DENK: Retikuläre Hyperplasie der Haut durch ein Hydantoin-Derivat. Derm. Wschr. *152:* 257–262 (1966).

(29) LAUGIER, P., N. HUNZIKER et V. ELLENA: Les réticuloses hyperplasiques réactionnelles. Schweiz. med. Wschr. *101:* 1045–1051 (1971).

(30) LEWANDOWSKY, F.: Über einen eigentümlichen Naevus der Brustgegend. Arch. Derm. Syph. (Berl.) *131:* 90–94 (1921).

(31) LÖHR, J., und H. WILLEBRAND: Maligne Entdifferenzierung bei der Neurofibromatose v. Recklinghausen. Diagnostik *6:* 297–299 (1973).

(32) LOEWENTHAL, L. J. A.: Connective tissue naevi and collagénome éruptif. Dermatologica (Basel) *114:* 81–90 (1957).

(33) MACH, K.: Zur histologischen Differentialdiagnose der Retikulosen der Haut. Dermatologica (Basel) *132:* 1–15 (1966).

(34) MADSEN, A.: De l'épithélioma basocellulaire superficiel. Etudes histologiques de l'architecture de l'épithélioma en coupes horizontales en série. Acta derm.-venereol. (Stockh.) *22*, Suppl. *7:* 1–161 (1941).

(35) MARGHESCU, S., und H. ZIETHEN: Über die nodöse Erscheinungsform der Skabies. Derm. Wschr. *154:* 793–798 (1968).

(36) MCPEAK, CH. J., T. CRUZ and A. D. NICASTRI: Dermatofibrosarcoma protuberans: An analysis of 86 cases – five with metastasis. Ann. Surg. *166:* 803–816 (1967).

(37) MESSERLI, F. H., H. U. FUNK und W. SCHÜRCH: Renovaskuläre Hypertonie bei Neurofibromatose. Schweiz. med. Wschr. *103:* 372–377 (1973).

(38) MIKUZ, G., und A. PROPST: Über vasculäre Neurofibromatose. Virchows Arch. path. Anat., Abt. A *356:* 173–185 (1972).

(39) MISGELD, V., N. ALBRECHT und W. HÖFER: Mammäre Leiomyomatose unter dem Bild einer Lymphangiosis carcinomatosa. Fortschr. Röntgenstr. *112:* 649–654 (1970).

(40) MISGELD, V., und W. THIES: Beitrag zur Kenntnis des Chordoms. Hautarzt *21:* 309–312 (1970).

(41) MUSGER, A.: Hautretikulosen. Med. Klin. *62:* 1157–1160 (1967).

(42) NICKEL, W. R., and W. B. REED: Tuberous sclerosis. Special reference to the microscopic alterations in the cutaneous hamartomas. Arch. Derm. (Chic.) *85:* 209–224 (1962).

(43) NIKOLOWSKI, W.: Infraumbilicaler Mucoepidermoidtumor des Urachus. Arch. klin. exp. Derm. *208:* 646–658 (1959).

(44) NIX, TH. E., and C. J. YOUNG: Congenital umbilical anomalies. Arch. Derm. (Chic.) *90:* 160–165 (1964).

(45) NÖDL, F.: Strukturbesonderheiten im Stroma des Basalioms Type Pinkus. Arch. klin. exp. Derm. *235:* 173–179 (1969).

(46) NÜRNBERGER, F., und G. W. KORTING: Zum Vorkommen saurer Mucopolysyccharide in Neurofibromen und Neurofibrosarkomen. Arch. klin. exp. Derm. *235:* 97–114 (1969).

(47) PASTINSZKY, J., und Zs. CSATÓ: Über Hautveränderungen bei Osteopoikilie (Buschke-Ollendorff-Syndrom). Z. Haut-u. Geschl.-Kr. *43:* 313–323 (1968).

(48) PINKUS, H.: Premalignant fibroepithelial tumors of the skin. Arch. Derm. Syph. (Chic.) *67:* 598–615 (1953).

(49) PRAKKEN, J. R.: Connective tissue naevi. Brit. J. Derm. *64:* 87–96 (1952).

(50) SAVIĆ, B., und E. NOACK: Zur Ätiologie des Tietze-Syndroms. Med. Welt *20* (N.F.): 2148–2149 (1969).

(51) SCHORR, W. F., J. M. OPITZ and C. N. REYES: The connective tissue nevus-osteopoikilosis syndrome. Arch. Derm. (Chic.) *106:* 208–214 (1972).

(52) SCHULZ, K. H., M. JÄNNER und O. WEX: Akute Retikulose bei einem Säugling. Dermatologica (Basel) *135:* 392–402 (1967).

(53) SPRENG, A.: Ein Fall von Neuroblastoma sympathicum embryonale Typus Pepper oder congenitalem Sympathogoniom. Schweiz. med. Wschr. *66:* 1192–1194 (1936).

(54) STECK, M. W. D., and E. B. HELWIG: Cutaneous remnants of the omphalomesenteric duct. Arch. Derm. (Chic.) *90:* 463–470 (1964).

(55) STECK, M. W. D., and E. B. HELWIG: Cutaneous endometriosis. J. Amer. Med. Ass. *191:* 167–170 (1965).

(56) TAYLOR, H. B. and E. B. HELWIG: Dermatofibrosarcoma protuberans. Cancer *15:* 717–725 (1962).

(57) UNDEUTSCH, W.: Zum Problem der malignen Entartung der Neurofibromatosis Recklinghausen. Derm. Wschr. *136:* 1145–1153 (1957).

(58) WALTHER, H.: Pflastersteinartiger Naevus der Lumbosakralgegend bei Morbus Pringle. Derm. Wschr. *124:* 940–943 (1951).

(59) WEICKER, H.: Klinik und Therapie der Sympathogoniome an Hand von fünf eigenen Beobachtungen. Mschr. Kinderheilk. *98:* 3–15 (1950).

(60) WEPLER, W.: Über die sogenannte Tietzsche Krankheit. Dtsch. med. Wschr. *79:* 137–139 (1954).

(61) WÜST, G. P., und G. HERMES: Das metastasierende Mammakarzinom des Mannes und seine Behandlung. Med. Welt *22* (N.F.): 249–254 (1971).

(62) ZAK, F. G., and E. RUBIN: Histiocytic medullary reticulosis. Amer. J. Med. *31:* 813–814 (1961).

Appendix: Gynecomastia

The most frequent benign change of the male breast is **gynecomastia,** which has no relation to cancer of the breast. However, in the presence of a pronounced clinical condition of the male breast it is necessary to exclude cancer. Gynecomastia is not a disease in itself but is a multietiologic syndrome characterized by hyperplasia of the epithelium of the ducts or of the myoepithelial cells. Histopathologically, the so-called tubular gynecomastia is more frequent than the lobular type, the latter consisting of formation of lobulated glands caused either by hepatic decompensation* or, more frequently, by protracted estrogen medication, for instance, for treatment of cancer of the prostate. Clinically, gynecomastia usually occurs bilaterally, but it is not infrequently also unilateral. General adiposity in a man may result in an increase in circumference of the entire chest; such gynecomastia due to local deposition of fat should not be called true gynecomastia. Almost half of all boys develop a mild physiologic swelling of the breasts during puberty, the so-called *puberty macromastia.* Gynecomastias were apparently observed more frequently during war and postwar periods than in normal times, and were again seen especially often when food became more abundant; in addition, gynecomastia associated with enlargement of the parotis is observed in lipophilic dystrophic individuals as part of a congenital malformation known as "leprechaunism." The main cause of gynecomastia is probably a marked disturbance of the equilibrium between androgen and estrogen in men past the twenty-fifth year of life; these disturbances are known as the hepaticotesticular syndrome or the Silvestrini-Corda syndrome (liver decompensation is responsible for about 15 per cent of all

---

* Alcohol abuse. (Tr.)

cases of gynecomastia). Compared with the rather frequent occurrence of hepatogenic gynecomastia, marked endocrinopathies are responsible much more rarely for such enlargements of the male breast (for instance, tumors of the adrenals or hypophysis); also, one should not overestimate numerically the paraneoplastic nature of gynecomastia associated with bronchial cancer. In connection with diseases of the genitals, the symptomatic gynecomastias caused by the Leydig cell tumor of the testes should be emphasized. In addition, bilateral gynecomastias belong to the classic signs of primary *hypergonadotropic hypogonadism*. The *Klinefelter syndrome* includes azoospermia, bilateral testicular hypoplasia, increased values of urinary gonadotropin, the sex chromatin constellation of type XXY, impaired perception of red and green, and gynecomastia. Histological examination of the testes shows mostly focal proliferation of the Leydig intermediate cells. The *Gilbert syndrome* (choriogenic gynecomastia) is the name given an endocrinopathia with gynecomastia due to a high degree of secretion of prolan from testicular tumors. Gynecomastias caused by trauma, for instance after fracture of the skull or injuries to spinal nerves, are as rare as those seen in isolated cases of various skin diseases (mycosis fungoides, erythrodermas, relatively often in leprosy). In contrast, the gynecomastias caused by drugs (and these are often observed also by dermatologists) are more frequent; these occur not only after administration of digitalis and hemodialysis, but also after dermatologically used drugs such as vitamin D_2 urethan, INH, derivatives of nitrogen mustard "LOST"),* and others.

All this leads to the urgent advice that every case of gynecomastia of long duration in a patient after the age of 25 should undergo a comprehensive analysis regardless of the frequent finding of hepatogenic estrogenicity.[1-11]

(1) Bässler, R., und A. Schäfer: Elektronenmikroskopische Cytomorphologie der Gynäkomastie. Virchows Arch. path. Anat., Abt. A *348:* 356–373 (1969).
(2) Freeman, R. M., R. L. Lawton and M. O. Fearing: Gynecomastia: an endocrinologic complication of hemodialysis. Ann. Int. Med. *69:* 67–72 (1968).
(3) Hornstein, O.: Zur Klinik und Histopathologie des männlichen primären Hypogonadismus. II. Kastratismus und sogenanntes Klinefelter-Syndrom als Krankheitsformen mit bekannter Ätiologie. Arch. klin. exp. Derm. *217:* 149–195 (1963).
(4) Korting, G. W.: Temporäre Gynaekomastie als psychosomatisches Mangelsymptom beim geschlechtsreifen Manne. Dermatologica (Basel) *98:* 174–181 (1949).
(5) Korting, G. W.: Leitsymptom: Gynäkomastie. Hautarzt *12:* 529–533 (1961).
(6) Nieschlag, E., und M. Rohr: Gynäkomastie und Potenzverlust als Leitsymptom bei vier Fällen von Leydig-Zell-Tumor. Therapiewoche *20:* 3351–3356 (1970).
(7) Posternak, Fr.: Gynécomastie et cancer bronchique: syndrome paranéoplasique ou non? Schweiz. med. Wschr. *100:* 501–506 (1970).
(8) Riddick, Le Roy, R. H. Brodkin and R. C. Gibbs: Palmar and plantar keratoderma with hyperpigmentation and gynecomastia. Acta derm.-venereol. (Stockh.) *51:* 69–72 (1971).
(9) Schmitt, G. W., I. Shehadeh and C. T. Sawin: Transient gynecomastia in chronic renal failure during chronic intermittent hemodialysis. Ann. Int. Med. *69:* 73–79 (1968).

---

* "LOST" stands for LOmmel and STeinkopf, who developed a derivative of dichlorodiethyl sulfide mustard gas for war purposes during the Second World War. The Germans had stored enormous quantities of this poison gas near the Italian city of Bari; when Allied bombers hit this depot the gas spread into Bari and many people died, resulting in "the Bari catastrophe." (Tr.)

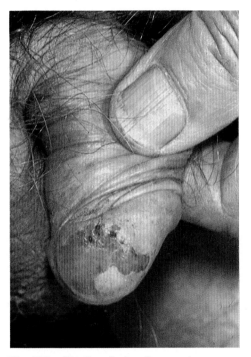

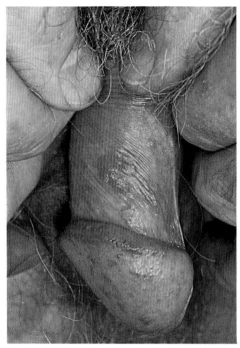

Fig. 745a. Erythroplasia: glans penis.

Fig. 745b. Erythroplasia: inner side of the prepuce.

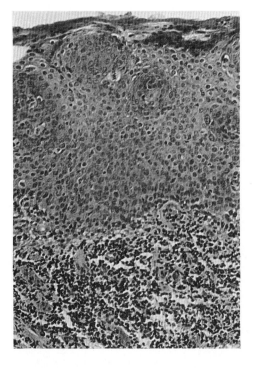

(10) SCHULTHEISS, FR.: Gynäkomastie als Digitalisnebenwirkung. Hippokrates *19:* 806–807 (1962).
(11) SCHWARTZ, I. S., and S. L. WILENS: The formation of acinar tissue in gynecomastia. Amer. J. Path. *43:* 797–807 (1963).

H. Tumors Found Predominantly in the Genital Region

Some of the tumor formations of the genital region have been discussed in other chapters: ulcerations (Chapter 33), abscesses and fistulas (Chapter 14), and recurrent and persistent swellings (Chap-

Fig. 746. Erythroplasia: parakeratosis, acanthosis with irregular order of cells, missing basal layer, subepidermal infiltrate. Hematoxylin and eosin, 155 × .

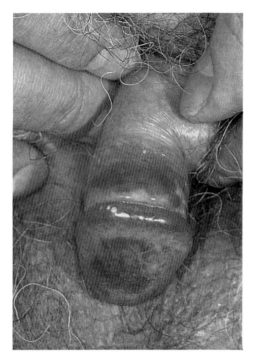

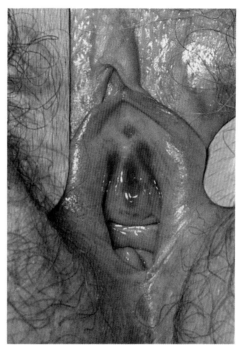

Fig. 747. Chronic plasmacellular balanitis. Fig. 748. Chronic plasmacellular vulvitis.

ter 10); these will not be discussed further in the following section.

1. Bowen's disease of the transitional mucous membranes and mucous membranes proper (erythroplasia) will be discussed here again, because when present in the genitoanal region its malignant character often is not correctly evaluated. Such underestimation results in delayed or insufficient therapeutic measures, and finally the growth of the tumor cannot be controlled. In erythroplasia there is a circumscribed, only slightly elevated, light red to meaty red, erythematous area that is also shiny, velvety, and finely granular (Fig. 745a, b). Exceptionally, several areas of erythroplasia may occur simultaneously. Pronounced elevation, induration, or verrucous transformation point to the presence of infiltrative growth. Histologically, one sees at first a carcinoma in situ with parakeratosis, bulky, block-shaped acan-

thosis, atypical epidermal cells, numerous dyskeratoses, and well-marked round cell infiltration of the corium (Fig. 746). After varying periods of time, this in-situ phase is followed by a breakthrough of the atypical cellular epidermal masses into the corium with rapid lymphogenous metastasis.[18]

2. Chronic plasmacellular balanoposthitis (Fig. 747) must be differentiated diagnostically from Bowen's disease; in the female the rather rare corresponding disease is chronic plasmacellular vulvitis (Fig. 748). Even more rare are similar changes in the conjunctivae. Chronic plasmacellular balanoposthitis is not shiny red but chocolate brown because it contains a large amount of hemosiderin. Its surface remains smooth and does not become coarsely granular as in erythroplasia. The individual lesions have markedly sharp borders and sometimes show no tendency to enlarge for several

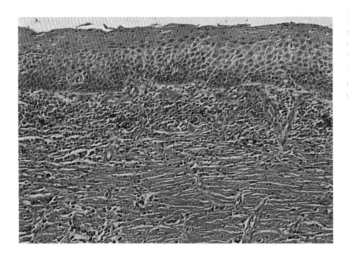

Fig. 749 a. Chronic plasma-cellular balanitis: subepidermal plasma cell infiltrate; extravasates of erythrocytes, deposits of hemosiderin. Hematoxylin and eosin, 100×.

months. A moist environment is an important prerequisite for the development of such a chronic inflammatory condition. Histologically, the mucosa shows chronic inflammatory changes interspersed with many erythrocytes and plasma cells. Signs of malignant transition are always absent (Figs. 749a, b).[23, 24, 44]

3. Extramammary **Paget's disease** has a strong similarity to Bowen's disease or an eczema. After the breast, the second most frequent location is the genital region in males also. The perianal or the perineal region is not infrequently the site of a Paget lesion also. In accordance with the concept that Paget's disease develops from the excretory duct of the apocrine sweat glands, the manifestations are confined to the regions of their physiologic occurrence. It should also be kept in mind that extramammary Paget's disease occurs more than coincidentally in conjunction with a second cancer of other organs. A therapeutically quite stubborn pruritus may precede the appearance of visible cutaneous changes for some time. Afterward, sharply limited erythematous patches without special infiltration can be observed. Because of the pruritus these patches will soon show excoriations and

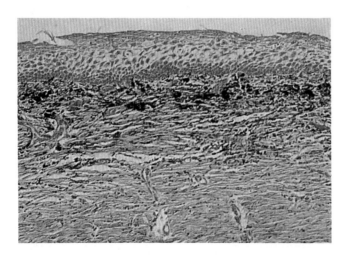

Fig. 749 b. Chronic plasma-cellular balanitis: same slide with positive iron reaction. Berlin blue reaction, 100×.

Fig. 750. Condylomata acuminata of the anal region.

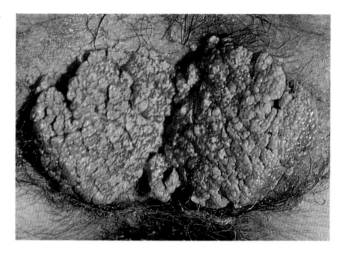

sometimes moist erosions. Confusion with an eczema can easily occur if impetiginization takes place as well. An important macroscopic difference in Paget's disease is the sharp border and the absence of isolated papules or vesiculopapules at the margin as compared with an eczematous reaction. Only after many months will this eczematoid condition of Paget's disease develop into a nodular, vegetating, and infiltrating growth; inspection alone will then raise the suspicion of a malignant tumor. For the histologic findings see Chapter 21, B3.

In exceptional cases extramammary Paget's disease may develop in multicentric fashion, although the individual areas may be close together. Even large plaquelike or vegetating lesions seldom advance to the small labia and the vaginal mucosa. Because the so-called Paget cells may at times contain an abundance of stored melanin granules, macroscopic and histologic similarities exist with preblastomatous circumscribed melanosis or a superficial spreading melanoma.[9, 22, 27, 28 36, 38, 41]

4. Condylomata acuminata are doubtless the most important pseudocancerosis of the genital region. The lesions resemble acanthomas followed by hyperkeratosis;

they are caused by the papovavirus. Frequently these condylomata grow especially well in constantly moist areas; however, there is not that close connection with a gonorrheal infection as was supposed for a long time. In men condylomata acuminata are found primarily on the glans

Fig. 751. Gonorrheic tysonitis.

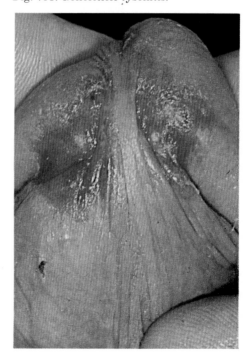

penis, the prepuce, and occasionally in the navicular fossa of the male urethra. In women the most important localizations are the vestibule of the vagina, the small labia, and, depending on the degree of involvement, either a part of or the entire vagina. Recently there has been an increasing frequency in both sexes of condylomata acuminata of the perianal region that spreads into the rectal mucosa (Fig. 750). Widespread and therapy-resistant condylomata are seen in patients receiving immunosuppressive medication or in patients with lowered immune resistance due to an underlying malignancy. The individual condyloma acuminatum starts as a skin-colored or red, pinhead-sized soft papule. After further growth, nodular, cauliflowerlike masses of various sizes arise from a small base. The clefts between the filaments in combination with the moist surroundings encourage rapid bacterial invasion with maceration. Enlargement of the regional lymph nodes does not occur regularly but may be the result of a secondary infection. In contrast to syphilitic lymphadenitis these lymph glands are painful. Perforation of the prepuce may occur as a complication (see also Chapter 33, C 13).

5. Papillomatosis penis (hirsuties papillaris penis, pearly penile papules) is a harmless atavistic anomaly which may be mistaken for beginning condylomata acuminata. These papillomas are seen in about 8 per cent of all males; they consist of pearly white, closely aggregated, small villosities of the corona of the glans penis (Fig. 571). The diameter of each papule is about 0.5 to 3.0 mm. Histologically, the papillary folds of each lesion show numerous blood vessels surrounded by dense connective tissue in their vicinity. Terminal rami of the nerve networks are absent.[3, 11]

The differential diagnosis should consider *ectopic sebaceous glands*, but these are not located on the corona of the glans penis, preferring the outer part of the foreskin or the penile skin instead. Also, these glands always have a smooth surface and are freely movable with the skin. Gonorrheal infections of the preputial (Tyson's) glands, **tysonitis**, result in highly inflammatory tumors that may grow as large as peas (Fig. 751). After perforation pus containing many gonococci is excreted.[17]

6. Condylomata lata are secondary syphilitic lesions that must be strictly separated from condylomata acuminata. The syphilitic condyloma does not show a papillomatous surface but one like a mushroom cap and the lesion arises

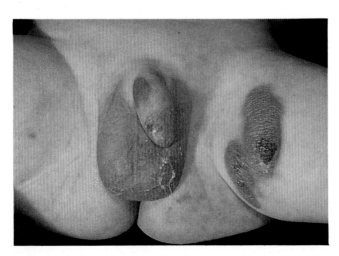

Fig. 752. Infantile gluteal granuloma.

from a broad base. The diagnosis should not be difficult because in most cases other specific cutaneous changes of secondary syphilis would be present simultaneously (indolent lymphadenopathy, macular or papular exanthems, and so on). Otherwise, darkfield examination for *Treponema pallidum* performed with specific secreta and the results of serum reactions have to be considered. One should not overlook the possibility that condylomata lata and condylomata acuminata may exist side by side in rare cases. In infants Jacquet's erythema (erythema papulosum posterosivum) has to be considered in the differential diagnosis (see also Chapter 18, A2). However, in contrast to syphilitic papules, the circumanal region in this disease remains uninvolved and the gluteal region shows lesions only at some distance. In addition, there are other signs of irritation such as erythemas, vesicles, and erosions.

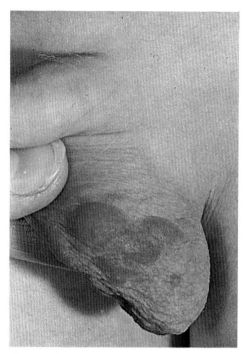

Fig. 753. Scrotal lymphocytoma.

7. Pseudosyphilis papulosa is the name given to acanthomas caused by external irritation. They are located in the anogenital region and resemble condylomata lata. These benign acanthomas are seen in many cases of urinary incontinence, malformations (e.g., ectopia of the bladder, hypospadia or epispadia), and also in the vicinity of fistulas of the ureter. Clinically these lesions consist of large papular elements of various sizes that either rise above the vicinity like tablets or are semispherical (Fig. 193). Their surface is smooth, rarely macerated, and there is no pruritus. If the continuous wetting with urine can be stopped, the acanthomas will regress completely within a few days.[19, 25, 39]

8. Granuloma gluteale infantum is limited to the areas in which diapers come in contact with the skin. It is preceded in many cases by candidiasis. Subsequently, hemispherically protruding blue-red or brown-red infiltrates of firm consistency develop. Usually several infiltrates of varying sizes (about 1 to 6 cm in diameter) are present at the same time. The surface is shiny and has an orange-peel-like aspect in places (Fig. 752). Under diascopic pressure a yellow-brown lupoid color is apparent. There are no bleeding points, and the epidermal cover over the infiltrates always remains closed. Ulcerations, liquefactions, or pustules are usually not observed. This is a purely cutaneous disorder, since there are no changes of the internal organs or disturbances in the general well-being. The cause of the disease is at present still unknown, but a reaction to detergents or rinsing agents is suspected. Histologically, polymorphonuclear infiltration amply interspersed with eosinophils and plasma cells is present. There are in addition vascular proliferations, several microabscesses, and gram-positive inclusions of leukocytes. In the differential diagnosis reticulosis of infants, vegetating pyoderma, bromoderma

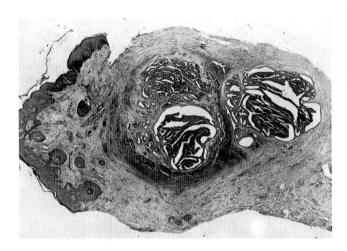

Fig. 754a. Hidradenoma papilliferum: cystic tumor surrounded by a fibrous capsule and without connection with the epidermis. Hematoxylin and eosin.

tuberosum, and mast cell tumors must be considered. If the dermatosis is located on the scrotum it should be kept in mind that quite often *lymphadenosis benigna cutis* may be present in this location (Fig. 753).[7, 37, 40]

9. It is possible that massive **trichomonas** infections cause **granulomas** of the vaginal mucosa. They are brown-red, edematous, and indurated infiltrates, which protrude flatly over the level of the surrounding mucosa. The surface may show shallow ulcerations. Since these clinical findings are unspecific and resemble primary syphilitic lesions, the differential diag-

nosis must always rule out syphilis initially. Evidence of *Trichomonas vaginalis* in the secretion and healing under exclusive trichomonacidal therapy are helpful for the diagnosis. In spite of this, it is important to retest the serologic findings for syphilis some time after healing.[35]

10. A not infrequent tumor of the female genitals is the **hidradenoma papilliferum**. Clinically, this adenoma of the apocrine sweat glands appears as an intradermal or subcutaneous, almost always solitary, pea- to bean-sized, firmly elastic overlying tumor. Larger tumors lead occasionally to pressure atrophy of the over-

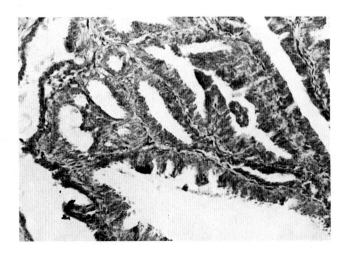

Fig. 754b. Hidradenoma papilliferum: close-up of *a* showing tufts covered with one layer of cylindric cells from the lumen of the tumor.

lying epidermis, so that at the height of the protuberance of the tumor a light red granular papilloma becomes visible. Cysts, pyogenic granulomas, and cutaneous endometriosis should be considered in the differential diagnosis. Histologically, the syringocystadenomatous nevus has similar features. The usual finding in this vulvar tumor is a tubulopapillary adenoma, which is well demarcated from the corium and which as a rule has no connection with the intact epidermis. Branching and winding villi grow into narrow cystic cavities. The villi are separated from each other by connective tissue septa (Fig. 745a, b).[1, 6, 15]

11. Nodular-ulcerating vulvar changes suggest primarily a **vulvar carcinoma** originating in the epidermis (see Chapter 33, C14). The vulva may also be the site of primary metastases of other genital carcinomas (cervical cancer, Fig. 755, and

uterine cancer). Without histologic examination the classification of such metastases is impossible.[12]

12. Carcinomas of the apocrine sweat glands are extremely rare and are occasionally associated with Paget's disease. They occur most often in the axillae and on the nipples, and, next in frequency, in the genital area (in women and men). They are firm, fast growing nodes. Some tumors soon ulcerate extensively. The localization suggests the diagnosis, but histologic confirmation is needed.[2]

13. Several benign and malignant neoplastic growths occur in the genital region only in exceptional cases. Since we may have to refer to them in the differential diagnosis, the chapters containing exact data are mentioned here. **Syringomas** may occur on the large labia and the penis. As a rule they become conspicuous only if

Fig. 755. Cutaneous metastases of a cervical carcinoma.

Fig. 756. Penile cyst of cylindrical epithelium.

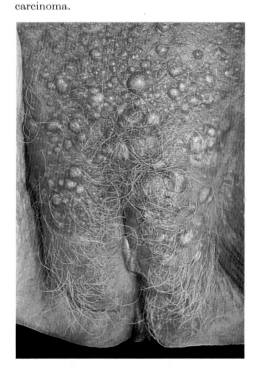

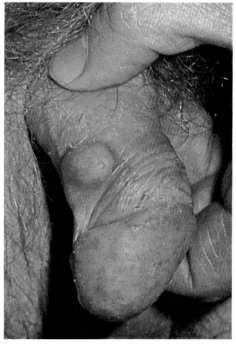

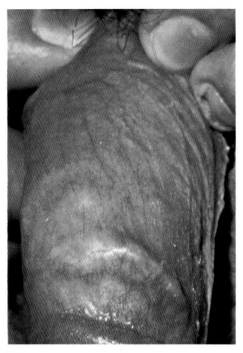

Fig. 757. Lines of phlebitis in the sulcus coronarius.

they reach an especially large size or occur as multiple growths (see Section C10). Also, in **generalized neurofibromatosis** tumors occur on the vulva and vagina relatively often (see Section G3). In males neurofibromas occur in the testicles and epididymis. This may explain the low fertility of these patients. Other very rare tumors in this location are **juvenile melanoma** (see Section B2), **myoblastomyoma** (see Section F2), and **dermatofibrosarcoma protuberans** (see Section G1). For **sebocystomas** on the scrotum and labia, see Chapter 32, B5, and for cutaneous **endometriosis,** see Section G21. [4, 13, 30, 32, 43]

14. So-called **cylindrical epithelial cysts** are rather typical tumors of the male genitals. Their characteristic site is almost exclusively near the raphe. Because of their serous contents they have a certain transparency (Fig. 756). The covering skin

is movable. In the differential diagnosis lymph varicosities and atheromas should be considered first.[14, 31]

15. Occasionally, firm cords with no symptoms appear spontaneously in the sulcus coronarius. These nonvenereal **cordlike lymphangitides** correspond to the so-called Mondor phlebitis. The overlying skin can be easily lifted and no inflammatory signs are present (Fig. 757). Although superficial ulcerations are possible, palpation of the characteristic cords alone rules out a syphilitic primary lesion. Etiologically, this disorder may arise from a chronic-inflammatory and sclerosing closure of a lymph vessel due to long-lasting stasis.[10, 21]

16. Penile induration (Peyronie's disease) appears chiefly between the ages of 40 and 60. It is frequently associated with other connective tissue fibroses such as Dupuytren's contracture, knuckle pads, mammary fibrosis, and others. The patient first notices a curvature of the penis at an erection. On palpation a longitudinal hard streak, plaque, or node can be felt. These partly bone-hard fibroses are firmly located in the tunica albuginea and may extend from the root of the penis to the glans. The overlying skin, on the other hand, always remains movable. The chronic progressive fibrosis finally leads to a contortion and flexion of the penis so that an erection is associated with violent pain or finally becomes impossible.

17. Fibrous indurations of the penis or scrotum may occur also in the course of fatty tissue necroses. Since these are predominantly artefacts, the physician sees only the scarred final stages. In some patients such **sclerosing lipogranulomas** have developed from injections of paraffin or mineral oil. In contrast to penile induration, cordlike indurations are absent and the fibrosis is usually firmly attached to the covering skin.[34]

18. Since the partially exophytically growing **carcinomas of the penis** ulcerate rather early, they are described in detail in Chapter 33, C12.

19. Among the enlargements or swellings of the testicles and epididymis, those in the form of inflammations are usually seen by the dermatologist. Most important of these is **acute epididymitis,** which shows uniform signs regardless of etiology. The patient complains of sudden violent pain in the testicles. Fever and leukocytosis are present. There are leukocytes and bacteria in the urinary sediment; a urethral smear may show gonococci. Careful lifting of the scrotum relieves the patient's pain. Some patients also complain of pain radiating into the lower abdomen. Palpation shows a unilateral, extremely painful enlargement of the epididymis, but a distinct separation of testicle and epididymis is not always possible in the acute inflammatory stage. Bilateral epididymitides are extremely rare. Etiologically, gonorrhea plays a major role and this should be confirmed by a smear. It should not be forgotten that tuberculous epididymitis may also have an acute onset.

20. A similar acute event is **testicular torsion,** which, in contrast to epididymitis, occurs most often in childhood and progresses without fever and leukocytosis. The patients, however, complain of nausea. The pain also starts suddenly and radiates to the lower abdomen. The affected side of the scrotum is distinctly red, extremely painful, and edematously enlarged, so that even after a short time the testicle and epididymis cannot be separated from each other. Elevation of the scrotum does not relieve the pain. Inflammatory urinary findings are absent.[5, 8]

21. Acute **orchitis** also begins with unilateral pain and fever. It usually occurs in adults in the course of an infectious disease (mumps, typhoid, influenza, or

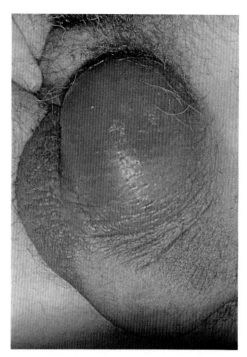

Fig. 758. Abscess in orchitis and epididymitis.

Bang's disease). The massive swelling of the testicle does not permit a definite separation of the epididymis (Fig. 758). No leukocytes or bacteria are found in the urinary sediment.[26]

22. Slowly increasing testicular enlargements principally suggest a malignant tumor. Malignant testicular tumors occur most frequently between the twentieth and fortieth years of life. Since inflammatory changes are usually lacking, the patient at first notices only an indefinite feeling of heaviness. Pressure on the enlarged testicle does not lead to the typical pain, accompanied by nausea, caused by compression of the testicle. Frequently, only metastases call attention to a possible testicular tumor, since the usual clinical signs (swelling, drawing pains, or a feeling of heaviness) do not constitute definite early manifestations. At the time of the diagnosis 20 to 75 per cent of the patients already have metastases. **Seminomas** represent dysgerminomas of the seminal epithelium, whereas **teratomas** originate from ectopic embryonic cells. Two-thirds of all malignant testicular tumors are seminomas. Both sides are involved in about 1 per cent. Seminomas are inactive hormonally, whereas malignant teratomas excrete increased amounts, mostly of chorionic gonadotropin. **Leydig cell tumors** excrete androgens. In addition, the testicles may be the site of **distant metastases** of various primary tumors (such as retothelsarcomas or bronchial or prostatic carcinomas).[20, 33]

23. It goes without saying that a testicular tumor must be differentiated from a **hydrocele** which develops slowly into a firmly elastic swelling adjacent to the testicle. The diagnosis is easily confirmed by transillumination. In slowly growing hydroceles, however, the wall of the hydrocele may be so scarred that transparency is no longer obtained. In such doubtful cases an exploratory puncture can be performed from below. Evidence of a hydrocele does not rule out the presence of a testicular tumor, since an exudate may occur as a sign of the tumor.

24. Spermatoceles, which are cysts in the area of the epididymis, cause discomfort only if they are large. Usually they are discovered by accident. They may cause drawing pains. Some patients state that the tumor, whose existence they had known, becomes smaller after an ejaculation. With careful palpation the point of origin is easily located at the epididymis or at the transition from testicle to epididymis. Small spermatoceles have a nodular surface, whereas larger spermatoceles have a smooth one. In doubtful cases the suspected "tumor" can be punctured, and spermatozoa will be found in the fluid from the puncture.[29]

Firm, nodular thickenings of the epididymis itself result from *chronic, unspecific inflammation or tuberculosis of the*

epididymis. Both disorders can be differentiated from spermatoceles by palpation alone. The type of chronic inflammation should be investigated by special bacteriologic methods.

(1) BACHMANN, F.: Gutartige und bösartige Schweißdrüsentumoren der Vulva. (Hidradenome und Hidradenokarzinome). Zbl. Gynäk. *92:* 945–954 (1970).
(2) BAES, H., and D. SUURMOND: Apocrine sweat gland carcinoma. Report of a case. Brit. J. Derm. *83:* 483–486 (1970).
(3) BUSCHKE, A., und M. GUMPERT: Die Papillen an der Corona glandis in vergleichend-anatomischer und ethnologischer Beziehung. Arch. Frauenheilk. (Leipzig) *11:* 43–55 (1925).
(4) CARNEIRO, S. J. C., H. L. GARDNER and J. M. KNOX: Syringoma of the vulva. Arch. Derm. (Chic.) *103:* 494–496 (1971).
(5) CHAPMAN, R. H., and A. J. WALTON: Torsion of the testis and its appendages. Brit. Med. J. *1972/*I: 164–166.
(6) CRAMER, H.: Zur Histogenese und Klinik des Hidradenoma vulvae. Geburtsh. u. Frauenheilk. *14:* 1135–1142 (1954).
(7) DELACRÉTAZ, J., D. GRIGORIU, H. DE CROUSAZ, B. TAPERNOUX, P.-A. NICOD et E. GAUTIER: Candidose nodulaire de la région inguino-génitale et des fesses (granuloma glutaeale infantum). Dermatologica (Basel) *144:* 144–155 (1972).
(8) DIETZ, O., R. FIEDLER und A. HAASE: Erkenntnisse bei der Symptomatik der Hodentorsion. Militärmed. *12:* 334–337 (1971).
(9) FENN, M. E., G. W. MORLEY and M. R. ABELL: Paget's disease of vulva. Obstet. Gynec. *38:* 660–670 (1971).
(10) FISCHER, H. R.: Nicht-venerische Kranzfurchenlymphangitis. Z. Haut- u. Geschl.-Kr. *9:* 370–373 (1950).
(11) GLICKSMAN, J. M., and R. G. FREEMAN: Pearly penile papules. Arch. Derm. (Chic.) *93:* 56–59 (1966).
(12) GRIMMER, H.: Hautmetastasen eines Portio- und Adenocarcinoms des Uterus. Z. Haut- u. Geschl.-Kr. *34:* [XLV]–[XLVIII] (1963).
(13) GRIMMER, H.: Krankheiten des äußeren weiblichen Genitale. Abrikosoff-Tumor. Z. Haut- u. Geschl.-Kr. *45:* [125]–[130] (1970).
(14) GROPPER, H., und W. NIKOLOWSKI: Cylinderepithelcysten des Penis. Arch. Derm. Syph. (Berl.) *199:* 212–220 (1955).

(15) HASSENPFLUG, K.-H.: Hidradenoma papilliferum vulvae. Z. Haut- u. Geschl.-Kr. *34:* [XLIX]–[LII] (1963).

(16) HEITE, H.-J., und H. H. SIEBRECHT: Beitrag zur Pathogenese der Induratio penis plastica. Derm. Wschr. *121:* 1–10, 25–34 (1950).

(17) HYMAN, A. B., and M. H. BROWNSTEIN: Tyson's »glands«. Ectopic sebaceous glands and papillomatosis penis. Arch. Derm. (Chic.) *99:* 31–36 (1969).

(18) HYMAN, A. B., and M. LEIDER: Erythroplasia of the female genitalia. Arch. Derm. (Chic.) *84:* 381–385 (1961).

(19) JANSEN, L. H., and F. B. G. GROOTHUIS: Pseudosyphilis papulosa. Arch. Derm. (Chic.) *84:* 639–641 (1961).

(20) JONAS, U., R. AY und R. TSCHOLL: Leydig-Zell-Tumor. Vergleichende Symptomatologie bei Manifestation im Kindes- und Erwachsenenalter. Urologie [A] *11:* 71–77 (1972).

(21) KANDIL, E., and I. M. AL KASHLAN: Non-venereal sclerosing lymphangitis of the penis. A clinicopathologic treatise. Acta derm.-venereol. (Stockh.) *50:* 309–312 (1970).

(22) KAWATSU, T., and Y. MIKI: Triple extramammary Paget's disease. Arch. Derm. (Chic.) *104:* 316–319 (1971).

(23) KORTING, G. W., und H. THEISEN: Circumscripte plasmacelluläre Balanoposthitis und Conjunctivitis bei derselben Person. Arch. klin. exp. Derm. *217:* 495–504 (1963).

(24) KUMER, L.: Über die chronische hämorrhagische Vulvitis (Lipschütz). Derm. Wschr. *97:* 1002–1005 (1933).

(25) LIPSCHÜTZ, B.: Untersuchungen über nicht venerische Gewebsveränderungen am äußeren Genitale des Weibes. Arch. Derm. Syph. (Berl.) *131:* 104–127 (1921).

(26) LUDWIG, G., und M. NURI: Differentialdiagnose der Hodenschwellung. Med. Welt 23 (N.F.): 1593–1597 (1972).

(27) LÜDERS, G.: Zur Pathologie und Genese des extramammären Morbus Paget. Arch. klin. exp. Derm. *232:* 16–32 (1968).

(28) MURREL, T. W., and F. H. McMULLAN: Extramammary Paget's disease. A report of two cases. Arch. Derm. (Chic.) *85:* 600–613 (1962).

(29) NIKOLOWSKI, W.: Über Spermatozelen. Klinische Befunde und Punktionsergebnisse. Z. Urol. *42:* 110–133 (1949).

(30) NÖDL, F.: Juveniles Melanom der Vulva. Z. Haut- u. Geschl.-Kr. *44:* [11]–[16] (1969).

(31) RUPEC, M., und F. VAKILZADEH: Die sog. Cylinderepithelcyste des Penis. Z. Haut- u. Geschl.-Kr. *43:* [69]–[70] (1968).

(32) SCHREIBER, M. M.: Vulvar von Recklinghausen's disease. Arch. Derm. (Chic.) *88:* 320–321 (1963).

(33) SIGEL, A.: Moderne Diagnose und Therapie der malignen germinalen Hodentumoren. Dtsch. med. J. *19:* 730–736 (1968).

(34) SNAPPER, I., and D. SELD: Factitious genital sclerogranuloma. Arch. Derm. (Chic.) *98:* 30–34 (1968).

(35) SÖNNICHSEN, N., und I. STILLER: Über ein durch Trichomonaden bedingtes Granuloma der Vulva. Z. Haut- u. Geschl.-Kr. *41:* 202–204 (1966).

(36) STEIGLEDER, G.-K.: Pseudo-Paget des Skrotums. Dermatologica (Basel) *117:* 165–172 (1958).

(37) STÖGMANN, W.: Granuloma glutaeale infantum: eine neue – waschmittelbedingte ? – Säuglingsdermatose. Umweltmedizin *1:* 24–26 (1973).

(38) STRAUSS, G.: Histochemische Untersuchungen bei Pagetscher Erkrankung der Vulva. Z. Krebsforsch. *61:* 632–648 (1957).

(39) SUNDHAUSSEN, E.: Pseudosyphilis papulosa Lipschütz. Hautarzt *23:* 551–553 (1972).

(40) TAPPEINER, J., und L. PFLEGER: Granuloma glutaeale infantum. Hautarzt *22:* 382–388 (1971).

(41) TCHANG, F., T. OKAGAKI and R. M. RICHART: Adenocarcinoma of Bartholin's gland associated with Paget's disease of vulvar area. Cancer *31:* 221–225 (1973).

(42) VÖLTER, D., und W. STAEHLER: Die Induratio penis plastica. Med. Welt 23 (N.F.): 213–214 (1972).

(43) ZALLA, J. A., and H. O. PERRY: An unusual case of syringoma. Arch. Derm. (Chic.) *103:* 215–217 (1971).

(44) ZOON, J. J.: Balanoposthite chronique circonscrite bénigne à plasmocytes. Dermatologica (Basel) *105:* 1–7 (1952).

I. Tumors Found Predominantly on the Extremities

In order to prevent repetitions, it is again necessary to refer to the chapters on juxta-articular nodes (Chapter 8, A), pain-

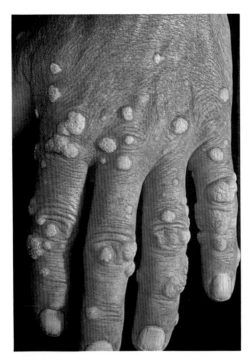

Fig. 759. Common warts.

ful tumors (Chapter 38, A), and tumors containing pigment (Chapter 38, B). Light-provoked cancerous and precancerous cutaneous changes (senile keratosis, squamous cell carcinoma, and keratoacanthoma, among others) have already been partially discussed in this chapter, Section C – tumors found mainly on the face.

1. Common tumors found predominantly on the hands are probably **verrucae vulgares.** Children, adolescents, and young adults with peripheral vascular dysfunction (moist cool hands and feet, acrocyanosis, perniosis, and others) are especially prone to infection with the virus of warts. In general, the diagnosis of common warts is not difficult if typical, pea-sized, gray-yellowish tumors are present; these have a firm hyperkeratotic surface with fine fissures once they reach a certain size (Fig. 759). On the soles the wart cannot grow as an exophytic tumor because

of the constant pressure; instead, it grows into deeper tissues (thorny wart). The surface therefore remains smooth, but its gray-yellow color points to the massive hyperkeratosis. Plantar warts occur mostly on areas of pressure such as the heels and balls of the toes; they often cause considerable pain on pressure. So-called mosaic warts develop from the confluence of single plantar warts that form more superficial verrucoid plaques. Plantar warts occasionally contain single point-sized blue-black and brown-black pigmented spots in the hyperkeratosis. These represent minute hemorrhages growing upward; they may occur if the pressure is especially intense.

In the differential diagnosis a number of cutaneous changes must be considered. They have already been discussed in other chapters and are therefore mentioned here only briefly. Verrucae planae juveniles always occur as multiple growths and favor the backs of the hands as well as the face. They always remain flatly elevated papules of 1 to 2 mm at the most. Their surface is never so "wartily" fissured as that of common warts (see also Chapter 38, C11). Senile warts may in exceptional cases occur on the backs of the hands, but this happens only in individuals over the age of 35. Senile warts on the backs of the hands also remain small and, therefore, appear only as small brown spots (see also Chapter 38, B7). Keratosis senilis also occurs on the backs of the hands, but always remains a flat hyperkeratosis with basal erythema. It never occurs in children and adolescents but appears first in advanced age. On the feet the distinction between common warts and common clavi may occasionally become difficult. The latter are always located on distinctly pressure-exposed points. In contrast to warts they have a smooth rather than a rugged surface (see also Chapter 8, C2). Palmoplantar arsenical hyperkeratoses as single keratoses remain clinically indistinguishable from common warts. However, multiple lesions often appear, and the patient's history reveals intake of arsenic. Because of possible malignant transformation of arsenical hyperkeratosis, a histologic examination should be undertaken in doubtful cases (see also Chapter 28, D5). If plantar warts show hemorrhagic points, as they occasionally do, some similarity with pseudochromohidrosis plantaris may exist (see also Chapter 4, A2). The differentiation of a large, hemorrhagic, dark black wart from a melanoma is difficult, especially if it occurs on the heel. If the clinical findings, history, and a paring from the lesion do not permit a definite diagnosis, the tumor should be completely excised under local ischemia and further therapeutic procedures should be determined after the result of the frozen section analysis has been obtained.[17, 19]

2. If there is an extensive number of closely agminated warts, the possibility of a massive development of common warts (verrucosis generalisata) or, next in frequency, **epidermodysplasia verruciformis** should be considered. Although the development of these warts also begins in childhood, the lesions remain unchanged with no tendency to spontaneous regression, as would be the case in a high percentage of common warts. The favorite locations are the backs of hands and

fingers, the extensor surfaces of the forearms, and the neck; the lesions occur symmetrically. Involvement of the trunk, however, is not unusual. The single lesions suggest either atypical common warts or verrucae planae juveniles, which are slightly more protuberant. The closely agminated disseminated papular types tend to form confluent areas. After a course of years, transition to a squamous cell carcinoma or Bowen's disease is possible even at an early age. The histologic findings also greatly resemble those of flat juvenile warts. Besides irregular but decisive acanthotic epidermal widening, massive vacuolization of the rete cells and the granular layer is striking. The widened stratum corneum has a loosened basket-weave-like texture. Inoculation experiments and electron-microscopic examinations have determined the viral etiology of epidermodysplasia verruciformis. The recovered viral particles are probably identical with the virus of warts. Because of the clinical findings and the course, both of which distinctly differ from those of warts, a special susceptibility of the patient must be presumed. It is important for the differential diagnosis that in dyskeratosis follicularis the lesions may be distributed like those of epidermodysplasia verruciformis. If the differentiation is not pos-

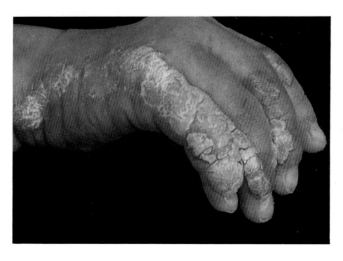

Fig. 760. Incontinentia pigmenti: streaks of hyperkeratosis after blisterous stage.

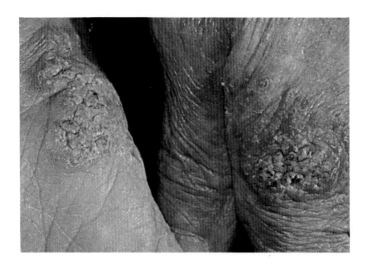

Fig. 761. Tuberculosis
cutis verrucosa.

sible from the distinctive form of the
papule, nail changes and the typical interruptions of the dermal papillae on the
palms and soles will be helpful.[13, 14, 15, 34]

3. Nodular, verrucous cutaneous changes on the legs, dorsum of the foot, and
extensor surfaces of the toes occur in
children suffering from **incontinentia pigmenti** (Bloch-Sulzberger type). The verrucous hyperkeratoses occur in a streaklike or reticular form, corresponding to the
preceding blisters and hyperpigmentations
(Fig. 760). For further details see Chapter
24, E9).[10]

4. Tuberculosis cutis verrucosa is usually
observed on the distal extremities and can
easily be mistaken for common warts. In
contrast to lupus vulgaris it appears initially, not as the characteristic lupus spot
but with a distinctly elevated, firm, brown-
red papule whose surface remains smooth
at first. Additional nodules are added by
peripheral apposition, and as a rough hyperkeratosis develops, the lesion assumes a
wartlike aspect (Fig. 761). The probe
phenomenon remains negative and under
diascopic pressure no lupoid infiltrates are
visible. The whole lesion is surrounded by
a red halo. After removal of the central
hyperkeratosis, drops of purulent secretion

can be expressed by tangential pressure.
As the lesions enlarge, their wartlike
aspect is lost, since central healing with
scars then becomes recognizable. In the
differential diagnosis, besides common
warts, chronic vegetating pyodermas,
mycoses, hyperkeratotic lesions of Bowen's
disease, and infections from atypical
mycobacteria should be considered.

5. Among cutaneous infections with
causative organisms of the atypical mycobacteria group, the so-called **swimming
pool granuloma** is often transmitted by
the aquatic *Mycobacterium balnei seu
marinum* and *Mycobacterium ulcerans*. In
the patient's history, superficial injuries
from scratches while bathing or cleaning
fish tanks play a role. Therefore, the
cutaneous changes are most frequently
located on the hands, forearms, legs, and
feet. Some time after such minimal injury, aggregated papules, which assume a
hyperkeratotic surface, appear. On the
other hand, the papules may break down
with pus, leaving shallow ulcerations. In
the area of lymph drainage from the primary lesion, additional specific lesions often
develop. Histologically, they contain epithelioid cell granulomas with Langhans'
giant cells and "fibrillary necroses." In
contrast to tuberculosis cutis verrucosa,

Fig. 762. Accessory rudiment of finger.

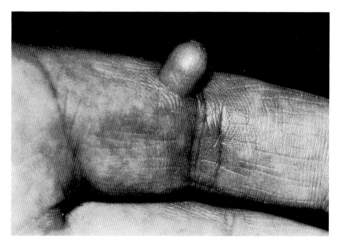

acid-fast mycobacteria are found only rarely. If the history and clinical findings do not permit distinction from tuberculosis cutis verrucosa, the decision has to be based on bacteriologic data derived from a culture.[30, 32, 45]

6. On the base or in the middle of the proximal phalanx of the little finger there may be a pea- to bean-sized tumor, which is a sign of **rudimentary polydactylia** (Fig. 762). Such appendices to fingers are usually found on both hands and are already present at birth. In many cases anlagen to nails are present also. In contrast to acquired fibrokeratomas, the finger rudiments have their own pattern of papillary ridges. Histologically, they contain numerous nerve fibers, tactile corpuscles, and occasionally cartilaginous tissue.[5]

7. Acquired digital fibrokeratomas may look very similar to finger rudiments; they are, however, tumors which may develop any time during the course of life. In addition, they may be located on the sides and flexor aspects of any finger. The individual tumor has a wide base and is surrounded by a small, inconspicuous, scaly collar (Fig. 763). It may be hemispherical or have the shape of a pastille,

but it simulates a finger rudiment 1 to 2 cm long. The surface is covered on all sides by normal skin, which has no papillary furrows. There is often a small, firmly attached hyperkeratosis on top, which looks like a small cornu cutaneum. Histologically, the whole tumor consists

Fig. 763. So-called acquired fibrokeratoma.

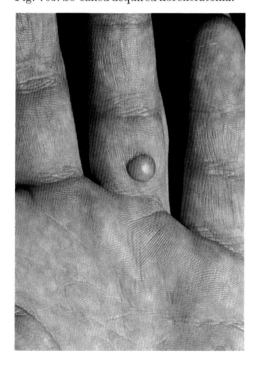

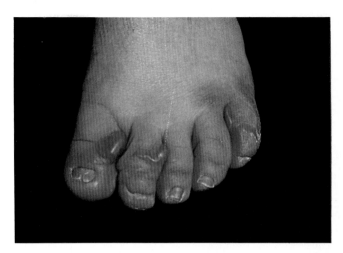

Fig. 764. Recurrent digital fibromatosis.

of connective tissue surrounded by epidermis, which is irregularly acanthotically widened and partly covered by ortho-hyperkeratosis. The elastic fibers are rarefied or are missing completely, and the same is true of the nerve fibers.[3, 9, 43]

8. One of the connective tissue tumors which occurs exclusively on the fingers and toes is the **recurrent digital fibromatosis of childhood.** The changes are either present at birth or begin within the first year of life. Usually, several toes or several fingers are affected. Clinically, the tumors are hemispherically protuberant nodes of soft-elastic consistency, about 1 to 2 cm in size. They always have a wide base, and the color varies between red and red-brown. The individual nodes usually remain well movable on their base, but the overlying skin is firmly adherent. Typical sites are the extensor or lateral sides of the fingers and toes (Fig. 764). Their size increases only slowly, and some of the tumors have a tendency to grow into the tendons and osseous tissue below. Surgical removal is often followed by local recurrence, but in no case are metastases present. Spontaneous regression, on the other hand, is not rare. Histologically, this is poorly demarcated tumor of fibroblasts, histiocytes, and

collagenous tissue, which varies in maturity. Reticular fibers are lacking, and capillaries with small lumina are numerous. Characteristically, there are three to ten large inclusion bodies near the nucleolus in the cytoplasm of the large, bulky squamous cells. They are especially well demonstrated with phosphotungstic acid – hematoxylin or methyl green pyronine stain*. The inclusion bodies probably do not represent virus particles but deposits of metabolic products.[12, 26, 27, 37]

9. The **juvenile aponeurotic palmoplantar fibroma** starts with indefinite, rapidly growing subcutaneous indurations or formations of nodes. The individual nodes can hardly be separated from their surroundings. They are firmly fixed to their base, and although the overlying skin can easily be lifted up, it also remains free from secondary changes. The tumors may be present at birth or may appear as late as the twentieth year of life. Although the lesions favor the palm (thenar and hypothenar eminences) and the middle of the soles, other regions of the body may be affected also. Local recurrences may occur even after exten-

---

* Unna-Pappenheim stain. (Tr.)

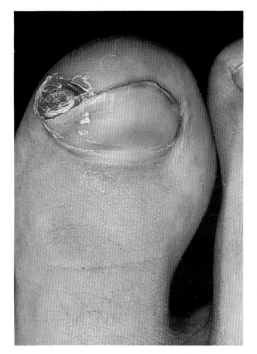

Fig. 765. Soft tissue tumor above exostosis of the ungual phalanx.

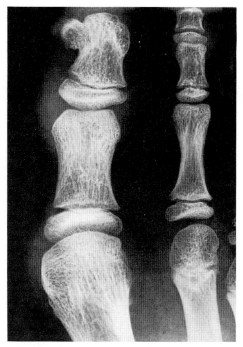

Fig. 766. Radiograph of the exostosis of the distal phalanx of the toe.

Fig. 767. Luxuriantly growing flesh.

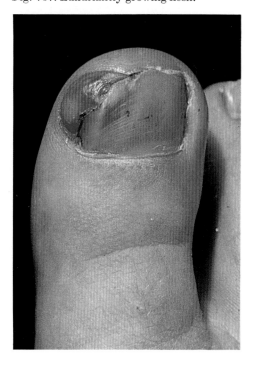

sive surgical intervention. On the other hand, spontaneous regressions are possible; metastases do not take place. Radiographic examination of the tumors may at times show finely stippled areas of calcification. Histologically, the lesions contain proliferations of fibroblastlike cells arranged in columns, rows, or whorls. In spite of considerable nuclear polymorphism, mitoses are absent. The subcutis and musculature are diffusely infiltrated by these cell formations. Within these cellular proliferations chondroid or osteoid metaplasia may take place.[4, 18, 23, 36]

10. Exostoses of the phalanges of the toes may be accompanied by tumorlike thickenings of the subungual or paraungual tissue. These tumorlike reactions usually develop some time after trauma at the site of the exostosis and result in thickening of the tissue or formation of

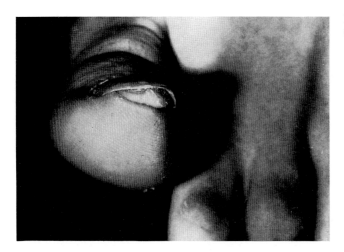

Fig. 768. Subungual chondroma.

calluses (Figs. 765, 766). As a rule, additional chronic inflammatory changes, including deformities of the nailplate, take place. Secondary infections result in chronic paronychia. The differential diagnosis includes pyogenic granuloma, soft tissue granuloma (Fig. 767), glomus tumor, melanoma, and other benign and malignant tumors. However, when examined radiographically, none of these tumors show a corresponding exostosis.[6, 31]

11. Solitary chondromas of the hands and feet (sometimes also at subungual sites) are extremely rare (Fig. 768). They are firm tumors of various sizes; in the smaller type (about 2 to 3 cm) the skin can be lifted up and the origin from the capsule of a joint or the tenosynovial sheath can be found by palpation. In larger tumors it is not possible to distinguish definitely between the tumor and the surrounding tissue. Histologic examination will make a definite diagnosis possible only if hyaline cartilage or poorly differentiated chondroid tissue is found. In contrast to the systemic type of chondroma, the localized type includes

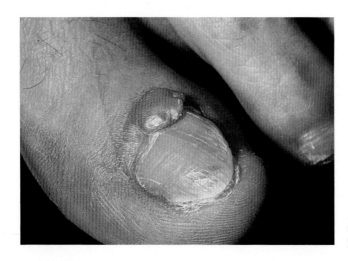

Fig. 769. Periungual fibromas in Pringle-Bourneville's phakomatosis.

mainly benign tumors; malignant degeneration is exceptional.[24]

12. A patient with subungual or periungual fibromas should be examined for other signs of **Pringle-Bourneville's phakomatosis,** such as depigmentations, Pringle tumors, or lumbosacral connective tissue nevi. Like the various histologic aspects of adenoma sebaceum, the periungual Koenen tumor may have either an angiofibromatous or a fibromatous character. The periungual fibromas that are part of this phakomatosis develop relatively late; however, about half of the patients are affected. The lesions are fairly hard, partly cockscomblike, red-brown or meaty red tumors (Fig. 769). These tumors are seen subungually only in a few cases, as most of them arise from the paronychium. The resultant nail changes have a similar appearance.[20, 28]

Solitary periungual fibromas may remain as the residuum of a common injury (Fig. 770) and have no connection with a systemic disease like Pringle-Bourneville's phakomatosis.

13. The **eccrine poroma** is a tumor that also occurs frequently on the palms and soles. Its clinical macroscopic appearance, however, offers so few characteristics that a diagnosis can be made only by histologic examination (see also Section B 7).

14. For **squamous cell carcinoma** see Section C17. A special type of squamous carcinoma peculiar to the foot is the *"epithelioma cuniculatum,"* which shows numerous formations of crypts. The deep crypts are filled with macerated masses of keratin, resulting in marked fetor from this tumor. According to the descriptions of this tumor so far available it is locally invasive but does not metastasize; one may therefore suppose that the tumor represents a pseudoepitheliomatous hyperplasia corresponding to papillomatosis cutis carcinoides.[1, 40]

15. **Multiple herniations of fat of the heels** (piezogenic papules of the feet) are a harmless anomaly. They are present in adults of both sexes and usually are not noticed by the patient because they cause no trouble. However, some patients experience pain after prolonged standing, although such pain cannot be definitely ascribed to the herniated areas. As a rule these changes are not visible if the patient is in the supine position, but upon standing there are easily visible protrusions on the sides of the heel. In the presence of especially numerous protrusions the

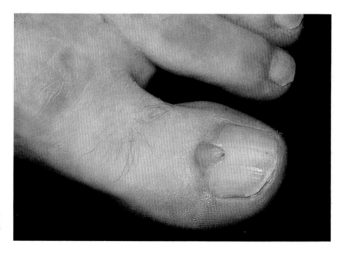

Fig. 770. Post-traumatic periungual fibroma with nail impression.

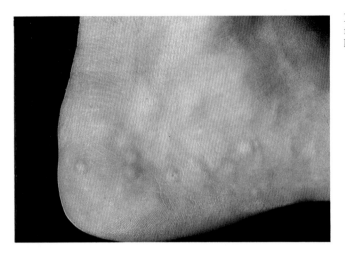

Fig. 771. Multiple hernias of fatty tissue in the area of the heel.

condition resembles a bag of peas (Fig. 771). The tumors are soft, not painful upon pressure, and can easily be pushed back. Histologically, they are "sliding" hernias of the subcutaneous fatty tissue.[7, 35, 44]

16. Histiocytoma (nodulus cutaneus) is a relatively frequent tumor of the extremities but is of only minor importance (Fig. 772). It often occurs as a multiple tumor favoring the legs. The patients cannot state the time of its appearance exactly in most cases; however, many maintain that such a histiocytoma developed slowly after an insect bite or after a small mechanical injury from a prick or tear. Subjectively, a mild pruritus is present within the tumor area. Clinically, one sees a fairly hard, more or less reddish-yellow nodule which either is not elevated at all or is only slightly higher than the surrounding skin. The histiocytoma is firmly attached to the epidermis, and when the surrounding skin is pressed together, the lesion sinks down in plaque-like fashion. If the tumor contains many blood vessels, extravasation may account for considerable deposits of hemosiderin in the histiocytes of the tumor tissue.

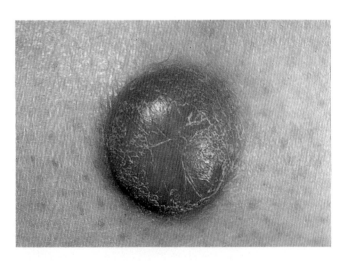

Fig. 772. Unusually large tumorous histiocytoma.

Even macroscopically, these histiocytomas have a very dark color and must be included as histiocytomas storing hemosiderin (see Section B5) in the differential diagnosis of pigmented tumors. Histologically, histiocytomas have an abundance of histiocytes, in contrast to the fibrillary-fascicular structure of hard fibromas and the more loosely and finely fibered structure of soft fibromas. Also in contrast to hard fibromas, histiocytomas have a potency for storage (among other substances, double refractive lipids and hemosiderins). In addition, not infrequently Touton type giant cells or giant cell reactions to a foreign body and vascular neoplasias with endothelial swelling *("sclerosing angiomas")* are characteristic of the cutaneous changes. The overlying epidermis becomes either atrophic because of pressure or widened by bulky acanthosis. Even basal cell epitheliomatouslike proliferations or even true buds of basal cell epitheliomas have been observed overlying histiocytomas. The differential diagnosis includes, in addition to the previously mentioned hard fibromas (Section G2), disseminated connective tissue nevi (Section G25), rheumatic nodules (see Chapter 8, F), and nevoxanthoendotheliomas (see Chapter 32, B1).[2, 11, 25, 29, 38]

17. Pseudosarcomatous nodular fasciitis consists of rapidly growing nodes, which therefore come early to the attention of the patient; this rapid growth contrasts with the markedly slow development of a histiocytoma. The primary manifestation of nodular fasciitis may begin at any age; however, there is a distinct increase in frequency between the twentieth and fiftieth years of life. With rare exceptions the disease begins as a solitary nodule favoring the extremities, especially the forearms. Although the general health is unimpaired, such a tumor may reach a diameter of 1.5 to 3.0 cm within a few weeks. The isolated, hard, subcutaneous tu-

mor is usually firmly attached to the underlying fascia; however, the overlying skin can easily be lifted up. After some time spontaneous regression will take place, unless the tumor has been surgically removed owing to suspected malignancy. The nodular fasciitis is not accompanied by regional lymphadenopathy, metastases, or local recurrences. Clinically, the diagnosis can only be suspected, as in all other subcutaneous growths; only histologic examination can furnish the final diagnosis by showing a tumor derived from the fascia and infiltrating into the musculature and the subcutaneous fat. However, the corium is seldom infiltrated. The tumor is composed of vascular tissue consisting of large, spindle-shaped fibroblasts, whose nuclei show a distinct nucleolus together with numerous but not atypical mitoses. Fifty per cent of the tumors have multinucleated giant cells. The fibroblasts are embedded in a mucoid ground substance interwoven with reticular fibers. The edge of the tumor may show an inflammatory infiltrate of various degrees of intensity. The differential diagnosis includes primarily a fibrosarcoma, which can usually be excluded when atypical mitoses are absent and vascularity and a mucoid ground substance are present[21, 33, 42]

18. Leiomyosarcomas of the skin, like leiomyomas, are derived mostly from the arrector muscles. In contrast to leiomyomas, they lack the pain accompanying these benign tumors. Leiomyosarcomas may occur at any age; however, they are seen somewhat more frequently after the sixtieth year of life. The tumors favor the lower extremities primarily; however, other parts of the body may be involved also. A single lesion may reach a size of 9.0 cm in diameter. In most cases the tumors arise from the subcutaneous fat and are movable against their base, while the overlying cutis remains definitely fixed to the tumor. Sometimes superficial

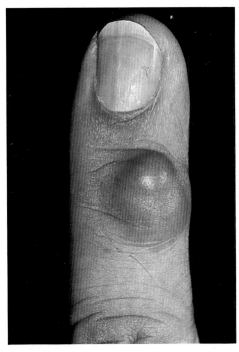

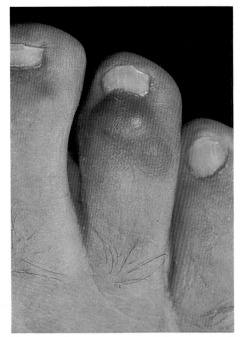

Fig. 774. Synovioma containing giant cells on the fourth toe.

Fig. 773. Synovioma containing giant cells on the finger.

Fig. 775. Lupoid foreign body granuloma.

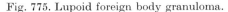

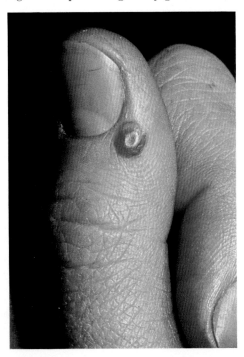

ulcerations, which may bleed easily, have been observed. Operative removal is followed by a high rate of local recurrence. Some leiomyosarcomas metastasize rather early into the regional lymph nodes or via the blood stream into the lungs. Histologically, at least part of the tumor retains the structure of a myoma; otherwise, anaplastic groups of cells with shapeless nuclei and many mitoses predominate.[12, 39, 41]

19. Since synoviomas are derived from the synovial membrane of the articular capsule, the tendon sheaths, or the bursae, they are found primarily on the extremities. Synoviomas at other locations, e.g. breast or lumbosacral region, are highly exceptional. Benign and malignant synoviomas can be differentiated according to the histologic findings and the clinical course. The two types of tumor may occur with or without giant cells. The clinical picture does not permit a differentiation between these four types of synoviomas. The malignant type has a tendency to local recurrences on the one hand and to lymphogenous or hematogenous (lung) metastases on the other hand. A patient with a synovioma complains at first about stinging or drawing pains near the joints; however, in the beginning sympathetic articular effusions or impairment of mobility is lacking. Because the growth of even the malignant synoviomas proceeds extremely slowly and the formation of the tumor cannot be recognized immediately, chronic inflammatory conditions are the most noticeable sign. The periarticular tumor of the fingers, when finally recognizable, attains a size of 0.5 to 1.0 cm, whereas at the larger joints much larger tumors measuring 5 to 8 cm in diameter have been observed (Figs. 773, 774). Some of the tumors show definite fluctuation; the overlying skin remains freely movable. A biopsy is necessary to establish the proper diagnosis. The differential diagnosis must include, besides chronic inflammatory changes, the presence of a ganglion, chondromas, and tumorlike reactions over an exostosis. A distinction from Heberden's nodes should not be difficult (see Chapter 8, B1). However, the diagnosis of a synovial cyst requires a histologic examination (see Chapter 8, B2). Even the painful periarticular foreign body granulomas may present a certain similarity to a synovioma (Fig. 775). In the absence of a definite history indicating exposure to a foreign body, a histologic examination will be necessary.[8, 22, 46]

(1) AIRD, I., H. D. JOHNSON, B. LENNOX and A. G. STANSFELD: Epithelioma cuniculatum. A variety of squamous carcinoma peculiar to the foot. Brit. J. Surg. 42: 245–250 (1954).
(2) BANDMAN, H.-J.: Ein Beitrag zur morphologischen Pathologie des Dermatofibroma lenticulare bzw. des Histio-

cytoms. Arch. klin. exp. Derm. 204: 584–603 (1957).
(3) BART, R. S., R. ANDRADE, A. W. KOPF and M. LEIDER: Acquired digital fibrokeratomas. Arch. Derm. (Chic.) 97: 120–129 (1968).
(4) BARTÓK, I.: Ein Fall von juvenilem aponeurotischem Fibrom. Zbl. Allg. Path. 110: 217–221 (1967).
(5) BREHME, H.: Über rudimentäre Polydaktylie bei Bantu-Negern. Humangenetik 15: 81–83 (1972).
(6) COHEN, H. J., S. B. FRANK, W. MINKIN and R. C. GIBBS: Subungual exostoses. Arch. Derm. (Chic.) 107: 431–432 (1973).
(7) COHEN, H. J., R. C. GIBBS, W. MINKIN and S. B. FRANK: Painful piezogenic pedal papules. Arch. Derm. (Chic.) 101: 112–113 (1970).
(8) GEILER, G.: Die Synovialome. Morphologie und Pathogenese. Springer, Berlin, Göttingen, Heidelberg 1961.
(9) GEISER, J. D.: Le fibrokératome digital acquis. Dermatologica (Basel) 143. 21–28 (1971).
(10) GERTLER, W.: Melanoblastosis cutis systematisata – Carol (Incontinentia pigmenti Bloch-Sulzberger) mit Initialexanthem und Hyperkeratomen der unteren Extremitäten. Derm. Wschr. 131: 183–185 (1955).
(11) GROSS, R. E., and S. W. WOLBACH: Sclerosing hemangiomas; their relationship to dermatofibroma, histiocytoma, xanthoma and to certain pigmented lesions of the skin. Amer. J. Path. 19: 533–551 (1943).
(12) HAIM, S., and B. GELLEI: Leiomyosarcoma of the skin. Report of two cases. Dermatologica (Basel) 140: 30–35 (1970).
(13) JABŁOŃSKA, S., W. BICZYSKO, K. JAKUBOWICZ and J. DABROWSKI: On the viral etiology of epidermodysplasia verruciformis Lewandowsky-Lutz. Electron microscope studies. Dermatologica (Basel) 137: 113–125 (1968).
(14) JABŁOŃSKA, S., W. BICZYSKO, K. JAKUBOWICZ and H. DABROWSKI: The ultrastructure of transitional states to Bowen's disease and invasive Bowen's carcinoma in epidermodysplasia verruciformis. Dermatologica (Basel) 140: 186–194 (1970).
(15) JABŁOŃSKA, S., and B. MILEWSKI: Zur Kenntnis der Epidermodysplasia verruciformis Lewandowsky-Lutz (positive Ergebnisse der Auto- und Heteroinokulation). Dermatologica (Basel) 115: 1–22 (1957).

(16) Jaschke, E., und B. Wohlfarth: Rezidivierende Digitalfibrome im Kindesalter. Z. Haut- u. Geschl.-Kr. *48:* 317–323 (1973).

(17) Kaffarnik, H., und R. Juchems: Verrucae vulgares und neurozirkulatorische Asthenie. Arch. klin. exp. Derm. *224:* 138–143 (1966).

(18) Keasbey, L. E., and H. A. Fanselau: The aponeurotic fibroma. Clin. Orthop. *19:* 115–131 (1961).

(19) Keining, E., und K. Halter: Verrucae planae-artige seborrhoische Warzen. Arch. Derm. Syph. (Berl.) *188:* 482–489 (1949).

(20) Knoth, W., und W. Meyhöfer: Zur Nosologie des Adenoma sebaceum Typ Balzer, der Koenenschen Tumoren und des Morbus Bourneville-Pringle. Hautarzt *8:* 359–366 (1957).

(21) Konwaler, B. E., L. Keasbey and L. Kaplan: Subcutaneous pseudosarcomatous fibromatosis (fasciitis). Report of 8 cases. Amer. J. Clin. Path. *25:* 241–252 (1955).

(22) Krakovic, M., und K. A. Lennert: Zur Klinik der Synovialome. Med. Welt *23* (N. F.): 215–218 (1972).

(23) Lichtenstein, L., and R. L. Goldman: The cartilage analogue of fibromatosis. A reinterpretation of the condition called »juvenile aponeurotic fibroma«. Cancer (Philad.) *17:* 810–816 (1964).

(24) Lichtenstein, L., and R. L. Goldman: Cartilage tumors in soft tissues, particularly in the hand and foot. Cancer (Philad.) *17:* 1203–1208 (1964).

(25) Mascaro, J.-M., et N. D. Toan: Prolifération à type d'épithélioma basocellulaire sur histiocytofibrome. Bull. Soc. franç. Derm, Syph. *73:* 480–482 (1966).

(26) McKenzie, A. W., F. L. F. Innes, J. M. Rack, A. S. Breathnach and M. Gross: Digital fibrous swellings in children. Brit. J. Derm. *83:* 446–458 (1970).

(27) Mehregan, A. H., H. Nabai and J. E. Matthews: Recurring digital fibrous tumor of childhood. Arch. Derm. (Chic.) *106:* 375–378 (1972).

(28) Nickel, W. R., and W. B. Reed: Tuberous sclerosis. Arch. Derm. (Chic.) *85:* 209–226 (1962).

(29) Niemi, K. M.: The benign fibrohistiocytic tumours of the skin. Acta derm.-venereol. (Stockh.) *50:* Suppl. 63 (1970).

(30) Nürnberger, F., und R. Denk: Schwimmbadgranulom. Med. Welt *19* (N. F.): 1747–1748 (1968).

(31) Pambor, M., und H. Neubert: Tumorartige Begleitreaktionen der Haut bei Exostosen der Zehenendphalangen. Derm. Mschr. *157:* 532–537 (1971).

(32) Philpott, J., A. Woodburne, O. Philpott, W. Schaefer and C. Mollohan: Swimming pool granuloma: A study of 290 cases. Arch. Derm. (Chic.) *88:* 158–162 (1963).

(33) Röckl, H., und E. Schubert: Fasciitis nodularis pseudosarcomatosa. Hautarzt *22:* 150–153 (1971).

(34) Ruiter, M., and P. J. van Mullem: An intranuclear virus in epidermodysplasia verruciformis. Dermatologica (Basel) *136:* 270–272 (1968).

(35) Schubert, E., E. Schilling und J. Metz: Multiple Fettgewebshernien der Ferse (Sogenannte »painful piezogenic pedal papules«). Hautarzt *24:* 111–114 (1973).

(36) Schweizer, P., A. Flach, und G. Müller: Zur Klinik der juvenilen Fibromatose. Dtsch. med. Wschr. *95:* 1303–1308 (1970).

(37) Shapiro, L.: Infantile digital fibromatosis and aponeurotic fibroma. Case reports of two rare pseudosarcomas and review of the literature. Arch. Derm. (Chic.) *99:* 37–42 (1969).

(38) Steigleder, G. K., H. Nicklas und Y. Kamei: Die Epithelveränderungen beim Histiocytom, ihre Genese und ihr Erscheinungsbild. Derm. Wschr. *146:* 457–468 (1962).

(39) Stout, A. P., and W. T. Hill: Leiomyosarcoma of the superficial soft tissues. Cancer (Philad.) *11:* 844–854 (1958).

(40) Swanbeck, G., and L. Hillström: Analysis of etiological factors of squamous cell skin cancer of different locations. I. The lower limbs. Acta derm.-venereol. (Stockh.) *49:* 427–435 (1969).

(41) Tappeiner, J., and P. Wodniansky: Solitäres Leiomyom-Leiomyosarkom. Hautarzt *12:* 160–163 (1961).

(42) Türk, G.: Die Fasciitis nodularis. Münch. med. Wschr. *114:* 278–282 (1972).

(43) Verallo, V. V. M.: Acquired digital fibrokeratomas. Brit. J. Derm. *80:* 730–736 (1968).

(44) WOERDEMAN, M. J., and E. VAN DIJK: Piezogenic papules of the feet. Acta derm.-venereol. (Stockh.) *52:* 411–414 (1972).

(45) ZELIGMAN, I.: Mycobacterium marinum granuloma. A disease acquired in the tributaries of Chesapeake bay. Arch. Derm. (Chic.) *106:* 26–31 (1972).

(46) ZIPPEL, H.: Zur Diagnose, Differential-diagnose und Therapie der Synoviaiome. Zbl. Chir. *94:* 958–975 (1969).

K. Tumors Favoring No Particular Body Region

1. Lipomas, as benign tumors of the subcutaneous fatty tissue, do not favor any definite body area. They usually occur as multiple growths and are to a certain extent symmetrically distributed. Notable is the fact that a certain disposition to the formation of lipomas exists in some families. The development of multiple lipomas may begin as early as the second decade of life and often progresses in spurts thereafter. Most patients experience no symptoms, but there are explicitly painful lipomas, which have already been discussed in Section A5 of this chapter. Clinically, the tumors vary in size but rarely exceed a diameter of 5 cm. Either they are deeply situated in the subcutaneous tissue and are evident only by palpation or they elevate the cutaneous surface like a calotte. Their surface may be irregularly nodular. Palpation usually gives the impression of a firm-elastic, lobular, "granular"-appearing tumor. Skin lying above the lipoma is unchanged in color and can be easily lifted. Moreover, the whole tumor remains well movable against its surroundings. An angiolipoma is a lipomatous variety that is especially rich in vessels and looks red-brown or blue-red through the skin. Differentiation from a subcutaneous hemangioma is therefore necessary, but often this is possible only

by excision of the tumor. Another variety is circumscribed lipomatosis of the fingers or toes, a tumor that may lead to or suggest gigantism of these parts of the extremities. In such cases the typical lobulation of the lipoma is no longer palpable, but the tense elastic consistency remains. If only a single tumor or a few tumors of this description exist, subcutaneous metastases of internal malignant tumors must be considered, especially if growth is rapid. In general, however, metastases appear firmer on palpation than do lipomas. In doubtful cases, histologic proof of the diagnosis should be attempted. Multiple lipomas occur also in combination with other benign tumors in Gardner's syndrome (see Chapter 24, E5 and Chapter 38, C6) and in generalized neurofibromatosis (see Chapter 24, E7 and Chapter 38, G3). Also, there are multiple lipomas in the Richner-Hanhart syndrome (see Chapter 28, C3) in addition to palmoplantar keratoses. Congenital lumbosacral lipomas point to an underlying spina bifida or meningocele (see Chapter 38, G27).[12, 15, 30]

2. Congenital, generalized fibromatosis is a very rare disorder which in most instances is already manifest in utero. It consists of multiple, poorly demarcated tumors of about 0.5 to 2 cm in size. According to their location in the cutis or in the subcutaneous fatty tissue they are visible as protrusions or are evident only by palpation. They are not always distinct nodular formations but may be only firm plaquelike infiltrates. Almost always similar tumor formations exist in the internal organs, such as the heart, gastrointestinal tract, kidneys, lungs, striated muscles, and skeleton. Most of the children die after a few weeks from the sequelae of cardiac, pulmonary, or intestinal complications. Spontaneous regression of the tumors can be seen in exceptional cases. The histologic substrate of this form of fibromatosis consists

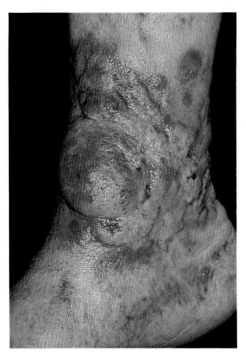

Fig. 776. Reticulosarcoma.

of bandlike or whorl-like spindle-shaped fibroblasts. Increased or pathologic mitoses are absent. The cellular nuclei stain partially hyperchromatically. In the tissue of the tumor a dense rete of pale collagenous and reticular fibers may be present. Vessels at the margins of the tumors show subintimal cell proliferations and fibroses which may lead to complete closure of the lumina.[1, 13]

3. Exophytic tumors growing extensively and in clusters in older adults suggest first a **reticulosarcoma.** This is valid above all in the case of a protruding tumor which is initially localized and quickly becomes nodular or notched and protuberant. The node is red, yellowish, or brownish, but with increased vascularization it turns bluish-red. Owing to its development from the subcutis, the node is not movable on its base (Fig. 776). More rarely, this tumor of the lymphoreticular connective or fatty tissue develops from

simultaneous multiple small, partly regressing nodules, which, however, soon unite to become a large nodular infiltrate. If the course is very rapid, erosions or ulcerations of the surface appear. In contrast to the usually firm to boardlike consistency, if the regression of the tumor is pronounced, a carbunclelike softening may occur in the deeper lying regions. Pronounced perifocal elephantiasic thickening indicates early involvement of regional lymph nodes. Because of its matrix a reticulosarcoma is the most common tumor of the lymph nodes, of which the nodes of the throat and palate are the most important for the dermatologist. The most common locations of reticulosarcoma on the skin are the scalp, fingers, toes, and ankles. Metastases of reticulosarcoma occur predominantly by lymphatic spread and occasionally also hematogenously, if no development to reticuloendotheliosis (generalized lymph node swelling, enlarged spleen, tumorous cachexia) ensues. In addition, invasion of neighboring organs from a contiguous sarcomatous lymph node may attract attention clinically. Histogenetically, reticulum cell sarcomas are divided into syncytial, afibrillar, fibril-forming (pronounced net of reticular fibers with tumorous cells that are appended like pussywillows), and types with mixed cells.[7, 14, 17]

If a primary tumor is not present but multiple autochthonous development can be assumed, the picture is that of a *reticulosarcomatosis.* In such cases a differentiation from reticuloendotheliosis may be necessary. Reticuloendotheliosis is usually generalized or disseminated, i.e., limited to certain cutaneous areas either as multiple, pea- to bean-sized, pale or dark red nodes or initially as eczemalike, later plaquelike, palm-sized infiltrates. In contrast to the previously mentioned tendency to disintegration of reticulosarcomatosis, the individual lesions of reticuloendotheliosis remain solid and are confined to the skin for a long

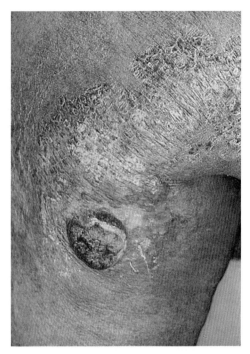

Fig. 777. Sarcoma on area of lupus vulgaris previously treated roentgenologically.

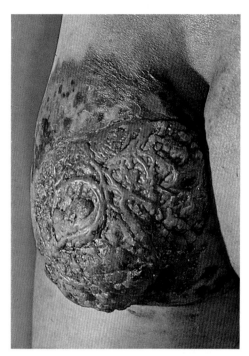

Fig. 778. Lupus vulgaris (hypertrophic).

time. In reticuloendothelioses, furthermore, changes of blood protein (e.g., with marked elevation of the ESR) can be expected sooner than in reticulosarcomatosis. Hematologically, dissemination of monocytes is somewhat characteristic of terminal reticuloendotheliosis.[17, 33]

4. Fibrosarcoma of the skin (dermatofibrosarcoma protuberans) favors the trunk. For this reason it was discussed in Section G1 of this chapter. The following paragraph discusses primarily those fibrosarcomas that develop subsequently to long or excessive exposure to ionizing radiation. Typical examples are the so-called roentgen sarcoma of lupus vulgaris treated with x-rays (Fig. 777) and, likewise, similar sarcomatous developments in xeroderma pigmentosum. But a fibrosarcoma is not found under every radiated and exophytically growing lupus vulgaris. Figure 778 shows such a tumor form of lupus vulgaris with no evidence of any malignant transformation. On the other hand, fibrosarcomas may originate from the fasciae or connective tissue of the subcutis and only secondarily infiltrate the entire skin. They are hemispherically protruding nodes with a firm to soft consistency. The color of the skin remains unchanged or is occasionally slightly brown-reddish. After longer duration there is a distinct tendency toward ulcerations or central breakdown, so that fluctuation becomes evident. In contrast to reticulosarcomas, fibrosarcomas clearly disintegrate more slowly but bleed much more easily. Some fibrosarcomas form distinct mucus, so that there are fluent transitions to myxosarcoma.[6, 7, 11, 23, 32]

5. Myxomas are also nodose, flat protuberances with a subcutaneous localization. The protruding surface usually remains unchanged or is at most some-

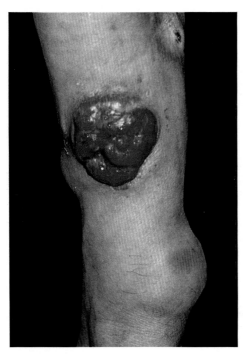

Fig. 779. Myxosarcoma.

sizes with increased and atypical mitotic figures are surrounded by mucoid material. Between the spindle cells tumorous giant cells with coarse or multiple nuclei may be present.[16, 21]

6. The various forms of **plasmacytomas** occasionally show specific cutaneous changes, but for the most part the accompanying paraproteinemic, paraproteinuric, and osseous changes are more important. Many patients complain only of rheumatoid difficulties initially.

Nonspecific, nontumorlike cutaneous manifestations of this systemic disorder include such general symptoms and signs as pruritus, erythemas, cyanoses, symptomatic ichthyoses, symmetrical, vesicular and lichenoid, partly petechial rashes, lichenifications, and herpes zoster eruptions if there is a focus in the spine. Specific extramedullary manifestations that develop in the skin usually occur as disseminated, lenticular papules and tumorlike infiltrates on the nose, lips, and cheeks, and also on the extremities and trunk. Some are very hard tumors, others are moderately firm, and the rest may even be soft tumors (Fig. 780), whose etiology must be decided definitely by histologic examination. Such a plasmacytoma rarely remains solitary for many years. Specific plasma cell proliferations are apt to develop on the mucosae, where they appear as blue-red, gray-yellowish, or dark brown tumor infiltrates that may ulcerate. On the soft parts of the oral cavity plasmacytomas may remain single for a long time. On the other hand, these plasmacytomas of the oral cavity are either a partial expression of a systemic myelomatosis or a pathologic manifestation that is associated with tumors of the neighboring osseous parts. Especially typical are the pillowlike or occasionally petechial swellings at both sides of the raphe palati and the tumorlike maxillary or mandibular gingival hyperplasias. The conjunctiva and the genital mucosa may

what reddened. The tumor may occasionally drain, simulating regression. Myxomas, which are easily mistaken for fibromas, lipofibromas, or lipomas, have no preferred locations; reports have listed the face, trunk, genitals, and also the extremities as sites. The *myxosarcoma* was formerly considered etiologically related to a lipoplastic sarcoma, since it may show fatty deposits in connection with regressive tumor changes. In spite of a distinct local tendency toward recurrences, distant metastases occur only rarely. Single tumors, which often reach the size of a hen's egg, are extremely firm. They can be moved on their base only minimally, if at all. The skin over the nodes can be easily lifted at first, but becomes firmly attached with further growth of the tumor. Finally the epidermis is pierced by the tumor, resulting in a "naked" papillary tumor (Fig. 779). Histologically, spindle cells of various

Fig. 780. Solitary plasmacytoma of the skin in nonhomogeneous pigmentation.

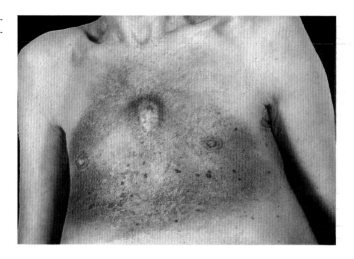

also be the sites of extramedullary plasmacytomas. Ocular changes (hemorrhages of the fundus, "fundus paraproteinemicus") and the presence of a primary systemic amyloidosis often complete the picture of a plasmacytoma.

7. Waldenström's macroglobulinemia is a systemic disease with specific tumorlike cutaneous infiltrates. The diagnosis of this entity is verified by immunoelectrophoresis (increased gamma M-macroglobulins), by ultracentrifugation of the serum (molecular weight of over 1,000,000), and by examination of the bone marrow (increase of small lymphoid reticulum cells and mast cells in the tissue). In contrast to the plasmacytoma, in macroglobulinemia skeletal pains or radiologic osseous changes recede almost completely into the background, and an abnormally high sedimentation rate (125 in the first hour) and the so-called Sia reaction (a few drops of serum added to distilled water show flocculation) are important clues. Symptomatic macroglobulinemias, however, occur not only with plasmacytoma, reticuloses, carcinoses, and sarcomatoses but also with congenital syphilis and some liver diseases. In addition, about 3 per cent of all people over 70 years of age have an

M-component indicative of a benign gammopathy. Especially important in connection with the cutaneous lesions are tumorlike, small nodular or plaquelike and sometimes ulcerating infiltrates; either they rise exophytically above the skin or they can be palpated only as plaquelike infiltrates, for instance around the orbit of the eye or the mouth. The tendency toward purpuric exanthemas or at least the occurrence of petechiae within the infiltrates is also diagnostically important. These clublike or plaquelike circumscribed infiltrates may have an erythematous epidermis in places, and in a periorbicular location they may give the appearance of a leonine facies. The lesions have a jellylike consistency and look like large lacrimal sacs or like a chain of sausages; they are easily movable against the subcutis.

Histologically, such tumorigenic cutaneous lesions of macroglobulinemia show an apparently multiple autochthonous accumulation of cells with a tendency either to penetration or to destruction of the surrounding tissue. The separate cellular elements are considered to be either atypical lymphocytes or reticulum cells with a partly plasmacytoid modulation-Electron microscopy shows that the grow-

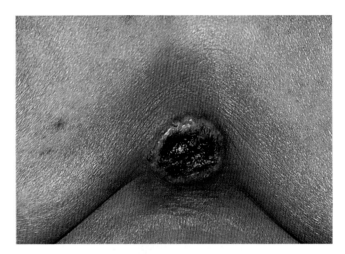

Fig. 781. Extramedullary manifestation of an osteomyelosclerosis syndrome.

ing tumor cells are round lymphoid cells of various sizes containing much ribonucleic acid and ergastoplasma.* [5, 8, 29, 31]

* A cellular organelle of protein synthesis. (Tr.)

8. The **osteomyelosclerosis syndrome** sometimes shows nodular cutaneous infiltrates (Fig. 781). Their spongy consistency as well as the formation of a few pustules may suggest at first a bacterial granuloma as a complication of the basic disease. Histologically, or using a touch smear,

Fig. 782. Metastasis of a bronchial carcinoma on the nose.

Fig. 783. Metastasis of a seminoma on the leg.

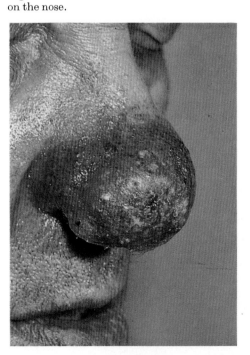

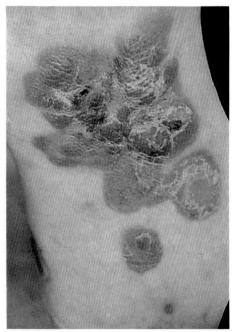

precursors of erythrocytes and granulocytes can be seen as signs of extramedullary myelopoiesis. In contrast to erythremia (better known as polycythemia vera) and chronic myelosis (myelocytic leukemia), the erythroblasts remain PAS-negative and the neutrophil granulocytes are more than 50 per cent phosphatase-positive. The patients show a pronounced splenomegaly, and after a preliminary period of polycythemia they develop severe anemia. The peripheral blood smear shows immature white cells, although the leukocyte values are about normal; precursors of erythrocytes may also appear in the peripheral blood. Examination of the bone marrow shows either complete absence of the marrow or only a few remnants.

9. Cutaneous metastases of visceral malignancies or so-called secondary cancers of the skin are rare (Figs. 782, 783). Generally they are estimated to occur in about 1 to 4 per cent of all cutaneous tumors. The most frequent cutaneous tumor is a metastasis from a breast cancer. A favorite site of a hematogenous distant metastasis is the hairy scalp, whereas the facial location appears more seldom. In spite of this rare occurrence, furunculoid or basal cell epithelioma-like nodular formations of the face should raise the possibility of a distant metastasis. Usually such secondary cutaneous tumors present as nodular or cystic formations, which frequently appear simultaneously in several places. The histologic appearance of such cutaneous metastatic cancer originating from internal organs is scarcely any more recognizable than the clinical picture with regard to the original site of the tumor. As a rule it is almost impossible to draw definite conclusions about the primary tumor. Such metastatic lesions are found in different layers of the subcutis or the corium. In addition, because these malignant cells are found in the capillaries or as carcinomatous infarcts in the lymph

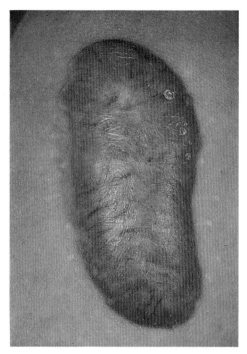

Fig. 784. Keloid following vaccination.

ducts, inflammatory changes within the surrounding tissue are usually absent. These metastases generally do not show any primary affinity to the epithelium.[2, 4, 10, 19, 20, 34]

10. The **keloid** (Fig. 784) is a sharply circumscribed plaquelike hyperplasia of the connective tissue of various thicknesses which is elevated above the surrounding tissue. Such a keloid develops weeks or months after a trauma (vaccination, burn keloids) or in connection with an inflammatory process (acne nodes, especially the so-called keloid-acne type). A keloid may also appear as an apparently spontaneous growth, frequently with special formations of claw or pincerlike projections. Thin, cordlike, reticulated formations of keloids may occur on the sites of former alterations (scars after herpes zoster or variola). The surface of these hard, firm, infiltrated patches is smooth

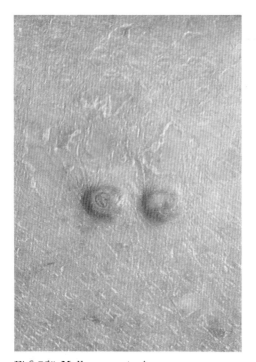

Fig. 785. Mollusca contagiosa.

Fig. 786. Molluscum contagiosum: deep depression of the epidermis with numerous molluscum bodies. Hematoxylin and eosin, $63 \times$.

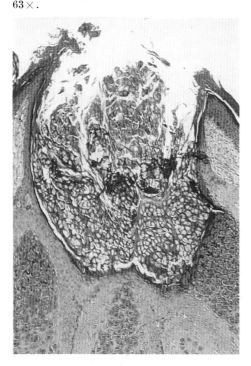

in most cases; they are freely movable with the skin over the subcutis. Older and partly regressed keloids sometimes show a somewhat slack wrinkled surface. Older and firmer keloids also show a rather white-reddish or ivory color; younger keloids a more saturated or brownish red tint. Fine hairs or comedones are rarely found on keloids, but telangiectases, pruritus, and other paresthesias are present more often.

Keloids almost always have a history of trauma and therefore can be found on any part of the body except the palms and soles. However, the upper half of the body is favored (face, middle of chest, ears). Young people (especially females) have a special predisposition toward formation of keloids, as do blacks. The tendency to form keloids is subject to temporary variations in an individual. A person may develop a keloid in one part of the body, while an identical, concurrent trauma fails to cause a keloid in another part.

Hypertrophic scars, in contrast to keloidal scars, do not extend beyond the border of the scar and they develop more quickly, but there are no other clinical differences. Although keloids are rather typical, a small singular keloidal node without a previous history of trauma is difficult to distinguish from a hard fibroma, a leiomyoma, or a keloidlike circumscribed scleroderma.

Histologically, one sees a finely fibered, almost avascular transformation of the collagen within the numerous beginning fibrocytes; the lesion is present in the middle and deep layers of the corium and from there extends into the epidermis. The elastica is rarefied or completely absent, and an argentaffin fiber formation does not exist with keloids. Especially significant is the initial mucoid penetration with metachromatic substances such as acid mucopolysaccharides (glycosamino-glycanes). As these substances disappear there is a decrease in the number of cells and an increase of collagen (thick and hyalinized bundles of collagen which show a reddish tint when stained by hematoxylin and eosin).[9, 18, 28]

11. Molluscum contagiosum is caused by a virus of the paravaccinia group, and it may occur either singly or in multiples on any part of the body except perhaps the palms and soles. Multiple mollusca appear as tumors of various sizes, probably as an expression of different lengths of duration; their diameter ranges from 1 to 2 mm up to 5 to 10 mm. The color fluctuates from skin colored to a faintly reddish tinge. The semispherical surface of the smaller firm mollusca has a smooth appearance (Fig. 785). Larger tumors show a slight central umbilication with a rough surface. Scratching the surface with a scalpel permits the expression of a mushy fatty mass without bleeding. Histologically, unmistakable, purely epidermal changes are seen. The epidermis shows an enormous, circumscribed, bulky, peglike thickening, and consists of epithelial masses containing large inclusion bodies (the so-called molluscum bodies, Fig. 786).[24, 27]

(1) BEATTY, E. C., Jr.: Congenital generalized fibromatosis in infancy. Amer. J. Dis. Children *103:* 620–624 (1962).

(2) BENZ, K., und R. JANZEN: Beitrag zur Problematik der Hautmetastasen beim Prostatakarzinom. Dtsch. med. J. *22:* 490–494 (1971).

(3) BLUEFARB, S. M.: Cutaneous manifestations of multiple myeloma. Arch. Derm. Syph. (Chic.) *72:* 506–522 (1955).

(4) BROWNSTEIN, M. H., and E. B. HELWIG: Patterns of cutaneous metastasis. Arch. Derm. (Chic.) *105:* 862–868 (1972).

(5) BUREAU, Y., H. BARRIÈRE, P. LITOUX et L. BUREAU: Maladie de Waldenström avec manifestations cutanées à type de lymphoréticulose diffuse du visage. Presse méd. *71:* 2101–2103 (1963).

(6) GENTELE, H.: Malignant, fibroblastic tumors of the skin. Acta derm.-venereol. (Stockh.) *31:* Suppl. 27 (1951).

(7) GOTTRON, H. A.: Sarkom der Haut. Hautarzt *4:* 1–11, 49–56 (1953).

(8) GOTTRON, H. A., G. W. KORTING und W. NIKOLOWSKI: Die makroglobulinämische retikuläreHyperplasie der Haut. Arch. klin. exp. Derm. *210:* 176–201 (1960).

(9) GRAUL, E. H.: Zur Klinik des Keloids. Strahlentherapie *98:* 119–132 (1955).

(10) HOEDE, N., und R. GEBHARDT: Ungewöhnliche Metastasierung eines Bronchialkarzinoms. Med. Welt *21* (N. F.): 369–371 (1970).

(11) HOEDE, N., und H. THEISEN: Tumorförmiger Lupus vulgaris papillomatosus. Med. Welt *22* (N. F.): 324–326 (1971).

(12) HOWARD, W. R., and E. B. HELWIG: Angiolipoma. Arch. Derm. (Chic.) *82:* 924–931 (1960).

(13) HOWER, J., F.-J. GÖBEL, J. R. RÜTTNER und K. WURSTER: Familiäre kongenitale generalisierte Fibromatose bei zwei Halbschwestern. Schweiz. med. Wschr. *101:* 1381–1385 (1971).

(14) KIM, R., R. K. WINKELMANN and M. DOCKERTY: Reticulum cell sarcoma of the skin. Cancer *16:* 646–655 (1963).

(15) KLEINE-NATROP, H. E., G. BELLMANN und C. SEEBACHER: Riesenwuchs eines Fingers bei angeborenem Lipom. Hautarzt *19:* 432–434 (1968).

(16) KNERLER, CH., and L. ROWE: Myxosarcoma of the skin. Arch. Derm. (Chic.) *72:* 173–175 (1955).

(17) KNOTH, W.: Zur Cyto- und Histogenese und zur klinischen Einteilung der reticulohistiocytären Erkrankungen der Haut. Arch. klin. exp. Derm. *209:* 130–170 (1959).

(18) KORTING, G. W.: Über keloidartige Sklerodermie nebst Bemerkungen über das etagenmäßig differente Verhalten von einigen sklerodermischen Krankheitszuständen. Arch. Derm. Syph. (Berl.) *198:* 306–318 (1954).

(19) KORTING, G. W.: Siegelringzellen ausbildende Magencarcinommetastasen der Haut in massiver Aussaat. Z. Haut- u. Geschl.-Kr. *34:* [VII] – [X] (1963).

(20) KORTING G. W., und K.-H. HASSENPFLUG: Aggregierte Seminom-Metastasen der Haut. Z. Haut- u. Geschl.-Kr. *34:* [LIII] – [LVI] (1963).

(21) KORTING G. W., und F. NÜRNBERGER: Zur Frage des Lipidgehaltes von Myxosarkomen. Arch. klin. exp. Derm. *230:* 172–182 (1967).

(22) LEINBROCK, A.: Das Plasmocytom und seine pathologischen Hautveränderungen. Hautarzt *9:* 249–259 (1958).

(23) MACKENZIE, D. H.: The differential diagnosis of fibroblastic disorders. Blackwell, Oxford 1970.

(24) MEHREGAN, A. H.: Molluscum contagiosum. A clinicopathologic study. Arch. Derm. (Chic.) *84:* 123–127 (1961).

(25) MIKHAIL, G. R., A. C. SPINDLER and A. P. KELLY: Malignant plasmacytoma cutis. Arch. Derm. (Chic.) *101:* 59–62 (1970).

(26) MISGELD, V.: Solitäres Plasmocytom der Haut. Hautarzt *21:* 265–270 (1970).

(27) NASEMANN TH.: Licht- und elektronenoptische Untersuchungen zur Morphologie des Molluscum contagiosum-Virus und dessen Einschlußbildungen, sowie Beiträge zur Klinik, Serologie, Histopathologie und Pathogenese des Molluscum contagiosum. Hautarzt *8:* 301–309, 352–359, 397–405 (1957).

(28) NIKOLOWSKI, W.: Pathogenese, Klinik und Therapie des Keloids. Arch. klin. exp. Derm. *212:* 550–569 (1961).

(29) ORFANOS, C., und G. K. STEIGLEDER: Die tumorbildende kutane Form des Morbus Waldenström. Dtsch. med. Wschr. *92:* 1449–1454 (1967).

(30) REICH, B.: Elephantiasisartige Extremitätenverdickung mit Wachstumsvermehrung infolge Lipombildung. Dtsch. Z. Chir. *247:* 555–557 (1936).

(31) RÖCKL, H., H. BORCHERS und F. SCHRÖPL: Lymphoretikulose der Haut mit Makroglobulinämie als Sonderform der Makroglobulinämie Waldenström. Hautarzt *13:* 491–499 (1962).

(32) SCHNEIDER, W.: Sarkome und Carcinome in ihren Wechselbeziehungen auf röntgenbestrahltem Lupus vulgaris. Strahlentherapie *80:* 335–366 (1949).

(33) SONK, C. E.: Primäre Reticulumzellsarkomatose der Haut. Acta derm.-venereol. (Stockh.) *37:* 129–139 (1957).

(34) WALTHER, H. E.: Krebsmetastasen. Schwabe, Basel 1948.

Index

Page numbers in *italic* type refer to illustrations. Page numbers followed by (t) indicate tables.